Spain's Journey in Medicine

Miguel A. Cuesta • Francisco Mateo Vallejo
Editors

Spain's Journey in Medicine

From Moorish Surgery to Modern Research

Springer

Editors
Miguel A. Cuesta
Department of Surgery
Amsterdam University Medical Centre (UMC)
Amsterdam, The Netherlands

Francisco Mateo Vallejo
Surgeon Specialized in Minimally Invasive
Surgery for Gastrointestinal Cancer
Jerez de la Frontera, Spain

ISBN 978-3-032-12220-9 ISBN 978-3-032-12221-6 (eBook)
https://doi.org/10.1007/978-3-032-12221-6

This Springer imprint is published by the registered company Springer Nature Switzerland AG
The registered company address is: Gewerbestrasse 11, 6330 Cham, Switzerland

To my wife Carmen Padules, *for her love, support, and patience.*
—Miguel A. Cuesta

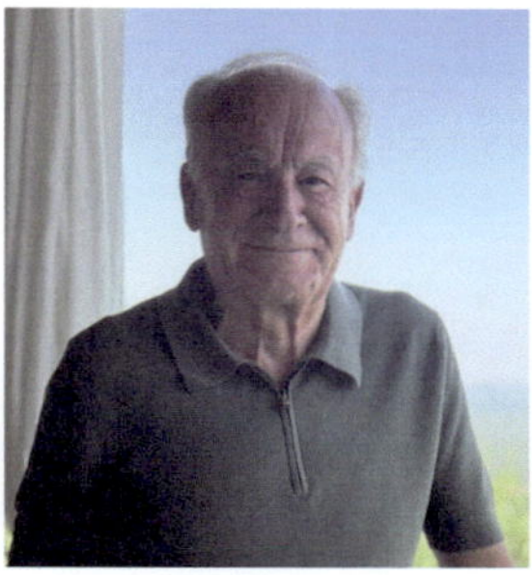

To my beloved Rosa, my companion through the journey of life,
whose love and patience have been my steadfast refuge.
To my children, *who have found their own paths*
amid the trials of this world,
and to all those I hold close to my soul,
with enduring love and gratitude.
—Francisco Mateo Vallejo

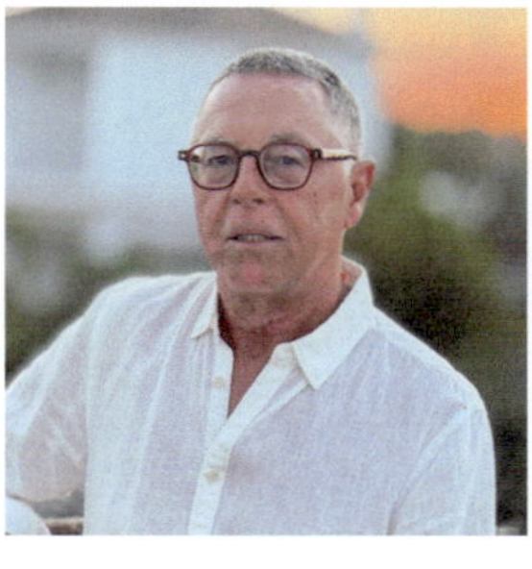

Preface

Some of the most transcendental contributions in the field of medicine and biology have come from the work of scientists in the United Kingdom, Northern Europe, Japan, the United States, and Italy, whose visionary minds have left an indelible mark on the history of human knowledge. Spain, however, has produced lesser-known but also significant contributions to the universal scientific community. Often, these feats of knowledge have been the work of scientists who, like Santiago Ramón y Cajal, undertook their first works almost alone. Others, on the other hand, had to leave our country for foreign institutions, where knowledge flourished far from their homeland.

This book aims to take the reader by the hand, whether a specialist or just a curious reader, and guide them through a journey through the valuable contributions of Spanish doctors, biologists, and scientists to the international medical community. Discoveries that have marked the advancement of medicine in various fields are unfolded here, intertwining fascinating stories that transport us from the Islamic-Jewish era and the splendor of the Renaissance to the idealistic fervor of the Lutheran Reformation. Throughout these pages, the great philanthropic Balmis expedition that sailed the oceans to bring the newly discovered vaccines to the ends of the earth are also evoked.

We will look at the birth of the first surgical schools in Spain, the discovery of new anatomical structures, and the invention of laryngoscopy, conceived in Paris to reveal the secrets of the voice of opera singers. We will explore the dawn of vascular surgery at the hands of San Martín and Goyanes and move on to the pioneering discoveries in neuroscience by Ramón y Cajal and his Spanish Neurological School, with figures such as Pío del Rio Hortega and Fernando de Castro followed years later by Rafael Yuste and his BRAIN project. We will dive into the enzyme findings of Severo Ochoa and his school, essential for the synthesis of RNA and DNA, the search for the genetic code, and the contributions of world-renowned cardiologists, such as the Brugada brothers and Valentín Fuster. The important role of Carlos Jiménez Díaz, teaching us that without knowledge of basic sciences one cannot be a good clinician. Furthermore, important works of pioneers in urology, with Joaquín Albarrán and the Gil Vernet saga, ophthalmology with the Spanish A B and C, Arruga, Barraquer, and Castroviejo, and traumatology and war surgery with Fidel Pagés, discoverer of the epidural anesthesia, and Josep Trueta, are also described.

In turn, we will evoke the research on the origin of life by Joan Oró, the contemporary studies on morphogenesis, genetics and cellular aging by García Bellido and Izpisúa Belmonte and the spread of quinine as a treatment for malaria and discoveries in neuroendocrinology. The book concludes with the work of three great oncologists of international prestige: José Baselga, Joan Rodés and Josep Llovet.

In order to give visibility to the role of Spanish women researchers in science, we highlight four women scientists of international stature: Margarita Salas, Gabriella Morreale, Carmen Gil Fernández, Sara Borrell and Magdalena Ugarte, who have contributed significantly to the development of universal medicine through their work. We also highlight the transcendental work of the National Transplant Organization in the consolidation of one of the most efficient transplant organization in the world, the well-thought-out Primary Care organization, and the global projection of Spanish Group of Minimally Invasive Surgery.

There are many reasons that have led us to publish this book. First and foremost, the love and passion for our profession, which has driven us to live it with dedication and to devote the best years of our lives to it.

We are also motivated by a feeling of national pride, because many Spaniards have contributed to the advancement of science—not only in medicine but in various disciplines—and yet their legacy remains in the shadows, little recognized within and beyond our borders. With this book, we wish to vindicate their memory and give voice to these fascinating stories that unfold throughout the 42 chapters of this work, a journey through the history of science in Spain, intertwined with the great universal history.

In order to bring this book to fruition, we have contacted a large number of prestigious professionals, with more or less experience in writing, who, in addition to their daily work, have delved into the lives of many of our characters. We would like to thank them for their commitment and dedication. Without them, this work would not have been possible.

The contributors include journalists, doctors, philosophers, relatives of the biographers, and even some who have written their own biography, as is the case of Antonio Gómez-Pan.

As editors, we have tried to maintain a common thread in terms of the structure, the number of photographs, the length of the chapters, and the bibliography cited, with the aim of offering a book that is faithful to reality and of interest to readers.

We are proud that the book is published by Springer, which has distinguished itself by publishing books on Medicine and Science.

The reader may wonder what criteria were used to select the characters and why some great influential physicians have not been included.

Our choice has followed objective criteria, giving priority to those scientists whose contributions were pioneering and innovative at the global level, beyond their impact at the national level. This has been the spirit that has guided our work, and we trust in the public's understanding of the inevitable omissions, for which we apologize.

One of the main objectives of our work is to encourage new generations of doctors and scientists to develop their curiosity and ideas, reading this book, as there are still many fields to explore, innovate, and research. Curiosity is an essential pillar in the life of a doctor or biologist, as countless opportunities for discovery present themselves to us on a daily basis. To take advantage of them, it is essential to be well prepared from university, to carry out diverse studies and to develop doctoral theses in different areas such as statistics, epidemiology, basic sciences, or everyday clinical practice. All this enriches professional life, and these biographies can be a source of inspiration.

Two themes emerge from this book and should be chosen as areas for special dedication and funding: neurological sciences and biochemistry. Finally, it is essential to reflect on funding and support for science in Spain. The lack of a stable and comprehensive policy in this area is unacceptable. The flight of young talent abroad, not only to the United States but also to nearby European countries, due to the ineffectiveness or inadequacy of organization and funding mechanisms, represents a serious loss of human resources. This situation must change. Our governments, regardless of their political leanings, must be aware of this reality and act accordingly. As reflected in the chapter index, some of the scientists portrayed worked in Spain, especially the older ones. However, those closer to the twentieth and twenty-first centuries, although they have proudly carried their Spanish identity around the world, have been forced to emigrate in order to develop professionally. It is regrettable that our talents continue to leave, forced to depend on other countries in order to prosper. Although Spain cannot compete with America in terms of technological investment, in a globalized world it is crucial to find strategies to work together and avoid the loss of national talent. As Margarita Salas has said: "A country without science is a country without development".

Amsterdam, The Netherlands — Miguel A. Cuesta
Jerez de la Frontera, Spain — Francisco Mateo Vallejo

Contents

About the Editors and Contributors

About the Editors

Miguel A. Cuesta Doctor of Medicine and Surgery. Emeritus Professor of General and Digestive Surgery at the Department of Surgery. Amsterdam University Medical Centre (UMC), Amsterdam, The Netherlands, where he specialized in Minimally Invasive Oncological Surgery of the Digestive Tract. Knight of Honour (Ridder van de Orde van de Nederlandse Leeuw), bestowed by His Majesty King Willem-Alexander of the Netherlands in 2018. Honorary member of various surgical societies in Spain, Germany, Poland, Japan, Chile, Peru, and several Spanish autonomous communities. In November 2021, he received the Career Achievement Award in Surgery from the European Association for Endoscopic Surgery (EAES) in Barcelona.

Francisco Mateo Vallejo Doctor of Medicine and Surgery; specialist in General and Digestive Surgery. Associate Professor and Academic Coordinator of Surgery at the University of Cádiz. Particularly dedicated to Minimally Invasive Oncological Surgery of the upper digestive tract. Former Head of the Department of Surgery at the Hospital of Jerez. Full Member of the Royal Academy of Medicine and Surgery of Cádiz.

Contributors

Rolando Pérez Álvarez Science Research Centre, Universidad Autónoma del Estado de Morelos, Cuernavaca, Mexico

José Borrell Andrés Emeritus Professor, Researcher CSIC, Madrid, Spain

Josep Brugada Professor of Cardiology, Universidad de Barcelona, Barcelona, Spain

Pedro Brugada Professor of Cardiology, Free University of Brussels, Brussels, Belgium

Medical Centre Brugada, Aalst, Belgium

Hospital Medical Helicopters, Puerto Banús, Málaga, Spain

Ramón Brugada Professor of Cardiology. Universidad de Girona, Girona, Spain

Sara Sánchez Canto Ophthalmology Department, Hospital Universitario San Agustín, Avilés, Spain

Juan Bernal Sols-Morreale Institute of Biomedical Research, Consejo Superior de Investigaciones Científicas and Universidad Autónoma de Madrid, Madrid, Spain

Roger Corcho Philosopher, and Science Popularizer, Barcelona, Spain

Miguel A. Cuesta Department of Surgery, Amsterdam University Medical Centre (UMC), Amsterdam, The Netherlands

Fernando de Castro Soubriet Myelin Dynamics & Repair Lab, Madrid, Spain

Centro de Neurociencias, Cajal-CSIC (former Instituto Cajal), Madrid, Spain

Manuel Doblas Dominguez Vascular surgeon. Former Head of the Department of Vascular Surgery, Hospital of Toledo, Toledo, Spain

Carlos Márquez Espinós Anaesthesiologist and historian of Medicine. Department of the History of Medicine, University of Cádiz, Cádiz, Spain

Luis A. Fariña Urologist. Department of Urology, Ribera Povisa Hospital in Vigo, Vigo, Spain

Damián García-Olmo Professor of Surgery, Universidad Autonoma de Madrid (UAM), Madrid, Spain

Department of Surgery, Head of the Department of Surgery, "Fundación Jiménez Díaz" University Hospital, Madrid, Spain

Víctor García Gil Architect, AUG-Architects, SLP, Castellón de la Plana, Spain

Antonio Gómez-Pan Professor in Endocrinology, Madrid, Spain

Carmen Padules González Registered Nurse and Researcher, Centro de Salud Cerro del Aire, Madrid, Spain

Susana Pérez Holgueras Head of the Science Culture Unit, Fundación madri+d, Regional Goverment of Madrid, Madrid, Spain

Antonio San José Journalist, Political Analyst, Madrid, Spain

Carlos Pera Madrazo University of Córdoba, Emeritus Professor of the Department of Surgery. Liver and Pancreas Transplantation Unit at the Reina Sofía University Hospital, Córdoba, Spain

Eva Maranillo Alcaide Professor of the Department of Anatomy and Embryology, Faculty of Medicine, Rovira i Virgili University, Reus, Tarragona, Spain

Antonio Martín Mateos Specialist in Otorhinolaryngology, Puerta del Mar Hospital, Cádiz, Spain

Rafael Matesanz Former Director, National Organization of Transplants, Madrid, Spain

Raquel Salazar Méndez Ophthalmology Department, Hospital Universitario San Agustín, Avilés, Spain

Nacho Meneses Journalist newspaper "El País", Madrid, Spain

Miguel Pocoví Mieras Professor of Biochemistry and Molecular Biology, University of Zaragoza, Zaragoza, Spain

Lluís Montoliu Department of Molecular and Cellular Biology, Spanish National Research Council (CSIC), National Centre for Biotechnology (CNB), Madrid, Spain, and Centre for Biomedical Network Research on Rare Diseases (CIBERER) of (ISCIII), Madrid, Spain

Isabel Adrados Morán Professor of Anatomy and Embriology, Faculty of Medicine, Complutense University, Madrid, Spain

Daniel Moreno Moreno Department of Philosophy, IES Miguel Servet, Zaragoza, Spain

Miguel Ángel Piris Pinilla Department of Pathological Anatomy, Fundación Jiménez Díaz, Madrid, Spain

Arturo Prada Oliveira Department of Anatomy, University of Cádiz, Cádiz, Spain

Carlos Vaquero Puerta Professor of Surgery, University of Valladolid, Valladolid, Spain

Antoni Roca Rosell Professor of History of Science and Technology. Polytechnic University of Catalonia, Barcelona, Catalonia, Spain

Julio Virseda Rodriguez Former Head of the Department of Urology, Hospital of Albacete, Albacete, Spain

Iole Ferrara Romeo Institute of Medicinal Chemistry (IQM-CSIC), Spanish National Research Council (CSIC), Madrid, España

Jose Sanudo Former Head of the Department of Anatomy and Embryology, Faculty of Medicine, Complutense University of Madrid, Madrid, Spain

José María Gil-Vernet Sedó Gil-Vernet Urology Centre, Barcelona, Spain

Juan José Rodríguez Sendín Family Medicine and Communitarian Medicine, General Council of the College of Physicians of Spain (CGCOM), National Commission of Deontological Ethics (CGCOM), Madrid, Spain

Estrella Mateo Torres Specialist in Anaesthesia and Resuscitation, Madrid, Spain

Joan Oró Trilla President of the Foundation Joan Oró, Lleida, Spain

Francisco Mateo Vallejo Surgeon Specialized in Minimally Invasive Surgery for Gastrointestinal Cancer, Jerez de la Frontera, Cádiz, Spain

Pedro Mestres Ventura Autonomous University of Barcelona, Barcelona, Spain

Director of the Department of Anatomy at Saarland University, Saarbrücken, Germany

Faculty of Science, University of Luxembourg, Esch-sur-Alzette, Luxembourg

Inmaculada Yruela Guerrero Senior Research Scientist, Experimental Station Aula Dei (EEAD), Spanish Research Council (CSIC), Zaragoza, Spain

1

Muslim-Jewish Medicine in Al-Andalus: Abulcasis and Maimonides: The Andalusian Physicians Who Integrate Surgery into Medicine in the 10–12th Century

Carlos Pera Madrazo

Medicine and Surgery

The term "medicine" derives from the Indo-European root "med", which originates from the Greek Word "mèdomai", meaning "to care for", "to measure" or "to think". In antiquity, diseases were explained as being caused by supernatural forces, rewards or punishments from the gods, and medicine sought to cure them by magical and sacred means, being clearly separated from surgery. In ancient Greek, surgery is related to two words: "keiros" (hands) and "ergos" (work). Surgery was considered a craft that was performed with the aid of a knife.

Later, the Greek world developed its humoral theory, which explained disease as an imbalance between the four bodily humors: blood, black bile, yellow bile and phlegm. Treatment aimed to restore this humoral harmony through a set of guiding principles, thereby facilitating the natural process of healing. Hippocrates of Cos (460–370 BC), the true father of medicine, and later Galen of Pergamon (129–216 AD), established these therapeutic principles, which persisted until the eighteenth century. In their compendia,

C. P. Madrazo (✉)
University of Córdoba, Former Head of the Department of Surgery. Liver and Pancreas Transplantation Unit at the Reina Sofía University Hospital, Córdoba, Spain

M. A. Cuesta, F. Mateo Vallejo (eds.), *Spain's Journey in Medicine*,
https://doi.org/10.1007/978-3-032-12221-6_1

always separating medicine from surgery, they considered the latter as a profession that was only used when medicine was ineffective or as a first choice for those improper doctors, the "surgeons".

The "surgeons" of the time were, in general, poorly trained people who only performed abscess drainage, tooth extractions, bloodletting and little else. The separation between medicine and surgery continued in the Roman world (medici clinici and medici chirurgici). In the Byzantine world, in Alexandria, Paulus of Aegina (625–690) wrote his seven-book "Hypomnema" or "Memorandum", with the sixth book devoted to soft tissue surgery and traumatology (dislocations and fractures). From then on, there was a great silence in the medical world during the Middle Ages, until the arrival of Islam in Al-Andalus (711–1492) and the appearance of the great figure of Abulcasis in the tenth century.

The Legacy of the Physicians of Al-Andalus

Al-Andalus was the Muslim-ruled territory of the south of the Iberian Peninsula. The Muslims, since the invasion from North Africa, controlled this large area of Spain between 711 and 1492. In today's Andalucía, name derived from Al-Andalus, remnants of Muslims culture are present in everyday life. From the Arabic names of cities and places to the brilliant arquitecture with monuments such as the Alhambra of Granada, the mosque of Cordoba and many others in towns and cities across Andalucía, the culture developed in many other aspects such as philosophy, literature, and transmission of the old Greek culture to Occident, aspects that are considered essential to the current culture of today's world. The Muslims together with the Jewish and Christians people developed as part of these activities, the Medicine as science.

This chapter describes the integration of Surgery, until then unscientific work carried out by barbers, into the science of Medicine, until then based on the principles of Galen.

The physicians who were significant in the *Muslim West*, among them Abulcasis and Maimonides, were not only of Arab origin, but also Jewish; therefore, what gives unity to this Arab medicine of the Middle Ages is the language: Arabic. We intentionally speak of the *Muslim West* or *Western Muslim World* as their work was carried out not only in the Iberian Peninsula (Al-Andalus) but also in the Maghreb (North Africa), and in the case of the Cordoban Jew Maimonides in Egypt, as his family fled the religious fundamentalism of the Almohads who ruled, at the time, in Al-Andalus and the Maghreb. Their writings spread not only throughout the Islamic and Jewish world, but also to the whole of the medieval Christian world, since Al-Andalus was to its Almoravid, Almohad and finally Christian conquerors what Greece was to Rome:

> *Græcia capta ferum victorem cepit (the victor, Rome, was in turn conquered by the defeated Greece),*

which could be paraphrased as: Al-Andalus conquered, reconquers its fierce conquerors (É. Levi Provençal).

The historical context in which these figures carried out their work was conditioned by the successive Muslim conquest of the Iberian Peninsula. When the caliphate of Damascus fell in AD 750, a prince of the Marwanid house, the Umayyad prince, future ʿAbd al-Raḥmān" I (known as the immigrant), went to seek his fortune at the farthest reaches of the Muslim world.

> At that time, Morocco was a desirable and attractive dominion; yet, upon his arrival, the Umayyad prince soon realized that their tribes were not only insufficiently Islamized, but also under the influence of Kharijite religion—this being the third major branch of Islam, alongside Sunnis and Shiites, whose faithful maintained that caliphal authority derived from the community itself, which ought to choose the worthiest individual, "even if he be a black slave"

Consequently, ʿAbd al-Raḥmān turned his attention to Spain, where he overthrew the already weakened authority of the Arab governor and established the Umayyad dynasty in AD 756—less than half a century after Ṭāriq's landing at Tarifa in AD 711 (start of the Muslim invasion in Spain).

Abulcasis, Father of Modern Surgery. Rescues and Renews Surgery as a Science (Fig. 1.1)

Abu'l Qasim Khalaf ibin 'Abbas al-Zahrawi or Abulcasis (936–1013)

> is known in the West by multiple Latinized forms of his name, more than fourteen: *Albucasis, Albucasim, Abulcasis*, etc.; and others that refer to his *nisba*, his place of birth, such as: *Ezzahrawi, Zaharawius, Alcarani, Alsahrawi*, etc.

Although we know a great deal about his medical and surgical work (in Arabic and translated into Latin), especially his Volume Thirtieth, we know very little about his life. And the little information we have comes from the text of Leo the African: "About some distinguished men among the Arabs" (*De viris quibusdam ilustribus apud árabes)*

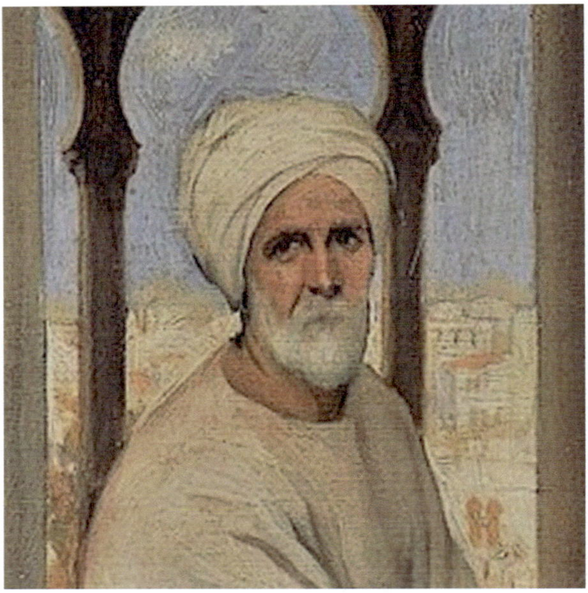

Fig. 1.1 Abulcasis. Foundation Hamdi

> *Ezaharagui was the physician of Mansor, close adviser of Cordoba and eminent among the learned, who composed a book similar to Avicenna's Canon in the art of Medicine, indeed a very useful one, which even now Muslim physicians still use. He lived for one hundred and one years. He died in the year of the "War of Cordoba," in the year 404 of the Hijra* [1].

We know, doubtful data, that he could live 101 years, dying in the 44th year of the Hegira coinciding with the Cordoban wars, the *fitnas* [2]. He was the physician and advisor to Almanzor (Mansori), Muslim Andalusi leader and statesman in the court of Caliph Hisram II, and that he wrote his treatise on Medicine following the guidelines of the *Canon of Medicine* (5-volume encyclopedia written by the Persian doctor Avicenna in 1025) [3, 4]. In the manuscript Velliüddin (Süleymaniye Library) in Istanbul it is stated about Abulcasis: "God bless him- was extremely ascetic. He cared charitably for the sick for half of his time and wrote a treatise over forty years dedicated to his sons [disciples]" [5].

His father had been also a doctor and Albucasis went to study at the famous school of Medicine in Baghdad [6].

At the time, Abulcasis was not recognized in the Arab world of his time, his name does not appear in the Diwane (official list of physicians at the court of the caliphs Abderraman III and Al-Haken II), and his compatriot Averroes [7] (1126–1198) practically ignored him.

Although we know little of his biography, we know his work very well.

His "Book of Medical Practice" has 30 volumes that include anatomical descriptions, classifications of diseases, nutritional and surgical information, as well as sections related to medicine, orthopedic surgery, ophthalmology, pharmacology, among others. However, it is particularly notable for its references to surgery.

Arabic manuscript known as *Kitâb al-Tasrîf li-man 'ajiza 'an al-ta'âlif*, or *Kitâb al-Tasrîf, which* we could translate as: "Book of medical readiness for those who are not able to learn by themselves" or "Book of medical practice", were collected by Spink and Lewis [3] in their work "*Abulcasis on surgery and instruments*". In the Christian world, his work it is known by its Latin name "Concessio ei data qui componere haud valet". Most of the Latin manuscripts that are preserved today are a copy of Gerard of Cremona's, translated from the Arabic at the Toledo School of Translators. Three and other five, *among which is the oldest surviving* manuscript of the Surgery of *Abulcasis, (Khuda Bakhsh 2146, also known as Bankipore 17),* dated 8 March 1188, is kept in *the Khuda Baksh Library in Patna, India.*

In Spain, surprisingly, only two manuscripts of Volume XXX (The Surgery) are preserved, one in the Library of the Royal Monastery of San Lorenzo de El Escorial [8] and the other in Granada in the Abadía del Sacromonte (Fig. 1.2). There are other manuscripts dedicated to other medical and pharmaceutical topics throughout the European world.

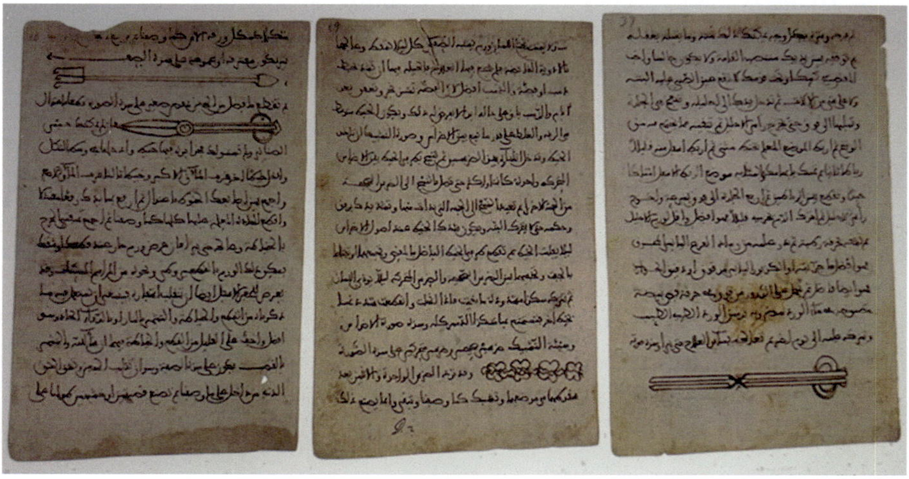

Fig. 1.2 Abulcasis. Manuscript of San Lorenzo de El Escorial. Depicted tissue forceps and scissors

The work of Abulcasis remained for almost six centuries, for both physicians and surgeons, one of the most important practical guides in the Islamic and medieval European world. Finally, they were translated into English in 1973 by Spink and Lewis [3].

The most important on the subject of this chapter is the Volume Thirtieth, dedicated to Surgery, knowledge that spread throughout the Islamic world, and from the twelfth century onwards to the Christian world through its translation by Gerard of Cremona in Toledo [8] although there are many different versions [9, 10].

Centuries later, Abulcasis' books were taken up by Gulielmus de Salicetum (1210–1280), Guy de Chauliac (1290–1368) and Fabrizius de Aquapendente (1537–1519). It was first printed in Venice, together with Guy de Chauliac's *Cirugía parva (*1497). Other Venetian editions are those of 1499; 1500—the most cited of them all; 1520; 1532; and 1540. The first modern Latin edition is by Channing's (1778).

The Thirtieth Volume

The thirtieth volume, dedicated to Surgery comprises three books: the first "Concerns the use of cautery"; the second deals with "Incisions, perforations, venous sections, extractions of arrows and other similar things", and the third refers to "Fractures and dislocations". It is important to emphasize that Books I and II from this Volume describe everything from head to toe and only Book III alters this order of presentation. It should also be noted that Abulcasis insists on the knowledge of Anatomy, as well as on the need for professional ethics, as other Andalusíes surgeons did later (Abenzoar) [11].

The Use of Cautery

Cauterization was a well-established treatment modality at the time and, for some authors, the definitive treatment for most conditions.

> Cautery is a technique used to destroy tissue with a burning or caustic instrument, useful for removing small tumors or for closing blood vessels to stop bleeding.

Abulcasis questions the effectiveness of cautery in its classical conception, while advising his disciples that they may resort to this method with caution and only after other treatment modalities have failed. Although he questions the traditional applications of cautery, he also envisages other therapeutic possibilities. Not only does he use it in a similar way to acupuncture—in its classical form- but he also applies it as though it were a modern electric scalpel: that is, for the purpose of coagulate. He insists that the operative field must be dry, and that the bleeding vessel should be clamped or compressed with the fingers before applying the cautery. Moreover, he uses it to perform incisions, thereby emphasizing his preference for iron cautery, which when heated first turns red—the ideal moment for coagulating—and then yellow, making it suitable for opening an abscess, for example. In fact, he rejects gold cauteries, because it melts quickly when heated. He designed various types of cautery, such as the half-moon cautery, which he used to treat eyelid ptosis, as the healing of the scar caused the eyelid to retract. He also developed a specific cautery for the treatment of inguinal hernias, different to that of Paul of Aegina.

> In the text he describes how it should be done: for this purpose the patient should be relaxed, and the hernial contents reduced in the abdominal cavity, and then the surgeon with the index finger will prevent it from coming out again, and taking the cautery described by him, with the right hand he will apply it, causing a deep burn until it reaches the bone [pubis] In this last, as in the design of the cautery, he also disagrees with Paul of Aegina, since the latter does not make such a deep burn. Afterwards, for forty days he did not allow the patient to make any effort, administering laxatives to facilitate defecation; in this way he achieved a firm cicatricial scar that prevented hernial recurrence (of course such a maneuver entailed the burning of the cord and testicular atrophy). As an anecdote I would like to point out that in the miniature corresponding to this chapter of the Codex nova series 2641 of the *Wien Österreichische Nationalbibliothek*, the patient is shown on a pair of stretchers tied with a rope, and we suppose, lulled to sleep with mandrake, although nothing is made clear about the latter.

Instruments

His most important personal contributions, according to Spink and Lewis [3] on instruments are to be found in Book II, the most important of which are the following: the scissors for tonsillectomy, with their jaws arranged as if they were pincers, also describing how to use them; the lancet for debriding abscesses in fearful persons, which hides its blade with an ogive-shaped sheath; the design of a new trocar for paracentesis, to avoid injuring the viscera; the possibility that he introduced the use of straight scissors and the syringe in surgery [12], the design of an instrument to remove stones; his original conception of the vaginal speculum and that of an instrument designed to remove dead fetuses, precursor of Chamberlen's forceps (1631). His innovations also include the use of animal gut as a suture material (catgut), which was in use until a few years ago and was banned in the wake of the bovine spongiform encephalopathy (mad cow disease) epidemic. The use of this material is understandable because it was popular among Arab sailors, for mooring the rigging of sailing ships, due to its resistance to water.

Contributions to Dentistry and Surgery of Oral Cavity

It is worth mentioning his contributions to dentistry and surgery of the oral cavity, which are not dealt with in the classical texts, such as the treatment of dental plaque, for which he designed an instrument called the *mijrad* (scraper). He also deals with the extraction of roots and broken pieces, with the design of a forceps in the shape of a stork's beak, which is very useful for extracting roots. And, Abulcasis adds, if the operator does not succeed, he must try to do so with the nail puller, which he draws, and which is very similar to the one used today. It is also very original the way of interlacing loose teeth with silver or gold thread, better with the latter because silver oxidizes, according to the author. At the end of this chapter he explains his technique of replacing teeth with carved animal bone. Also interesting is his treatment of the ranula (a saliva-filled cyst that develops under the tongue), which consists, as today, of laying it open, and for which he uses his straight, fine-tipped scissors. To conclude these comments on Book II, we will refer to an instrument he designed for the extraction of foreign bodies from the throat. The instrument is also found in Aetius and Paul of Aegina, but its originality lies in its design, as it is made of lead and, being malleable, it can be adapted to the anatomy of each individual.

Ophtalmology

His contributions to ophthalmology are also very interesting and are included in both Book I and II of this volume. In Book I we would like to highlight "*De cauterizatione fistula que est in lacrimali oculo*": "On the cauterization of the fistula located in the lacrimal (tear) duct of the eye." In the treatment of this condition, Abulcasis prefers to perforate with a drill, the design of which is original. And perhaps the most novel aspect is his fine curved scissors for removing superfluous skin, which are not mentioned in classical literature and which Guy de Chauliac copied from him, and the three-pronged retractor used to elevate the eyelid, the tips of which are protected with small spherical ends to prevent injury. He described also the treatment of the *pannus (inflammation of the cornea)* secondary to trachoma, in which he describes fine hooks for pulling the *pannus*. In the treatment of cataracts, he prefers the takeoff of the crystalline lens (which consisted of introducing a needle into the eye and with a movement detach the opacified crystalline lens and it was placed into the vitreous humor) and provides for this two instruments of great interest: the first one, *the miqdah*. It is a needle ending in a small heart-shaped spatula; if the "reclining needle" cannot enter the eye because the sclera is hard, he proposes a scalpel which he calls *al-barid*, which allows the *miqdah* to enter. It is interesting that he refers in this chapter to the aspiration of cataracts by Rhazes in Mesopotamia and also by al-Mwsilî in Mosul. We would also like to mention his comments on distichiasis [10].

On the Wounds of Abdomen

Of great interest to us is chapter LXXXV "on the wounds of the abdomen, frequent on the battlefield, with the exit of the intestine and the way of suturing them". This chapter contains all the specifications he gives on the closure of a wound in the abdomen (comparable with the closure as we surgeons do it today).

Fractures and Dislocations

Book III is the shortest of his *Treatise on Surgery.* Its structure of exposition differs from that of the preceding two books. In it, the comments are made under two major headings: cranial injuries, and fractures and dislocations in general. These are again divided into chapters which are described in the classic order from head to toe. It is preceded by an introduction in which it is emphasized that traumatology is an important part of surgery, but that unfortunately it is practiced by the ignorant and by those who have never read a page of the classic books on the subject. According to the author, his aim in writing it was to simplify and to set out briefly and clearly what he has learned from his experience and from reading the classics. Like the other two books, it is also enriched with illustrations.

The section concerning cranial wounds is drawn from Hippocrates and adds nothing substantially new to the body of doctrine contained in the classical treatises. What is noteworthy, however, are the various instruments depicted therein, ranging from chisels, and trephines to a speculum designed by Abulcasis himself to protect delicate structures—referred to in the text as the menigophilax.

Under the heading of "Fractures and dislocations" a series of chapters are written which, fundamentally, follow the work of Paul of Aegina and, like this author, omit fractures of the calcaneus.

Among the points of interest developed in the introduction of this book is the description of a diet for the traumatized person. The aim of this diet is the consolidation of fractures and the recovery of the injured person. Another point that stands out is the need to carry out reduction manoeuvres with great care to avoid pain, and that these should be carried out on a flat surface to facilitate alignment. And it is worth highlighting the different ways of making a bandage and obtaining fixation; and it is here where he comments that, in order to harden the bandage, flour and egg white should be added. He was therefore the true precursor of Larrey's French plaster.

In this Book III is the drawing of the traction table for treating spinal fractures (In the S. Nova code of the *Wien Österreichische Nationalbibliothek* the drawing of the traction table has become famous).

As a curiosity and anecdote we can mention fractures of the genitals, which do not appear in any of the classical treatises and where such curious things are stated as: "When the male organ is fractured, insert the penis in a goose neck, wrap and bandage it and leave it to rest for three days until it heals" [13].

Maimonides (Fig. 1.3)

Maimonides referred to himself as "Moses, son of Rabbi Maimon the Spaniard". Moses b. Abd 'Allâh Maimûn al-Qurtubi al-isra'îlî, Maimonides, was born in Cordoba in 1135 into a Sephardic family of judges. He is also known as *Moses ben Maimon*, or by his Hebrew acronym, *Ramban.*

The arrival of the Almohads in the Iberian Peninsula in 1145 AD forced his family to emigrate due to the intransigent religious conditions of the new rulers; at first, they thought the situation would be temporary and settled in Almería in 1148. He was then 12 years old. Christian rule lasted only ten years, and in 1157 the Almohads again imposed Islam on Almería, and the Banû Maymûn

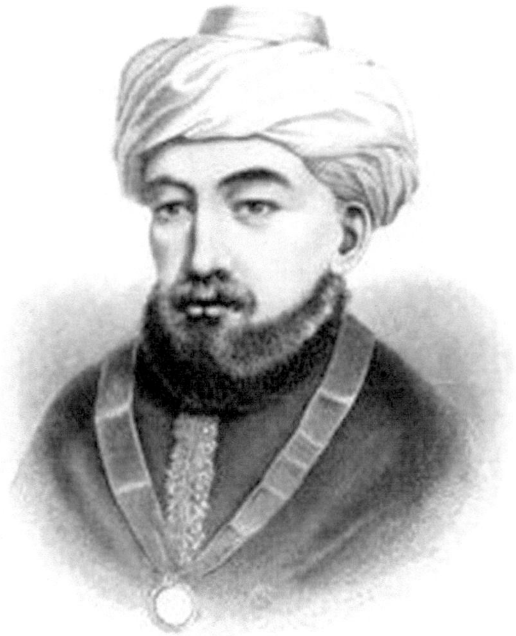

Fig. 1.3 Maimonides

were forced to leave. It seems that between 1157 and 1160, still on the run, they stayed in the Jewish quarters of Lucena and Granada. By this time Maimonides had already written much of his legal and theological work, but not his medical work, It is believed that it was then that he met and became friends with the Tibbonides family, the translators of Granada. In 1160 they left for Fez which, although under Almohad rule, his family thought they could pass unnoticed. However, in 1165 the situation in Fez became untenable (a well-known teacher rabbi of Maimonides, *Yhuda b. Sasan*, was executed for refusing to convert to Islam, and then it was Maimonides who escaped the same fate, thanks to the intervention of a Muslim theologian who vouched for him). The family was again forced to emigrate by ship to St. John of Acre in Palestine, and after a brief stay in Jerusalem and Hebron (at that time Palestine was the scene of fighting between Crusaders and Muslims)—they moved to Egypt, first in Alexandria, and then permanently in Al-Fustat, a place near the new city of Cairo.

In Egypt, the family, which was engaged in commerce, went bankrupt, and Maimonides was forced to seek a profession to make a living, and he chose medicine; a science which he learned from the sons and disciples of *Ibn Zhur* during his stay in Morocco.

The period in which he lived was the culmination and at the same time the end of the intellectual period known as the "Golden Age" of Jewish-Arabic culture

His monumental work is a book of laws completed in Egypt in 1168, *Sefer hamaor* (book of enlightenment), which is a commentary on the Mišnà. Another important work is a book of laws, the *Mišné Torah*, in fourteen volumes, which is a systematic synthesis of all the religious and moral laws of Judaism, reaching back to the time of the author's life. His philosophical book *Moré nevochim*—Guide for the Perplexed—is the most famous work outside of the Jewish sphere and aims to give a philosophical vision of his time in the form of a reconciliation between the wisdom of the Bible and philosophy.

At the end of his life he wrote ten medical works which have been revised in recent years and, for the most part, printed for the first time. His ten medical texts written mainly in Arabic are: Treatise on the Regimen of Health (a compendium of the most important recommendations to be followed in order to maintain health and avoid illness. He recommends that those suffering from illnesses such as neurosis or paranoia should turn to philosophy and ethics). The Book of Asthma, (written in Arabic on behalf of a nobleman who suffered from it); Poisons and Antidotes; Treatise on the Cure of Haemorrhoids (Risâla fî l-bawâsîr), Treatise on Coitus (Maqalâ fi l-yîmâ') which includes a series of recipes for foods and medicines that act as aphrodisiacs. It recommends some attitudes and feelings that benefit sex, such as laughter, happiness, rest and sleep, if it is not excessive. Furthermore, he wrote about Medical Responsibilities; Commentaries on the aphorisms of Hippocrates; Names of materia medica; *Compendium Galeni* (seven volumes); and Medical aphorisms of *Moses*.

According to him, when treating the sick, we encounter two unknown factors: (a) the reciprocal influences between the soul and the body of the sick person and, (b) the concurrence of scientific knowledge, the intuitive capacity to establish a diagnosis and the power of influence that the doctor has over the patient. All of these are different for each physician. In his work *Maqâla fîl-rabw*, the Treatise on Asthma, he says: "always and above all, medical care is of great importance, not only during the illness, but also at all times", "medicine is governed by a coincidence of logic, medical expertise and intuition". And it was this treatise on asthma that was one of the most influential works for Süssmann Muntner [14]. It describes the disease in detail and recommends practical treatments for its management. But perhaps most importantly, it emphasized the importance of "prevention", as it anticipates some of the principles of modern medicine. However, Carmen Peña et al. do not consider it as such and cite it among the minor works such as: Risâla fî l-bawâsîr (Epistle on haemorrhoids) and the Maqalâ fi l-yîmâ' (Epistle on coitus) [15]

References

1. De Ezaharagui lived for one hundred and one years. He died in the year of the "War of Cordoba", in the year 404 of the Hegira.
2. The 404th year of the Hegira runs roughly from 27 July 1013 to 5 July 1014. The first *fitnahs* took place between 1009 and 1031, their end coinciding with the abolition of the Caliphate.
3. Spink MS, Lewis GL. Abulcasis on surgery and instruments (a definitive edition of the Arabic text with English translation and commentary). London: The Wellcome Institute of the History of Medicine; 1973.
4. Almanzor built a new caliphate city, Medina al-Zahira, whose exact location is not known, but it is known that it was built between 979 and 987 and that it was sacked and destroyed in April 1009.
5. This manuscript. was used by Spink and Lewis, among six others for the final composition of their Arabic text and is a *katabah*^{u} *li-nafsihi*^{i} copy.
6. Castejón R. La higiene de Albucasis: Un manuscrito inédito de origen cordobés (by Mr. Eugenio M.O. Dognée, translated by D. Rafael Castejón). 1925. Córdoba: Publications of the Academia de Ciencias Médicas de Córdoba.
7. Averroes *(Ibn Rushd*, 1126–1198) was an Andalusian jurist, philosopher and physician born in Córdoba, whose work had a profound influence on medieval philosophy and medicine in both the Islamic and Christian worlds.
8. Cano Ledesma A. Indexing of the Arabic manuscripts of El Escorial. Biblioteca La Ciudad de Dios, 1996. Real biblioteca del Escorial, Catalogues. Ediciones Escurialenses. Real Monasterio del Escorial.
9. The chapters change from book I to II, and some have not been found. Therefore, the Introduction; the first 16 chapters of Book I; 44 chapters of Book II; and the complete Book III are missing.
10. Irblich E. Einfluß von Vorlage und Text im himblick auf kodicologische Erscheinungformen am Beispiel der Überlieferung der, Chirurgie "des Abu'l Qâsim Halaf Ibn ^{C}Abbâs al-Zaharâwî von 13. Jarhundert bis 1500 (Tafeln XXXVII-XXXVI) Colloquium des Comité International de Paléographie, 15-18 September 1981. 1982. München: Arbeo-Gessellschaft.
11. Abenzoar (1091/95-1161/2), also known as Ibn Zuhr or in its Latinized form Avenzoar, was born in Peñaflor (Seville). His legacy in surgery and clinical practice is remarkable. His most famous work is the *Kitab al-Taysir* (the Book of Simplification), among eight others. It was translated into Hebrew and Latin. He is considered to be the introducer of dissection, which he practiced on sheep. He maintained a professional relationship with Averroes.

12. The use of scissors in surgery was known as early as the Bronze Age. We have had the opportunity to see them carved on a wall, together with other surgical instruments, the temple of Kom Ombo on the Nile (2nd century BC, although its construction was completed in the 1st century BC). But the use of fine-tipped straight-cut scissors for ophthalmology and blunt-tipped scissors for circumcision are original to Abulcasis , as is the one already described for tonsillectomy.

13. Pera Madrazo C. Albucasis and Al-Gâfiqî, two examples of Andalusian physicians in Médicos cordobeses de aayer y de hoy. Fernández Dueñas A, Casal Román M, editors (Rafael Castejón Collection). 2018. Córdoba (ISBN:978-84-120060-1-8)
14. Muntner S. Medieval Hebrew Medicine in Historia Medieval de la Medicina (Tomo III) Laín Entralgo P. Director. 1972. Barcelona: Salvat Editores SA
15. Peña C., Girón F., Barchin M. La prevención de la enfermedad en el Al-Andalus del siglo XII en la Medicina en el al-Andalus coordinada por Alvares de Morales C. Y Molina E. 1999. (Fundación el Legado Andalusí). Junta de Andalucía Consejería de Cultura.

2

Miguel Servet (Michael Servetus): Between Heresy and Science. Discovery of the Minor Circulation

Francisco Mateo Vallejo and Daniel Moreno Moreno

My name is Miguel, and I wish to use these few remaining days of my life to bear witness to the course of events that have led me to my present situation. I am confined within a filthy cell in a prison in Geneva, and, thanks to an acquaintance, I have managed to obtain a quill and some ink in order to set down, succinctly, this brief account of my life in these final moments (Fig. 2.1).

I was born in Villanueva de Sigena on 29 September in the year of our Lord 1511, a small Aragonese village located in the Monegros region. Its location is marked by the existence of a fertile plain irrigated by the river Alcanadre, as well as by the Monastery of Santa María de Sigena, under whose protection the village was founded. My father, Antón Serveto, was a man of low nobility, employed as a notary for the nuns of the monastery. My mother, Catalina Conesa Zaporta, originally from Barbastro, came from a family of Jewish converts (Fig. 2.2).

I had two brothers: Pedro, who continued with my father's notary's office, and Juan, who, at the age of 15, was ordained a priest, working in the village of Poleñino. I learned my first letters from my father and from the nuns who lived in the monastery. I continued my studies to become a clergyman in the monastery of Montearagón, near Huesca.

F. M. Vallejo (✉)
Surgeon Specialized in Minimally Invasive Surgery for Gastrointestinal Cancer, Jerez de la Frontera, Cádiz, Spain

D. M. Moreno
Department of Philosophy. IES Miguel Servet, Zaragoza, Spain

M. A. Cuesta, F. Mateo Vallejo (eds.), *Spain's Journey in Medicine*,
https://doi.org/10.1007/978-3-032-12221-6_2

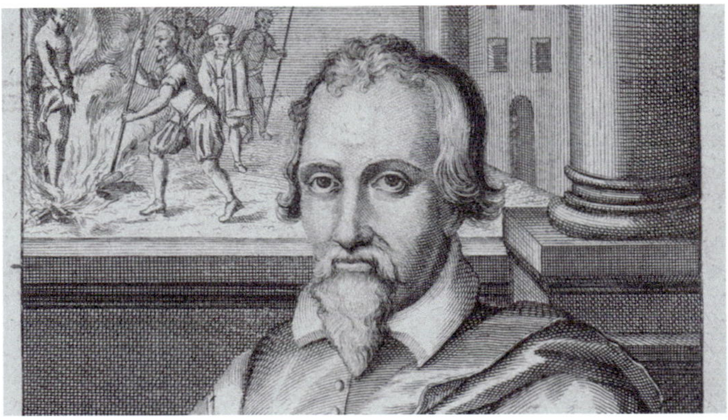

Fig. 2.1 Miguel Servet

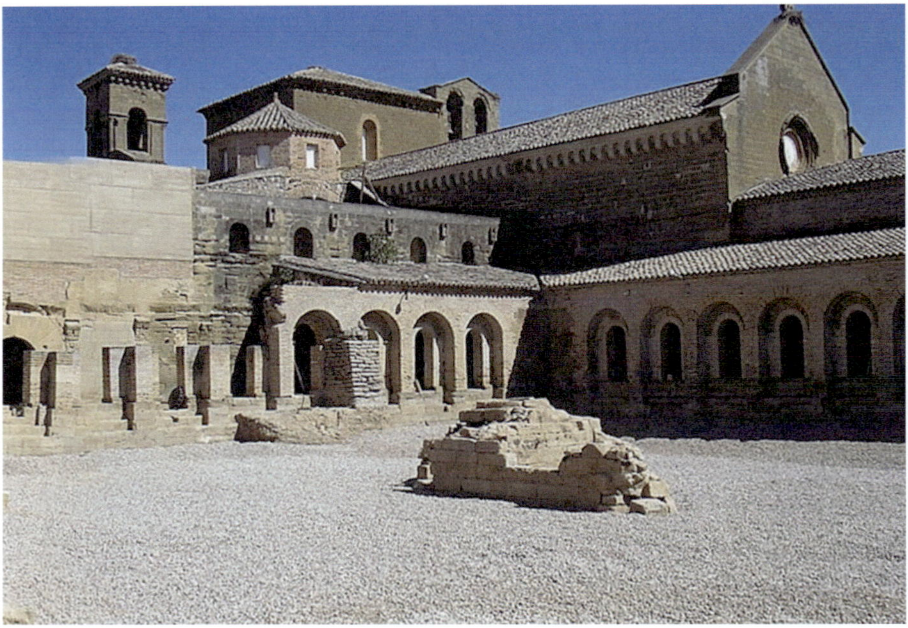

Fig. 2.2 Royal Monastery of Santa María de Sigena

I was 14 years old when my father, through some acquaintances, put me in contact with a Franciscan Father from Huesca who accepted me as a disciple. Later, grateful for my services, he appointed me as his personal secretary. His name was Fray Juan de Quintana, member of the court of the Crown of Aragon and part of the council of King Fernando II. After entering his service, he became inquisitor and personal confessor to our Emperor Carlos V (Charles V), which allowed me to travel with him to various cities, not only in Spain but also in the rest of Europe. I was at his side for two years, during which time I studied theology and deepened my knowledge of Latin and Greek.

At 17 years of age, my father, following the advice of my teacher sent me to study theology and law at the University of Toulouse, in Languedoc, known for its quality of teaching.

At the same time, the ecclesiastical reform of Martin Luther was spreading rapidly. Thanks to the recent discovery of the printing press, the "*95 theses of Luther*" were spread and vividly discussed among teachers and students, remarking the different views on theological doctrines.

Like many of my peers, I was fed up with the excesses of the Church, its ostentation of wealth and its economic interests, such as the sale of papal bulls and indulgences, which allowed those who possessed them to enter more easily into the Kingdom of Heaven and to obtain forgiveness of sins in exchange for money or goods. Luther rejected the authority of the Pope as God's representative and proposed a return to the origins of Christianity, both in poverty and in following the Bible as a source of spirituality. He opposed the veneration of images of saints and, while accepting the theory of the Trinity, considered God the Father and God the Son to be two distinct entities.

In this atmosphere of reaction against the Pope and his Church, the former rector of the university in Toulouse, Ramón Sabunde, has published *"Theologia Naturalis, sive Liber Creaturarum"*. In this work he defended the possibility of understanding the Scriptures through the contemplation of nature.

As these thoughts took root in me, my theological ideas became more and more consolidated and distanced from those considered orthodox by the Roman Catholic Church.

A historical event helped to consolidate the ideas that had germinated in me in Toulouse. In 1529, Juan de Quintana asked to accompany him to Bologna for the coronation of the emperor Carlos V. The choice of Bologna was mainly due to the fact that the king was not sure that he would be well received in Rome after the sack of Rome he had carried out there on 6 May 1527.

In the last days of July 1529, we left Barcelona by sea, accompanied by a large retinue of nobles, clergy, military and service personnel. We disembarked in Genoa on 12 August and, from there, arrived in Bologna in early November.

On our arrival, the city was bustling with activity; a large number of merchants, street artists and petty thieves had taken advantage of the arrival of such a royal expedition and the Pope Clement VII, who had arrived already on 23 October. The city was crowded, and it was common to see merchants, maids and military men milling about, busy with their chores or going to the taverns, which had proliferated due to the increase in population during the festivities. Much money had been spent on beautifying and decorating the town, including a fountain in the shape of an eagle, flanked by two lions from which red wine, white wine and water flowed. Bread, cheese and meat were also distributed to the delight of the townsfolk.

Both the papal retinue and our own were housed in the Public Palace. The monarch and the Pope occupied adjoining rooms to facilitate their meetings and ensure privacy. Meanwhile, I devoted the first few weeks to my duties as secretary to Friar Juan de Quintana, which took up most of my time. However, this did not prevent me from observing the papal retinue and appreciating their taste for good food and drink, as well as their generally relaxed life.

Although I assumed that our stay in Bologna would not be too long, in the end, the monarch decided that the coronation date should coincide with his birthday, 24 February of the following year.

The place chosen for the coronation was the immense basilica of San Petronio, located in the city's main square. This choice was no coincidence, given the large number of aristocrats, nobles and papal acolytes who were to form part of the entourage at this royal event (Fig. 2.3).

The basilica dedicated to the patron saint of the city was 132 metres long by 60 metres wide and was fitted out for the event with richly decorated

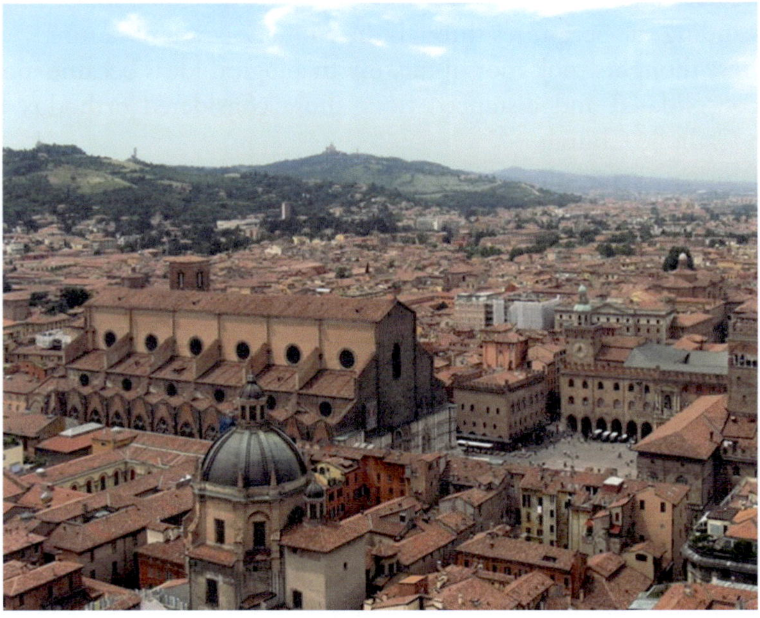

Fig. 2.3 Basilica of San Petronio, Bologna

tribunes. To make the way between the monarch's and the pope's apartments and the basilica more attractive, the king had a wooden bridge built to take him directly from his rooms to the high altar, in full view of the people and all his guests.

Two days before the coronation, on 22 February, the monarch received from Clement VII the Iron Crown of Lombardy, which accredited him as King of Italy, in an almost private ceremony in the Palazzo d'Accursio.

On 24 February, the day of the coronation, the emperor paraded across the wooden bridge, richly attired and wearing the iron crown on his head. Beside him were the Dukes of Urbino, Savoy and Bavaria, while the Marquis of Monferrato carried the golden crown, the sword, and the scepter. We were below, as part of the procession, and, by a twist of fate, after the Marquis had passed, there was a great crack and the footbridge collapsed, falling on the crowd and causing shrieks, alarm and confusion. I would later know that several people had been killed and injured when they were crushed by the collapsed structure.

Inside the basilica, before the high altar, the emperor knelt before the Pope, who handed him the golden scepter, the sword with which he was to pursue all the enemies of Christ, the golden apple, symbol of piety, virtue and constancy in his reign, and finally the imperial crown, which was placed on his head.

When the ceremony was over, both the emperor and the Pope went in procession through the streets of the city, followed by all the nobles and great men who accompanied them. The sight of the pope on the gestatorial chair, carried on the shoulders of many people above the heads of the rest of mortals, wearing a miter richly decorated with precious stones and treating everyone as if he himself were God, has led me to reflect on the meaning of religion and what it has become. Add to this the luxury and the disposition towards good food and drink, while the rest of the population suffers need and want, and I become increasingly critical of Christian practices.

I believe that all these ideas that are swirling around in my mind need to be expressed so that I can share them with those who I believe think like me. During those days, I got to writing:

> He does not deign to set foot on the ground so as not to sully his holiness! He is carried on the shoulders of men and worshipped as if he were God, which no wicked man has ever dared to do since the world began. I have seen with my own eyes how the princes carried him with pomp on their shoulders, with crosses flashing in their hands, and how all the people worshipped him on their knees along the streets. They went so far that those who could kiss his feet or sandals consid-

ered themselves more fortunate than the rest, and proclaimed that they had obtained numerous indulgences, by which long years of hellish sufferings would be reduced to them. O Beast, the vilest of beasts, the most shameless of harlots!

When all the coronation celebrations were over, Juan de Quintana informed me that the monarch had called a meeting in Augsburg to discuss the issue that most concerned Catholicism at the time: the spread of Lutheran doctrine. In this German city the Imperial Diet of the Holy Roman Empire was seeking to re-establish the unity of Catholicism in the face of the Lutheran Reformation. Carlos V, as the highest representative of Catholicism, had to be there.

On 25 June 1530, Philip Melanchthon presented to the emperor what became known as the *"Augsburg Confession"*, a catalogue of 28 items defining the ideas of the Lutheran Church. These confessions were not only written by him; they had been written in collaboration with Luther, Johannes Bugenhagen, Justus Jonas and John of Saxony. In response, Catholic theologians presented a refutation known as the *"Confutatio Augustana"*, which was delivered to the Holy Roman Emperor at the Diet of Augsburg, where he had no choice but to accept them, given his links with powerful people who had access to power and richness.

In October 1530, I left for Basel, a more liberal city, where one of the most radical reformers, Johannes Oecolampadius, lived. I got a job as a printer's proofreader in Conrad Roesch's printing workshop, which gave me access to all the works printed there, and I lived in the house of Oecolampadius, who welcomed me with great joy, or so it seemed to me at first.

During the days I spent with him, Oecolampadius even confessed to me that due to his contradictions with the Catholic Church he had become a supporter of Protestant doctrine, being the main introducer of Protestantism in Basel.

We talked a lot about Erasmus of Rotterdam, with whom he had worked on the Greek translation of the New Testament, his knowledge of Hebrew, and his knowledge with Melanchthon and Luther.

The time spent in his house was very enriching, as we discussed theological issues, and he recommended that I improve my knowledge of Hebrew.

However, what were at first amiable, if heated, discussions soon turned into disagreements, and it was our differences on the dogma of the Trinity that finally broke our harmony. My conviction about the dogma of the Trinity is that it does not exist in tradition or in early Christian writings. It was not until the Council of Nicaea, where Constantine I introduced it as an official doctrine of Christianity, that it became symbolic and detached from the earliest texts. I question, therefore, not only the traditional understanding of the Trinity, but also the baptism of newborn babies, as I believe it should not be done until they have the use of reason to freely decide whether they want to do so.

At first, Oecolampadius confessed to me, he was impressed by my intelligence and erudition, but as our theological differences emerged, he was dismayed, especially by my anti-Trinitarian ideas.

During that period of time my work in the printing house consisted in acting as proof-reader of publications, and although I got on well with Charles Roesch, who never objected to my doing that work, it was another matter when I asked him to publish a book I had just finished. I believe that the ideas contained in its pages were not to his liking, or at least feared criticism from many theologians and the Inquisition. Although Basel had always been known for its tolerance of critical and liberal ideas, at that time it was almost impossible to publish anything that departed from the more conservative theological norms.

Although he told me that he would not publish it, he was kind enough to put me in touch with another publisher friend of his, Johannes Setzer, who had a printing house in Haguenau a few kilometers from Strasbourg. Thanks to him, the book could be put on sale in 1531 under the title *De Trinitatis erroribus libri septem*, ("On the Errors of the Trinity") which contained, in essence, all my ideas against the mystery of the Trinity, because for me concepts about which there are doubts should not be imposed as truths.

I took it upon myself to distribute copies of my book among my closest friends, hoping that my ideas would be well received. Instead, what I found was severe criticism: I was declared as Arian and an Anabaptist; an Arian for not recognizing Jesus as having the same divine characteristics as God the Father, and an Anabaptist for not considering it proper for infants to be baptized without the use of reason to decide. These are only similarities with a small part of my theological theory, but they do not constitute its basis. I differ on many other issues. Erasmus did not even answer me, and others, like Martin Bucer, said of me that I deserved to have my entrails torn out!

Oecolampadius even threatened to denounce me. I believe that the ideas defended in this book have brought me more enemies than friends! I learned later that the copy sent to Juan de Quintana outraged him and, at the behest of the Inquisition, he tried to send my brother to make me see reason. The ecclesiastical authorities in Strasbourg and Basel immediately condemned my work and forbade its sale.

However, these criticisms did not discourage me and a year later, in 1532, I published my second book, *Dialogorum de Trinitate libri duo.* (Dialogues on the Trinity).

I began the work by revising what I had written in the first book, not because I had changed my mind or for fear of the reactions generated by my first book, but to complete my Christology by explaining how faith in Christ justifies, how the New Testament surpasses the Old, and how the Holy Spirit shows Himself in faith and charity, the former as a door, the latter as perfection.

In Spain, the Inquisition was already on my trail, and the University of Toulouse was demanding my capture. On 17 June 1532, the Toulouse Inquisition published a search and seizure list of 40 possible heretics, including my name, so I was forced to change my surname to Miguel Villanueva, or Villeneuve to the French.

In my situation, and after the furious criticism of my two books, I decided to change my life quickly and went to Paris. In the French capital I spent two years studying subjects such as grammar, rhetoric and dialectics, arithmetic, geometry, astronomy and music at the Collège Calvi. At the Sorbonne I had the opportunity to listen to renowned professors such as John Mayor and the physician Nicolas Cop. The speech given by the latter on 1 November 1533 at the Sorbonne was my first approach to Calvin. It seems that much of the speech, or at least its basis, was written by him, and it cost them both an order of imprisonment by the parliament of Paris. They both disappeared from the city, but I had already some contact with Calvin, and we intended to meet again before the end of the year.

Calvin summoned me to a secret meeting in the rue Saint Antoine, but he made the mistake of quoting me by my surname of Servet, so I decided not to attend, fearing that it was a trap given my arrest warrant.

At the beginning of the following year, I moved to Lyon, which had become an important publishing centre thanks to the printing house of the Trechsel brothers. After applying, I managed to work with them and began revising an edition of *Ptolemy's Geography*, which took me away from the theological subject for a year, allowing the waters, after the publication of my second book, to calm down. The fact that I was chosen to revise *Ptolemy's Geography* was due to my knowledge of both mathematics and classical languages.

This book had been edited and published on many occasions, as it was very useful and sold well thanks to the voyages and navigations that were made on in those years, which generated great profits. I set to work and began to revise it in detail, correcting errors I found in longitudes and latitudes, and accompanying the description of the lands with comments on the customs and inhabitants of each area. It was published in Lyon in 1535 under the title

Claudii Ptolomaei Alexandrini Geographicae enarrationis, libri Octo, ("Of Claudius Ptolemy of Alexandria, the Explanation of Geography"). It was such a success that a second edition was published in 1541.

During my stay in Lyon, I made friends with a person who was to set the course for my later years: Symphorien Champier. Thanks to his knowledge of medicine and his broad culture, he was able to bring out in me the doctor who had not yet blossomed. I was his friend, disciple, proofreader and amanuensis, helping him in the drafting and publication of several of his writings. In 1536 I published my first work with medical elements entitled *In Leonardum Fuchsium apologia* ("A defence of Leonhart Fuchs."). Apart from defending Champier against the attacks of Leonhart Fuchs, I wrote disquisitions on syphilis and the use of scammony, a plant used as a purgative.

The following year, on Champier's advice, I moved to Paris to study medicine. Enrolled at the University of Paris in 1537 and 1538, I lived with great scientists of the time and worked alongside Andreas Vesalius, a fellow student and friend. With him I carried out dissections, anatomical preparations and autopsies.

In 1537 I published one of my most successful books, *Syroporum universa ratio*, ("The Universal Method of Syrups") which deals with syrups, describing formulas for digestion, laxatives, diuretics, invigorants, relaxants, emetics and various mixtures for purging. I divided the book into seven chapters, in which I included a theoretical part on the different humor's decoctions and other procedures detailing the uses of the compounds.

Because of the need to earn income to support myself, I began to give classes at the College of the Lombards on astronomy and the sidereal influences on the human organism, known as judicial astrology. My students included court nobles, ecclesiastics of renown and, among them, my later friend and patron Pierre Palmier.

I wrote a short eight-page booklet on astrology entitled Quendam Medicum Apologetica Disceptatio Pro astrologia, ("A Certain Physician's Apologetic Disputation in Defense of Astrology"). I decided to publish it in bad time, as some Parisian medical doctors, including the dean of the Faculty of Medicine in Paris, Jean Tagault, read it and started legal proceedings against me. Although the judgement concluded that I could continue my lectures on the influence of the stars, I was condemned to hand over all copies of the Apologetica and admonished to respect and obey my teachers and preceptors. I decided to discontinue the course and leave for Charlieu, near Lyon.

There I lived in the house of a physician named Rivoire, treating his clientele and studying to complete my knowledge of medicine, until I obtained my doctorate in medicine in Montpellier in 1540. From then on, I earned my living as a qualified physician, first in Charlieu and then in Vienna in the Dauphinat, where I lived quietly from 1541 to 1553 as a personal physician in the service of Archbishop Pierre Palmier. As I have already mentioned, the archbishop had been one of my pupils in the classes I taught in Paris and we had become good friends, so I stayed in his archbishop's palace with luxuries and high remuneration.

In 1542, the *Pagninus Bible of Santes Pagninus* was edited by Melchior Novesianus, published by Hugues de la Porte and corrected by me. Thanks to this first revision, my reputation grew, and I was hired by the Compagnie des Libraires de Lyon to correct and edit *Pagninus Bible* in seven volumes. Apart from revising the annotations in Hebrew, Latin and Greek, I added to the Bible a preface and notes recommending the study of Hebrew culture and language for a better understanding of the text. This edition was published in 1545.

During my stay at Archbishop Palmier's house, he advised me not to publish anything, as he already knew of my unorthodox ideas; however, I had time to start writing one of the books of which I am most proud, *Christianismi restitutio* [1]. Published in 1553 without author or publisher to avoid destruction by the Inquisition, the printers were unaware that I was working on it, and the original sheets were destroyed as soon as they were printed. In this work I criticize the corruption of the Church of my time and advocate a return to the origins of Christianity. I also expand on my interpretations of the dogma of the Trinity and the divinity of Christ.

In the book, as for the soul and the vital spirit, I defend my theory that it enters the human body with the first inhalation through the nose and spreads to the rest of the body through the blood. The communication between the air and the blood does not take place as hitherto supposed in the heart. According to Vesalius, in his work *De humani corporis fabrica, libri septem*, the blood flows through the septum from the right to the left ventricle, through small pores, and it is there that it changes color from dark red to bright red.

I believe that this theory, which originally came from Galen, is wrong and that there is no such passage of blood between the ventricles. The blood would pass from the right ventricle to the lungs via a long circuit through the pulmonary artery, where it would mix with the air and acquire its bright red color. This mixing should occur in fine communications that allow the blood to pass from the arteries to the veins. It would then pass through the veins back to the heart to be distributed to the rest of the body from the left ventricle.

In the left ventricle of the heart there is not enough space for such copious mixing, nor for the blood to change its color. Finally, the interventricular septum, which lacks orifices, is not suitable for such communication and transformation, although I do not rule out the possibility of some leakage. Furthermore, the size of the artery to the lung is disproportionately large to nourish it, suggesting that the blood reaching the lungs does not stay there to nourish them, but must continue its circuit to the veins and, through them, return to the heart [2, 3] (Fig. 2.4).

Years before it was printed, in 1546, I sent a manuscript copy to Calvin, and we began a correspondence that would eventually become my misfortune. We exchanged numerous letters between that year and the next; although they initially dealt with theological matters related to our appreciation of religion, they soon became the subject of theological disputes and personal

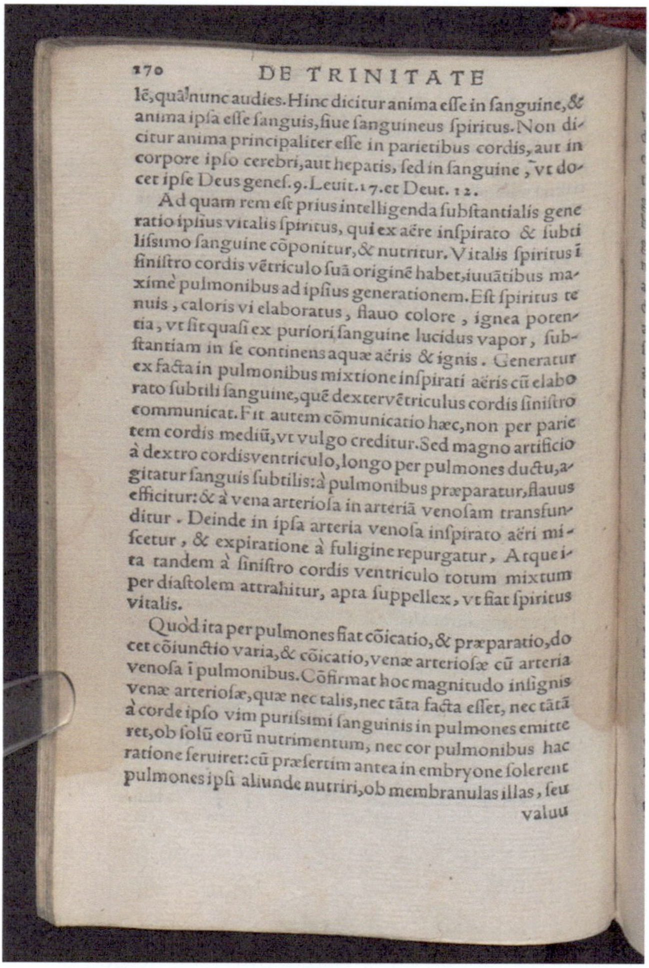

170 DE TRINITATE

lẽ,quãnunc audies. Hinc dicitur anima eſſe in ſanguine,& anima ipſa eſſe ſanguis, ſiue ſanguineus ſpiritus. Non dicitur anima principaliter eſſe in parietibus cordis, aut in corpore ipſo cerebri, aut hepatis, ſed in ſanguine, vt docet ipſe Deus geneſ. 9. Leuit. 17. et Deut. 12.

Ad quam rem eſt prius intelligenda ſubſtantialis generatio ipſius vitalis ſpiritus, qui ex aëre inſpirato & ſubtiliſsimo ſanguine cõponitur, & nutritur. Vitalis ſpiritus ĩ ſiniſtro cordis vẽtriculo ſuã originẽ habet, iuuãtibus maximè pulmonibus ad ipſius generationem. Eſt ſpiritus tenuis, caloris vi elaboratus, flauo colore, ignea potentia, vt ſit quaſi ex puriori ſanguine lucidus vapor, ſubſtantiam in ſe continens aquæ aëris & ignis. Generatur ex facta in pulmonibus mixtione inſpirati aëris cũ elaborato ſubtili ſanguine, quẽ dexter vẽtriculus cordis ſiniſtro communicat. Fit autem cõmunicatio hæc, non per parietem cordis mediũ, vt vulgo creditur. Sed magno artificio à dextro cordis ventriculo, longo per pulmones ductu, agitatur ſanguis ſubtilis: à pulmonibus præparatur, flauus efficitur: & à vena arterioſa in arteriã venoſam transfunditur. Deinde in ipſa arteria venoſa inſpirato aëri miſcetur, & expiratione à fuligine repurgatur. Atque ita tandem à ſiniſtro cordis ventriculo totum mixtum per diaſtolem attrahitur, apta ſuppellex, vt fiat ſpiritus vitalis.

Quòd ita per pulmones fiat cõicatio, & præparatio, docet cõiunctio varia, & cõicatio, venæ arterioſæ cũ arteria venoſa ĩ pulmonibus. Cõfirmat hoc magnitudo inſignis venæ arterioſæ, quæ nec talis, nec tãta facta eſſet, nec tãtã à corde ipſo vim puriſsimi ſanguinis in pulmones emitteret, ob ſolũ eorũ nutrimentum, nec cor pulmonibus hac ratione ſeruiret: cũ præſertim antea in embryone ſolerent pulmones ipſi aliunde nutriri, ob membranulas illas, ſeu

valuu

Fig. 2.4 Page from the book "Christianismi Restitutio" where the lesser circulation is explained on the chapter "On the Divine Trinity"

attacks, flooded with insults and serious accusations of heresy on Calvin's part. We exchanged as many as thirty letters! In some of them, he called me a blasphemer, a thief, a sacrilegious and a heretic. I included this correspondence as part four of the book *Christianismi restitutio*, which was still awaiting publication.

I had reasons, or so I believed, to attack Calvinist doctrine, and that is why he did not like my annotations to one of his works, *Institutio Christianae religionis*. After reading them, Calvin flew into a rage and, through a figurehead, Antoine Arneys, denounced me to the authorities of Vienna of the Dauphinate.

This led to my trial and imprisonment on 4 April 1553. The next two days were spent interrogating me; I denied having written the theological books, insisting that I had only written the medical ones. To be truthful, I must admit that the attitude towards me in the prison where I was held was benign. I was allowed to walk around the prison garden, which led to a platform from which it was easy to jump onto a patio whose door was always open. I believe that having contributed to the cure of the daughter of Antoine de la Court, one of my captors, may have influenced the treatment I received, as I was given great freedom of movement and was almost allowed to escape.

On 7 April, I asked my jailer for the key to the garden, and after jumping into the courtyard, I left as quickly as possible in the direction of the Rhône bridge, escaping in the early hours of the morning. I later learned that, despite my escape, the execution was carried out: on 17 June 1553, an auto da fe was held at the door of the palace, burning an effigy of me and a number of books, most of them blank. For the next four months I wandered around the lands near Lyon, not wanting to ask how I could reach Italy, fearing that I would be recognized and imprisoned again. Then I made the unwise decision to head for Geneva.

On the 13th of August I arrived at the "Auberge de la Rose" on the shore of the lake where the city is located, and, as it was Sunday, I could not take the boat to Zurich. My restless spirit played a trick on me, and I had no better idea than to go to the church where Calvin was officiating, and he recognized me and had me arrested. Calvin looked for a front man to accuse me and found him in Nicolás de la Fontaine, his secretary. According to the laws of Geneva, the accused and the accuser were to be in prison together until the claim was proved; and if it was not confirmed, the punishment fell on the accuser. Calvin therefore did not act as accuser, but sought out someone who owed him favors and worked in his service.

Nicolás accused me of having written thirty-eight heretical propositions and of having defamed Calvin and the church of Geneva. To add to my charge, he also incriminated me for the escape from the prison of Vienna of the Dauphinate.

After several days of arguing at the trial with my accuser, who had little theological knowledge, Calvin decided to send Germain Colladon to get my indictment; however, seeing that he could not obtain a clear advantage either, he decided to present himself in order to exert more pressure on the jury. We both appeared before the judges on 17 August, and amid disputes and controversies we were on trial until 15 September, at which time I decided to write a letter to the judges, in which I described my plight, in a flea-ridden cell, shirtless and in tattered tights, while Calvin only wished to have me burnt at the stake.

Despite all that I wrote and testified—despite the many explanations I offered for every accusation made against me—on 26 September I was sentenced to death. Here I am now, awaiting the fatal day appointed for 27 October on the hill of Champel. They say that Calvin has taken pity on me and asked that, instead of burning me, they should cut off my head, which the judges have refused. I cannot deny that I would prefer that end to the stake, but, even so, death awaits me shortly. I ask God's forgiveness if I have erred in any way; I have only tried to make the voice of a man who longs for a more just church heard.

Epilogue

On 27 October 1553, Servetus burned with a copy of his work *Christianismi restitutio* added to the green wood. His execution on the hill of Champel was carried out by Calvinists from Geneva.

This biographical and novelistic portrait of Servetus' life draws on the work of researchers and experts in the field, and the chronology and details of his various wanderings in sixteenth-century Europe are well supported.

The sixteenth century in Europe was a period of struggle between the power of the Church and the Empire, against freethinkers who found their place neither with one nor the other. The society of the late 14th and early 15th centuries threatened to upset the feudal organization, the established political power and the religious orthodoxy of the Roman Church.

In 1507, Pope Julius II authorized the sale of indulgences to finance the construction of St. Peter's Basilica in Rome, thus allowing lords, in exchange for a high price, to obtain forgiveness for their sins.

When in 1517 the sale of indulgences began in the vicinity of Wittenberg, Martin Luther, an Augustinian friar, professor of theology at the University of

Wittenberg and preacher in that city, wrote the *Questioning of the Power and Efficacy of Indulgences*, known as *"The 95 Theses"*, thus initiating the Protestant Reformation.

His ideas were joined by many freethinkers of his time, as well as artists who, to a greater or lesser extent, defended them or used them to attack the orthodox customs of Church and State. People such as Melanchthon, Oecolampadius, Calvin, Cranach, Holbein and Servetus himself were attracted to this movement.

Several factors contributed to the bellicosity in relations between many of the freethinkers of the time. First, their personal character, which, as we shall see, became psychopathological in some cases. Secondly, their constant struggle against the powerful Church, as the vast majority of them were excommunicated, persecuted by the Inquisition and subjected to imprisonment or finally executed. This resulted in a struggle for survival that led them to quarrel among themselves in an attempt to save their lives.

Luther came from a family where he suffered mistreatment, as well as in the school where he studied. He became arrogant over the years, so self-confident that he bordered on arrogance; he became authoritarian and fell into subjectivism. He became incapable of understanding those who held different views, and of questioning his own ideas, which he imposed in a tyrannical manner. He lacked charity towards his adversaries, to whom he reacted violently and whom he disqualified with the coarsest and foulest invective, to the point of becoming obsessed with them and did not hesitate to break the unity of the Church.

As José María Serra de Martínez [4] says, Johannes Calvin was gloomy, taciturn, moody, restless and strange; hard on others and on himself, always inclined to accusation, suspicion, intrigue and rancor. In addition, his illnesses—gout, tuberculosis and chronic migraine—made him selfish, irritable and unstable; his selfishness made him taciturn and proud; his irritability made him stern, cruel and tyrannical; and his instability of character made him restless, turbulent and belligerent.

Servetus himself was a stubborn, arrogant, argumentative, idealistic, multifaceted, uncompromising and true to his principles, so much so that it would lead him to the stake.

However, Servetus, in the medical field, is best known for his description of the pulmonary circulation. This discovery appears in the chapter entitled "On the Divine Trinity", where he deals with the Holy Spirit because for Servetus the air that we breathe and that renews the blood when it unites in the lungs is the spirit, and in believers who feel regenerated that air is the Holy Spirit, which makes them children of God.

His book *Christianismi restitutio* is theological, and his description of the circulation of the blood is based on his perception of how the soul reaches the body and extends to the heart. His worldwide fame is due to his description of the lesser circulation of the blood. William Wojtyla (1666–1727) and the Enlightenment scholars G.W. Leibniz, Voltaire, and B. J. Feijóo made decisive contributions to this fame.

Up to that time, the physiology of the circulation followed the doctrines of Galen and Vesalius. The lung was regarded as a coolant of cardiac heat, with no role in respiration. Galen thought that venous blood flowed from the liver, where it was formed, to the inferior and superior vena cava, and from there to the periphery of the body.

He did not consider it possible that the blood could return to the heart, because the function he attributed to it was to transport nutritive substances. Therefore, only a small amount of venous blood would pass from the vena cava to the heart and lungs, and from there to the arterial system.

However, Galen made a serious mistake, which became the basis of later erroneous doctrine: as the size of the pulmonary vessels is smaller than that of the vena cava and the aorta, he did not believe it possible for all the blood to pass through the lungs and had to devise an alternative route, which would consist of passing through the interventricular septum through supposed pores or perforations.

Servetus was not only correct in describing the passage of blood from the heart to the lung through the pulmonary arteries, but also in describing the arterio-venous communications and the absence of transudate or passage of blood between the interventricular walls. He had experience with the human anatomy from his dissections during his Medicine's study.

The important contribution of Michael Servetus regarding the lesser circulation of blood in 1553 likely went unnoticed at that time due to the massive destruction of his theological book "Cristianismi Restitutio." It was a Spanish anatomist, Juan Valverde de Amusco [5–7], who, three years later, in 1556, published in Rome, in Spanish, his significant book "Historia de la composición del cuerpo humano," (History of the composition of the human body) using "De humani corporis fabrica" by Andreas Vesalius as a reference, often correcting it and making numerous new contributions [8]. This treatise by Valverde is notable for its anatomical drawings and modern language, being the most reprinted, translated, and well-known anatomy book in Europe during the sixteenth century. Among his important contributions are the anatomy of the eye, the ear, the palm of the hand, and especially the detailed description of the lesser circulation of blood, as we know it today. It is likely that Valverde was unaware of Servet's publication and probably based his description on joint knowledge acquired with his teacher Realdo Colombo, who, however, published it years later than Valverde, in 1559 (Fig. 2.5).

Servetus was executed twice and burned three times: the first time he escaped, and only a representation of himself in wood and straw was burned. The second ended his life on the hill of Champel on 27 October 1553. However, he was to be burned in effigy a third time.

In 1902, the Barcelona essayist and author Pompeu Gener proposed at the International Congress of Freethinkers, held in Geneva, that a monument be erected in Servetus' honor in the city where he was executed.

The city of Geneva did not support the idea, but merely placed a commemorative plaque defending freedom of conscience but atoning for Calvin's error. Finally, in 1908, the statue of Servetus in prison, the work of the

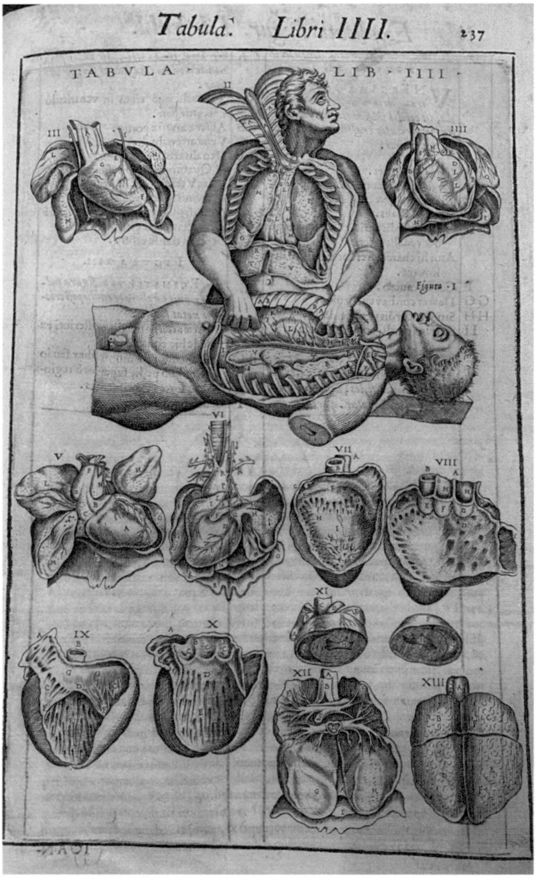

Fig. 2.5 Illustration of the anatomical diagram of the pulmonary lesser circulation. Book "Historia de la composición del cuerpo humano" by Juan Valverde de Amusco

Genevan Clotilde Roch, was erected in Annemasse, a few kilometers from Geneva, but on French territory. However, this statue would not survive another modern inquisition: that of Nazism. On 13 September 1941, the French Vichy government, a collaborator of the Nazi occupation, removed and melted down the bronze sculpture to obtain metal to make cannons.

The statue was finally restored in 1960 in a park in Annemasse. There are now two more copies of the sculpture: one on the very hill where Servetus was burnt, next to the Memorial Plaque, in Geneva, and another in front of the main building of the Hospital Clínico Universitario "Miguel Servet" in Zaragoza (Fig. 2.6).

To read about Michael Servetus in English:

"Restoration of Christianity" An English Translation of "Christianismi Restitutio" by Michael Servetus (1511–1553). Translated by Marian Hillar and Christopher A. Hoffman. 2007. Book News, Inc., Portland (OR).

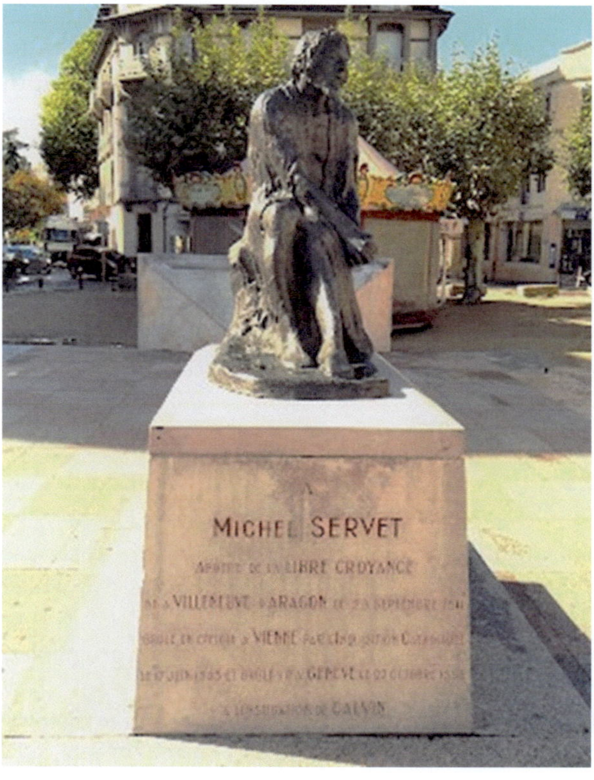

Fig. 2.6 Statue of Miguel Servet in Annemasse

An English translation of Servetus's major work, which led to his condemnation. (Three parts of the book are separately publish in English: On the Holy Spirit, On the Mysteries of the World and On the Trinity and the Bible (Lynn Gordon Hughes and Justo Hernandez, editors) and Peter Zerner as translator (Blackstone Editions, 2024 and 2025).

"Hunted Heretic: The Life and Death of Michael Servetus, 1511-1553" by Roland H. Bainton: A classic and detailed account of Servetus's life, his religious views, and his fatal confrontation with Calvin.

"Out of the Flames: The Remarkable Story of a Fearless Scholar, a Fatal Heresy, and One of the Rarest Books in the World" by Nancy and Lawrence Goldstone: A narrative focusing on Servetus's intellectual achievements and the dramatic events leading to his burning at the stake in Geneva.

"Michael Servetus: A Translation Of His Geographical, Medical And Astrological Writings": This collection includes his non-theological works, offering insight into his broader scientific and intellectual pursuits including among others, the description of the lesser circulation from Christianismi Restitutio. With introductory notes and context by Charles Donald O'Malley.

"The Life of Michael Servetus" by William Hamilton Drummond: An 1848 biography focusing on the events of his entrapment, imprisonment, and execution by Johannes Calvin.

"Michael Servetus: His Life and Teachings" by Carl Theophilus Odhner: A classic work providing a comprehensive overview of Servetus's life and theological ideas.

Historia de Los Heterodoxos Españoles by M. Menéndez Pelayo (1880). English and Spanish Edition. Kessinger's Rare Reprints. 2010.

Michael Servetus Institute of Studios Sijenenses. *Michael* Servetus. https://miguelservet.org/

References

1. "Restoration of Christianity". An English translation of "Christianismi Restitutio" by Michael Servetus (1511–1553). Translated by M Hillar, Christopher A. Hoffman. 2007. Book News, Inc, Portland.
2. Lesser circulation. Michael Servetus: A translation of his geographical, medical and astrological writings. Edition by CD O'Malley.
3. Josep Lluís Barona Vilar. The historical significance of the discovery of the minor circulation. Asclepio. 1992;44(2):3–27.

4. de Martínez JMS. Juan Calvino (pathological case). In: Vilamala, editor. Las Sectas Library, vol. 3. Barcelona; 1932. p. 55–61.
5. Valverde De Amusco J. Historia de la composición del cuerpo humano. Printed in Rome by Antonio Salamanca and Antonio Lafrerii 1556.
6. İlhan Bahşi, Zeynep Simgül, Büyükbeşe Saliha, Seda Adanir. Juan Valverde de Amusco (1525–1588): who was the great anatomist of the renaissance. Childs Nerv Syst. 2022;38:1051–4.
7. Arráez-Aybar LA, Reblet C, Bueno-López JL. Review Juan Valverde de Amusco: pioneering the transfer of post-vesalian anatomy. Anatomia. 2023;2:450–71.
8. Vesalius A. De Humani Corporis Fabrica. 1543. In: O'Malley CD, editor. Andreas Vesalius of Brussels, 1514–1564. Berkeley: University of California Press; 1964.

3

Dionisio Daza Chacón: The Most Relevant Spanish Surgeon of the Renaissance, in the Spanish Empire

Carlos Vaquero Puerta

Dionisio Daza Chacón can be considered one of the most prestigious European surgeons of the Renaissance. In the service of Emperor Carlos V (Charles V) and his son Felipe II (Philip II), he participated in important changes in the development of surgery, contributing with new concepts and new methods. He learned his skills on the battlefield as a military surgeon, participating in the numerous European wars in which the Spanish Crown was involved. His documentary contribution was made in an extensive work that he wrote in the last period of his life in the Spanish Romance language and not in the classical Latin. This fact, although possibly fundamental for training and transmitting his knowledge to his Hispanic colleagues and peers, possibly deprived him of a more international projection, which other contemporary surgeons of lesser value, but with better support in transmitting their knowledge, did have (Fig. 3.1).

The Spanish Empire in the XVI century, also known as the Hispanic Monarchy of the Austrias, was a huge colonial empire that spanned across the globe, creating a period of great power and influence of Spain. The empire faced numerous conflicts with France, England, the Ottoman Empire and the Dutch Republic (the 80 years' war). The histories in this chapter described the work of surgeons in the court of the Spanish kings and in the battle fields in North Europe.

C. V. Puerta (✉)
Professor of Surgery, University of Valladolid, Valladolid, Spain

M. A. Cuesta, F. Mateo Vallejo (eds.), *Spain's Journey in Medicine*,
https://doi.org/10.1007/978-3-032-12221-6_3

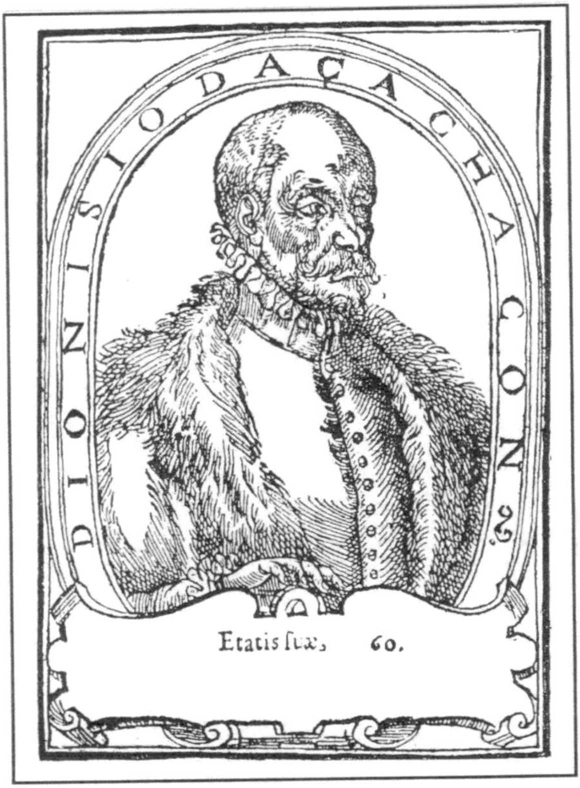

Fig. 3.1 Engraving preserved from Dionisio Daza Chacón of the Practica y Theorica de Cirugia en Romance y Latin (Practical and Theoretical work in Surgery). (Printed by Bernardino de S. Domingo, Valladolid, 1584)

Dionisio Daza Chacón was born in Valladolid in 1503, with roots in Avila and Portugal. He was the son of the physician Bernardino Daza Chacón and Lucía de Castro, of the parish of San Miguel de Valladolid, being the grandson of Arnal Chacón, physician to King Felipe I el Hermoso (Philip I the Handsome), who granted him the title of hidalgo by on 30 July 1492. His young brother, Bernardino Daza was a prestigious jurist of the time, who in 1544 published the so-called "*Institutiones imperiales, or Principles of Civil Law", a* reference work in his field.

He had studied grammar and philosophy in Valladolid, where he began medical training with the graduate Arias and bachelor Torres, completing them in Salamanca with the prestigious surgeon Ponce el Chico.

After completion of his medical studies in 1530 when he was 20 years old, returned to Valladolid, where he completed his surgical training at the Hospital de La Corte in Valladolid with the surgeon Luis Herrera, and for a term of 13 years they do not demand further references of his professional life.

In 1543 he decided to embark from the Cantabrian port of Laredo to Flanders as a military doctor, accompanying the army commanded by the Master of the Field Don Pedro de Guzmán, made up of three thousand men who disembarked in the port of Encusa (Enkhuizen). The war in Flanders between France and the Spanish Habsburg monarchy, heiress to the Burgundian house was still in full swing. This military contingent moved towards the city of Landresi (Landrecies), with the aim of besieging it, with another group of six thousand men, mainly made up of English archers, who joined the Imperial army formed by the fifteen thousand Walloons and Burgundians captained by the Duke of Ariscot, by what Daza had to carry out intense work, taking into account the bloody clashes resulted in a large number of casualties; and on the other hand, the limited number of surgeons available to treat them. On 12th December of that year, the Emperor arrived in the war field and the army was reorganized, so Daza Chacón was transferred to a field hospital in Valenciennes, which was considered a reference point for the care of all the wounded.

The following year, after the 4th Imperial Diet of Espira (Speyer), or imperial agreement of 1544, the army moved to Saint Dizier, a town controlled by the French, to besiege it, where the Emperor's forces had up to one hundred thousand troops, for which a surgical care group was created, directed by Daza Chacon and made up of eight surgeons. Here he coincided with a prestigious Flemish anatomist and surgeon serving also in the army of Emperor, Andreas Vesalius, whom he considered to be an excellent professional, and from that moment on they would share surgical activities.

With the signing of the Peace of Crépy-en-Laonnois, signed the 18th of September of 1544, between Carlos V and Francis I, king of France, a period of peace was established with the French, and it was then that Daza Chacón travelled to Brussels, with the imperial court, later returning to Madrid in 1545, accompanying the emperor's secretary, Don Juan Vazquez de Molina. He then left Madrid to live in Valladolid, but remained in his native city for little more than a year, because in 1547 he travelled by land to Augsburg, the former Roman *Augusta Vindelicorum*, finding on arriving the city, that the population, suffered an epidemic of plague, so that he had to remain isolated, for three and a half months attending to the sick in one of the hospitals created specifically to treat the Spanish soldiers, with a capacity of one hundred beds. There was a second hospital reserved for German patients.

The following year, 1548, he returned to Spain, this time accompanying Archduke Maximilian, the future Emperor of Germany, who was travelling to Valladolid to marry the eldest daughter of Carlos V, the Infanta Maria. After his return from Germany, Daza Chacón joined the service of the Infanta Doña Juana in 1552, accompanying her on her journey to Portugal to marry

Prince Juan Manuel of Portugal, initially passing through Toro to do it by proxy in this town. They returned to Spain in 1554, and it is known that in 1555, he resided in Valladolid, and it was in 1557, when the surgeon of the Hospital de La Corte, Luis de Herrera died, being Daza Chacon assigned to the task after an open competition with other prestigious opponents.

After working at the Hospital de La Corte and at the Royal Palace, on 4 July 1561 Daza Chacon was appointed surgeon to the monarch Felipe II (Philip II) and his son the Prince Don Carlos.

As Felipe II's surgeon, Daza Chacón had a salary of 60,000 maravedís (one maravedi is equal to 10 euro's cents), to which were added in 1564 another 20,000 maravedís in aid of the cost.

Because his growing prestige, in 1568, by order of the king, Daza was at the service of Don Juan de Austria, bastard brother of Felipe II, "*in charge of an excursion against the Berbers, to cleanse the islands and coasts of the Mediterranean sea from the corsairs who infest them*".

A year later, he was asked again to take part in the crusade against the Berbers and later against the Turks of the Ottoman Empire, under the command of Don Juan de Austria, embarking with the fleet in Cartagena, going first to Barcelona, then to Genoa, Naples and Sicily, and finally to Corfu to take part in the battle of Lepanto before returning to Spain in 1573.

He continued in Spain in the service of the Court and the King, and it was in 1580, at the age of 70, when he was allowed to retire due to his delicate health, maintaining his salary after 37 years of service.

In the last years of his life he moved to Madrid, where he died on 6th October 1596, after making a will, although others suggest that he died in his native town of Valladolid, which is not certain [1–4].

Little is known about his personal life, only that he married the widowed Ana de Losada, having no children.

It is important to point out important facts about his biography, such as the fact that Daza Chacón coincided in time with Ambroise Paré, a surgeon in the French army in the service of Francis I of France, who was in war with the Hispanic monarchy. Daza Chacón had the profile of a Latin surgeon, trained at university, who acquired knowledge in Latin, although he considered transmitting his knowledge and teachings especially in the Spanish Romance language so that they could reach the greatest number of professionals, as there were many who did not speak the scientific language of the time. On the other hand, Ambroise Paré has been better known at a historical and international level, without the slightest doubt of the validity and importance of his contributions in the field surgery, both in the treatment wounds and in the design of surgical material or prostheses derived from armors. His origins, in contrast to Daza's, were humble, the son of a prostitute, and he can be described as a barber surgeon and did not publish in Latin either. Some historians have pointed out that the two knew each other, one as surgeon of the Spanish army and the other in French army. On the other hand, both were born and died at the same time.

The greatest amount of information on the biography of Daza Chacon is available from the publication of his work or treatise on surgery, considering that he wrote it with reference to the clinical cases he dealt with, providing a great deal of information on complementary data, such as who was treated, where, under what conditions and also references to his own personal situation and circumstances.

His Most Relevant Surgical Performances

Throughout his extensive professional life as a surgeon, he attended both the illustrious figures and the humble patients, most notably soldiers. It was said of him "*he treats the poor as well as the rich, and slaves as well as the free*". In them he was able to apply his knowledge and obtain the information supporting his contributions to surgery. Many of these experiences and contributions were described in his work *Practica y Theorica de Cirugia* (Practice and theory of Surgery) [1]. The references of three of them can be considered very striking and illustrative.

One of the most well-known instances of his medical practice was his attendance, alongside his colleague and friend Andreas Vesalius, to Prince Charles—son of King Philip II and Doña María Manuela of Avis—on 19 April 1562. Prince Charles, heir to the throne of Spain, had been born in Valladolid on 8 July 1545, though his mother tragically passed away four days after childbirth.

Known to suffer from malaria as a child, at 18th years of age, the Prince had suffered a fall down a staircase while pursuing María Garcetas, the daughter of the palace gardener, at his residence—the Archbishop's Palace of Alcalá de Henares, which had been adapted as the Prince's House. Don Carlos suffered a serious cranial injury, which was initially treated by Doctors Vega and Olivares, both royal physicians, as well as by Daza Chacón, who served as Royal Surgeon.

Due to the severity of the injuries and the high status of the patient, various other physicians also took part in his treatment, including Juan Gutiérrez (referred to as the Portuguese Doctor) and Pedro de Torres. These physicians diagnosed a cerebral lesion that had become infected, leading to disagreements among the attending medical professionals—most notably between Doctor Torres, and later Mena and Andreas Vesalius—regarding the most appropriate course of treatment. The Prince's condition deteriorated into one of extreme gravity, yet ultimately, the crisis was resolved after trepanation that had been recommended by Daza Chacón. It is said that the recovery was due in part to the intercession of the remains of the Franciscan Fray Diego de Alcalá, who was later canonized as a result of this event.

Don Carlos passed away six years later under historically unclear circumstances in Madrid, on 24 July 1568, at the age of 23.

Some maintain that it was Daza Chacón who served as the surgeon attending to Miguel de Cervantes, then author of Don Quixote of the Mancha, in 1571 at the sea battle of Lepanto, in the Ionic Sea against the Turkish empire. He treated the injuries of his thorax, arm, and hand. Cervantes's wounds were inflicted aboard a galley, yet he received medical care at the hospital in Messina. The injury caused by an arquebus resulted in a contused wound typical of the projectile fired by such a weapon, involving damage to soft tissues and possibly affecting more vital structures, with the likelihood that the lead ball remained lodged within, thereby causing the sustained trauma. The final outcome, as Cervantes himself would later recount in various documents, was far from satisfactory, leaving him with a useless, claw-like hand. Indeed, following this injury, Cervantes came to be known as El Manco de Lepanto— "The one-handed man of Lepanto" [5].

Don Juan de Austria, bastard son of Carlos V, was an illustrious military man. The care of Don Juan in 1578, when he was in a state of depression and also sick with typhoid fever, is also well known. The soldier's condition worsened at the end of September, when he was in his camp around the besieged town of Namur in Belgium. According to reports of Dionisio Daza Chacón, an unresolved anal piles operation with postoperative bleeding and the weakening caused by typhus triggered his death.

His Work

Dionisio Daza Chacón, despite having the profile of a Latin surgeon, cultured, educated in the humanities and fluent in the Latin language, preferred to write in the Spanish language of the time, in the so-called Spanish romance.

He wrote his work at an advanced age, a compendium of all his knowledge and contributions to surgery, initially published in Valladolid in 1580 under the title: Practica y Teorica de Cirugía en Romance y en Latín. His work reached great diffusion for two reasons, to be written in romance Spanish and second because breaks with the tradition expressing his personal experience in a vivid form. After the first edition, there is a second one in 1584 in Valladolid and a third in two books in Madrid, the first in 1609 and the second in 1619. The second is dedicated to the treatment of the wounds. Both parts were re-edited several times. His style is precise direct and sober, similar to the direct style of today's surgeons.

Two major theme stand out in his work, the treatment of the wounds and of the tumors. In his treatise he does not talk about the treatment of fractures, which is strange in today's eyes, being a war surgeon. The reason is that at that time fractures and luxations were treated by a kind of traumatologists, a category of doctors inferior to the surgeons. Fifty years later, Felipe III ordered that fractures be included in the treatment of surgeons (Figs. 3.2 and 3.3).

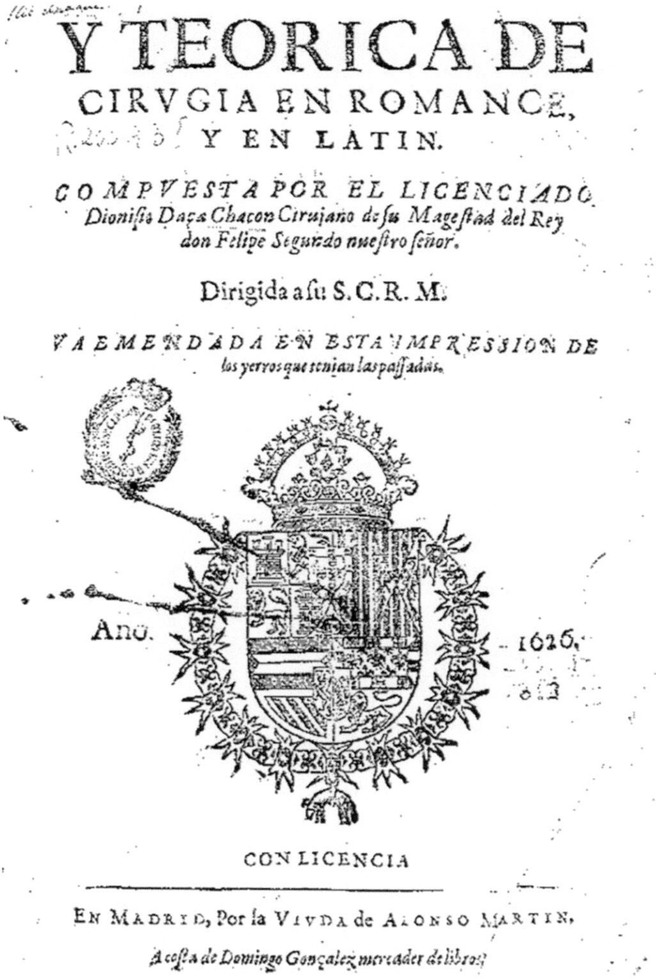
Y TEORICA DE
CIRVGIA EN ROMANCE,
Y EN LATIN.

COMPVESTA POR EL LICENCIADO
Dionisio Daça Chacon Cirujano de su Magestad del Rey don Felipe Segundo nuestro señor.

Dirigida a su S.C.R.M.

VA EMENDADA EN ESTA IMPRESSION DE
los yerros que tenian las passadas.

Año. 1626.

CON LICENCIA

EN MADRID, Por la VIVDA de ALONSO MARTIN,
A costa de Domingo Gonçalez mercader de libros.

Fig. 3.2 Image of the title page of Practica y Theorica de Cirugia en Romance y Latin. (Printed by Bernardino de S. Domingo, Valladolid, 1583)

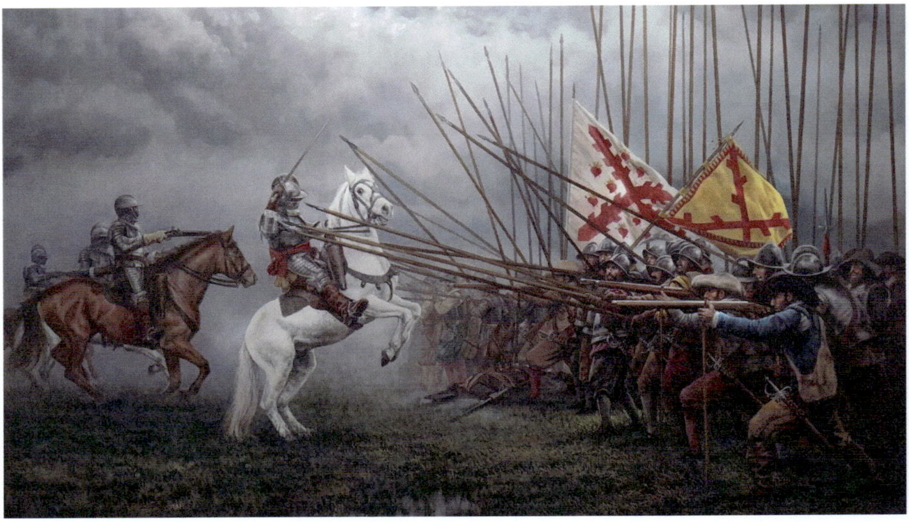

Fig. 3.3 Battle of the Tercios of Flanders. (Painting from José Ferre-Clauzel)

His Contributions

In evaluating the surgical contributions of Daza Chacón, it seems evident that these were firmly grounded in his practical experience as a military surgeon, and particularly in the treatment of war wounds. Through this he acquired extraordinary knowledge and expertise, derived from the care provided both on the battlefield and within the field hospitals established to treat the injured.

His education, which may be regarded as both academic and humanistic, was initially based on knowledge gained from more experienced surgeons, as well as the hands-on practice obtained within hospitals. It should also be noted that, at the time, the transmission of knowledge at university was carried out through the reading of lectures by professors. The Chair of Surgery did not exist in Spanish universities during his era; surgical training was typically acquired alongside experienced professionals during their daily practice or in certain institutions with a strong focus on surgical teaching, such as the renowned Monastery of Guadalupe or others, particularly in Valencia. In Valladolid, during the time of Dionisio Daza y Chacón, the primary educational institution was the Hospital de la Corte (Royal Court Hospital).

In the course of his surgical career, he made notable contributions, including the treatment of traumatic aneurysms by ligating the vessel proximal to the aneurysmatic sac, followed by an incision into the latter. He addressed treating bleeding by lesions in blood vessels using techniques considered innovative at the time, such as ligation, as opposed to the then common practice of cauterization. Particularly noteworthy is his approach to amputations and the reconstruction of the residual limb through the transposition of a cutaneous flap to cover the wound.

Moreover, he conducted studies on malignant tumors, offering valuable insights, and proposed new practical approaches to cranial trepanation as a solution to various cranial pathologies. Additionally, he contributed to the understanding of inflammatory processes affecting the kidneys, bladder, and genital organs. Within intestinal pathology, he distinguished between conditions of the small and large intestines. He described the treatment of nasal polyps by ligating the neck of the polyp. His work also encompassed the treatment of thoracic wounds, offering both practical experience and proposals for closing the thoracic cavity, which later served as a precursor to future surgical innovations.

However, his most significant contributions undoubtedly lie in the field of wound management. He rejected the classical belief in the salutary nature of 'laudable pus' in the healing process, instead introducing a classification of wounds as either simple or complicated, with corresponding therapeutic approaches.

The siege of the fortress of Saint Dizier in 1544 represents a pivotal moment in the evolution of war wound treatment, especially in the treatment of firearms wounds. It marked a departure from traditional doctrines, which regarded such wounds as toxic or poisonous by gunpowder considering the pus produced by infection as beneficial. Daza Chacón, alongside Andreas Vesalius, Ambroise Paré and influenced by the Italian surgeon Micer Bartolomeo—historically identified as Bartolomeo Maggi—implemented new practices that eschewed cauterization, treating them as blunt wounds leading to quicker recoveries reducing pain and mortality. For this shift of paradigm he carried out clinical, pathological and experimental studies to prove this. Also describes blast injuries wounds, and special wounds such as vascular, thoracic and abdominal. In vascular wounds recommends ligation, closure of thoracic wounds and classifies abdominal wounds into simple and complicated wounds (with intestinal lesions), considering that the latter cannot be cured [6, 7].

To conclude by pointing out that Daza, on the basis of his conceptual positioning of medicine, maintained that the surgeon, apart from technical skills and abilities has knowledge, must have training and knowledge and therefore will have superiority over the mere practitioner. He was a man open to adopting new criteria, as opposed to the classical postulates maintained in the

Middle Ages. He gave truly original descriptions of his actions and their practical application, based on his extensive experience of his professional practice.

To read more in English about D. Daza Chacón:

Dionisio Daza Chacón (1503–1596?). Charles Donald O'Malley. 1971 pp. 160–170- In BA.AF (Heischkel-Artelt). Germany.

References

1. Daza Chacón D. Práctica y Theórica de Cirugía en Romance y Latín. Valladolid: Imprenta Bernardino de S. Domingo; 1584.
2. Soriano de la Rosa C. The surgical work of Daza Chacón. Publications of the Seminar on the History of Medicine. University of Salamanca. 1958. Vol. II, no. 1, p. 50.
3. de Heredia B, de Onís JM. Dionisio Daza Chacón, renaissance surgeon: his contribution to the treatment of wounds. Inaugural lecture of the 1971–72 academic year at the University of Valladolid. 1971. Editorial Sever Cuesta. Valladolid.
4. Riera Palmero J. Dionisio Daza Chacón (Valladolid, 1510 - Madrid, 1596). Rev Esp Invest Quir. 2004;7:85–92.
5. Mejia-Rivera O. Shaking palsy and other neurologic illness in the Quixote. Acta Med Colomb. 2023; 48.
6. Vaquero C, Cenizo N, Del Río L. San Norberto E. Dionisio Daza Chacón. Spanish Renaissance surgeon. Rev Iberoam Cir Vasc. 2018;6:27–31.
7. Vaquero C, San Norberto EM, Brizuela JA, Estévez I, Flota C, Fidalgo L, García-Rivera E, Diez M. Renaissance surgery. The treatment of war wounds. Anal Real Acad Med Cir Valladolid. 2018;55:137–48.

4

Quinine: Discovery and Diffusion of Quinine Throughout the World for the Treatment of Malaria

Miguel A. Cuesta and Carmen Padules González

Born from the bark of the cinchona, a tree native to the Andean rainforests, quinine was, for more than three centuries, the only substance available to treat malaria, a terrible disease that still affects millions of people around the world. Considered the substance that has brought the most relief to human suffering, quinine began to be displaced a couple of decades ago by the introduction of synthetic compounds. However, it has experienced a recent resurgence in the face of early manifestations of resistance to modern drugs. In May 2001, Dr. G. Stork of Columbia University announced the first stereoselective synthesis of quinine (Fig. 4.1).

M. A. Cuesta (✉)
Department of Surgery, Amsterdam University Medical Centre (UMC), Amsterdam, The Netherlands

C. P. González
Registered Nurse and Researcher, Centro de Salud Cerro del Aire, Madrid, Spain

M. A. Cuesta, F. Mateo Vallejo (eds.), *Spain's Journey in Medicine*,
https://doi.org/10.1007/978-3-032-12221-6_4

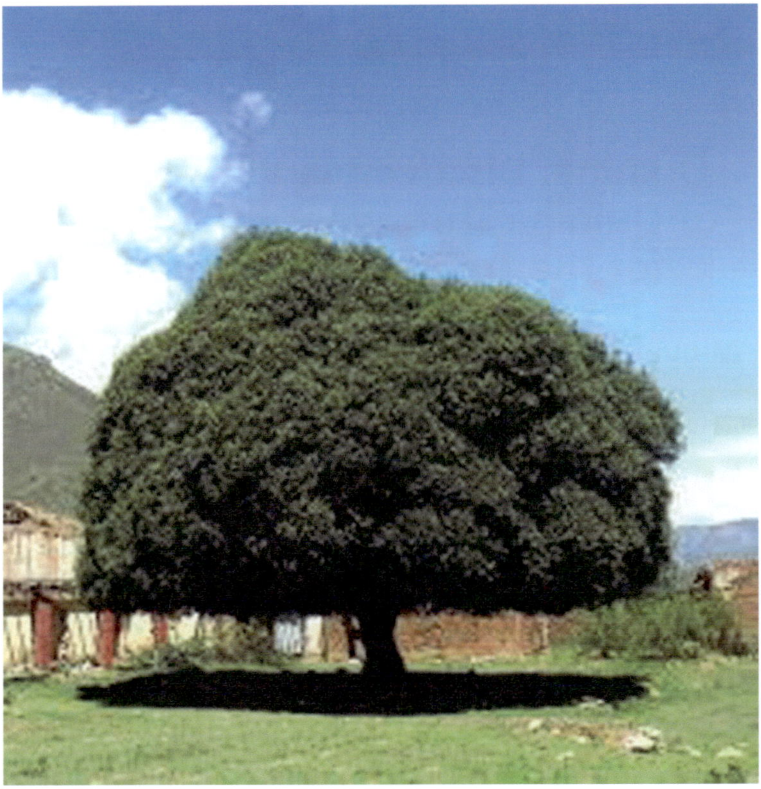

Fig. 4.1 Quinine's tree

History of Quinine

Let's go back in time; what seem to be facts could be legends. However, throughout history, some of these events have been of significant importance, especially after the discovery of quinine's great curative potential for malaria in the Viceroyalty of Peru, in the XVII century, which led to its spread to Europe and the rest of the world via Spain.

Malaria, a disease known for thousands of years, is a parasitic disease that causes high fevers, chills, muscle aches and anaemia. It is caused by a parasite, which is transmitted to humans through the bite of infected female Anopheles mosquitoes. After infection, single-celled parasites of the genus Plasmodium, called sporozoites, travel through the bloodstream to the liver. There they mature and produce another form of parasites, known as merozoites. These parasites enter the bloodstream and infect the red blood cells, multiplying inside them. After 48–72 hours, the red blood cells break, releasing the parasites, which re-infect more red blood cells.

The first symptoms usually occur 2–4 weeks after infection, although they can appear as early as 8 days or up to a year later. Symptoms occur in cycles of three or four days. In Spain, malaria was almost always known as "tercianas" or "fiebre tercianas" (tertian fever: 3-day cycles of fever and chills), which is relatively mild and caused by Plasmodium malariae. Less frequently, there is the much more severe quartan fever, which is caused by Plasmodium falciparum or Plasmodium vivax, causing an intermittent fever every four days.

Both forms of malaria were endemic and were treated with cinchona tree bark powder, or quinine, until the mid-twentieth century. Later, other treatments were added, such as chloroquine, and at the end of the century, artemisinin. Today, treatments containing artemisinin derivatives are the global standard for malaria treatment. The main component of artemisinin is isolated from the plant *Artemisia annua*, a plant that has been described in traditional Chinese medicine.

Malaria can also be transmitted from mother to fetus and through blood transfusions. Although mosquitoes in temperate climates can carry malaria, the parasite tends to disappear during the winter.

Malaria is a major health problem in most tropical and subtropical countries. The US Centers for Disease Control and Prevention (CDC) reported that in 2020 there were approximately 241 million cases of malaria, with about 627,000 associated deaths. Malaria is a significant risk for travelers to hot climates, so it is recommended that prophylactic treatment be initiated prior to travel.

It is important to note that the first and best remedy against malaria, discovered in the former Viceroyalty of Peru, is quinine, found in the bark of the cinchona tree. Quinine is the most potent of the four alkaloids found in the bark of *Cinchona* trees (quinine, quinidine, cinchonine and cinchodine). There are approximately 23 species of these trees, all of which are distributed throughout the eastern Andes. Initially used by indigenous peoples for the treatment of fevers and chills, its use against malaria in the seventeenth century has represented the greatest contribution of the traditional medicine of these peoples to universal medical science, bringing great benefits to the world's population.

Its rapid expansion, the varied effectiveness of the different species and their therapeutic uses led to numerous scientific expeditions to Peru and South America to investigate its various species and barks, with the aim of adapting them to other continents.

A Fascinationg Story

There is evidence that in the New World, before the arrival of the Spanish, the indigenous people, especially the yachak or shamans, used cinchona bark from immemorial time to treat fevers. The only evidence found in the archives suggests that the inhabitants of the Palta culture were the discoverers of the "cascarilla tree" and used it effectively in the field of natural medicine. From Loxa (present-day Loja in Ecuador), in colonial times, the bark was taken to Lima, from where its therapeutic fame spread and quickly transcended to Spain.

Although it was part of the traditional medicine, legend has it that the Indian Pedro de Leyva, chief of Rumishitana, devoured by fevers, stumbled forward and fell almost dying on the bank of a pond in the middle of the Peruvian Andes. Sweating and consumed by an intense thirst, he approached the water, brushed aside the leaves and branches that had fallen into the backwater and took a few bitter sips. Then the fever subsided. The sick man had been saved by the miraculous mixture of water with the bark of the tree that grew around the pond.

This seventeenth century story, compiled by the Peruvian traditionalist Ricardo Palma, recounts the facts behind the anti-malarial properties of the cinchona tree [1].

The narrative unfolds as follows: "In 1629, Doña Francisca Enríquez de Rivera, second wife of the IV Count of Chinchón, Don Luis Jerónimo Fernández de Cabrera y Bobadilla, had fallen seriously ill with malaria and was on the verge of death. Despite numerous bloodlettings in an attempt to cure her of the fever, there was no success. Since her arrival in Lima a couple of years before, her life had been spent between audiences, dictating rules of coexistence between Spaniards with indigenous peoples, banquets and parties. News of her illness spread throughout the viceroyalty, reaching as far as Loxa. In those days, the viceroy received a parcel sent by the corregidor of Loxa, Don Juan López de Cañizares. The package contained cinchona bark and was accompanied by a letter which read: "Your Highness, I humbly and respectfully send you, through my servant, some pieces of bark from the cinchona tree that grows in this district. It can be made more palatable by mixing it, once pulverized, with strong wine. And God willing, this will cure your countess of the deadly disease from which she suffers. Years ago, it saved me from a similar fever" (Fig. 4.2).

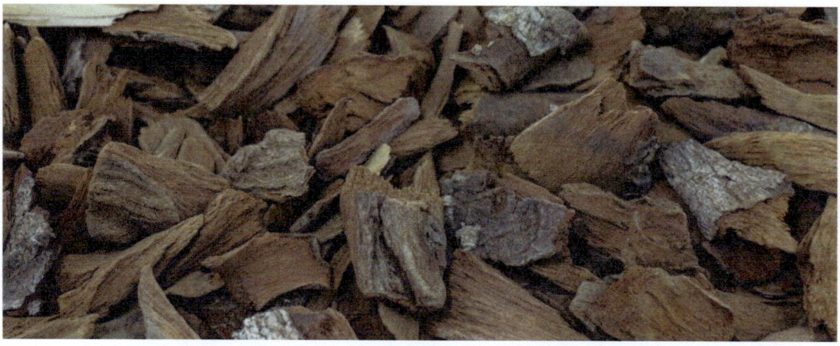

Fig. 4.2 Bark of the Cinchona oficinalis, quinine's tree

Juan López de Cañizares had been cured by an indigenous cacique from the village of Malacatos, on the banks of the river Malacatos, near Loxa, whose name has not been recorded.

It is now known that malaria did not exist in pre-Columbian America, suggesting that the parasite that transmits the disease arrived from Europe along with the Anopheles mosquito. The Andean people of the Viceroyalty soon realized that one of their traditional medicines, the bark of the cinchona tree (or quina), could offer relief from the symptoms of this disease, and they were the first to use this ground bark as a remedy for malaria.

The viceroy, however, reacted with many doubts and preferred to take certain precautions. According to the chronicler Antonio Hernández Morejón, doctor and historian of the 18th–19th century: "The viceroy was convinced that no one better than the corregidor could administer the remedy, so he called him to Lima and ordered him to carry out the tests himself in the hospitals with other patients before giving it to the vicereine. In fact, accompanied by the hospital doctors, he carried out what the viceroy had instructed him to do, and in a few days all the patients who had taken the remedy were free of fever. With such evident and happy results, the viceroy decided that it should be administered to his consort, who, desiring his improvement, did not hesitate to take it. Thus, within a few days, she was free of the fever and recovered the health that had been lost for many months" (Fig. 4.3).

Grateful, the vicereine declared herself the protector of the new remedy, which she personally distributed to all those suffering from tertian and quartan fevers, hence the name "polvos de la condesa" (the countess's powder) by which the treatment was initially known. As a result of his wife's cure, the viceroy accepted the request of Jaime de Alloza, rector of the University of San Marcos, founded in 1548 in Lima, to establish the professorships of Primas and Vespers of Medicine.

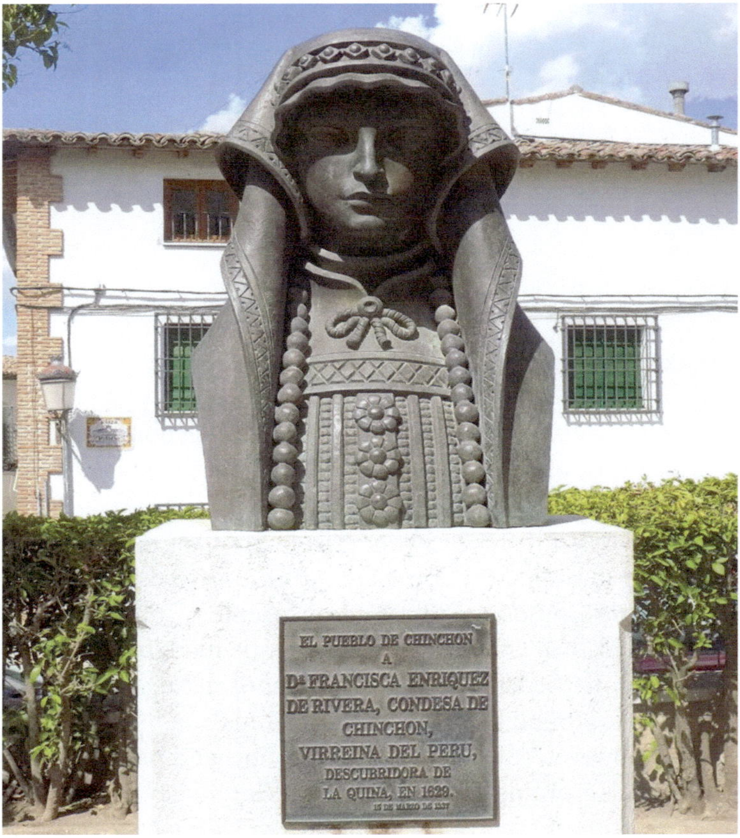
EL PUEBLO DE CHINCHON
A
Dª FRANCISCA ENRIQUEZ
DE RIVERA, CONDESA DE
CHINCHON,
VIRREINA DEL PERU,
DESCUBRIDORA DE
LA QUINA, EN 1629.

Fig. 4.3 Monument in Chinchón (Spain) to the countess of Chinchón

During the colonial period, there were initially publications of a journalistic nature—which did not reach the European scientific sphere—in which the first descriptions of the cinchona tree stand out. In the news bulletins published in 1611 by the physician Nicolás Monardes, it is already mentioned in his "*Historia Medicinal de las cosas que se traen de nuestras Indias Occidentales que sirven de medicamentos*" (*Medicinal History of the things brought from our West Indies that serve as medicines*). A second reference to the species whose bark was used to cure fevers was made in 1638 by Fray Antonio de Calancha, an Augustinian who mentions it in his "*Crónica Moralizada del Orden de San Agustín en el Perú*" (*Moralized Chronicle of the Order of Saint Augustine in Peru*), where he speaks of a "*tree that the Indians call the fever tree, whose bark, made into powder, is paid in silver and is used as a drink to cure fevers and tertian fever*".

In turn, the Counts of Chinchón returned to Spain in 1640, bringing with them their physician, Juan de Vega, who brought back a quantity of cinchona, selling it in Seville for 100 reales a pound. The Jesuits began to market the bark, and its use then spread from Spain to, Italy, France, the Netherlands and England. It is said that the religious recommended that the extractors plant five trees for every one that was cut, arranging them in the shape of a cross.

Its virtues were recognized in Europe in 1642, when it was brought to Rome by two Jesuit fathers, Father Bernabé de Cobo and Father Alfonso Masías Venegas.

Moved by a spirit of charity, Jesuit missionaries distributed the miraculous powders to the sick and poor, becoming the first to use them to treat orderly the malaria, which is why they became known as "*Jesuit powder*". Although the introduction of quinine by the Jesuits in Spain and later in Rome is poorly documented, both fathers introduced it to the Jesuits in Rome, where malaria affected popes and cardinals. A few years later, in 1650, in Rome itself, the general of the Order of Jesus at the papal court gave a certain quantity of quinine to Cardinal Juan Lugo, who added a new name: "*cardinal's powder or Lugo's powder*". It was this cardinal who introduced its widespread use in the mid-seventeenth century in Rome, which at that time, surrounded by swamps, was a malaria-endemic area. His doctor, Sebastiano Bado, is considered to be the author of one of the first botanical-scientific descriptions of quinine, "*Anastasis corticis peruviae, seu chinae defensio*" ("The Resurrection of the Peruvian Bark, or the Defense of the China's tree") where he echoes the letter of an Italian merchant, Antonio Bolli, where he mentions in 1663, the bark of Peru or China-Chinae as the species used to combat fever, also telling the story of the Countess of Chinchón. It is said that the great Linnaeus took this story of the Countess from Bado's book.

In 1668, the English apothecary Robert Talbor prepared a remedy for malaria that looked like wine and whose formula he kept secret. He opened an office in London specializing in curing fevers and did very good business. He cured several noblemen of malaria, including King Charles II of England himself, which earned him a knighthood and an official court physician. In 1679, he travelled to France, where King Louis XIV offered him compensation and a title in exchange for revealing the formula for his medicine. It was eventually revealed that the secret consisted of six units of infused rose leaves, two ounces of lemon juice and cinchona bark.

In 1699, Dr. Diego Herrera [2] wrote the treatise "*De Cortice chinae, et de Loxa, etsi diversorum arborum uniformis virtutis*", ("On the Bark of China's tree and of Loxa, though from different trees, of uniform virtue") the manuscript of which was found in Lima in 1737 by the French naturalist

Charles-Marie de La Condamine [3]. In 1742, La Condamine explored the Loxa area for the first time, and the following year he published in Paris his report "*Sur l'arbre du quinaquina*" (About the cinchona tree), which is considered one of the first scientific works on this plant.

The Spanish botanist Hipólito Ruiz López (1754–1816), was appointed by Carlos III of Spain to lead the "*Royal Botanical Expedition to the Viceroyalty of Peru*" (1777–1816), along with José Antonio Pavón Jiménez (1754–1840), Juan José Tafalla Navascués (1755–1811), Juan Agustín Manzanilla and the French naturalist Joseph Dombey [4]. Together they explored the central coast, the highlands, the central jungle (now Pozuzo, Huánuco and Chinchao) and the Upper Marañón river in Peru. For ten years, they studied botany, describing numerous plants and tree species, including several species of cascarilla quinine tree.

In 1792, Hipólito Ruiz published the book "*Quinología o tratado del árbol de la quina o cascarilla*" (*Quinology or treatise on the cinchona tree or cascarilla*), translated into Italian (Rome, 1792), German (Göttingen, 1794), and later into English (London, 1821). These translations were responsible for the scientific dissemination of quinine throughout Europe (Fig. 4.4).

The first plant of the cinchona tree to reach Spain was sent by the Ruiz y Pavón expedition to the Herbarium of the Royal Botanical Garden in Madrid. The first specimen of this plant is preserved there, which was collected, studied and catalogued for conservation (Fig. 4.5).

The branches are dried on a sheet of paper on which the pressed plant has been arranged in two dimensions, with the leaves, stems and fruit or flowers in view, together with all the data on their collection (the day, the place and the environment).

The story of the vicereine's cure persisted, and in 1753, Carl Linnaeus, creator of the classification of living things or taxonomy, received information from the tree.

The binomial nomenclature system (1735) is based on the use of a first term, with its initial letter written in capital letters, indicating the genus, and a second part, corresponding to the specific name of the species described, written in lower case letters.

He received the cinchona plant from the botanist José Celestino Mutis from New Granada, now Colombia, and then created the genus "*Cinchona officinalis*" in memory of the countess. However, he introduced a spelling error by including it as Cinchona instead of Chinchona, although the Latin pronunciation is the same, and so it has persisted to the present day.

In those treatises it is described that the "*Cinchona officinalis*" gris de Loxa grows between 1400 and 3000 metres altitude, in regions with abundant

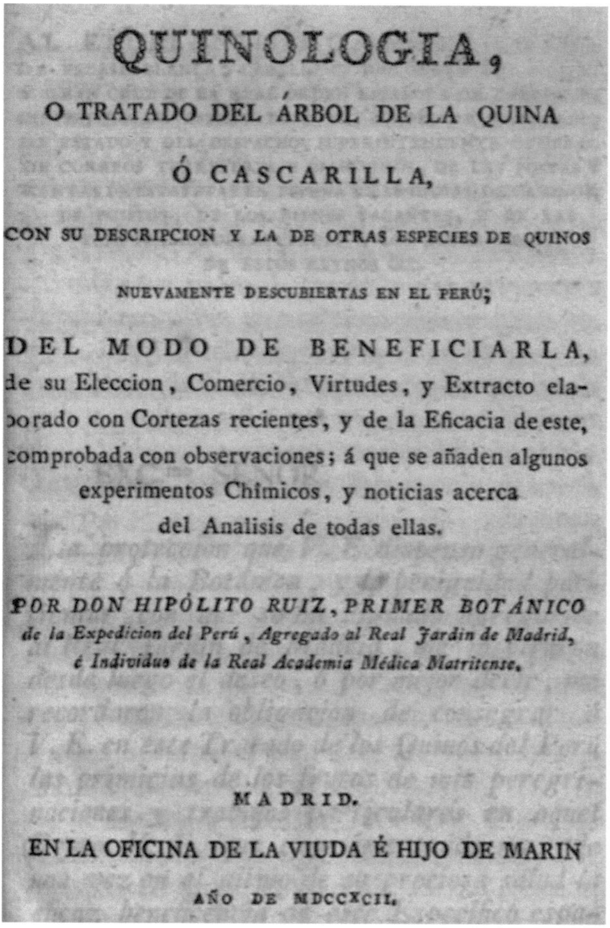

QUINOLOGIA,

O TRATADO DEL ÁRBOL DE LA QUINA

Ó CASCARILLA,

CON SU DESCRIPCION Y LA DE OTRAS ESPECIES DE QUINOS NUEVAMENTE DESCUBIERTAS EN EL PERÚ;

DEL MODO DE BENEFICIARLA, de su Eleccion, Comercio, Virtudes, y Extracto elaborado con Cortezas recientes, y de la Eficacia de este, comprobada con observaciones; á que se añaden algunos experimentos Chîmicos, y noticias acerca del Analisis de todas ellas.

POR DON HIPÓLITO RUIZ, PRIMER BOTÁNICO de la Expedicion del Perú, Agregado al Real Jardin de Madrid, é Individuo de la Real Academia Médica Matritense.

MADRID.

EN LA OFICINA DE LA VIUDA É HIJO DE MARIN

AÑO DE MDCCXCII.

Fig. 4.4 Cover of the book: Quinology of Hipólito Ruiz

rainfall, and is the only bark known to cure fevers. Over the years, new species of Cinchona were discovered in different places along the foothills of the Andes. Other species known at that time were the Red Chinchona ('*Cinchona pubescens*'), which is found further north, as far as Costa Rica; as well as the purple, orange, pink and yellow of Popayán, the '*Cinchona calisaya*'.

As a result of these discoveries, various European courts, especially the Spanish court, due to the great need they to treat their subjects with malaria, began to perceive the importance of scientific explorations to the Viceroyalty, not only to discover more properties of the cinchona tree, but also to study other botanical species with applications in medicine or industry. This was, in part, one of the reasons for organizing the great scientific expedition of

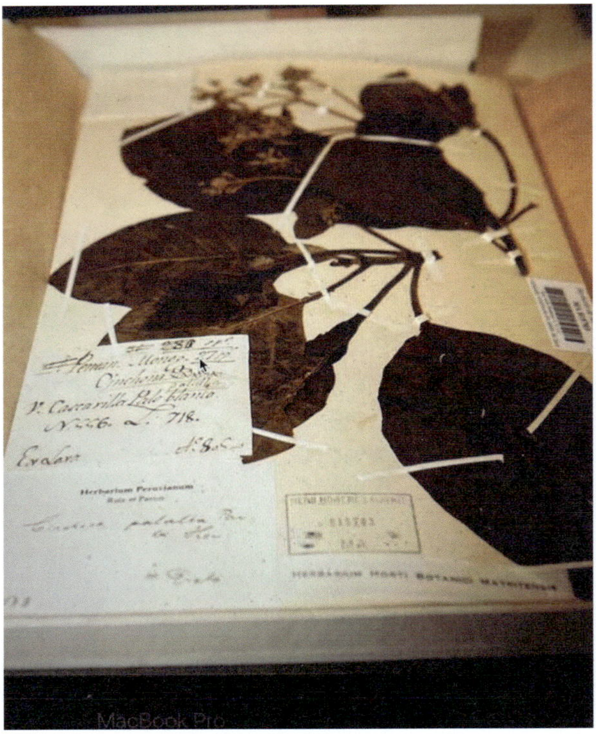

Fig. 4.5 First specimen of the cinchona plant in the Archives of the Royal Botanical Garden of Madrid

Alejandro Malaspina and José de Bustamante, in the time of Carlos IV, at the end of the eighteenth century. This scientific voyage around the world was financed by the Spanish Crown at the time of the Enlightenment. The expedition, which included the corvettes Atrevida and Descubierta, set sail from Cadiz on 30 July 1789, sailing along the coasts of all America, from Buenos Aires to Alaska, as well as the Philippines, the Marianas, Vavao, New Zealand and Australia. The expedition returned to Spain on 21 September 1794, having generated an enormous wealth of knowledge on natural history, cartography, ethnography, astronomy, hydrography, botany and medicine—all branches of knowledge of great geopolitical importance—as well as on the political, economic and social aspects of these territories.

Most of the collections are kept in the Museo de America, the Museo Naval de Madrid, the Real Observatorio de la Armada, the Real Jardin Botánico and the Museo Nacional de Ciencias Naturales.

The expedition, which had on board the cream of the Spanish Navy's astronomers and geographers, also included scientists and illustrators, such as the naturalists Tadeo Haenke and Antonio Pineda, the botanist Luis Née, and the painters and illustrators José del Pozo, José Guio, Juan Francisco Ravenet, Bunel and Fernando Brambila, as well as the chronicler Tomás de Suría.

One of the naturalists and botanists on the expedition was the discoverer of cinchona in Upper Peru: Tadeo Haenke (1761–1816), a naturalist originally from Bohemia in the service of the Spanish Crown [5].

Hired for Malaspina's expedition, he faced various vicissitudes, such as his late arrival in Cadiz, when the ships had already set sail, and the shipwreck in Montevideo of the vessel in which he was travelling. He finally reached Buenos Aires, where Viceroy Vértiz helped him to travel overland to Santiago de Chile. On the way, he collected around 1400 plants for study. In Santiago, he rejoined the expedition on 2 April 1790, continuing his work of botanical collection. Together with the expedition, he travelled the complete journey, and then disembarked in Callao in July 1793, where he separated from the expedition. He then explored the Peruvian Amazon region and went on to La Paz, before settling in Cochabamba in 1794. His observations and works on many aspects of the city and nature of Cochabamba form part of an archive which, in part, ended up in the Royal Botanical Garden in Madrid. Haenke's best known work is his "*Introducción a la historia natural de la provincia de Cochabamba y sus circunvecinas*" (*Introduction to the natural history of the province of Cochabamba and its surrounding areas*), first published in 1801 and republished several times. Many years later, it was discovered that the Bolivian cinchona described by Haenke contained the highest quinine content of all of them. A quarter of a century later, extracts and tinctures of cinchona bark were present in most European pharmacopoeias.

A contemporary of this expedition, the Cadiz-born José Celestino Mutis (1760–1808) was an exceptional character whose contributions to the world of botany and medicine have survived to the present day [6]. In 1783, the Archbishop-Viceroy Antonio Caballero y Góngora, proposed to the Crown that a "*Royal Botanical Expedition of the New Kingdom of Granada*" should be undertaken, in which Mutis travelled with other members of the expedition to La Mesa de Juan Díaz. Thus began the systematic exploration of the area of Mariquita, now in Colombia. During his work, he established contacts with many European naturalists, including Linnaeus. His news about American plants was well received in an information-hungry Europe (Fig. 4.6), however, his main commercial objective was cinchona. On one of his visits to the Sierra de Tena in 1772 in the company of Pedro Ugarte, he located some others cinchona trees, classifying and describing, after a long process of analysis and observation, the benefits of seven different species of cinchona trees. Such curative benefits generated great expectation among the wealthy society of the old continent, eager to obtain the plant. In May 1793, his "*Arcano de la Quina*" (*Arcanum of Quina*) began to be published in the newspaper of the

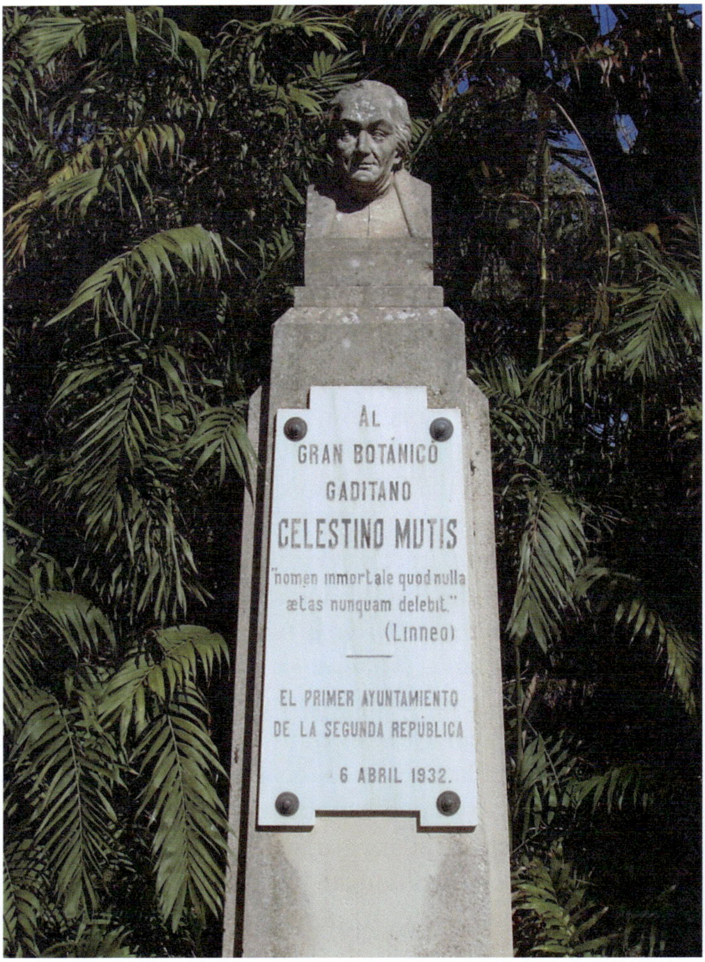
AL
GRAN BOTÁNICO
GADITANO
CELESTINO MUTIS
"nomen inmortale quod nulla
ætas nunquam delebit."
(Linneo)
EL PRIMER AYUNTAMIENTO
DE LA SEGUNDA REPÚBLICA
6 ABRIL 1932.

Fig. 4.6 Bust of Celestino Mutis. Parque Genovés in Cádiz

city of Santa Fe de Bogotá. In this publication, his interest in defending the commercialization of the quinas novo-granadinas, whose quality he praised in comparison with the other varieties marketed from the port of El Callao, is evident.

The main concern of J.C. Mutis was to promote the natural resources of the territory where he carried out his work, not for the direct benefit of the people located at the Court, but with the cultural and economic development of the American territory in mind. The archive and the materials collected by Mutis have been kept in the Royal Botanical Garden in Madrid since 1817.

Another important expedition was undertaken by the Prussian naturalist and scientist Alexander von Humboldt, who, accompanied by the French naturalist Aimé Bonpland, made a journey to Peru from 2 August to 24 December 1802 [7]. During their stay, they travelled from Ayabaca to Jaén, near the border with Ecuador, and continued on to Cajamarca and Lima. In his first letter to his brother, he went into great detail about how amazed he was by the nature: "How numerous are also the smallest plants not yet examined! And what colors the birds, the fish, even the crabs have. So far, we have been running around like crazy; in the first three days we have not been able to decide anything, because people keep changing one topic to get interested in another".

During this trip, Humboldt met Celestino Mutis, with whom he exchanged ideas about the area's botany and the cinchona tree species. In 1807, he wrote a memoir on cinchona forests. In this book, he recommended the cultivation of the cinchona tree for the first time, since harvesting their bark was leading to the depletion of the species. He even described methods for building nurseries and managing the saplings of cut trees.

The appearance of new species generated, at the end of the 18th and beginning of the nineteenth century, a great controversy about which of the species discovered was the "good" or the "original" one. These issues were of great importance to European governments, especially to the Spanish government, which led to the sending of new botanists and naturalists on successive scientific expeditions, such as those of J. Tafalla and F.J. Caldas, as well as the Royal Botanical Expedition to New Spain (Mexico, 1787–1803) by Sessé y Mociño, whose archives are also preserved in the Botanical Garden of Madrid.

The controversy was based on two reasons: what name to give to the new botanical discovery, a discovery that gave prestige to the naturalist, and the economic reasons related to the exports of the bark to Europe. The different species of cinchona trees, with their different concentrations of cinchona, were found in different geographical areas, and this aroused great commercial interests for their exploitation. Reports such as that of G. Bañares to the Crown, summarizing the many reports and memoirs sent by naturalists, helped to clarify concepts, smoothing out differences in this respect [8, 9].

In Search of the Active Ingredient

Because of its importance in the treatment of malaria, scientists began to study the components of cinchona bark in order to find its active ingredient, a goal that was only made possible by later advances in chemistry. The discovery was made by the French chemists Pierre-Joseph Pelletier (1788–1842) and Joseph-Bienaimé Caventou (1795–1877), who in 1820 discovered quinine, the alkaloid in the bark of the yellow chinchona, and proved it to be the active ingredient effective against malaria. Since then, quinine has established itself as the most bitter substance recognizable to the human tongue. Four years later, these two chemists also discovered caffeine, the basic principle of coffee.

As a result of these developments, quinine began to be used more and more frequently in large areas of Europe and America affected by the disease. For example, in 1832, Dr. John Sappington of Philadelphia purchased quinine to manufacture what became known as '*Dr Sappington's Fever Pills*'. He persuaded shepherds in the Mississippi Valley to ring bells every evening to remind people to take the malaria pills. This ingenious strategy brought him huge profits.

Monopolies and Seed Theft

Since quinine had to be obtained from the bark of the cinchona tree, which made it scarce and very expensive, from 1850 onwards European governments worked in two directions: on the one hand, looking for a synthetic substitute for quinine, and on the other, trying to break the quinine monopoly. This involved obtaining small trees or seeds to cultivate and adapt in other parts of the world.

The quina monopoly was in the hands of Ecuador, Peru and Bolivia, which, despite the high cost of extraction, exported it at a low price. However, it was the middlemen who made the product more expensive, so that it ended up costing its weight in gold. Quantification of the quinine content in cinchona bark made it possible to recognize the superiority of Bolivian varieties, which led to excessive exploitation of the cinchona forests in these areas. Faced with this situation, in 1834, Mariscal Andrés de Santa Cruz, leader of the Bolivian Republic, enacted a law limiting the exploitation and extraction of cinchona bark. At the time, Bolivia was probably one of the most prosperous nations in South America, thanks to the value of its quina and silver exports. However, the law remained a dead letter as world demand continued to grow.

As early as 1845, the great colonial powers of the time—England, France and Holland—sought to break the virtual monopoly on cinchona by attempting to establish plantations in their colonies in Africa and Asia. All of them failed in their first attempt. During these years, illicit acts of smuggling of wild cinchona seeds were intertwined with scientific studies, such as Weddell's 1849 study of the complex taxonomy, work that would be completed almost 100 years later by Stanley (1931). The French attempted to plant cinchona trees in Algeria, but their growth did not prosper.

The Englishman Clements Robert Markham (1830–1916), an employee of the East India Company, was commissioned in 1860 to obtain seeds and was in charge of a team of experienced botanists. Woolcock Pritchett went to the forests of Huánuco in search of the grey bark; Richard Spruce searched for the red chinchona in Ecuador, and Markham himself went to Carabaya (Puno) in search of the red chinchona, while the plants obtained were sent to Britain on a warship. In recognition of his work, Markham was honored as a Fellow of the Royal Geographic Society. In 1874, he published a memoir dedicated to the Countess of Chinchón: "*A Memoir of the Lady Ana de Osorio, Countess of Chinchón and Vice-queen of Perú (A. D. 1629-39)*", in which he made a mistake in putting the name of the sick Countess, wrong (as Ana Osorio was the Count's first wife) but somewhat positive, making a call for a correct transcription of the name of the tree. In 1880, he published the work "*Corteza peruana. Introduction of the cultivation of the chinchona in British India*". However, despite all Markham's efforts, the cultivation of cinchona in India failed [10, 11].

The colonial powers' efforts to seize quinine finally bore fruit in 1865, when an obscure British subject, C. Ledger, a Peru-based exporter of the bark, managed to take 12 pounds of cinchona seeds from the Alto Beni and sold them for $20 to Holland. The seeds were shipped to the island of Java, where plantations were established. By 1876, the quinine content of the bark reached 13.25%, and by 1930, Southeast Asia produced 90% of the world's production, estimated at 1 million pounds of quinine extracted from the new variety, named *Cinchona Ledgeriana*.

During that time, research into the treatment of malaria revealed how quinine works against the disease, interfering with the Plasmodium parasite by breaking down and digesting hemoglobin. Quinine binds to hemoglobin in red blood cells infected by the parasite, preventing the parasite from using it as a source for multiplication.

In the late nineteenth century, quinine became a common medicine for those travelling to Africa or Southeast Asia, where malaria was endemic among the population. The Scottish explorer William Balfour Baikie was the first to realize, during his expedition to Niger in 1854, that quinine served not only as a treatment for malaria, but also as a preventive measure.

When the French entrepreneur F. de Lesseps started the construction of the Panama Canal in 1883, he did not imagine that, a year later, malaria and yellow fever would be claiming the lives of 200 workers every month. Despite the availability of quinine, the project went bankrupt five years later. When the United States resumed work, it adopted preventive measures against yellow fever and malaria, using quinine as part of its strategy to complete the project.

Chemical Structure and Synthesis of Quinine

The long and laborious elucidation of the chemical structure of quinine was largely made possible by the work of the German chemist P. Rabe, who, around 1907, explored various synthetic routes. The presence of four asymmetric carbons, whose absolute orientation in space was unknown, implied the existence of 16 similar structures, of which only one corresponded to quinine [12] (Fig. 4.7).

With signs of an impending war in Europe, the Bolivian botanist M. Cárdenas conducted explorations in the Coroico river basin in 1937, with the support of the Kinabureau of Amsterdam, a private organization dedicated to the production and commercialization of quinine. Three years earlier, Cárdenas had discovered two new species of quinine while exploring the quinine-growing areas of the Boopi River in Alto Beni, as well as in Mapiri, Tipuani and Challana. The aim of his expedition was to prevent Nazi Germany from gaining access to quinine.

When the cinchona plantations in Asia fell to the Japanese Empire, the United States began to use Bolivian cinchona on a massive scale. However, this did not prevent some 60,000 American soldiers from dying during the war from malaria. During and after the war other options were explored, and the last years of the millennium were spent searching for new methods for the synthesis of quinine. In the 1990s, quinine was discovered to be useful as a potassium channel blocker in biological systems, opening up new prospects for treating diseases such as glaucoma, Parkinson's disease and rheumatoid arthritis. As the curtain of history fell on the millennium, quinine was still trading at US$2.70 an ounce and continued to be extracted from cinchona bark.

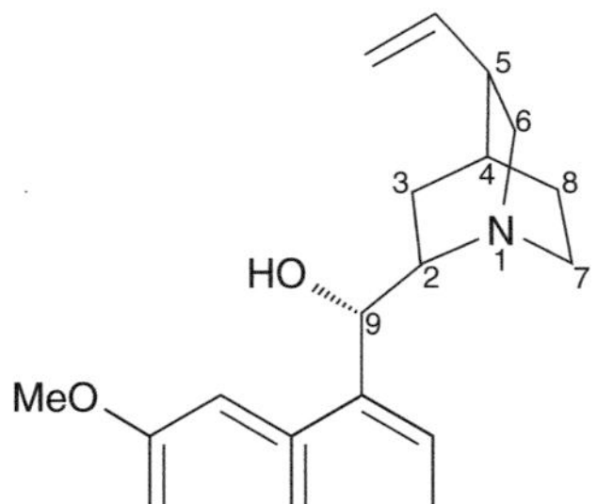

1

Fig. 4.7 Formula and technical name of quinine: (6-Methoxy—quinolin-4-yl)—(5-vinyl-1-aza- bicyclo [2.2.2]oct-2-yl)—methanol

In 1946, Gilbert Stork made progress in the development of intermediates to quinine; however, it was many years before he and his collaborators were able to publish their work entitled "*The First Stereoselective Total Synthesis of Quinine*", which appeared in 2001, using modern methods and concepts of organic synthesis [13]. However, for society, and because of its lag in the race to meet the demand for quinine, this synthesis is unlikely to be an alternative source for supplying the natural product. As Stork himself recognized: "The value of the synthesis has nothing to do with the commercial value of quinine; it is like the solution of an ancient theorem: it favors the advancement of science".

Although organic synthesis has evolved by leaps and bounds over the last half century, thanks to the availability of new methodologies, reagents, more sensitive analytical tools and digital techniques that allow structures to be visualized and their properties predicted, the synthesis of natural products remains a challenge to the ingenuity and tenacity of organic chemists. As Woodward summed it up: "The known but inaccessible structure represents to the chemist what to other people the unclimbed mountain, the unmapped sea, the uncultivated field, the uncharted planet…".

Other Uses of Quinine

At the same time, to facilitate travel for travelers in the nineteenth century, tonic water was suggested as a medicine. In 1858, a London entrepreneur, Erasmus Bond, patented the first "tonic drink with added air". In those years, quinine was added to tonic water, resulting in a drink that was extremely bitter and difficult to consume. To make it more palatable, it was mixed with sugar and lime, which not only made it drinkable, but also helped to combat scurvy on long sea voyages. Of course, gin was added, giving rise to the gin and tonic, which became a public favorite. It is known that it was in the Royal Botanic Gardens that gin and tonic was first prepared. *Oriental Sporting Magazine* describes it in 1868, mentioning that it was first consumed at the end of horse races in Lucknow, India, enjoyed as a cocktail while smoking a cigar.

In addition, quinine is an important ingredient in the production of other drinks that are a must in any self-respecting bar. Because of its bitter taste, small portions of quinine add an unmistakable flavor to many drinks, including Dubonnet, Elizabeth II's favorite drink, as well as to Cynar bitters and Spanish quinas used as restoratives, such as Quina Santa Catalina, for example, or to the Italian Barolo Chinato, a red wine with added quinine.

However, excessive consumption of quinine can cause alarming effects, such as nausea, ringing in the ears, blurred vision and confusion. According to the US Food & Drug Administration, the amount of quinine in carbonated beverages should not exceed 83 parts per million.

References

1. Palma R. El Correo del Perú, No. XLI, Año II, 19 octubre 1872. p. 323–4.
2. Herrera D. De Cortice chinae, et de Loxa, etsi diversorum arborum uniformis virtutis. Manuscript was published in Lima in 1737.
3. Charles M, La Condamine. Sur l'arbre du quinaquina (About the cinchona tree). Mem Acad Sci. 1738;4:226–43.
4. Hipólito Ruiz. Quinología o tratado del árbol de la quina o cascarilla. Madrid: Viuda e hijo de Marin; 1792.
5. Haenke T. Introducción a la historia natural de la provincia de Cochabamba y circunvecinas, first published in 1801.
6. Mutis JC. The arcanum of cinchona. Discourse containing the medical part of the four species of officinal cinchona, their eminent virtues and their legitimate preparation. Madrid: Imp Ibarra; 1828.
7. von Humboldt A, Bonpland A. Voyage aux régions Équinoxiales du Nouveau Continent. [Relation historique]: Fait en 1799, 1800, 1801, 1802, 1803 et 1804. F. Schoell, Paris; 1814.
8. Bañares G. Informe sobre la memoria hecha por el Dr. F.J. de Caldas del estado de las quinas en general y en particular de la de Loxa. 1808. Arch Gral Indias, legajo 1557.
9. Pérez JF, Artacho CJ, Diaz JF. La quinas de Caldas. UCM Madrid. Actas VIII Congreso de la Sociedad Española de Historia de las Ciencias y de las Técnicas.
10. Robert Markham C. A memoir of the Lady Ana de Osorio, Countess of Chinchón and Vice-queen of Perú with a plea for the correct spelling of the Chinchona Genus Legare Street Publishers Paperback 2022; 1874.
11. Miller LH, Rojas-Jaimes J, Low LM, Corbellini G. What historical records teach us about the discovery of quinine. Am J Trop Med Hyg. 2022;108:7–11.
12. David Amurrio D. Quinine. History and Synthesis. Rev Acta Nova. 2001;1(3). Cochabamba, Bolivia.
13. Gilbert Stork, R.A. Niu, A. Fujimoto, et al. The first stereoselective total synthesis of Quinine. J Am Chem Soc. 2001;123:8644–6.

5

Antonio de Gimbernat: The First School of Surgery in Spain and His Contributions to Inguinal Anatomy

Francisco Mateo Vallejo and Pedro Mestres Ventura

Antonio de Gimbernat y Arbós was born on 15 February 1734 in Cambrils, in the Baix Camp of the province of Tarragona, Catalonia, on the shores of Mediterranean sea (Fig. 5.1).

His parents, Antonio Gimbernat and Antonia Arbós, were farmers who belonged to a an upper-middle social class [1, 2].

When Antonio was six years old, the family suffered a sad misfortune: his father died suddenly, leaving a widow and six children, whose ages ranged from nineteen years old for the eldest to twenty months old for the youngest. Despite this tragedy, the family was able to continue their life without hardship, and the children received a proper education.

He started going to the public school in Cambrils, where received Latin instruction, that facilitated his admission as a pupil in the convent of the Franciscan Recollects Fathers in Riudoms, a town nearby Cambrils. He was subsequently admitted to the University of Cervera (Lleida) where he studied for five years, two years of Latin and three years of Philosophy.

F. M. Vallejo (✉)
Surgeon Specialized in Minimally Invasive Surgery for Gastrointestinal Cancer, Jerez de la Frontera, Cádiz, Spain

P. M. Ventura
Autonomous University of Barcelona, Barcelona, Spain

Department of Anatomy at Saarland University, Saarbrücken, Germany

Faculty of Science, University of Luxembourg, Esch-sur-Alzette, Luxembourg

M. A. Cuesta, F. Mateo Vallejo (eds.), *Spain's Journey in Medicine*,
https://doi.org/10.1007/978-3-032-12221-6_5

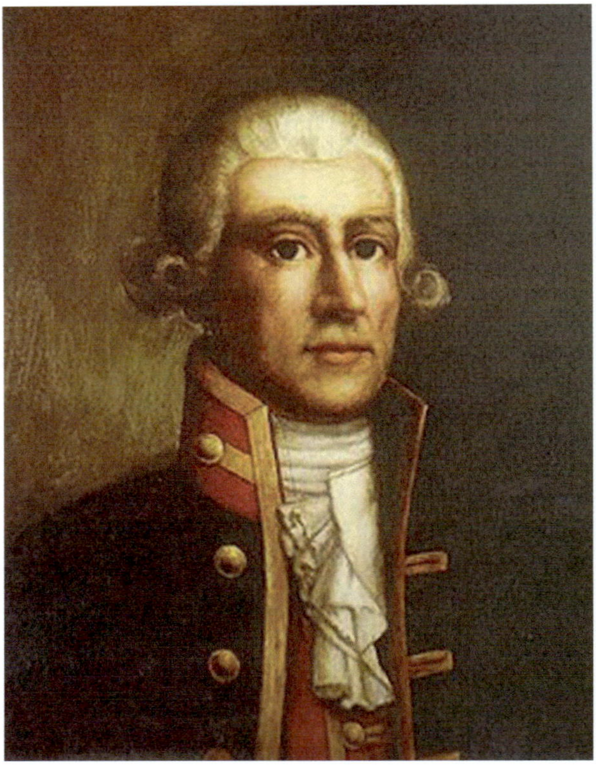

Fig. 5.1 Antonio de Gimbernat

In 1756, at the age of 22, after completing his studies, he decided to move to Cadiz to begin medical studies at the Real Colegio de Cirugía de la Armada (Royal School of Surgery of the Navy), founded by Juan de Lacomba and Pedro Virgili in 1748. The recent foundation of the Royal School of Cadiz and its rapid popularity aroused great interest among Cervera's students, who praised the modernity and quality of its teaching, as well as its connection to the Navy, which offered a more stable professional perspective than civilian life. The high number of Catalonians who chose to study there underlines the prestige of the institution in its early years (Fig. 5.2).

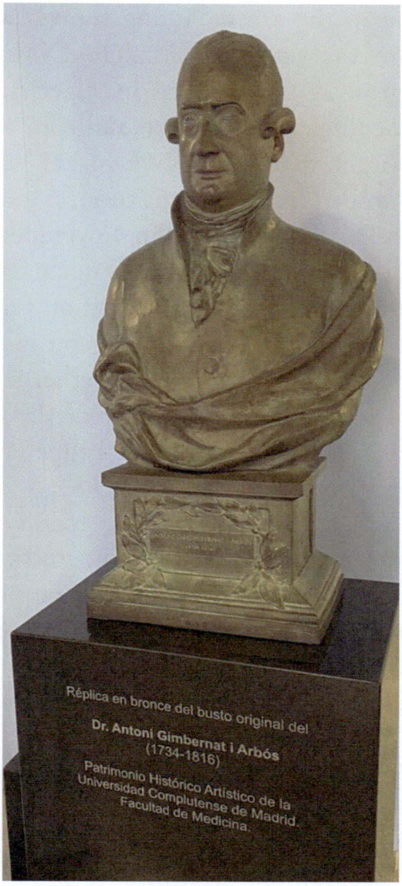
Réplica en bronce del busto original del
Dr. Antoni Gimbernat i Arbós
(1734-1816)
Patrimonio Histórico Artístico de la
Universidad Complutense de Madrid.
Facultad de Medicina.

Fig. 5.2 Brons's bust of A. de Gimbernat of 1788 , Universidad Complutense de Madrid, Facultad de Medicina

Pedro Virgili Bellver and the Creation of the Royal School of Surgery of the Navy in Cadiz

Pedro Virgili Bellver (1699–1776) was born in Villalonga del Camp (Tarragona) and grew up in a farming family. Although they owned some land and rented it, the family's finances were modest. Lacking sufficient means to study medicine, Virgili opted for surgery, becoming in January 1721, apprentice of the surgeon Gabriel Riera, of Tarragona.

In 1724 he enlisted in the army, joining the Calatrava Regiment, with which he took part in the siege of Gibraltar. During that time, he was appointed senior surgeon at the hospital in Algeciras, where he met and befriended Juan de Lacomba, French born surgeon, who captivated by his character, convinced Virgili, to join the Navy. In 1732 the Navy awarded him a scholarship to travel to Paris to extend his surgical training.

After a year's stay in Paris, he returned in November 1733 and joined the Royal Hospital of Cadiz. As a Navy surgeon he made several trips to America, always seeking to improve his training as expedition surgeon.

Upon his return in Cadiz, he worked as surgeon in the Naval Hospital in Cádiz under the orders of Juan de Lacomba. Together, they proposed a project for the creation of a Royal School of Surgery of the Navy to the Minister Marquis de la Ensenada, a project approved by Felipe V that finally opened by his successor Fernando VI on 11 November 1748.

The creation of the School responded to the necessity to improve the medical services on the Navy in general. At that time, most surgeons lacked solid academic training; their knowledge was acquired empirically or transmitted by tradition, far from the scientific advances that the Age of Enlightenment spread throughout Europe.

After a serious illness, Juan de Lacomba, died on December 18, 1748 [3] (Fig. 5.2).

The School with Virgili as its head, not only transformed the teaching of surgery, but also introduced important innovations. He emphasized the value of anatomy, promoted clinical practice and encouraged scientific publications in Spanish, breaking with centuries of exclusive reliance on Latin texts. Under his leadership, surgeons ceased to be viewed as mere technicians and achieved the prestige that had until then been reserved for physicians (Fig. 5.3).

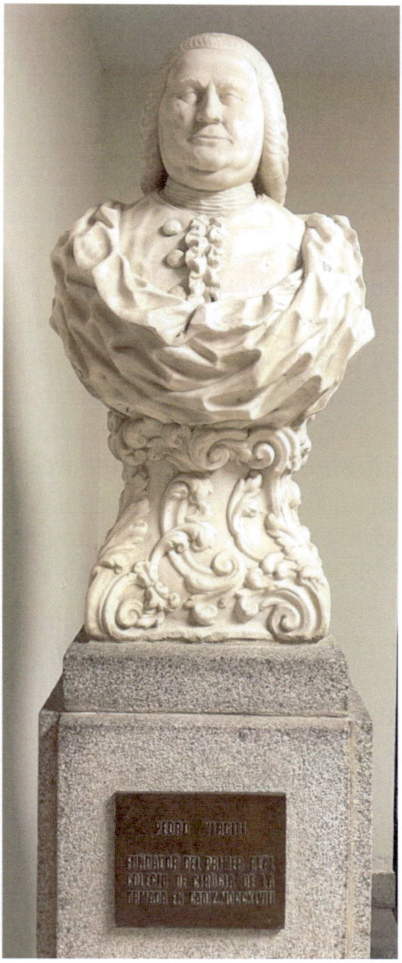

Fig. 5.3 Bust of Pedro Virgili in the School of Medicine in Cadiz

The Enlightenment and Independence War Against Napoleon During Gimbernat's Lifetime

The political situation and the various monarchs who succeeded each other in Spain throughout Gimbernat's life profoundly influenced his career.

This century was characterized by the influence of the Enlightenment movement on politics, culture and society. It was a transformative intellectual and cultural movement in eighteenth century Europe that championed reason, individualism, and progress. It challenged traditional authority and promoted ideas like natural rights, liberty, and separation of church and state.

The Enlightenment gave a pre-eminent role to science and progress as essential tools for improving the human condition. In Spain, although with its own particularities, this period witnessed important reforms and transformations that left a profound mark on the country. After a long period of the Bourbon monarchy, with great advances in economy and science, first the French revolution (1789) and then the Napoleonic invasion of Spain (1808–1814) brought great changes dominated by the chaotic and painful war of independence to expel the French. Napoleon had appointed his brother Joseph Bonaparte on the throne of Spain, sparking strong popular resistance. In Cádiz, a city that resisted French occupation, the first Spanish Constitution was promulgated in 1812, one of the most advanced of its time, establishing a representative government, national sovereignty, and limitations on monarchical power.

In 1814, after Napoleon's defeat, Ferdinand VII returned to the throne and annulled the 1812 Constitution, restoring absolutism. His repressive government generated deep tension with the liberal sectors, which aspired to re-establish the constitutional reforms.

Antonio de Gimbernat and the Royal Schools of Surgery of Cadiz and Barcelona

The prestige acquired by the Royal School of Surgery of Cadiz as a centre of excellence in surgical education was a great attraction, for many students from all over Spain (Fig. 5.4).

The first reference to his enrollment in the Royal School dates from May 1758, [4] and over the next two years, Gimbernat trained as a Practical student in Surgery, dedicated to anatomy, botany, mathematics, physics and

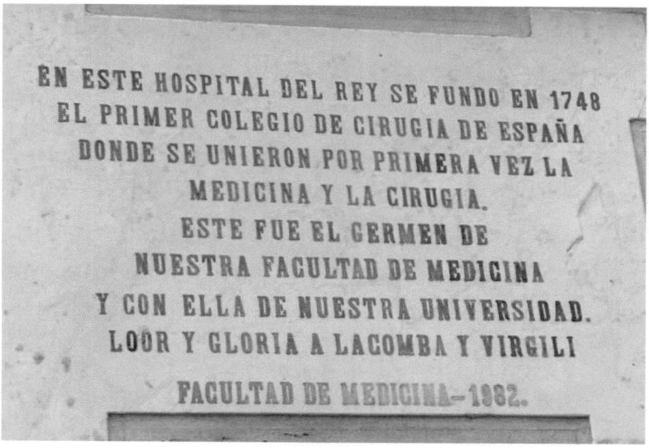

Fig. 5.4 Commemorative plaque, dated in 1982, in the School of Medicine in Cádiz, where Medicine and Surgery were first united. It mentions the origin of the Faculty of Medicine, honoring Lacomba and Virgili

chemistry. His true passion was the anatomical study of the cadaver, to which he devoted much of his time and effort. He was an outstanding disciple of Lorenzo Roland, master anatomist and son-in-law of Virgili, whom he substituted in his classes during his absences.

In 1748 Pedro Virgili conceived the creation of a new School of Surgery in Barcelona, which he and the monarch believed should be dedicated to the service of the army and the population of the surrounding region. Appointed in 1758 as first surgeon of the Royal Chamber, together with Pedro Perchet, surgeon of the General Hospital of Barcelona, Virgili presented the project to the King for the new School in Barcelona. Carlos III authorized the project and on March 29, 1764, the new School was inaugurated.

In the meantime, Gimbernat ended his studies in Cadiz in the summer of 1762, after successfully passing the final exam and obtaining the title de *Cirujano Latino* [2]. In 1766 he was appointed [5] as professor at the School, obtaining at the same time the position of senior surgeon at the Hospital de la Santa Creu, annexed to the building of the new School.

In 1763, Gimbernat married Eulalia Grassot Ballester, daughter of a Barcelona surgeon, with whom he had six children.

During his years in Barcelona, his research into the anatomy of the femoral region led him to create a new surgical technique for operating on inguinal hernias, an advancement whose legacy has been perpetuated to the present day.

Antonio de Gimbernat and His Trip Around Europe on a Grant from the King

In 1774, he received a commission from King Carlos III, to travel together with Mariano Ribas Elías, professor at the Royal College of Surgery in Cadiz, to visit the main medical centres in Europe with the aim of learning, studying, and evaluating advances in medicine and surgery. The final goal was to apply these experiences and knowledge in a third Royal School of Surgery, which the king wished to establish in Madrid.

In Paris, he attended the departments of the Hopitaux Hotel-Dieu and Charité, where they met Antoine Louis, Joseph Desault, and Francois Chopart, heads of the Académie Royale de Chirurgie.

In 1776, they visited different hospitals in London such as St. Thomas' Hospital, Guy's Hospital, and St. Bartholomew's Hospital, being as observers of surgical interventions performed by Samuel Sharp and other surgeons. They also followed a complete course on Surgery with John Hunter and others and about "medical material" with William Saunders.

On April 25,1777, a highly significant event took place for Gimbernat, when John Hunter was giving the 80th lesson on femoral hernias and the risks associated with the surgical technique used until then. Hunter maintained that, in order to dilate the opening of the hernia for its reduction, it was necessary to divide Poupart's ligament, a technique that entailed significant risks, such as damage to the epigastric artery, the spermatic cord or some other structure of the inguinal canal.

At the end of the lesson, Gimbernat requested the floor to present his own method. Using the same anatomical piece that Hunter had used in his explanation, Gimbernat detailed his procedure:

> *The grooved probe* is *introduced between the intestine and the hernial sac into the cavity, then directed obliquely inwards, and with it resting on the pubic ramus in a horizontal position, and its cannula turned sideways and inwards, the straight scalpel is introduced through this cannula, and the cut towards the pubis. In this way a portion of the aponeurotic expansion of Poupart's ligament is cut, together with its attachment to the pubic ramus, without in any way exposing any vessel, the spermatic cord or the ligament of Poupart. The incision thus made gives great liberty to introduce the intestine with the greatest ease, as I have already experienced on two occasions....* [6–11]

Hunter, surprised by the unknown Spanish surgeon's presentation, responded with a laudatory "You are right, Sir". In front of the entire student body, he assured that he would try the method as soon as he had the opportunity and that he would introduce it to the English surgical community. That he would use and recommend the technique in the future, adding that in honor of the Spaniard, he would call the lacunar ligament as Gimbernat's ligament. This generous and chivalrous gesture was decisive for Gimbernat's emergence from anonymity and achieve international recognition.

In this period, Gimbernat focused his attention on the study of healthcare organization and various surgical and medical problems, establishing contact with leading figures of the time, such as Herman Boerhaave, William Cullen and Peter Camper.

Finally, Gimbernat and Ribas concluded their European journey and returned to Spain in October 1778, where Gimbernat resumed his professional activity at the Royal School of Barcelona.

On learning of the brilliant scientific results of the trip made by Gimbernat and Ribas, Carlos III, initiated the steps for the creation of the Royal College of Surgery of Madrid.

Creation of the Royal College of Surgery of San Carlos in Madrid

In a letter dated March 1779, the Captain General of Catalonia informed him:

> *The King has learned with great pleasure of the progress and advances made by these doctors (Drs. Gimbernat and Ribas), and his Royal wish is that their light and observations should be used for the benefit and relief of his vassals, and he has ordered them to come to Madrid, where they are now, and his Majesty wishes them to continue attending at the General Hospital until the School of Surgery that his Majesty has planned and resolved to establish in this Court is established.*

A year later, in 1780, the order for the foundation of the Royal School of Surgery of San Carlos in Madrid was published, with Antonio de Gimbernat as its director.

Between 1780 and 1786, Gimbernat worked intensively on its construction, the training of the Royal School's medical staff, and on the development of its doctrinal and pedagogical framework.

Professionals selected to join the College were sent to France and England to complete their training. Concerning the building, the King ordered the Royal School to be located in the General Hospital of Madrid, being rebuilt by the famous architect Francisco Sabatini.

These reforms were concentrated in the basements of the hospital, where a meeting room, an anatomical amphitheater, a practice room, a library, an anatomical cabinet—an idea particularly appreciated by Gimbernat—and various adjoining rooms were installed.

The public inauguration of the Royal School did not take place until October 1,1787. That day, Gimbernat gave an inaugural lecture entitled *"Sobre el Recto Uso de las Suturas y su Abuso" (On the Right Use of Sutures and their Abuse)* (Fig. 5.5).

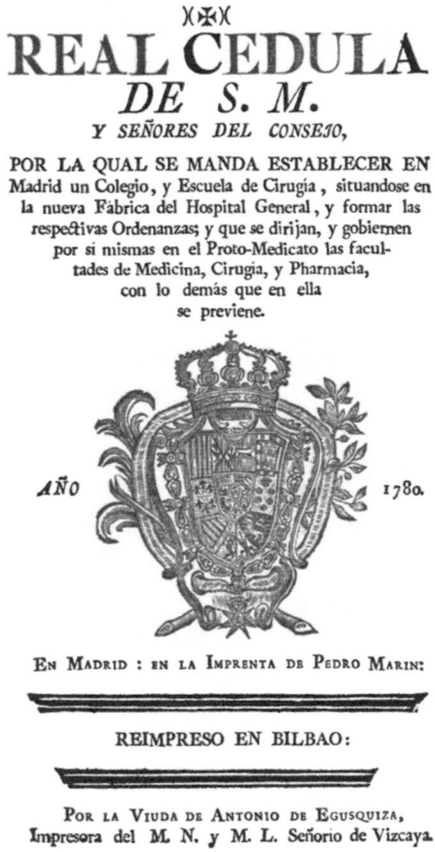
REAL CEDULA
DE S. M.
Y SEÑORES DEL CONSEJO,
POR LA QUAL SE MANDA ESTABLECER EN Madrid un Colegio, y Escuela de Cirugia, situandose en la nueva Fábrica del Hospital General, y formar las respectivas Ordenanzas; y que se dirijan, y gobiernen por si mismas en el Proto-Medicato las facultades de Medicina, Cirugia, y Pharmacia, con lo demás que en ella se previene.

AÑO 1780.

EN MADRID: EN LA IMPRENTA DE PEDRO MARIN:

REIMPRESO EN BILBAO:

POR LA VIUDA DE ANTONIO DE EGUSQUIZA, Impresora del M. N. y M. L. Señorio de Vizcaya.

Fig. 5.5 Royal document of Foundation of the Royal School of Surgery San Carlos, 1780, Madrid

The Gimbernat Ligament. Gimbernat Revolutionises Surgery for Crural Hernia

After the annual dissertation in October 1787 at the Royal School of Surgery of San Carlos about the use and abuse of sutures (Fig. 5.6), on October 9,1788, at the Meeting held again at the School of Surgery of San Carlos, A. Gimbernat read his famous dissertation on "Nuevo metodo de operar en la Hernia Crural", (*"New method of operating on femoral hernia")*. In this work, Gimbernat describes the anatomy of the crural arch, through which the iliac vessels pass, and femoral hernias are formed, Based on several years of personal experience, the dissertation was divided into two parts. In the first,

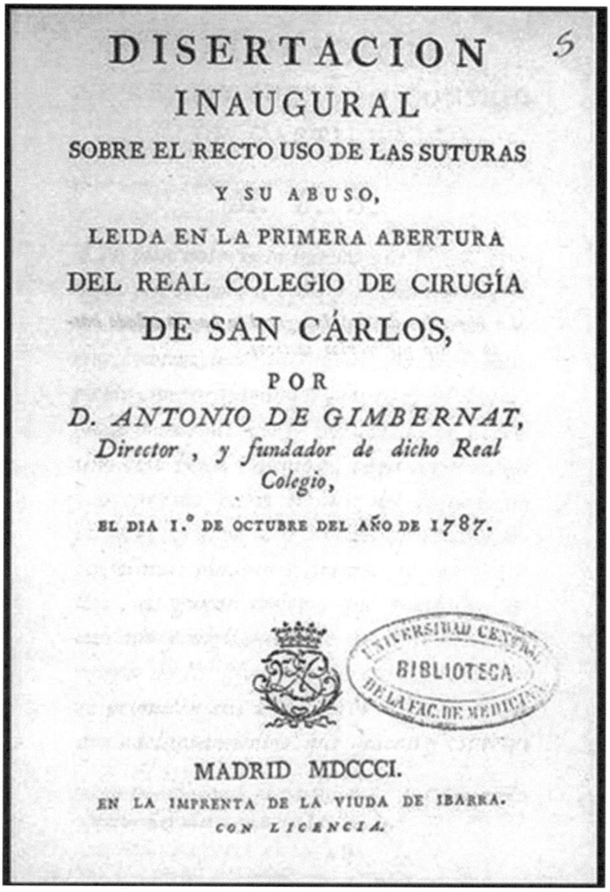

DISERTACION
INAUGURAL
SOBRE EL RECTO USO DE LAS SUTURAS
Y SU ABUSO,
LEIDA EN LA PRIMERA ABERTURA
DEL REAL COLEGIO DE CIRUGÍA
DE SAN CÁRLOS,
POR
D. ANTONIO DE GIMBERNAT,
Director, y fundador de dicho Real Colegio,
EL DIA 1.° DE OCTUBRE DEL AÑO DE 1787.

MADRID MDCCCI.
EN LA IMPRENTA DE LA VIUDA DE IBARRA.
CON LICENCIA.

Fig. 5.6 Inaugural lecture presented at the Real Colegio of San Carlos by D. Antonio Gimbernat about the use and abuse of sutures. (1st October 1787)

Gimbernat reviews the previous surgical techniques used to treat the femoral hernia. In the second, he offers a careful anatomical study of the inguinal region in which he described the ligament that was named after him by John Hunter, description that was accompanied by two beautiful drawings (Figs. 5.7 and 5.8).

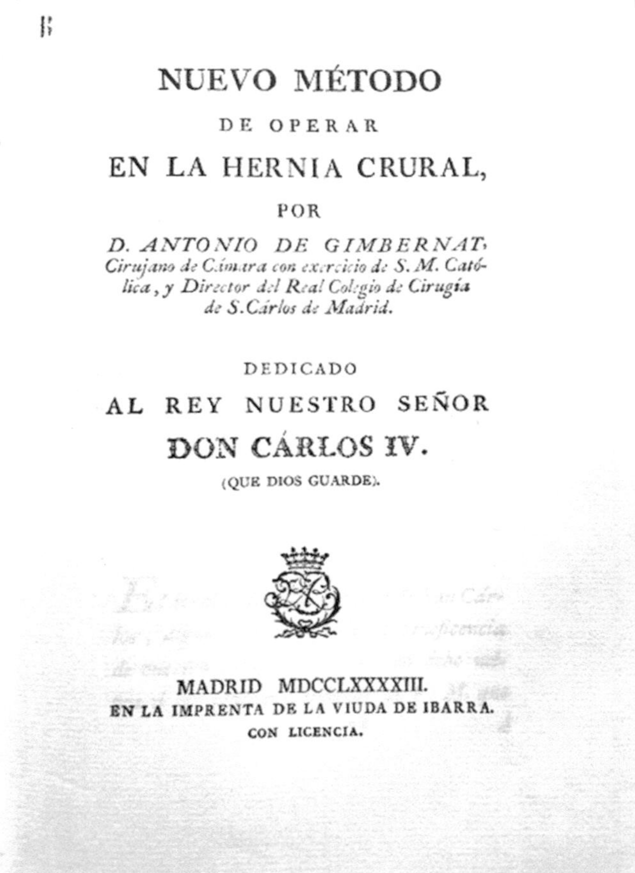
NUEVO MÉTODO

DE OPERAR

EN LA HERNIA CRURAL,

POR

D. ANTONIO DE GIMBERNAT,
Cirujano de Cámara con exercicio de S. M. Católica, y Director del Real Colegio de Cirugía de S. Cárlos de Madrid.

DEDICADO

AL REY NUESTRO SEÑOR

DON CÁRLOS IV.

(QUE DIOS GUARDE).

MADRID MDCCLXXXXIII.
EN LA IMPRENTA DE LA VIUDA DE IBARRA.
CON LICENCIA.

Fig. 5.7 Cover of the book of D. Antonio Gimbernat: "New Method to operate a crural hernia". 1793, Madrid.

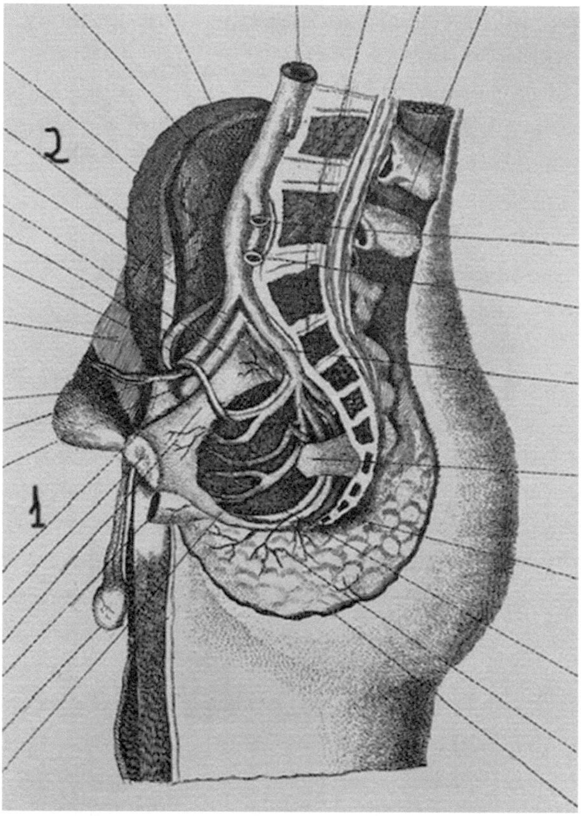

Fig. 5.8 Anatomical plate describing how to operate a crural hernia and the location of the ligament of Gimbernat. (the numbering is not the original)

Impact of Gimbernat's Work Abroad

During his travels in Europe, Gimbernat, thanks to his knowledge of several languages and his affable character, established strong relationships with numerous colleagues, which he maintained on his return to Spain [12].

In London, he befriended the Reverend Joseph Townsend, to whom he entrusted his method of operating on crural hernias. Townsend included this technique in his famous textbook for students, published in 1795 [13]. His English colleagues learned of his method soon after its appearance in 1793. The physician and scientific popularizer Thomas Beddoes translated the Gimbernat's work into English and published it in 1795, just two years after its difussion in Spain. In addition, Beddoes also made known a method devised by Gimbernat for the treatment of hydrocele, which was never published by its author. Thus, had it not been for Beddoes, this procedure would have been lost in time.

The impact of Gimbernat's method in Germany is particularly striking, as there is no record of him having contact with German colleagues during his lifetime. However, his work was translated into German by Professor Bernhard Schreger, Professor of Anatomy and Surgery at the University of Erlangen. Schreger enriched the publication with an extensive and detailed comparative study of the hernia operation techniques known until then, creating an exceptional book in which he expressed his admiration for Gimbernat and his method.

Years later, in 1827, the professor of anatomy Gilbert Breschet of the University of Paris published a French translation of Gimbernat's work, ensuring its dissemination in the European academic sphere.

Gimbernat's name has endured in the academic discourse of anatomists and surgeons to the present day. However, the elimination of eponyms in modern anatomical nomenclature has meant a significant loss, depriving future generations of a valuable historical reference [14].

Gimbernat's Activities Outside the Royal School of Surgery of San Carlos

In the following years, Gimbernat devoted part of his efforts to the creation of new Schools of Surgery that would follow the model of those already established in Cadiz, Barcelona and Madrid. The first two to be founded were those of Burgos and Santiago, in 1799. He also undertook new effort to establish similar institutions in Salamanca, Saragossa and other cities, with the aim of expanding surgical training.

Even at that time, the medical and surgical professions were kept separate and functioned as independent disciplines. In 1797, Gimbernat signed a provision stating that physicians could not practice surgery, and surgeons could not practice medicine, except in mixed cases where a physician and a surgeon must intervene jointly. However, this separation gradually began to be diluted. In 1799, the Higher Governing Board presented a proposal to associate the Royal Study of Practical Medicine with the Royal School of Surgery. The initiative was approved a few days later, and the institution was renamed the Real estudio de Medicina Práctica y el real Colegio de Cirugía de San Carlos (*Royal Study of Practical Medicine and the Royal School of Surgery of San Carlos.*

In this context, a General Board was created comprising the Chamber Physicians and the Chamber Surgeons, who, from then on, were called Chamber Physicians, with the status of physician-surgeons.

Spanish War of Independence (1808–1814)

The situation, both in Spain and in Antonio de Gimbernat's life, changed radically after the Napoleonic occupation of Spain in 1808. Although the French allowed teaching to continue at the Royal School, all physicians, surgeons and staff were forced to sign an oath of loyalty to the oppressive government. This requirement extended to all the Schools of Surgery in the country, with the sole exception of the Royal School of Surgery of Cadiz, the only Spanish enclave that remained outside French rule.

A few years later, Gimbernat's health had seriously deteriorated. He suffered from advanced cataracts and had difficulty moving without assistance, so he decided to undergo cataracts surgery.

The operation was performed by Professor José Ribes Mayor. However, that same night, impatient to know the outcome of the operation, Gimbernat uncovered the wound dressing. Whether due to this action or complications arising from the surgery, he ended up retaining only a slight degree of vision in one eye.

In January 1811, all the medical and pharmacological schools and the Royal Schools of Surgery were reorganized into a new institution created by King Joseph Bonaparte and called the Supreme Council of Health. Gimbernat was appointed director, thus becoming the highest authority in the country's health system. He swore loyalty to the invader and obliged the directors of the surgical schools to do the same. It is possible to assume that he accepted the position in order to protect the institutions and individuals under his direction from the new political power. Added to this was his well-known affinity with French culture, not only in the field of surgery, but also in other intellectual and scientific aspects, undoubtedly influenced his decision.

With the restoration of Fernando VII in 1814, and possibly in retaliation for his pro-French attitude, Gimbernat was relegated to the position of member of the recently re-established Higher Governmental Boards (Juntas Superiores Gubernativas), when he should have been president. At the age of 80 and with severe sight problems, he decided to resign and retire definitively from public life.

A memorandum found and collected by Usandizaga in 1948 [15] in the Palace Archives [16] provides evidence of Gimbernat's situation in his last years:

> *Mr. Antonio de Gimbernat, the first Chamber Surgeon ever, to Your Majesty, with the deepest respect, states: That, deprived of all salary by virtue of the employee classification judgment, he found himself in the most bitter and deplorable situation, deprived of the sole means of support on which he based his subsistence at the age of over 81, almost blind, and with an absolute physical disability, which has him separated from the rest of society. In such a deplorable state, it has become known that Your Majesty has been pleased to grant several members of the Royal Chamber, who are in the same situation as the exponent, a substantial annual allowance. Considering that the unhappiness in which the exponent finds himself is much greater than that of the aforementioned individuals, it is absolutely impossible for him to support himself by other means, due to his painful aggravation with the resulting ailments, since his poor eyesight and his advanced age, which do not even allow him to leave his house, he humbly begs Your Majesty, taking into account the afflicted fate of the exponent, and considering the particular circumstances already indicated, which distinguish his current situation, and using the paternal clemency and piety that shine so brightly in the Royal Spirit of Your Majesty, to deign to grant him, likewise, an allowance with which he may support himself and his relatives, ordering that he be paid and satisfied, from the same date as the other aforementioned members of the Royal Chamber. Thus, he hopes for the justified benevolence of Your Majesty, whose life may God preserve for the long years that Christendom and its subjects need and desire. Madrid, July 15, 1815.*

The situation in which he spent the remaining months of his life has been described in dark tones. Economic precariousness and physical weakness (blindness) have been pointed out as the personal circumstances that marked the end of one of the most outstanding figures of Spanish Surgery. Gimbernat died in Madrid on November 17, 1816.

References

1. Pagarolas Sabaté L. Els Gimbernat i el Cambrils del Segle XVIII. Published by Cambrils Town Council (in Catalan). 1985.
2. Mestres Ventura P. Antonio de Gimbernat i Arboç (1734-1816). 2022. Arola Editors (Tarragona).
3. González G, Antonio J, editors. El Real Colegio de Cirugía de la Armada en Cádiz, Reflexiones en el Aniversario de su Creación (1748-2023). Institute of

Academies of Andalucia. Regional Government of Andalucia, Department of University, Research and Innovation. Málaga; 2024.
4. Prada-Oliveira JA, et al. Gimbernat's stay in Cadiz and his discovery of the human anatomy. Eur J Anat. 2016;20(Suppl. 1):23–34.
5. Gimbernat Grassot, A. (1828) Sucinta Noticia del Sr. D. Antonio de Gimbernat, del Consejo de Hacienda, primer Cirujano de Cámara, fundador y primer director del real Colegio de Cirugía de San Carlos, presidente de la Real Junta Gubernativa de los reales Colegios de Cirugía. Barcelona: Imprenta de Valero Sierra y Martí.
6. de Gimbernat A. New method of operating on Crural Hernia. Dedicated to King Carlos IV. Madrid Imprenta: de la Viuda de Ibarra; 1793.
7. Loukas M, El-Sedfy, Tubbs RS, et al. Gimbernat y Arbós, Antonio de (1734-1816). World J Surg. 2007;31:855–7.
8. Miranda Efraín A. Don Antonio de Gimbernat. In Medical Terminology Daily 2012. In a moment in history. February 2012.
9. Matheson NM. Antonio de Gimbernat (1734–1816), Proc R Soc Med. 1948;42:407–10.
10. Honoring Don Antonio de Gimbernat. Anatomist and Surgeon (1734–1816). Eur J Anat. 2016; Edited by Mestres-Ventura P. 20(Suppl1). Accessed online: http://eurjanat.com/v1/data/pdf/eja.20s10001.pdf.
11. Salcedo y Ginestal E. Works by Don Antonio de Gimbernat. Preceded by a bio-bibliographical study of the same. Classic Library of Spanish Medicine. 6:192–3. Imp de Cosano. Madrid; 1926.
12. Mestres Ventura PJ. The impact of Gimbernat's work in the Europe of his age (18th century). Gimbernat: Revista de Historia de la Medicina i de les Ciències [Barcelona]. 2023;80:11–24.
13. Townsend J, editor. a guide to health; being cautions and directions in the treatment of diseases. Designed chiefly for the use of students. London: Printed for Cox; 1795. p. 416.
14. Pereira JA, López-Cano M. Components separation. Back-to-back: from anatomy knowledge to surgery and from surgical experience to anatomy. Eur J Anat Ed P Mestres. 2016;20:89–92.
15. Usandizaga M. Historia del Real Colegio de Cirugía de San Carlos de Madrid (1771-1828). Madrid: Consejo Superior de Investigaciones Científicas; 1948.
16. Arráez Aybar LA. Antonio Gimbernat y Arbós (1734-1816) director Perpetuo del Real Colegio de Cirugía de San Carlos in Madrid. An Inst Est Mad. 2016;56:179–202.

6

The Royal Philantropic Vaccine Expedition, The Balmis Expedition (1804–1812). The Smallpox Vaccine that Circled the Globe

Carlos Márquez Espinós

Smallpox, caused by a virus from the poxvirus family, is one of the most devastating diseases ever to exist in human history. Smallpox claimed the lives of more than 60 million people in Europe alone in the 18th century.

Throughout history, the disease occurred in periodic outbreaks and spread massively in America when the conquistadors arrived in the New World [1].

The vaccine to prevent smallpox had been discover by E. Jenner in 1798 when the Hispanic Crown (Carlos IV, 1788-1808), decided to finance and organize a philanthropic expedition to vaccinate as much as possible people in the Hispanic overseas (Fig. 6.1).

It was organized as a necessity in view of continuous epidemics that repeatedly ravaged America, with a consequent decline in the population. This medical expedition was defined as "Royal" because it was organized and financed directly by the Spanish Crown, and "Philanthropic" because it was motivated by the search for a benefit for the entire population of the Nation; a novelty in this health project is its philanthropy, since the spread of the smallpox vaccine transcended the utilitarian spirit of the Enlightenment in the context of social and political uncertainty plagued by the revolutions in America and Europe [2].

Finally in 1980, the WHO (World Health Organization) declared the eradication of smallpox, making it the first disease to be eliminated worldwide

C. M. Espinós (✉)
Anaesthesiologist and historian of Medicine. Department of the History of Medicine, University of Cádiz, Cádiz, Spain

M. A. Cuesta, F. Mateo Vallejo (eds.), *Spain's Journey in Medicine*,
https://doi.org/10.1007/978-3-032-12221-6_6

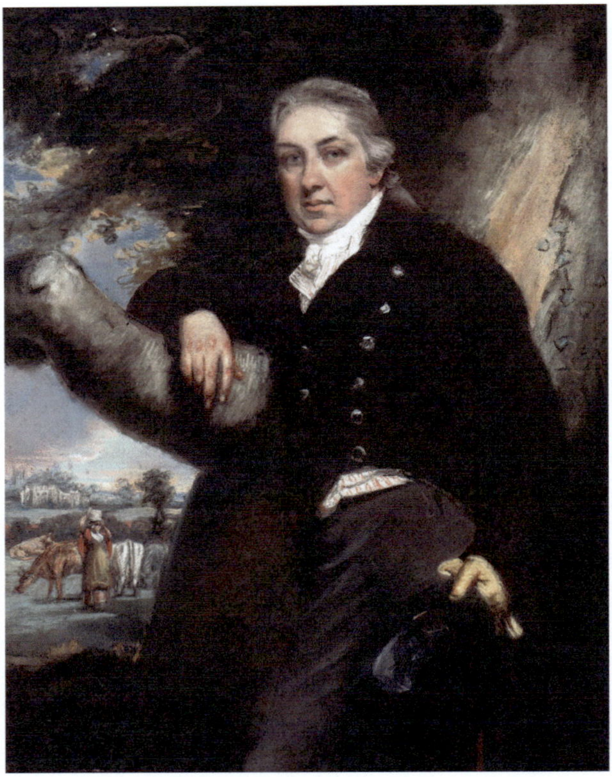

Fig. 6.1 Portrait of Edward Jenner (1749–1823) by John Raphael Smith. Private Collection

after an universal vaccination program, program that is considered one of the most important successes of modern medicine. This expedition was the first worldwide step towards this end.

Variolization

Important to the control of this disease was the introduction of variolization, a method used to protect people against smallpox, which preceded vaccination by a century. It involved the deliberate inoculation of the smallpox virus into healthy people, usually by introducing material from pustules of infected patients through small incisions in the skin. This procedure originated in China and India and became popular in Europe in the eighteenth century. Although it offered protection against severe forms of the disease, it had significant risks, such as the possibility of developing a severe infection and spreading the virus with a five percent mortality rate. Even so, it helped to reduce the danger of epidemics because it provided a new therapeutic tool to defend against the disease, and it was an innovative change of concept, as it is based on the empirical observation that those who have suffered a bout of smallpox and survived are forever free from it.

Vaccination

Vaccination was a process very similar to variolization and replaced it in the late 18th century, when an English country doctor Edward Jenner (1749-1823), observed that inoculated smallpox did not cause infection in those who had suffered from smallpox, so he used another form of smallpox, cowpox, to induce immunity without the risks of human smallpox. He published his work privately in *An inquiry into the causes and effects of the Variolae vaccine,* London, 1798, [3], illustrating the evolution of vaccination in colored plates, which is considered a milestone of medical progress (Fig. 6.2).

In 1796, during the height of the spread of the smallpox virus in Europe, Edward Jenner observed that milkmaids of dairy cows occasionally acquired a kind of "*cowpox*" or through continuous contact with these animals, and that it was a mild variant of the deadly "human smallpox", against which they were

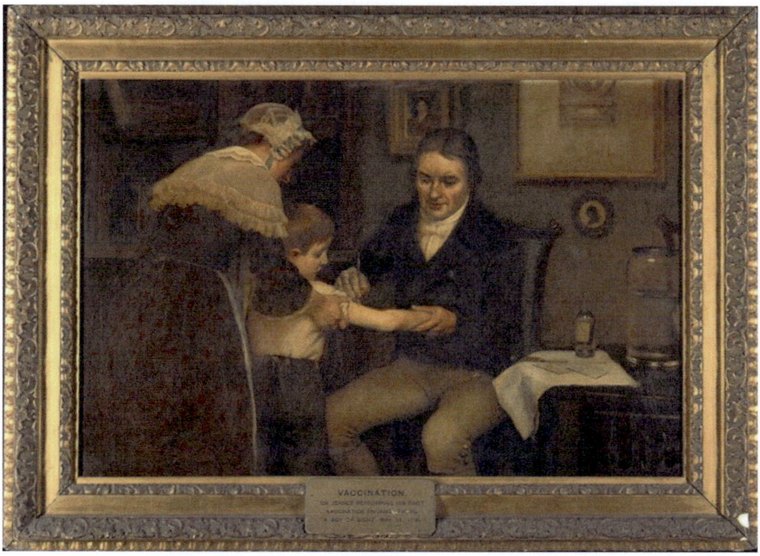

Fig. 6.2 Edward Jenner (1749–1823) performing the First vaccination to James Phipps, 14 May 1796, by Ernest Board

thus immunized. He adapted the variolization technique, extracting fluid from the udder pustules of a diseased cow to inoculate an 8-year-old boy, James Philips.

The little boy showed symptoms of cowpox infection, but much milder, and did not die. Other inoculated children responded surprisingly well and were immunized against human smallpox. But Jenner made another important discovery: he realized that this infection, with cowpox, could be transmitted from one person to another. At the site where the fluid had been introduced, the recipient developed pustules; and the fluid that accumulated could be removed and used to be administered as new vaccine to other people.

Thus, in 1798, Edward Jenner developed the smallpox vaccine, which began to be widely administered. The practice vaccination spread throughout all countries, as attempts were made to find cows with smallpox or to obtain Jenner's "vaccine" or lymph. In this context, the greatest effort to vaccinate an entire population was made by Spain which, in November 1803, launched what is considered to be the first mass vaccination campaign in the history, to take the vaccine from Spain to America and Asia.

Philantropic Vaccine Expedition

This expedition was part of the series of enlightened expeditions carried out by Spain in its American territories throughout the 18th century [4]. It was a philanthropic medical mission led by Dr Francisco Javier Balmis (1753-1819) between 1803 and 1806 and continued after by J. Salvany up to 1810, with the aim bringing the smallpox vaccine to overseas territories of the Spanish nation. This expedition, was one of the first global public health campaigns and a milestone in the history of medicine, being considered one of the most important medical feats in the history of Spanish medicine in the period prior to the independence of the Spanish territories in America [5].The objectives to be achieved with this expedition were:

1. Spread the vaccine from the Kingdom of Spain to all the overseas Spanish Viceroyalties in America and Asia.
2. Educate local health workers in the visited villages to continue in the practice of vaccination over time.
3. To establish Vaccination Boards (Juntas de Vacuna) in all territories as centres to conserve, produce and supply active vaccines to maintain the campaign on an ongoing basis.

The expedition's primary objective was the pursuit of public health by fighting smallpox epidemics [6]. Therefore, the expedition not only disseminated the vaccine throughout the Hispanic overseas territories, but also perpetuated it in those lands thanks to the establishment of the Vaccine Boards. These institutions managed the immunization of the population and were consolidated as health organizations after the independence of the territories, maintaining their public, hierarchical and central character [2].

Preliminaries and Preparation of the Expedition

The smallpox vaccine was introduced in Spain in 1799. After June 1802, when an epidemic broke out in the Viceroyalty of New Granada, the King Carlos IV consulted his Council of the Indias in January 1803 and, in March of the same year, it was declared advisable to spread the smallpox vaccine to

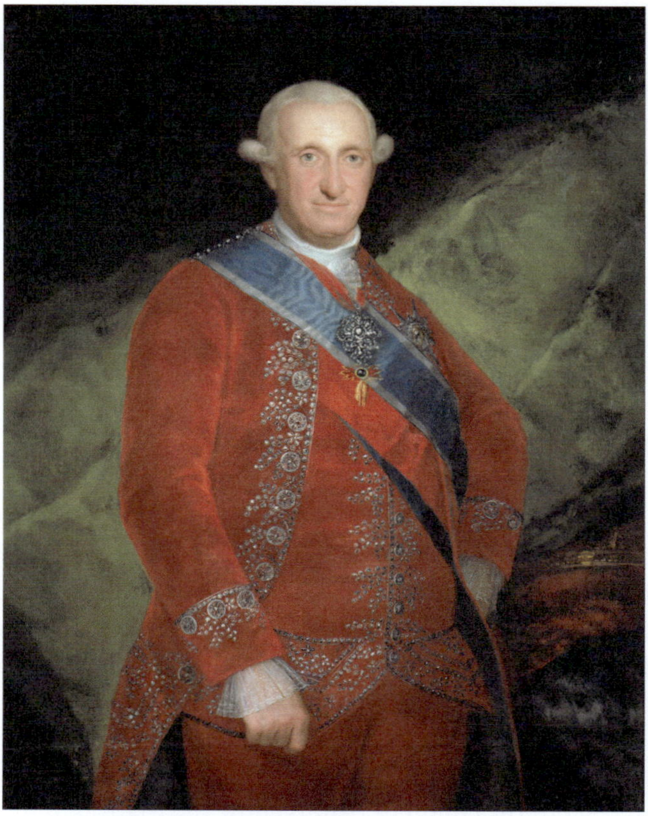

Fig. 6.3 Carlos IV. Francisco de Goya (1746–1828). Prado Museum, Madrid

stop the epidemic in the territory of New Granada (currently Panamá, Colombia, Venezuela, and Ecuador), in order to prevent it from spreading to the rest of America (Fig. 6.3). The Council of the Indias proposed an expedition as a way to spread the vaccine to overseas territories. The speed of the state bureaucracy was unusual. Only eight months elapsed from the time of the proposal on March 28,1803, until it began on November 30,1803 [7]. The doctor Francisco Javier Balmis presented the project "*Derrotero que debe seguirse para la propagación de la vacuna en los dominios de Su Majestad en América*" (*The route to be followed for the propagation of the vaccine in his Majesty's Dominions in America*), which was approved by the Board of Chamber Surgeons, formed by Antonio de Gimbernat, Leonardo Galli and Ignacio Lacaba and, consequently, he received the appointment of director of the "Royal Maritime Vaccine Expedition" [8].

Once the expedition had been decided, the problem lay in the financing and also in the legislation that would allow the project to be carried out. The Royal Treasury was responsible for all navigation and transport costs, but once the expedition reached American territory, it became dependent on the overseas authorities, who should finance the expedition's expenses with taxes collected from local production and church tithes.

Furthermore, the expedition's director demanded and obtained special legislation from the Crown to standardize all the Royal Expedition's actions. The legislation established rules of conduct for each members and the group that, in theory, should guarantee success. The responsibilities of each of the expedition members were clearly defined. Each member had specific functions, obligations, and responsibilities, so as to avoid overlapping efforts or leaving gaps [2, 8].

Components of the Expedition

They were as follows: Francisco Javier Balmis y Berenguer appointed as Director; the Catalan surgeon José Salvany y Lleopart was the second Director; two assistant surgeons accompanied them — Manuel Julián García Grajales and Antonio Gutiérrez Robredo, the latter being nominated by the expedition's Director; two medical practitioners — Francisco Pastor Balmis, the Director's nephew, and Rafael Lozano Pérez, who was selected due to his certification as a qualified surgeon; and three nurses — Basilio Bolaño, Pedro Ortega, and Antonio Pastor.

As the caretaker of the children, Balmis chose the Matron of the Foundling Home of La Coruña, Isabel Zendal y Gómez. Serving as carriers of health were a group of children, who played a vital role in transporting alive the vaccine across the globe, ensuring that the prophylactic chain — passed from arm to arm — remained unbroken.

The expedition achieved a remarkable technical feat: maintaining the vaccine in an active state throughout transoceanic voyages. This required that human recipients had neither previously suffered from smallpox nor been vaccinated, to avoid compromising the immunological process — thus making children the ideal candidates.However, only an active infection could be effective transferred to successive patients, as an human chain, so two children were vaccinated with cowpox at the beginning of the voyage, with two more infected at a intervals of nine to ten days, via arm-to-arm inoculation, and so on as it progressed across the Atlantic and beyond.

It took 22 orphaned children, from three to nine years old, (six from Madrid, 11 from Hospital de la Caridad de La Coruña and five from Santiago), to bring the vaccine through the Atlantic and other group of 26 Mexican children were required to cross the Pacific. On both journeys, the children were under the care of Isabel Zendal, who acted as nurse, overseeing the vaccination chain throughout the arduous transoceanic conditions. In this Philanthropic Expedition, the use of children was deemed a necessity, as there existed no other viable method of conveying the vaccine without it losing its properties during transit [7, 9, 10].

Criticism of this use of orphaned children (not slaves) for this philanthropic purpose can of course be analyzed and criticized, but it is well known that the situation was well considered and studied and that it was the only solution to save millions of lives, as was finally achieved with the life mission of all the components of the expedition.The rules of the expedition clearly indicated the care the children were to receive:

They shall be well cared for, maintained and educated until they have an occupation or a destiny to live with.

Previous projects and attempts to transport the vaccine alive had ended in failure. Initially, efforts were made to transport infected animals; however, the length of the journey and the extensive supply of fodder required rendered this impractical and expensive. Later, attempts were made to carry fluid extracted from the animals, in glass jars, lacquered, and wrapped in black cloth to protect it from air and sunlight. Nonetheless, the lengthy voyage — nearly two months — and the high temperatures of the Caribbean ultimately would cause the failure of this method [10].

Francisco Javier Balmis y Berenguer (1753–1819)

Born in Alicante, son and grandson of surgeons, he was appointed as expedition leader. He was a military surgeon, who has gained increasing recognition for his medical skills. In the early 1770s, he began his medical studies in the Royal Hospital in Alicante, working as a surgeon's assistant. In 1778, he obtained the degree of surgeon, working years later in La Habana and Mexico City as chief surgeon in the Hospital de San Juan de Dios (Fig. 6.4).

He had spent several years in the Americas, where he studied how natural remedies could be used to treat sexually transmitted diseases. This research led to the publication of a work titled "*Demonstration of the Effective, Newly Discovered Virtues in the Roots of Plants from New Spain*", which focused on agave and begonia species used to treat venereal and scrofulous conditions (Madrid, 1794).

After returning to Spain, he became a member of the Royal Academy of Medicine in Madrid and was appointed as royal court surgeon in 1795. When Edward Jenner introduced his smallpox vaccine, Balmis quickly became one of his earliest supporters. He translated to Spanish a French book on the topic, "Traité historique et pratique de la vaccine": "*Historical and Practical Treatise on the Vaccine*" (Madrid, 1803) by Jacques Louis Moreau de la Sarthe (1771–1826), and added an introduction based on his own experience and knowledge. This translation became a key guide for vaccination practices (Fig. 6.5).

For the expedition, Balmis included 2000 copies of this book to be distributed across the various Vaccine Boards that were being set up throughout Hispanic America. His legacy is closely tied to this ambitious and humanitarian effort, which was widely praised by people from different countries and

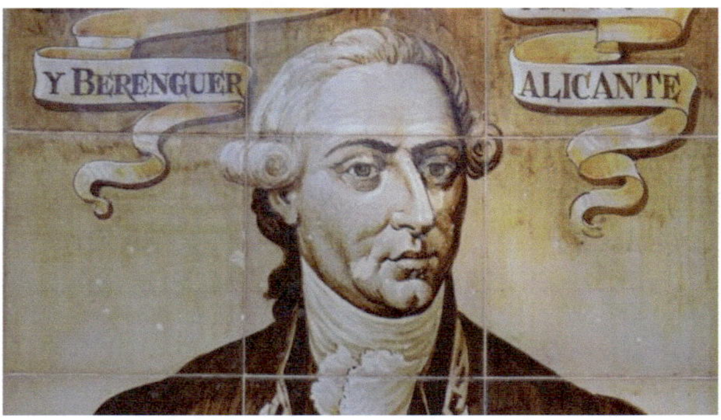

Fig. 6.4 Francisco Javier Balmis Berenguer

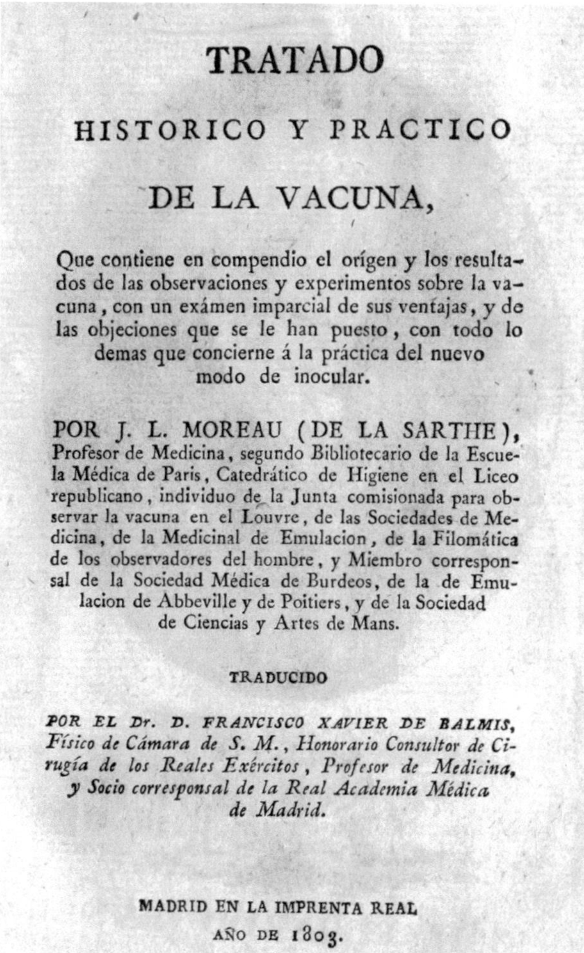

TRATADO

HISTORICO Y PRACTICO

DE LA VACUNA,

Que contiene en compendio el orígen y los resultados de las observaciones y experimentos sobre la vacuna, con un exámen imparcial de sus ventajas, y de las objeciones que se le han puesto, con todo lo demas que concierne á la práctica del nuevo modo de inocular.

POR J. L. MOREAU (DE LA SARTHE), Profesor de Medicina, segundo Bibliotecario de la Escuela Médica de Paris, Catedrático de Higiene en el Liceo republicano, individuo de la Junta comisionada para observar la vacuna en el Louvre, de las Sociedades de Medicina, de la Medicinal de Emulacion, de la Filomática de los observadores del hombre, y Miembro corresponsal de la Sociedad Médica de Burdeos, de la de Emulacion de Abbeville y de Poitiers, y de la Sociedad de Ciencias y Artes de Mans.

TRADUCIDO

POR EL Dr. D. FRANCISCO XAVIER DE BALMIS, Físico de Cámara de S. M., Honorario Consultor de Cirugía de los Reales Exércitos, Profesor de Medicina, y Socio corresponsal de la Real Academia Médica de Madrid.

MADRID EN LA IMPRENTA REAL
AÑO DE 1803.

Fig. 6.5 Cover of the translation into Spanish of the book: "*Tratado histórico y práctico de la vacuna*" (Madrid, 1803), from Jacques Louis Moreau de la Sarthe

backgrounds as one of the early milestones in the history of modern preventive medicine [11].

José Salvany Lleopart (1778–1810), born in Barcelona, entered the Royal School of Surgery in Barcelona in October 1791. He trained there until 1797, when he joined the army. He later pursued academic studies at one of the most prestigious universities in the Americas, the University of San Marcos in Lima, where, under the guidance of Hipólito Unanue, he obtained a doctorate in Medicine. He died in Cochabamba on July 21, 1810 [12] (Fig. 6.6).

Manuel Julián García Grajales Gil de la Serna (1775–1855), was born in Sonseca (Toledo), studied surgery for four years at the School of Surgery of

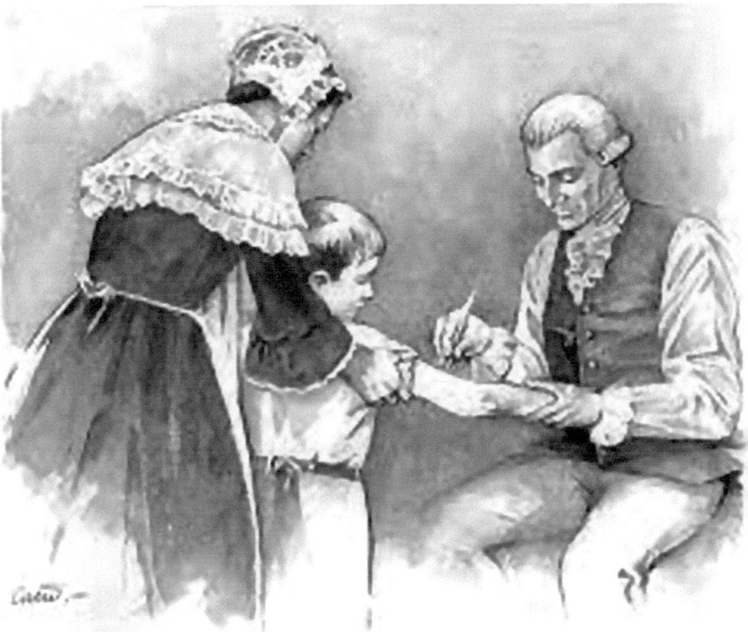

Fig. 6.6 J. Salvany vaccinating a child with the help of I. Zendal

San Carlos in Madrid., receiving later a bachelor's degree in medicine in 1802 from the Literary University of Toledo. Recruited by Balmis, under Salvany's command, he helped spread the vaccine along the Pacific coast up to the Captaincy General of Chile. In December 1824—shortly before the independence of Perú in Ayacucho—he returned to Spain [13].

Antonio Gutiérrez Robredo (1773–after 1833), originally from Madrid, also studied at the Royal School of Surgery of San Carlos. After serving in the army, he settled in Madrid, where he became familiar with the new practice of vaccination. It was at this time that he met Balmis, who invited him to join the expedition, remaining closely connected to him, serving as his spokesman during regional expeditions across New Spain (current Mexico). After completing his mission, he returned to Mexico where he began a career in private medical practice. After Mexico's independence and the expulsion order against Spaniards on December 20, 1827, Gutiérrez Robredo was not expelled and was reaffirmed in his teaching position. He continued as a full professor at the School of Surgery in Mexico until his retirement in 1833 [14].

One of the most notable members of the expedition was **Isabel Zendal Gómez (1773–early 19th century),** born in the town of Ordes (La Coruña).

A nurse by profession, she took care of the children who carried the smallpox vaccine, playing a vital role in the mission. Her work has been recognized by the World Health Organization, which considers her the first nurse to participate in an international humanitarian mission [15].

Precursors of Vaccination in America

S. Clavijo in his study in 1941, have asserted that any account of the history of the introduction and dissemination of the vaccine in Spanish America must acknowledge "two types of actions of equal significance, although differing in the chronological order of their implementation." The well-known expedition led by Balmis and Salvany, he argued, ought to be preceded in time by the efforts of various Spanish doctors, mostly naval surgeons, working in America, to introduce as early as possible the vaccine in the population [16].Recent studies have confirmed this perspective, emphasizing that the initial diffusion of the vaccine was driven by the personal and professional initiative of several surgeons attached to the Royal Navy and, consequently, connected to the Royal School of Surgery in Cádiz [17]. Prior to Balmis's arrival, the vaccinal fluid had already been introduced by Ángel Hidalgo in Cartagena de Indias and Santa Marta; by Alonso Ruiz y Moreno in Venezuela; by Bernardo de Cózar y Delgado in Cuba; by Miguel José Monzón y Farnel in Guatemala; by Anacleto Rodríguez Arguelles and Alejandro García Arboleya in Mexico; by Pedro Belomo y Cevallos in Peru; by Cristóbal Martín de Montúfar in the Río de la Plata; and by José María Gómez in the Chilean region of Coquimbo. However, these introductions of the vaccine did not have the necessary organizational character, which was essential to vaccinate the vast majority of the population.

Organization of the Spanish America and Asia

Spanish America was divided in four Viceroyalties: New Spain (Mexico, Central America, and territories north of the Rio Grande such as New Mexico, California, Texas and Florida; Caribbean territories, Filipinas and Pacific, capital Mexico City), New Granada (Venezuela, Colombia, Panama and Ecuador, capital Santa Fe de Bogota), Peru (Peru, capital Lima), and Rio de La Plata (Argentina, Bolivia, Paraguay and Chili, capital Buenos Aires). Within them were the general captaincies such as Santo Domingo, Guatemala, Yucatan, Puerto Rico, Cuba, Venezuela, and Filipinas.

Start of the Expedition

The expedition started from Madrid on September 7, 1803.

In La Coruña everything was prepared: the contract of the ship, the corvette Maria Pita, the staff, the materials and the children who were to carry the live vaccine. In addition, all routes and maps of America and Philippines, and contacts with the local authorities were reviewed.The expedition left the port of La Coruña on November 30,1803, aboard the corvette María Pita (Fig. 6.7). The expedition first landed on December 9 in the port of Santa Cruz de Tenerife, with the support of authorities the vaccine spread throughout the islands, where an intensive vaccination program began immediately. Hundreds of children were vaccinated along with many children from other islands of the archipelago who came to Tenerife to be vaccinated. On January 6, 1804, after completing the first phase of the mission, they departed from the Canary Islands to Puerto Rico, arriving on February 9, 1804. However, to the surprise of Balmis, the vaccine had already been introduced there by Francisco Oller Ferrer, a former student of the Royal School of Surgery in Barcelona and practicing physician on the island, who had imported the vaccine from the Danish island of Saint Thomas. This hindered the ability to locate children with the necessary immunological profile to continue the successive transmissions of the vaccine [18].The expedition reached Venezuelan soil on March 20, 1804, making Venezuela the first country it visited on the mainland. Although the original destination of the expedition was the port of La Guaira, the expedition arrived at Puerto Cabello (about 150 kilometers west of Caracas), where it was not expected. Despite this, Balmis and his expedition were well received, and some thirty children were immediately vaccinated. Balmis then decided to go to Caracas, dividing the expedition into three parts.

The first group, commanded by Balmis, left by land, is known to have passed through Maracay arriving in Caracas on March 28, 1804. The second group, commanded by Manuel Julián Grajales, travelled by sea on the coastguard ship "Rambli". It arrived in La Guaira where a large number of vaccinations were carried out, arriving in Caracas on March 31. The second man of the expedition José Salvany left Puerto Cabello for La Guaira, arriving in Caracas on April 5, which is when all the members of the expedition were reunited.

Balmis and his expedition were very well received in Caracas. From there the vaccine was sent to the rest of the country: Coro, P. Cabello, Ortiz, Santa Maria de Iripe, Tocuyo, Maracaibo, Cumaná, and Isla Margarita where the population was vaccinated.

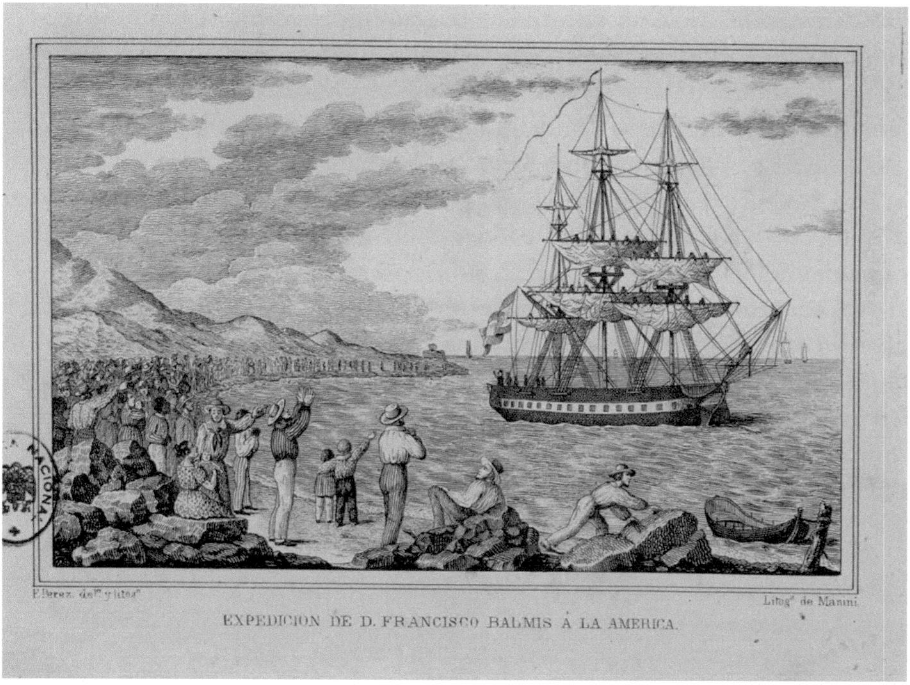

Fig. 6.7 The Corvette María Pita, leaving the port of La Coruña. Engraving of Francisco Pérez

On the other hand, a Junta Central de la Vacuna (Vaccine Board) was created in Venezuela, with the support of José Domingo Díaz and Vicente Salias, which was the first to be established in the Americas. whose regulations served as a model for other territories [19].

The Expedition Was Divided into Two Routes

Balmis Towards Northern America and Salvany to South America

Following the success of the vaccination campaign in Venezuela, Balmis sailed to New Granada (currently Colombia, Panamá, Ecuador and Venezuela), the only region that had recently suffered an outbreak of smallpox, and its viceroy had asked the king Carlos IV for the vaccination expedition.

However, in the face of the 1802 outbreak, the authorities in New Granada had already taken some initiative in a vaccination programme through Lorenzo Verges, a physician who had taken the initiative to implement public health measures to deal with the smallpox epidemic by administering vaccines. When Balmis arrived in New Granada, the response was similar to what he found in Puerto Rico. In the opinion of the authorities, the smallpox problem had already been solved and, little support was given to Balmis' expedition.

This led to a confrontation between Balmis and Verges, who criticized each other's methodological approach to vaccination. Verges died unexpectedly on 9 April 1804, which gave Balmis the opportunity to expand the vaccination campaign in this territory.

As the territory of New Granada was huge, Balmis realized that a single expedition could not cover the entire viceroyalty, therefore Balmis decided to divide the expedition into two groups. The division took place in March 1804, where Balmis assigned José Salvany the responsibility of taking the vaccine to southern America, while he would continue on to New Spain (Mexico), and then the Philippines and China (Fig. 6.8).

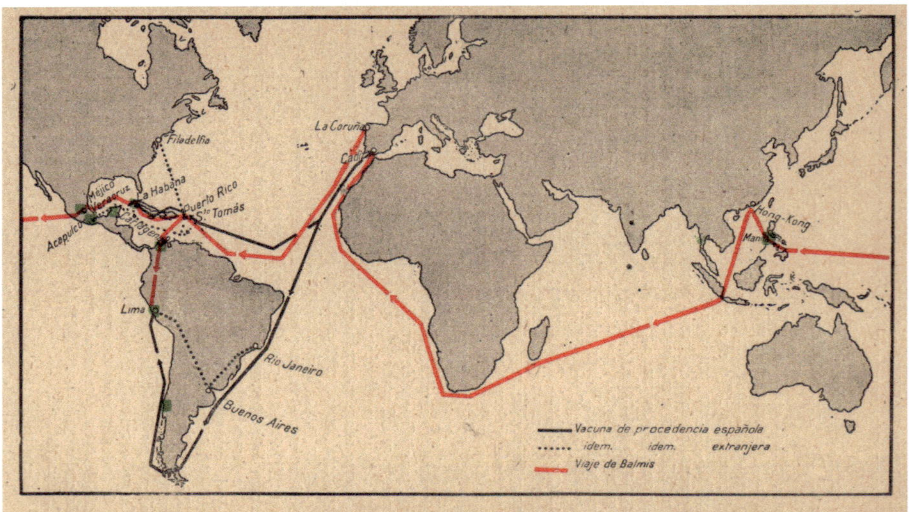

Zonas geográfico-marítimas, en las que los médicos de la Armada actuaron anticipadamente a la Expedición Española de la Vacuna a América (Expedición Balmis), logrando introducir y hacer prosperar el virus vacunal, por cuenta propia.

Fig. 6.8 Routes of the Balmis expedition through the Hispanic territories. From: S. Clavijo, Revista General de Marina. No. 1. Suplemento. 1941, p. 65

1. The expedition of Francisco J. Balmis (8/5/1804 to 4/9/1806)

The Balmis's group consisted of Balmis himself, Antonio Gutiérrez Robredo, Isabel Zendal, Francisco Pastor Balmis, and nurses Pedro Ortega and Antonio Pastor.

The expedition arrived in La Habana, Cuba on May 26 after a difficult voyage through the Caribbean that had affected the children's health. The physician Tomás Romay had started the vaccinations in Cuba with vaccine from Philadelphia. For this reason, the expedition decided to continue to Nueva España (current Mexico, Southeast of the USA and Caribean territories).

The expeditionary group landed at the port of Sisal, Yucatán, on June 25, and four days later they were in the city of Mérida. Three vaccination sessions were immediately held, attended by local surgeons to be instructed on the vaccination method. Several Vaccination Board were established from which the vaccine spread through the huge territory of the Viceroyalty.

The vaccine to Central America

Balmis commissioned Francisco Pastor to travel to the General Captaincy of Guatemala including Mérida, Villahermosa, Tabasco, Chiapas before joining him again in Mexico city. Furthermore, aware of the work that surgeon Monzón was doing in Campeche, Balmis appointed surgeon Antonio Gutiérrez to help that work. In fact, Gutiérrez used two young men vaccinated by Monzón to, in turn, vaccinate people in Isla del Carmen and Guatemala [20].

Balmis stayed short in Veracruz, because the program was good organized, returning to the city of Mexico on 9 August 1804.

From there, two groups were organized: the Balmis group and the group led by Gutierrez Robredo traveling different places of Celaya, Zacatecas, Durango, Guadalajara and Valladolid, establishing vaccine boards that were responsible for keeping the vaccine alive and the management of vaccination into the villages.

In the Spanish territories of New Mexico, Texas and California the expedition contributed to the spread of the vaccine and protection from the disease in the missions and indigenous communities. Although not known precisely, its impact was limited by distance and logistic challenges.The expedition arrived at the port of Acapulco on January 27, 1805, and set out on February 7, with the galleon Fernando de Magallanes (galleon of Manila, well organized maritime traject from 1565 to 1815), arriving in Manila in 15 mid-April. A Vaccine Board was again established in Manila as a center for disseminating the vaccine in the Philippine Islands.

First in Manila intramuros, extramuros, nearby provinces, further afield and the rest of the provinces in the archipelago.

In the Philippines, Balmis began to suffer from dysentery, and due to his fragile health, he decided not to return to the Americas after completing his stay in the Philippines. Instead, he opted to head east to the Portuguese possession of Macau (16 September 1805), so he split the group again. Balmis took the vaccine to Macau and Canton factory in China, where he was extraordinarily received by the authorities and following the Portuguese route, along Africa, returned to Spain in 1806 after stopping to vaccinate the people of Saint Helena, island in the South Atlantic after getting permission from the British authorities. He disembarked in Lisbon, having circumnavigated the globe with the vaccine. Once in Madrid, he was received with full honors by the court of Carlos IV on September 7, 1806. The remaining members of his group, led by Antonio Gutiérrez Robredo, with Antonio Pastor and Pedro Ortega organized the vaccination of the islands of Misamis, Zamboanga, Cebu and Mindanao, before returning with their children to Mexico via Acapulco. Isabel Zendal and her son settled in Puebla, Mexico. All the children remained in New Spain.

2. The expedition of José Salvany (8/5/1804 to 21/7/1810)

The other group led by José Salvany, was formed by himself as director, the physician Manuel Julián Grajales, the assistant Rafael Lozano Pérez, the nurse Basilio Bolaños and four children. The Expedition headed to South America and chronologically spans from the separation of the Expedition, on May 8, 1804, to the day of Salvany's death, on July 21, 1810.

Salvany's group traveled a much more arduous route than Balmis's group; they faced the distances, the harsh terrain, and the harsh weather conditions of the Andes and the jungle, and Salvany soon began to suffer the ill health that would plague him for the remainder of the journey.

They were entrusted with transporting the vaccine throughout South America (present-day Colombia, Ecuador, Peru, Bolivia, Chile, and Argentina). From Venezuela, it crossed the Andes to New Granada (Colombia) and then descended to the Viceroyalty of Peru. It traveled through Ecuador, Peru, and Bolivia between 1804 and 1809, where Salvany died in Cochabamba (Bolivia) in 1810, but his team continued the vaccination campaign.

The difficulties began when his brig, from Cartagena de Indias ran aground at the mouth of the Magdalena River (May 1804). In Cartagena with the support of the authorities they had created the Vaccine Board and from there expand the vaccination, sending the vaccine between glass to Portobello in Panama and Buenos Aires by Riohacha. During their journey, and faced with local outbreaks of smallpox, the group frequently split up to visit cities, towns, and settlements, often with the assistance of local missionary friars. They vaccinated and taught the technique to doctors and laypeople on their way across the western side of the South American continent.

Following the river from Cartagena, this group split in two,

(a) Through the Magdalena river: Salvany and Bolaños (visiting the areas of Ocaña, Nares, and Honda)
(b) Through the valley of Cucutá: Grajales and Lozano, (along the cities of Ocaña, Pamplona, Socorro y Vélez.

Both groups reunited in Bogotá in December, with support of the authorities and the church they vaccinated as much people as possible trying to reach every village or settlement. The established Vaccine Boards took care for the prevention of smallpox and other epidemics like the produce by yellow fever in New Granada.

In March 1805, they began their journey south through the Andes, to the Viceroyalty of Peru. Again, the group had to split to encompass more territory:

(a) Grajales and Bolaños crossed the sierras of Quindio through Naiva and La Plata, and,
(b) Salvany and Lozano, along the cities of Ibagué, Cartago, Trujillo, Llano Grande, Choco y Real Minas de Quilichas in the valley of Cauca.

Both groups reunited again in May of 1805 in Popayan, southeast of Bogotá.

From there, again two groups were organized:

(a) Salvany and Lozano, through the sierras, reaching Pasto, Tulcan, Ybarra, Otalvo, Cayambe, and Quito, affected by smallpox epidemic, and
(b) Grajales and Bolaños, along the coast reaching Tumaco, Esmeraldas, La Tola, Jipijapa and Guayaquil.

One group visited also Ambato, Riobamba and Cuenca in October 1805, whereas the other group visited Cumbe, Nabón, Oña, Loja, Piura and Lambayaque, arriving in December 1805, the latter city refusing the vaccine.

Then the whole group visited the coast and the interior, passing through Reque, Chepén, Chota and Cajamarca to Trujillo. After separating the group, they arrived in Lima in May 1806, with a new group of children to carry the vaccines.

In Lima both groups reunited finding that the vaccine had been delivered in small quantities to Lima from samples sent by overland mail from Buenos Aires, and that it was sold by traders (earning large sums of money from the fees they charged for vaccinations) and not administered philanthropically by medical staff. Therefore, they gave the vaccine to the doctors for mass vaccination, making a vaccination regulation for the whole viceroyalty. Salvany organized multiple campaigns, rest and study visiting some classes and conferences in the University de San Marcos. He created the position of vaccine inspector responsible for visiting every three years the vaccinations boards of the Viceroyalty of Peru.

In September 1807, Salvany travelled to Cuzco, Ica, Nazca, being forced to stop in Puno, on the shores of the Lake Titicaca, to recover from a heart problem, continuing afterwards to Arequipa where he arrived ill on December 8, 1807. Continuing his trip to Buenos Aires, in his last report (La Paz, April 1, 1809) he wrote that they was spreading the vaccination in the Viceroyalty of Rio de La Plata and indicating that nearly 200,000 vaccines had been administered in Peru. His more than 4000-kilometer journey ended in Cochabamba, present-day Bolivia, where he died in July 1810.

Vaccinations continued and the military doctor Santiago Granado was commissioned to administer the vaccines to the indigenous Jesuitic missions of Mojos, Chiquitos, currently in the east of Bolivia and Paraguay, who were suffering from epidemics.

The group of Grajales and Bolaños took the vaccine from Lima to the Captaincy General of Chili, arriving in Valparaíso in December 1807. Four years later, they sailed from southern Chile to the Peruvian port of El Callao, concluding the South American expedition in January 1812, returning finally to Spain [21, 22].

Final Considerations

Finally, in order to verify the status of the vaccine in New Spain and dictate the appropriate measures to perpetuate it, Balmis was commissioned by the Supreme Governing Board, on behalf of King Fernando VII, in 1809 to travel to Mexico. Upon landing in Veracruz in June 1810, he realized that the Vaccination Boards had not performed the work he had hoped and, as a result, the fluid had run out in several places. He reformed the regulations he had left in 1805 and in October 1810, he created a new one, leaving this task in the hands of the provincial intendants or governors and two physicians in charge of preserving the fluid and performing the vaccinations [21]. By then, the independence movement was underway in Mexico, and Balmis, always loyal to the Bourbon dynasty, pledged allegiance to the crown. In this endeavor, Balmis participated as a surgeon in the military campaigns against the Mexican rebels, in the Battles of Valladolid, and of Jalapa., returning in 1812 to Spain. He was appointed to medical positions and remained a respected physician. He died in Madrid on February 2, 1819.

The Royal Spanish Philanthropic Vaccine Expedition demonstrated the first attempts to resolve issues that remain essential to the introduction of universal vaccination campaigns: a strong and powerful world organization, with universal support of adequate research and technology transfer; public health professionalization of public health, evaluation of vaccine efficacy, and the safety and cost of vaccines. Worldwide vaccination should always be philanthropic [22]. "It is estimated that the Balmis Expedition directly vaccinated more than 500,000 people. It is also believed that the vaccination carried out by the Health Boards and public vaccination houses helped save millions more lives."

There has been much criticism in recent times about the expedition, especially for using children who were by no means slaves.

Neither Balmis's Expedition nor Jenner's work would be approved by current ethical standards of research. At no point were slaves used as a means of transporting the vaccine. The final destination of the children was carefully monitored, receiving an adequate education, ensuring them a future life as free men. The Expedition was a colossal sanitary planning project with a tangible legacy in global health. In addition to introducing the smallpox vaccine to protect populations, it contributed to the professionalization of public health and began an era of technology transfer. Should we then assume that Jenner was wrong when he said of the Expedition: *"I cannot imagine that in the annals of history there is a more noble and comprehensive example of philanthropy than this"?* We chose to side with Jenner's view.

Moreover, Alexander von Humboldt:

> This voyage will remain the most memorable in the annals of history

And L. Enjuanes:

> That medical milestone, the first humanitarian mission in history and the first mass vaccination campaign, is still present in Spanish culture, giving its name both to army health operations and to new hospital centres and biotechnology companies.
>
> This expedition is not exclusively a medical contribution, but also brought with it routes of communication and knowledge [23, 24]

References

1. Betrán Moya JL. Historia de las epidemias en España y sus colonias (1348–1919). Madrid: La Esfera de los libros; 2006.
2. Enjuanes, L. Prologue. La expedición Balmis. La primera lucha global contra las pandemias. Madrid: GeoPlaneta. 2022. pp.7–10.
3. Jenner E. An investigation into the causes and effects of Variolae vaccine. 1798. Translated by Juan Manuel Igea. Madrid: Calatrava ediciones médicas ejemplares; 2011.
4. Rodríguez González A. Spanish scientific expeditions in the 20th century. Madrid: Editorial EDAF; 2023.
5. Ramírez Martín SM. A health adventure. In: AA VV, editor. La expedición Balmis. The first global fight against pandemics. Madrid: GeoPlaneta. 2022; pp. 13–38.
6. Ramírez Martín SM. The legacy of the Royal Philanthropic Vaccine Expedition (1803-1810): the vaccine boards. Asclepio. 2004;56:33–61.
7. Ramírez Martín SM. The child and the smallpox vaccine on its way to America: the Royal Philanthropic Vaccine Expedition (1803-1806). Rev Complut Hist Am. 2003;29:77–101.
8. López Piñero JM. La Medicina en la Historia. Madrid: La esfera de los libros; 2002.
9. Balaguer Periguel E, Ballester Añón R. In the name of the children: the Royal Philanthropic Vaccine Expedition (1803–1806). Madrid: Asociación Española de Pediatría-Wyeth; 2003.
10. Ramírez Martín SM. The child and the smallpox vaccine on its way to America: the Royal Philanthropic Vaccine Expedition (1803-1806). Rev Complut Hist Am. 2003;29:84.
11. Andrade GE. A great inspiration for today's vaccination efforts: biographical sketch of Francisco Xavier Balmis (1753-1819). J Med Biogr. 2023;31:183–8.
12. Beláustegui Fernández, A. José Salvany y otros médicos militares ejemplares. Inicio de una lucha contra el olvido. Madrid: Ministerio de Defensa. 2006; 19–48
13. Beláustegui Fernández, A. José Salvany y otros médicos militares ejemplares. Inicio de una lucha contra el olvido. Madrid: Ministerio de Defensa. 2006; 67–108.
14. Beláustegui Fernández, A. José Salvany y otros médicos militares ejemplares. Inicio de una lucha contra el olvido. Madrid: Ministerio de Defensa. 2006; 109–132.
15. Gómez Vicente MA. Isabel Zendal Gómez. First nurse in on an international mission. Ministerio de Economía, Industria y Competitividad e Instituto de la Mujer y para la Igualdad de Oportunidades. 2017; Mujeres emprendedoras entre los siglos XVI y XIX. 90–110. Madrid.
16. Clavijo S. The orientation of Health in the Navy. Exemplary past. Active present. Consistent future. In: La Sanidad de la Armada en la Historia y en la Guerra de Liberación de España. Supplement to the Revista General de Marina; 1941. p. 15–88.

17. Pérez Pérez A. La Armada y la vacuna en Ultramar. A forgotten history (1801-1804). Madrid: Ministerio de Defensa; 2021.
18. Rigau-Pérez JG. The introduction of the smallpox vaccine in Puerto Rico, 1803–1804. In: Ramirez S, Valenciano L, Nájera R, Enjuanes L, editors. The Royal Philanthropic Vaccine Expedition. Two hundred years of the fight against smallpox. Madrid: C.S.I.C.; 2004. p. 77–87.
19. Esparza J, Yépez Colmenares G. Smallpox colonial Venezuela: epidemics, variolization and vaccination. In: Ramirez S, Valenciano L, Nájera R, Enjuanes L, editors. La Real Expedición Filantrópica de la Vacuna. Two hundred years of the fight against smallpox. Madrid: C.S.I.C.; 2004. p. 89–118.
20. Ramirez Ortega V, Rodriguez Sala ML. The participation of Novo-Hispanic surgeons in vaccination operations before, during and after the "Real Expedición Filantrópica de la Vacuna". Rev Comp Hist Am. 2009;35:187–207.
21. Mark C, Rigau- Pérez JG. The world's first immunization campaign: the Spanish smallpox vaccine expedition, 1803-1813. Bull Hist Med. 2009;83:63–94.
22. Tuells J. Ramirez S. Balmis et Variola. Alicante: Generalitat Valenciana. Conselleria de Sanitat. 2003.
23. Consorcio para el Parque de las Ciencias, Granada, España. Bicentenario de la Real Expedición. Archivado 3/6/2020 en Wayback Machine.
24. Tuells J, Franco-Paredes C. Letter to the editor.Deconstructing Balmis: a distorted story of enslaved orphans. J Gaceta. 2022;37.

7

Manuel Garcia: The Inventor of the Laryngoscope and Pioneer of Voice Physiology

Antonio Martín Mateos

Manuel García (1805–1906) occupies an exceptional place in the history of both music and medicine, having achieved an unprecedented convergence between the two disciplines by integrating the art of singing with the scientific rigour of anatomical and physiological study of the voice and singing. His long and prolific life established him as a pioneer in both artistic and scientific fields, demonstrating that curiosity and ingenuity can transcend any disciplinary boundary (Fig. 7.1).

The year 1854 marked a fundamental milestone in his career with the invention of the laryngoscope, a device that would revolutionize both medicine and the teaching of singing. Ingenious yet simple in design, this instrument made it possible, for the first time, to observe the larynx and vocal cords in action, revealing a previously inaccessible universe. His invention not only transformed vocal pedagogy and medical diagnosis, but also established a groundbreaking link between art and science. Considering his legacy as a seminal figure in both domains [1, 2].

A. Martín Mateos (✉)
Specialist in Otorhinolaryngology. Puerta del Mar Hospital, Cádiz, Spain

Royal Academy of Medicine and Surgery of Cádiz, Cádiz, Spain

M. A. Cuesta, F. Mateo Vallejo (eds.), *Spain's Journey in Medicine*,
https://doi.org/10.1007/978-3-032-12221-6_7

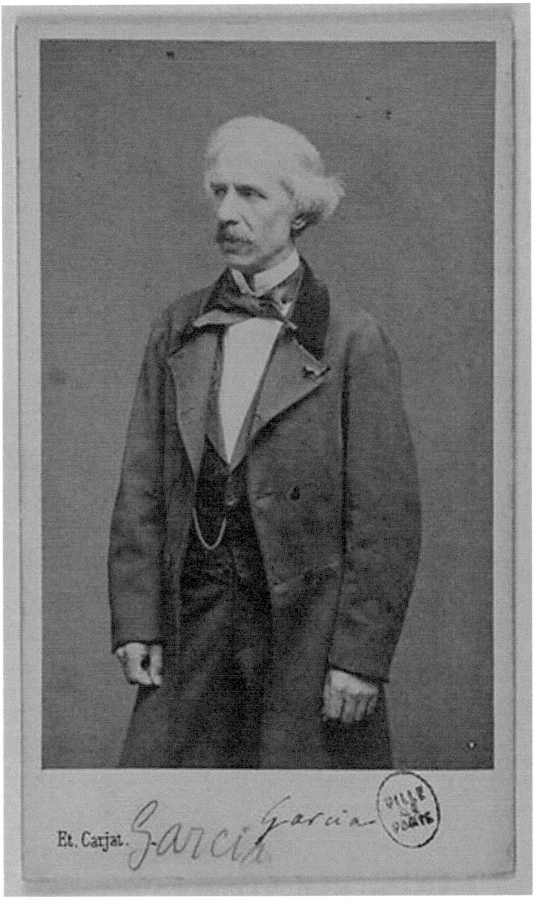

Fig. 7.1 Manuel García

Biography: Family History

Manuel Vicente Patricio Rodríguez Sitches, universally known as Manuel García, was born in 1805 in Madrid. He was the son of the renowned tenor Manuel del Pópulo Vicente García and the soprano Joaquina Sitches Briones.

His father, born in 1775 in Seville, was a famous maestro of the bel canto and favorite tenor of Gioachino Rossini, who left his mark on the most prestigious theatres in Europe. He excelled not only as a performer, but also as a composer, conductor, and impresario. His musical output was huge, but perhaps his most enduring legacy was his method of vocal instruction, structured with extraordinary rigour and precision (Fig. 7.2).

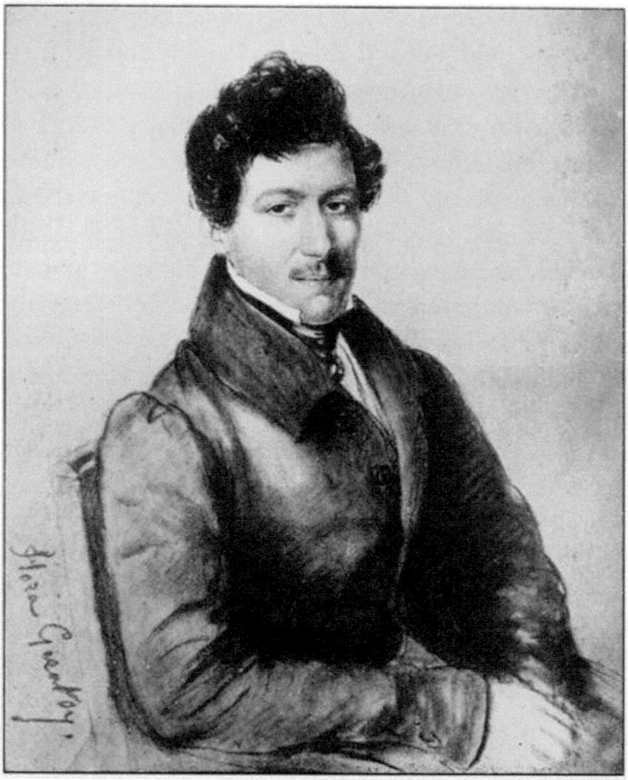

Fig. 7.2 Father of Manuel García: Manuel del Pópulo Vicente García

He married Joaquina Sitches, having three children from the marriage: Manuel Patricio (our character), María Felicia, and Pauline.

Joaquina Sitches, known in the artistic world as "La Briones", shone for her talent as a soprano, which enabled her to share the stage with the leading figures of her time, thus consolidating the García dynasty as one of the most influential in the history of music and bel canto. Manuel and his sisters raised in that environment.

María Felicia (1808–1836), known as Maria Malibran after her marriage to the banker François Eugène Malibran, possessed an expressive voice and an unmistakable dramatic presence that made her one of the most important sopranos of her era. Her brilliant career, tragically cut short by her premature death at the age of 28, only added to her legend, making her an enduring performer in the history of opera.

Pauline (1821–1910), the youngest of the siblings, known as Pauline Viardot after her marriage to the writer Louis Viardot, was a multifaceted artist: contralto, pianist, composer, and pedagogue. Ivan Turgenev, the Russian writer had a love story with her and followed Pauline and her husband to Paris and the Viardots estate in Courtavenel.

Manuel García's education was as unique as his later contributions to both music and science. His upbringing did not follow the conventional patterns of the time, as it was deeply shaped by the constant travel required by his parents' careers—primarily to Paris, Milan, Naples, London, and New York.

Although his father encouraged him to train his voice and study with the finest teachers and composers of the period, Manuel García began to find these rigorous studies tedious. Despite his musical talent, he did not appear to have a natural inclination for the opera stage. From an early age, his mind was drawn more towards science than to the performing arts.

On 7 June 1825, her sister Maria Malibran had the opportunity to make her official debut at the King's Theatre in London, portraying the role of Rosina in *Il barbiere di Siviglia*. Maria achieved a triumphant success, which was witnessed by her brother. Manuel would always maintain that his sister was the most natural and precocious genius he had ever encountered (Fig. 7.3).

That same year, 1825, the García family set sail from the port of Liverpool bound for New York. During the García family's stay in New York, the young María Felicia adopted the name by which she would become famous: María Malibran. after her marriage to the banker François Eugène Malibran, which took place during those months in the United States [3]. However, the marriage soon proved to be deeply unhappy. The situation culminated in her husband's imprisonment due to financial difficulties, which prompted Maria's return to Paris alone in September 1827.

Meanwhile, in Mexico—the family's next city of residence—Manuel García began to suffer from a growing fear of losing his voice, a fear that manifested with increasing frequency during performances. The rigours of the stage, adverse weather conditions, and cumulative strain all seemed to conspire against the continuation of his singing career. On the advice of his father, he left his family at the end of the opera season and set off for Paris in the early autumn of 1827. At the beginning of 1829, Manuel García made a public appearance in Naples, which marked his last serious attempt to establish himself as an opera singer. The performance was a failure.

The next day, Manuel collected the reports in the press, all of which agreed on the same verdict: he was not cut out for the opera stage. He sent them to his father, accompanied by a letter in which he wrote: "*As you can see, I will never be able to become an opera artist. From now on, I will devote myself to the occupation I love and for which I believe I was born*". With these words, he definitively ended his singing career.

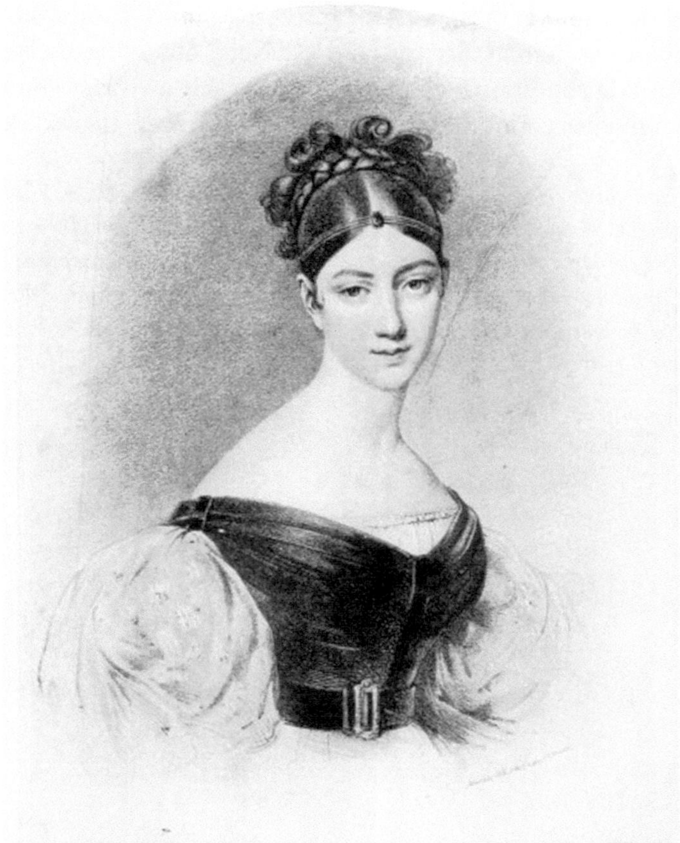

Fig. 7.3 Maria Malibrán

He himself attributed what he called the 'ruin' of his voice to the fact that he had continued his vocal training during adolescence, at the height of the pubertal transition, a critical period for the vocal cords. This practice, prolonged and poorly planned, would have compromised the full development of his vocal cords, as he would acknowledge years later.

Singing Teacher and Scientist

During the last months of 1830, Manuel García turned his attention to the study of the physiology and anatomy of the voice. By then he had already understood the importance of anatomical and physiological knowledge as an essential basis for the technical development of singing.

In order to explore these aspects further, Manuel conducted multiple experiments using animal larynxes and cadavers, observing their behaviour under controlled conditions. His sister, Pauline, left a vivid account of these experiments in an account full of wonder and tenderness (Fig. 7.4):

> *What do you think he brought? You'll never guess. The tracheas of all kinds of animals: chickens, sheep and cows. You'd think I would have been disgusted. But I wasn't. He gave me a pair of bellows, which I inserted into the windpipes, one after the other, and blew hard. My God, what extraordinary sounds they made! The windpipes of the hens clucked, those of the sheep bleated, and those of the bulls roared, almost as if they were alive.*

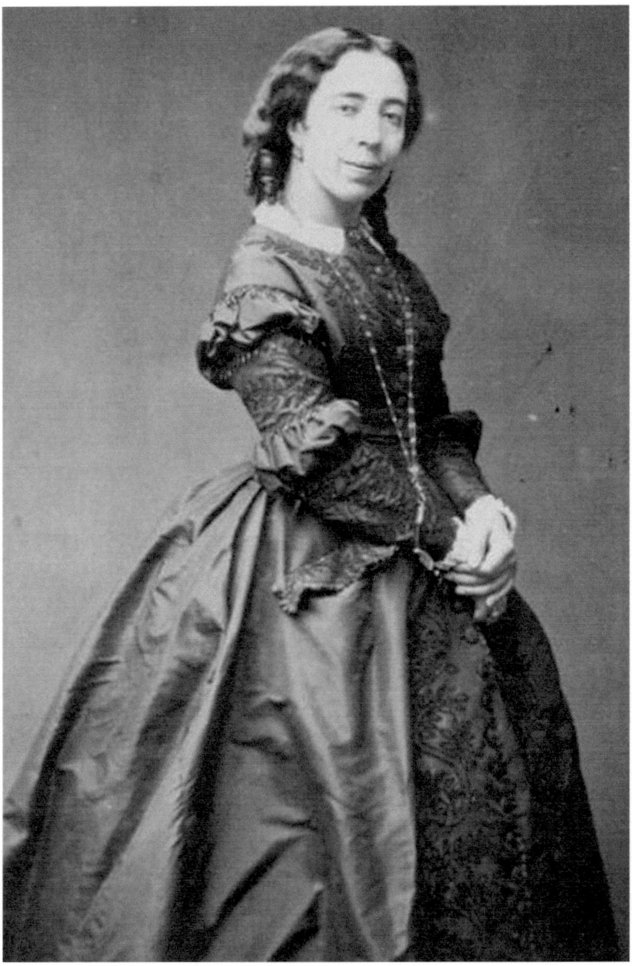

Fig. 7.4 Pauline Vardiot García

During this period, Manuel García began to develop his role as a vocal pedagogue, integrating his scientific knowledge into the teaching of singing in an innovative manner.

At the end of 1830, he joined his father in his work and immediately applied the knowledge he had acquired in the clinical and physiological fields. From that point onwards, he established a systematic practice that combined vocal evaluation with a preliminary medical assessment of each pupil. He regarded it as essential to carry out a functional examination of the voice, accompanied by an assessment of the larynx, and, if necessary, recommended specific advices or care to preserve the health of the vocal cords. This approach, clearly ahead of its time, reflects a holistic view of the vocal arts that anticipated modern principles of phoniatrics [4, 5].

Following the death of his father on 2 June 1832, at the age of fifty-seven, Manuel García became more independent in his pedagogical work and solidified his reputation as one of the most innovative singing teachers of his era.

Settled in Paris, he had access to a first-rate academic and cultural environment, with institutions such as the Paris Conservatoire and the Académie des Sciences nurturing his scientific interests. García aspired not only to teach the art of singing but also to prevent vocal damage—an ambition that clearly set him apart from most vocal pedagogues of his time.

He did not limit himself to imparting technical exercises but explained in detail to his students the anatomical and physiological functioning of the larynx, the mechanisms of phonation, breathing, and resonance, convinced that a rational understanding of these processes was essential for the healthy and effective development of the voice. This combination of art and science represented a significant innovation in nineteenth-century vocal pedagogy and laid the groundwork for future research in the field of phoniatrics.

His teaching proved so successful that, in 1835, he was appointed professor at the Paris Conservatoire—an important milestone in the institutional recognition of his method and the consolidation of his prestige as a master of singing.

That same year, he married Eugénie Mayer, a young pupil of his, who would go on to become one of the most acclaimed singers in Paris at the time. The marriage had four children. However, it came to an end in 1848, coinciding with a period of profound personal and professional transformation in Manuel García's life.

While the period from 1830 to 1836 had witnessed the stage triumphs of his elder sister and favorite pupil, Maria, the years that followed cemented the fame of his younger sister, Pauline Viardot, who had also been trained under his guidance. Following the death of Maria Malibran in 1836, the subsequent years of Manuel were marked by the steady rise of his prestige as a vocal teacher, accompanied by growing recognition in European musical and scientific circles.

Thanks to his intense research efforts, in 1840 he published his famous "*Mémoire sur la voix humaine*", presented to the Académie des Sciences in France. In this work, he compiled his discoveries on the anatomy and physiology of the voice, including fundamental aspects of the functioning of the larynx, vocal registers, and sound production.

This memoir represented one of the first systematic applications of scientific principles to the study of singing. It was examined by prominent members of the Academy such as François Magendie, Félix Savart, and Henri Dutrochet, who gave a favorable report during a public session held on April 12, 1841. The Academy expressed its appreciation to Professor García "for the skillful use he has made of his opportunities as a teacher of singing to arrive at a satisfactory physical theory of the human voice." [6].

That same year, 1840, García published the first part of his seminal treatise: "*École de García: Traité complet de l'art du chant*," the second part of which was published in 1847 under the full title: "*École de García. Traité complet de l'art du chant en deux parties*". This work marked a milestone in the history of vocal pedagogy, as it systematically laid out his belief that the art of singing should be grounded in a profound understanding of vocal physiology and a clear conception of how the voice is produced [7].

The year 1841 became an important year of Manuel García's teaching career, when among his pupils was the celebrated Swedish soprano Jenny Lind, universally known as "*the Swedish Nightingale*." The recovery of her voice—previously criticized and underestimated—thanks to García's technical guidance, was not only a clinical and artistic triumph, but also a powerful endorsement of his pedagogical method. In recognition of his outstanding contribution, he was later appointed a corresponding member of the University of Stockholm and, in 1847, was awarded the distinction of Knight of the Order of Merit of Gustav Vasa by King Oscar I of Sweden.

Between 1842 and 1848, the number of his students grew considerably, as numerous artists passed through his hands—artists whose successes stood as a testament to their master's method, teaching skill, considered as the foremost singing teacher of his time.

In 1848, the political upheavals that swept through Paris prompted Manuel García to relocate to London. His arrival in the British capital was met with enthusiasm, and he was soon regarded as the most distinguished vocal instructor in the city. His residence on George Street, in Hanover Square, became a renowned centre for vocal training, frequented not only by aspiring professional singers but also by members of the aristocracy and wealthy classes—a dynamic similar to that which had already characterized his time in Paris.

On November 10, 1848, shortly after his arrival, he was appointed professor at the Royal Academy of Music in London, an institution with which he would maintain a long and fruitful association. On July 5, 1869, he was appointed a member of the Academy's Management Committee, and in 1878 he assumed its directorship, thereby further consolidating its prestige.

It was precisely during his tenure as a teacher that Manuel García began to take an active interest in the possibility of observing the inner workings of the larynx, thinking about devising an effective method for visualizing the larynx during speech and singing.

This pursuit culminated in a landmark achievement for both medicine and vocal pedagogy: the invention of the laryngoscope. This instrument made it possible, for the first time in history, to observe the larynx and vocal cords during phonation, starting a new era in the functional study of the voice. Manuel García's contribution laid the foundation for the development of a new clinical discipline: laryngology.

Invention of the Laryngoscope and Its Clinical Impact

Despite the pioneering attempts of several clinicians to visualize the larynx using rudimentary optical devices, it was not until 1854 that Manuel Garcia—a singing teacher from outside the medical profession—could observe his own larynx during phonation.

Manuel was eager to see a healthy larynx in the very act of singing, feeling that his teaching remained confined to theoretical knowledge due to the impossibility of observing the larynx in action.

He devised a system that reflected the image of the larynx into his own eye using mirrors and sunlight. It consisted of two mirrors: a small one, placed inside the mouth, and a larger one, used to direct sunlight into the throat [8].

He recounted the story of his discovery in his own words:

Suddenly I saw the two mirrors of the laryngoscope in their respective positions as if they were actually present before my eyes. I went straight to Charriere, the maker of surgical instruments, and, on asking him if he happened to possess a small mirror with a long handle, he informed me that he had a small dentist's mirror which had been one of the failures of the London exhibition of 1851. I bought it for 6 francs. Having also obtained a hand mirror, I returned home at once, very impatient to begin my experiments.

On returning home, he placed the small mirror, previously heated in warm water and dried, against his uvula. Then, with the hand mirror, he projected a ray of sunlight onto the surface of the small mirror and immediately saw the larynx and vocal cords so wide open that he could see part of the trachea (Fig. 7.5).

Six months later, on March 22, 1855, his paper "*Observations on the Human Voice*", in which he set out his observations during phonation, was presented to the Royal Society of London. On May 24 it was commented by Professor Sharpey at a meeting of the Society held under the presidency of Lord Wrottesley and was published ("*Proceedings of the Royal Society; vol VII*). In his paper, Garcia documented his observations on the larynx and phonation. This work highlighted his ability to connect art and science, contributing to the understanding of vocal mechanisms. He described his method as follows:

It consists of placing a small mirror, fixed on a long handle suitably bent, in the throat of the person experimented on, against the soft palate and uvula. The person should turn towards the sun, so that the light rays falling on the small mirror are reflected on the larynx. If the observer experiments on himself, he should, by means of a second mirror, receive the rays of the sun and direct them to the mirror, which is placed against the uvula.

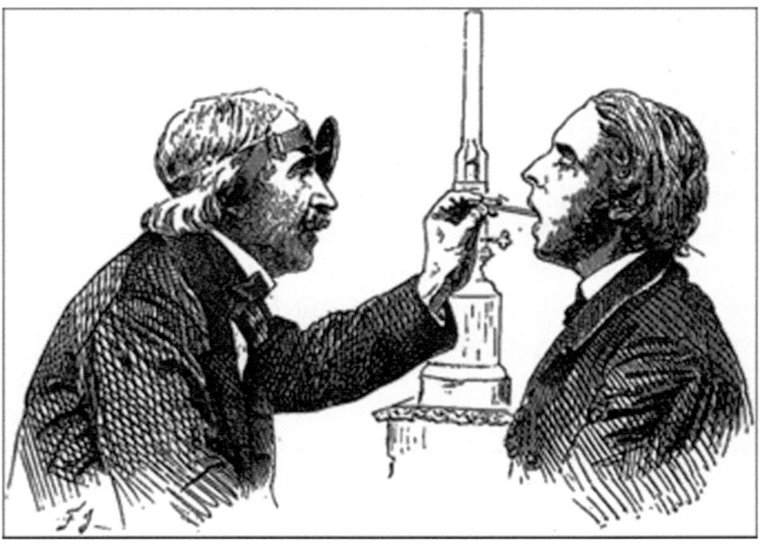

Fig. 7.5 Laringoscope of M. García

For García, the laryngoscope ceased to be useful once his initial investigations were completed. With the examination of the glottis (and the vocal cords), he had the satisfaction of proving that all his theories on voice production were absolutely correct. Beyond that, he saw little further value in it, except to satisfy the curiosity of those who wished to observe the forms and changes in the vocal cords when singing and speaking.

As for the subsequent use of the laryngoscope in other areas of research it was almost two years before any practical application was seen. The medical profession was slow to recognize the invaluable observational tool that the musician had provided, and initially, it was regarded by prominent figures as little more than a physiological novelty; indeed, as is often the case when someone outside the medical field makes a discovery, García's communication was initially met with indifference, if not disbelief, by physicians.

Until then, all observers had used sunlight reflected by a hand mirror, which imposed two major limitations: the dependence on natural light conditions and the need to occupy both hands during the laryngoscopic examination. Johann Nepomuk Czermak, based in Budapest, made significant improvements to the original design, incorporating a large, perforated concave mirror to reflect light from an artificial source. He also developed a system for supporting the mirror with an extension of the frame that was held in place by the teeth of the doctor. These innovations proved to be of paramount importance, as they both freed one hand of the examiner, enabling intralaryngeal manoeuvres, and eliminated the reliance on sunlight. For these reasons, Czermak can justifiably be regarded as the founder of the therapeutic laryngoscopy. Additionally, he was an outstanding disseminator of the technique, both through scientific publications, practical demonstrations, and the founding of the first laryngology schools.

In the issue of March 27,1858 of the *Wiener Medizinische Wochenschrift*, a publication by J. N. Czermak was dedicated to the use of the laryngeal mirror.

He wrote: "*Garcia's laryngoscope has given us access to a world we could only imagine before. His invention is a fundamental pillar in the study of the larynx*".

Later, with the invention of the electric light bulb, laryngoscopes began to incorporate electric lights, allowing them to be used in any environment, regardless of external lighting conditions. This innovation was a crucial step in making the laryngoscope a practical tool in the clinical setting. Subsequently, simple mirrors evolved to include more precise lenses that improved the clarity of reflected images. These advances allowed clinicians to observe the larynx in greater detail, resulting in more accurate diagnoses of larynx pathology and a better understanding of vocal physiology.

Thanks to the laryngoscope, physicians have transformed the diagnosis of numerous pathologies, like larynx cancer, it allowed the identification and treatment of tumors in early stages, it facilitated the detection and treatment of benign lesions, especially in voice professionals, it allowed the evaluation of vocal cord paralysis and inflammatory and infectious pathologies, and it facilitated the diagnosis and treatment of speech and voice disorders, such as dysphonia and aphonia, by allowing speech therapists to directly observe the functioning of the vocal cords.

Manuel Garcia's invention of the laryngoscope was a milestone that brought him international recognition. Despite not being a medical doctor, Garcia achieved remarkable recognition during his lifetime.

The improvements made by Johann Czermak generated controversy over who should receive primary credit for the invention of the laryngoscope. Although Czermak always acknowledged Garcia's priority, some medical historians suggested that the two should share the credit. Today, not without some controversy, Manuel Garcia is considered the actual inventor of the laryngoscope, Ludwig Turck the applicator of the laryngoscope to laryngeal pathology, and Johann N. Czermak who improved and simplified the instrument and popularized the procedure.

In 1865, the University of Königsberg recognized the magnitude of Manuel García's contribution by awarding him an honorary doctorate in Medicine. This honor was more than a simple gesture; it was an official recognition that him, although from the world of art, had left an indelible mark on the field of science. This recognition enhanced his reputation as an interdisciplinary innovator, connecting art and science.

Legacy in the Teaching of Singing

Manuel García revolutionized the pedagogy of the voice and singing by integrating anatomical and physiological studies with traditional vocal techniques, setting a standard that endures to this day. He emphasized that a singing teacher should understand both the artistic aspects and the scientific basis of the voice. His work "*Traité complet de l'art du chant*", which started an innovative pedagogical approach, can be considered his great legacy and a fundamental work in the history of vocal pedagogy [9] (Fig. 7.6).

The treatise includes a comprehensive description of the mechanisms of vocal production, such as respiration, phonation and resonance. García explains how the vocal cords, diaphragm, larynx and other organs are involved in the emission of sound. He also discusses concepts such as vocal registers, which were fundamental to his teaching method. He proposes a structured

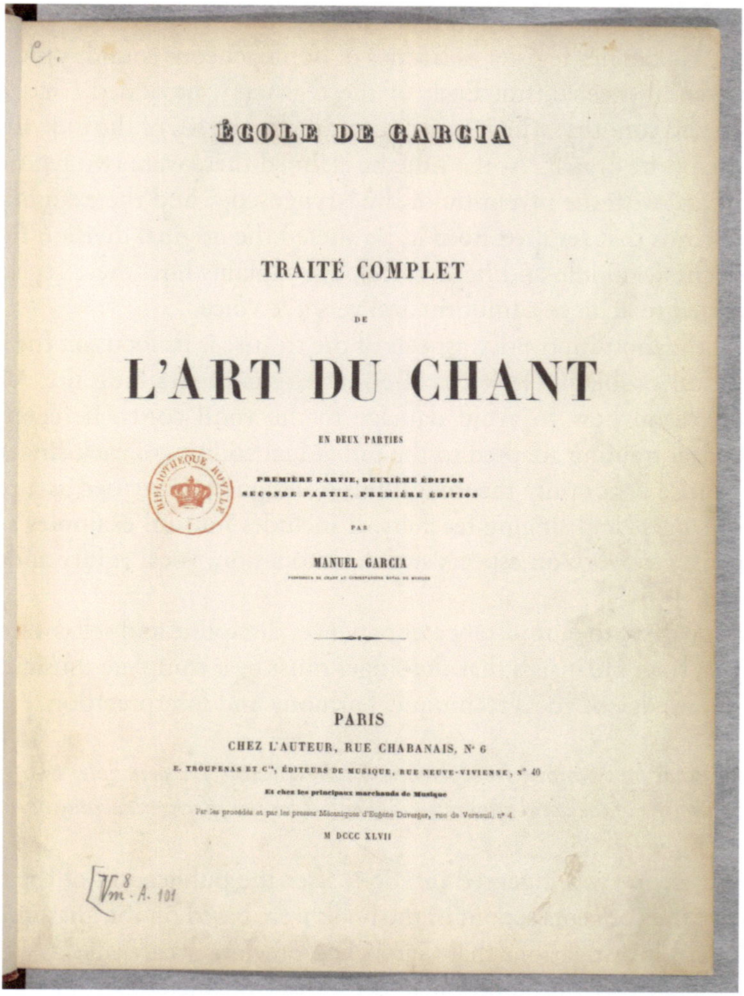

Fig. 7.6 Traité complet de l'art du chant. Manuel García. 1847

and progressive approach to learning to sing, based on technical exercises and specific practices. It includes a series of vocal exercises designed to develop technique, flexibility and stamina of the voice. These exercises are organized in such a way that the student progresses gradually, from the most basic to the most complex.

Breathing was considered by him to be the foundation of singing. He devotes an important part of the treatise to explaining how diaphragmatic breathing should be and how to control it in order to achieve an efficient vocal emission. He describes techniques to improve respiratory support and avoid vocal fatigue.

García clarified the confusion that existed until then between "timbre" and "register". He defines register as a series of homogeneous sounds produced by the same vocal mechanism. Each of the registers", he added, "has its own extension and sonority, which varies according to the sex of the individual and the nature of the organ". At the time he claimed there were two registers, but in later years, with the invention of the laryngoscope and the examination of the vocal cords that resulted from it, he altered the original division from two to three (chest, middle and head voice). He explains how these registers can be combined to achieve a uniform and versatile voice.

One of the most innovative aspects of the treatise is its focus on the prevention of vocal problems. It warns about the risks of straining the voice and offers advice on how to avoid damage to the vocal cords. It recommends gradual vocal training adapted to the individual abilities of each singer.

The treatise is not only theoretical but is designed to be used as a practical guide for singers and singing teachers. It includes musical examples and specific exercises to work on aspects such as intonation, vocal agility and artistic expression.

He emphasizes the importance of patience, discipline and self-awareness in learning to sing. He insists that the singer must be a complete musician, with a deep knowledge of vocal technique, harmony and interpretation.

Music cannot be separated from science. Understanding the principles that govern the functioning of the vocal apparatus is essential for the effective teaching of singing.

The laryngoscope was invented in 1854, after the publication of the treatise, so many of the concepts set out in the book were based on the anatomical and physiological investigations that Garcia had previously carried out.

The laryngoscope, in addition to its impact on medicine, revolutionized areas such as vocal pedagogy, speech therapy and acoustic research. Garcia, in his quest to understand the mechanisms of the voice, used his invention as a means to develop more accurate and effective teaching methods. This interdisciplinary approach made it possible to establish a connection between vocal anatomy and sound production, benefiting both music and science, transforming vocal teaching with a scientific approach.

In the field of vocal training, the device made it possible to study how vocal cords adapt to different vocal techniques, contributing to the improvement of educational programme for singers and speakers. Scientists specializing in acoustics found in the laryngoscope a key tool to analyze how the vocal cords produce sound and how it is modulated in the vocal tract. This breakthrough enriched the understanding of vocal physiology and its relationship to phonation.

Proof of his constant activity is the publication at the age of 89 of the book "*Hints on Singing*", which is a compilation of practical advice for singers. It is written in a more accessible and direct style, focusing on solving common problems and improving vocal technique. It includes reflections on breathing, vocal registers, expression and damage prevention. The book, written in English, was translated by his wife Beata Garcia, because, although he was fluent in English, he felt more confident in French. Manuel, in his seventy-fifth year, had previously married the young Beata in 1881, with whom he would have two daughters, Paula and Manuela, thus joining his previous offspring with Eugénie Mayer with four children: Maria, Eugénie, Gustave and Manuel.

On the occasion of his centenary, on 17 March 1905, he was the subject of an extraordinary tribute in London, during which he received many distinctions and tokens of recognition from leading personalities and institutions. Among the most important honors were the Royal Order of Alfonso XII, awarded by the King of Spain; the appointment as Honorary Commander of the Royal Victorian Order, awarded by the King of the United Kingdom; and the Grand Gold Medal for Science, awarded by the Emperor of Germany. He was also honored by various universities, scientific academies, professional societies, doctors, singing teachers, singers and former students, in a tribute that evidenced the magnitude and impact of his intellectual and artistic legacy. Manuel García died on 1 July 1906, and his remains were buried in the cemetery adjacent to St. Edward's Church, Sutton Place, near Woking, England.

Epilogue

We can consider Manuel García as an exceptional case of singer, singing teacher, scientist and researcher.

More than a medical instrument, Manuel García's laryngoscope is a symbol of interdisciplinary curiosity and human creativity. García not only solved practical problems in the teaching of singing, but also opened up new possibilities in medicine, demonstrating that art and science can converge in the pursuit of knowledge.

Garcia was noted for his ability to influence multiple disciplines. In the field of otorhinolaryngology, his laryngoscope became a fundamental tool for the diagnosis and treatment of laryngeal diseases. In speech therapy and phoniatrics, his focus on the prevention of vocal damage laid the foundations for the development of these disciplines. Finally, in music education, he revolutionized the teaching of singing, with developments in physiology setting standards that still persist today.

His life and work remind us that true innovation arises when curiosity and knowledge challenge established limits, he demonstrated that great innovations are born from the ability to look beyond conventional boundaries.

What makes his achievement all the more remarkable is that he had no formal medical training. His profound knowledge of anatomy and vocal physiology was the result of self-taught training, based on passionate reading, meticulous experiments and precise observations. The figure of Manuel García remains a testament to the power of human curiosity, hard work and a reminder that disciplinary barriers are only challenges to overcome.

References

1. The Garcia Centenary. Br Med J. 1905;66:681–9. Available at: http://www.jstor.org/stable/20284480
2. Mackinlay MS. *Garcia* the Centenarian and His Times. Edinburgh and. London: William Blackwood and Sons; 1908. Reprinted by Forgotten Books; 2012. Available at: https://www.gutenberg.org/files/37298/37298-h/37298-h.htm.
3. Moreno MA. Los García. A family for singing. Seville: Fundación Pública Andaluza Centro de Estudios Andaluces; 2018.
4. Díaz Marroquín L, Villoria MM. La práctica del canto según Manuel García. Madrid: Consejo Superior de Investigaciones Científicas; 2012.
5. Garcia MP. Observations on the human voice. Proc R Soc Lond. 1855;7:399–410. Available at:. https://doi.org/10.1098/rspl.1854.0094.
6. Garcia MP. Hints on singing, Garcia B, translator. London: E. Ascherberg; 1894. Available at: https://archive.org/details/hintsonsinging00garc/page/n1/mode/2up?view=theater.
7. Garcia MP. École de Garcia: traité complet de l'art du chant, en deux parties. 2nd ed. of part I, 1st ed. of part II. Paris: Troupenas; 1847. Available at: https://imslp.org/wiki/%C3%89cole_de_Garcia_(Garcia_Jr.,_Manuel).
8. Tilley H. The laryngoscope in medicine. Lancet. 1931;218:883–6. Available at:. https://doi.org/10.1016/S0140-6736(01)08870-5.
9. Radomski T. Manuel Garcia (1805–1906): a bicentenary reflection. Aust Voice. 2005;11:25–41. Available at: https://www.harmonicorde.com/Radomski%20Australian%20Voice.pdf

8

José Goyanes Capdevila: Performed the First Vascular Bypass in History on 12 June 1906, Published in "El Siglo Médico"

Miguel A. Cuesta and Manuel Doblas Dominguez

José Goyanes Capdevila was born in Monforte de Lemos (Lugo) on June 16, 1876, as the son of a judge Antonio Goyanes Meneses and Teresa Capdevila Martínez.

He studied at the secondary schools of Lugo and La Coruña, to enrolled at the Central University of Madrid, where he studied Medicine from 1893 to 1900. In 1901, he received his doctorate with cum laude for his thesis on thyroid surgery, entitled "*Influence of the Thyroid on Growth and Development During Childhood*".

He got the internship at the Hospital Clínico San Carlos de Madrid, working at the Departments of Clinical Medicine, with Prof. Manuel Alonso Sañudo, and Surgical Pathology, with Prof. Alejandro San Martín (Figs. 8.1 and 8.2). He also worked as assistant at the Anatomical Museum and, in 1902, as a resident of the Department of Surgery, continuing to work with his mentor San Martín, whose influence proved decisive in shaping his career.

M. A. Cuesta (✉)
Department of Surgery, Amsterdam University Medical Centre (UMC), Amsterdam, The Netherlands

M. D. Dominguez
Head of the Department of Vascular Surgery, Hospital of Toledo, Toledo, Spain

M. A. Cuesta, F. Mateo Vallejo (eds.), *Spain's Journey in Medicine*,
https://doi.org/10.1007/978-3-032-12221-6_8

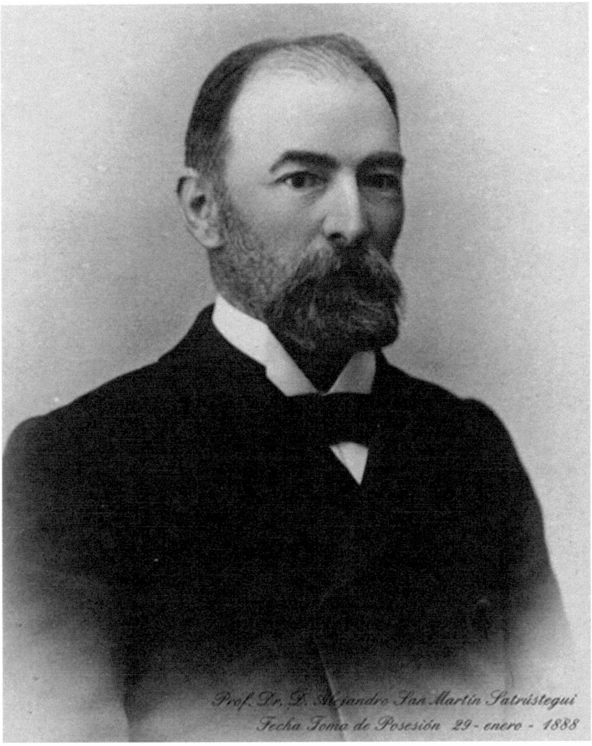
Prof. Dr. D. Alejandro San Martín Satrústegui
Fecha Toma de Posesión 29 - enero - 1888

Fig. 8.1 Alejandro San Martín y Satrústegui

In 1903, he married María Echegoyen, with whom he had six children, including José, a neurosurgeon, and Francisco, a vascular surgeon. In 1905, at 29 years of age, he was appointed Head of Surgery at the Hospital General de Madrid, a position he held for seven years (Fig. 8.3).

After the death of Eulogio Cervera, who managed a modest laboratory at the Rubio Institute, in Madrid, the Crown provided the necessary resources for the creation of the Prince of Asturias Institute, conceived as a healthcare facility dedicated to Oncology. Together with the Victoria Eugenia Pavilion, dedicated to research, these two institutions together formed the National Cancer Institute, which was inaugurated in 1922. Dr. Goyanes was appointed its first director, a position he held until 1935, when he was dismissed without notice, likely for political reasons. He was succeeded by the neurohistologist Pío del Río Hortega.

On July 18, 1936, while on holiday in San Rafael, in the province of Segovia, he was caught by the outbreak of the Civil War in the Nationalist zone. He spent the remainder of the conflict in Salamanca, caring for the war

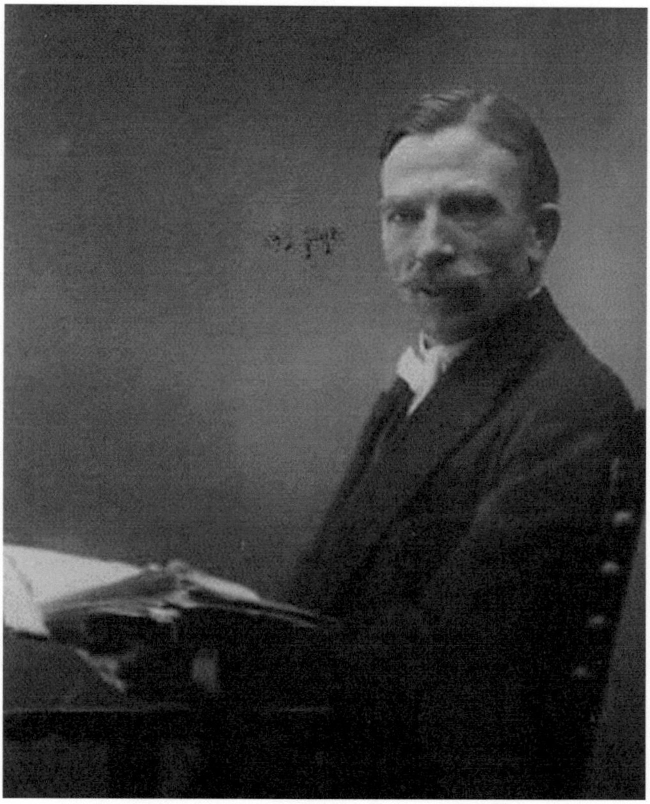

Fig. 8.2 José Goyanes Capdevila

wounded. After the war was over, he returned to Madrid, where he continued working as a surgeon until 1945, when he moved to Santa Cruz de Tenerife for family reasons. There, he devoted himself to writing medical and paramedical articles for *La Gaceta Médica Española.* He died in 1964, at the age of 88 [1–3].

José Goyanes was not only an innovative surgeon, an exceptional researcher, and a distinguished clinician, but also a great humanist, with profound knowledge of multiple languages, as well as Greek and Hebrew culture and medicine. As a medical historian, in addition to his works on Greek medicine, he conducted a historical review of Arab medical practices, including commentaries on the surgery of Abulcasis. He also explored in depth the life and thoughts of Michael Servetus, analyzed the psychosomatic types in *Don Quixote of the Mancha of M de Cervantes* and the criticism of doctors in the works of Quevedo, and critically examined J.W. Goethe's biological ideas, and

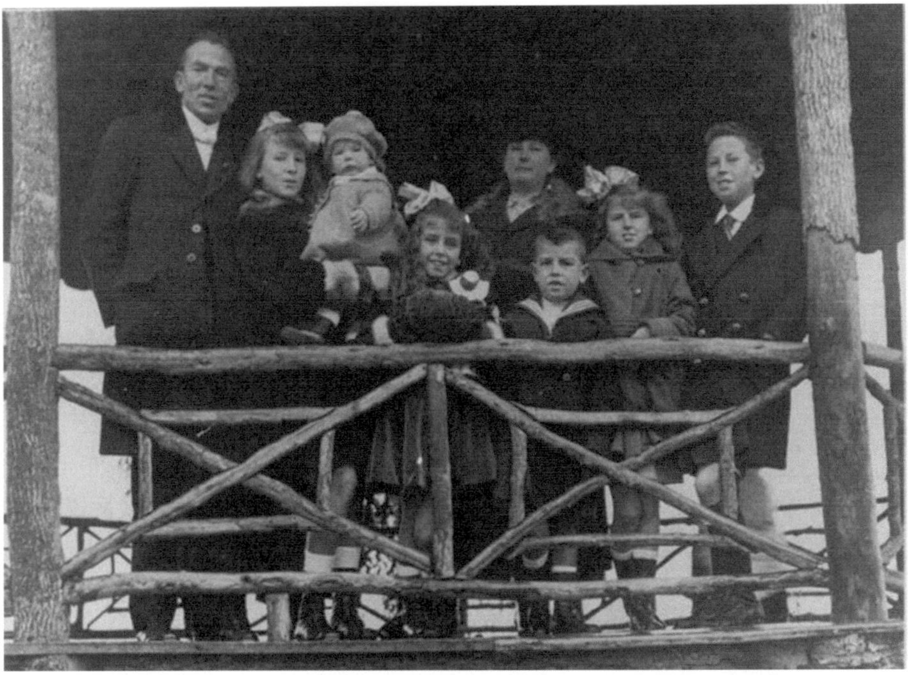

Fig. 8.3 The Goyanes's family in 1918

wrote biographical portraits of his mentors Alejandro San Martín, Santiago Ramón y Cajal, and Agustín del Cañizo [4, 5].

Throughout his career, Goyanes exchanged ideas and experiences with leading surgical figures of his time, such as E.F. Sauerbruch, the Mayo brothers (W.J. and Ch. H.), Rudolph Matas, and Alexis Carrel—the latter awarded the Nobel Prize in Medicine in 1912 for his advances in vascular techniques for organ transplantation. He also maintained close friendships with prominent intellectuals and cultural figures in Spain such as Miguel de Unamuno, José Ortega y Gasset, Gregorio Marañón, and Ramón Pérez de Ayala.

In recognition of his career, the book "*Homenaje a Goyanes*" was published by *La Gaceta Médica Española* between 1929 and 1930, featuring contributions from 87 leading national and international figures in science and culture [6, 7]. He was one of the founders of the Spanish Association of Surgeons in 1936 (Fig. 8.4).

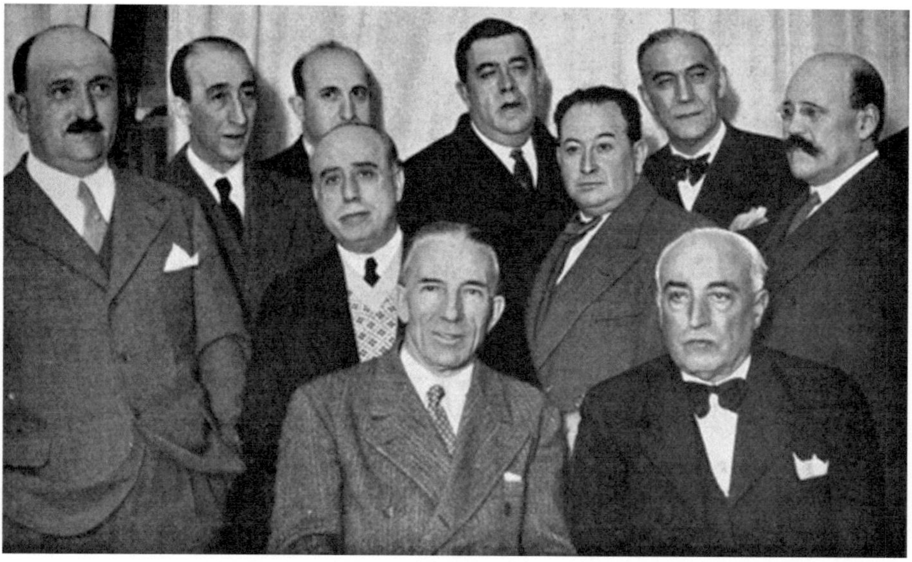

Fig. 8.4 Members of the First Board of the Spanish Association of Surgeons in 1936. J. Goyanes, the president below in the centre

The Surgeon

"*I was born and raised to be a doctor—or perhaps more precisely, a surgeon,*" José Goyanes once said of himself.

His mentor, Alejandro San Martín, played a fundamental role not only during his years as a resident at the Hospital but also along his early professional life. He collaborated closely with him, both personally and professionally, from 1904 through the 1930s at the Provincial Hospital of Madrid and the National Cancer Institute.

At these institutions, San Martín inculcated in him the fundamentals of surgical practice, awakened his interest in experimental research, and developed his ambition to innovate in the fields of vascular and oncological surgery.

During this period, Goyanes developed the three essential qualities of a surgeon: craftsmanship, scientific knowledge, and artistry. He was therefore described as "*a physician who also knows how to operate,*" and, following the teachings of Hippocrates, he upheld the principle that "*every surgeon is obliged to selflessly teach his science and art to students and physicians eager to learn.*"

Main Scientific Contributions

Status of Arterial Surgery

At the beginning of the twentieth century, vascular surgery was regarded as an almost prohibitive practice. Its origins date back to July 15, 1759, when the English surgeon Hallowell Lambert of Newcastle successfully sutured an injured humeral artery during a bloodletting procedure. However, throughout the eighteenth century and the first half of the nineteenth century, vascular surgery fell into obscurity, possibly due to the pessimism generated by the scientific communication of Conradus Assmann of Groningen in 1772–1773. In his experiments suturing femoral arteries in four dogs, Assmann observed that in three of the four re-explored cases, the artery had become completely obliterated, leading to widespread abandonment of such procedures. In the meanwhile some progress had been made in the management of venous injuries, B. Travers reported a lateral ligation of a femoral vein in 1816, and the experimental works to perform venous sutures and anastomosis.

Despite this, a few surgeons made sporadic attempts to treat stab wounds, though with limited success. This situation was reflected in the skeptical remark by Paul Broca in his treatise on the treatment of aneurysms: "*On revint à la ligature et il en était temps*" ("We returned to ligature, and it was high time"). However, by the end of the nineteenth century, this trend began to shift. A. San Martin responded to Broca with a new assertion: "*On revint à la suture et il en était temps*" ("We returned to suturing, and it was high time"), inspired by major advances that innovate surgery, such as Joseph Lister's introduction of antisepsis, and A. Jassinowsky's on arterial sutures experiments in his dissertation [8].

Attempts to deal with arterial aneurysm were marked by the endoaneurysmoorrhaphy technique by Rudolph Matas in New Orleans in 1888.

Rudolph Matas, named the Father of Vascular Surgery in U.S.A. was born on 12 September 1860 of Spanish emigrants parents (Narciso Matas and Teresa Jorda) from Catalonia to New Orleans [9].

In 1896, A. San Martín and J. Goyanes, studied different techniques of arterial suturing and arteriovenous anastomosis in dogs. Their contributions to vascular suturing were remarkably similar to those for which Alexis Carrel would later receive the Nobel Prize in Medicine—although San Martín and Goyanes's work predated Carrel's, It was published in scientific journals with limited audience.

Years later, Wieting published these techniques as if they were his own. In response, Spanish surgeons Guedea and Goyanes firmly asserted San Martín's undisputed priority in these pioneering techniques [10, 11].

At the end of the nineteenth century, prestigious surgeons once again attempted to repair injured arteries without resorting to ligation. San Martín identified several indications for arterial sutures:

> *Arterial sutures were born out of an excusable and even noble desire to conceal an operative slip; then they were applied to discontinuities anticipated by suspected tumoral adhesions; today they serve to correct accidental injuries to these vessels, and tomorrow, without doubt, they will be used to cure incipient traumatic aneurysms.*

Among the surgeons who implemented these ideas were the Spaniards Ortiz de la Torre, Goyanes, Ribera y Sans, and Ricardo Lozano.

During the late nineteenth and early twentieth centuries, two types of "end-to-end" arterial anastomosis were commonly used: the simple method and the invagination or "plug" method, the latter proposed by A. San Martin and J. B. Murphy. However, the so-called simple method, developed by Carrel in 1902—consisting of anastomosing the two vascular segments with a very fine continuous suture that "avoid the intima," ensuring ideal edge coaptation by placing three equidistant anchoring stitches—soon gained widespread acceptance.

Research on prosthetic sutures was also improving, with notable contributions such as those of T. Gluck and Erwin Payr, the latter employing a thin magnesium tube as a vascular prosthesis.

In clinical practice, the first cases of end-to-end arterial anastomosis were performed by J. B. Murphy in 1896. In March 1906, Goyanes performed the first ever recorded end-to-end anastomosis to repair a traumatic transection of the superior mesenteric artery, very close to the aorta.

For several years, Goyanes worked intensively with San Martín in the field of experimental surgery, conducting pioneering studies in vascular surgery at the *Casa de Salud "La Gallega"* in Madrid. He later continued this research at the Faculty of Medicine in Madrid and in the Physiology Laboratory directed by Professor Gómez Ocaña.

In July 1904, Goyanes conducted numerous experiments on dogs, documenting them with meticulous technical descriptions, detailed results, and even histological studies carried out by Dr. Tello in Ramón y Cajal's department. This experimental study was published in April 1905.

Goyanes' contributions to vascular surgery are numerous. As early as 1904, he pioneered the use of fine silk sutures for experimental vascular anastomoses. By the end of the nineteenth century, the use of catgut had been largely abandoned; however, the eminent American pharmacologist Guthrie is credited with introducing the silk for vascular sutures, recommending its clinical use to Carrel in the same year. Carrel himself expressed his appreciation in these words:

> *I am very glad of your discovery. I think this thread is splendid. Every improvement on the technique is very important. There is no improvement too small* [11].

Without seeking to claim priority for this technique, it is important to note that, in 1904, Goyanes was already routinely using fine silk in his experimental work, as documented in his study published in April 1905.

In addition, Goyanes made a significant contributions to aortic surgery by describing the importance of sequentially loosening the hemostatic clamps after completing vascular anastomosis—first the distal, then the proximal clamp—a practice that remains standard today. He also designed his own vascular clamp and performed the first experiments in dogs involving resection of an aortic segment and its replacement with a segment of the vena cava.

His research tested various types of arteriovenous anastomoses and venous grafting, designed by San Martín, including single side to side arteriovenous anastomosis, double side to side arteriovenous anastomoses and, most notably, the double end-to-end arteriovenous anastomosis—known as Goyanes' venous arterioplasty. This technique involved replacing an arterial segment with an adjacent venous segment, performing a double end-to-end anastomoses, without completely detaching the vein from the surrounding tissues.

During these experiments, Goyanes performed several procedures in which he interposed a "venous segment" approximately 6–8 cm long between the external iliac artery and the femoral artery. While the immediate results were satisfactory, the long-term outcomes were less encouraging.

This procedure corresponds to what is now known as a venous grafting, later as bypass, referred to in the medical literature as the Kunlin operation. In his first publication in 1948, Kunlin acknowledged Goyanes' contribution, stating that "*the first vascular graft in man was performed by Goyanes in 1906.*"

Following this experimental work, Goyanes decided to apply his findings to aneurysm surgery, based on the premise that "ideal surgery in the radical operation of aneurysms (total exclusion and/or resection) is conditioned by the immediate restoration of circulation." Immediate restoration of circulation was far superior to ligation or excision.

He implemented this concept in clinical practice and, on 1st September 1906, published in *El Siglo Médico,* the case of a popliteal artery aneurysm, in which he completely excluded the aneurysmal sac by endoaneurysmorrhaphy and restored the continuity of the femoropopliteal vessel through a double end-to-end anastomosis, using the popliteal vein from the same limb [12] (Fig. 8.5).

Goyanes described the technique as follows:

> *Diagnosis: Aneurysm of the left popliteal artery, probably fusiform and extensive in an arteriosclerotic patient, due to syphilitic infection and alcohol intoxication.*
>
> *Operation: Double ligation of the artery above and below the aneurysmal sac (circulatory exclusion of the aneurysm) and venous arterioplasty by double terminal arteriovenous anastomosis....*

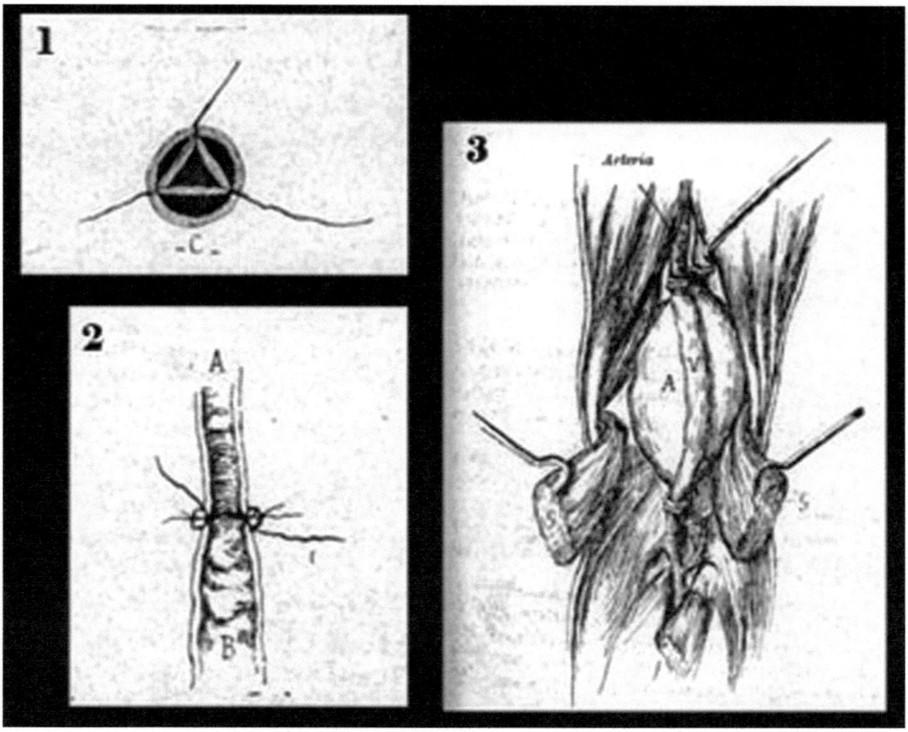

Fig. 8.5 Venous bypass for popliteal aneurysm. (Figures from the article in the Siglo Médico 1906). The subfigure 1 shows the type of anastomosis between the femoral artery and popliteal vein in a triangular fashion. The subfigure 2 shows the continuity after a end-to-end anastomosis between between the two structures and the subfigure 3 illustrates the whole anatomical picture with the popliteal aneurysm in situ and the femoro-popliteal bypass

... A wide incision along the entire length of the popliteal area over the tumour made it possible to reach the sac after sectioning the skin and the aponeurosis. The external saphenous vein circulating over the same aneurysmal sac was then isolated, and the popliteal vein, attached to the aneurysmal wall but perfectly permeable, and the external popliteal sciatic nerve (adhesions causing the pain) were discovered towards the outside. Once the vascular tumour was isolated, it was clearly seen to be fusiform, and it was also observed that its upper limit applied to the adductor ring, and the lower limit continued with a segment of popliteal artery of a few centimeters, the vein passing parallel to this segment.

The vessels below the aneurysm having been prepared....the femoral vessels were exposed, very close to the adductor ring. We now proceeded to the superior arteriovenous anastomosis, for which a hemostatic clamp with rubber bands was applied to the femoral artery and another one lower down to the vein (Dr. Ambrosio Rodriguez kindly compressed the femoral artery in Scarpa's triangle during the operation). The vessels were sectioned, the artery a little lower than the vein, and the peripheral end of the artery and the central end of the vein were ligated (the limb then became somewhat cyanotic). The central arterial end was now sutured to the peripheral venous end, using a cylindrical needle and fine silk, three perforating stitches were placed through the entire thickness of the vascular walls, passing the needle from the adventitia to the endothelial of the artery from the outside in and from the endothelial to the adventitia of the vein (from the inside out) to invert the vascular borders and achieve endothelial coaptation (U-suture of E. Brieau and M. Jaboulay, see 1).

Even with the three points equidistant on the anastomotic circumference and placed under tension, the calibre of the vessel was maintained, converting its cylindrical shape into a prismatic one (according to A. Carrel's technique), as can be seen in 2; a continuous suture was then performed, also perforating and with coaptation of the intima between each two angular points to knot the threads at the level of the latter.

After completing the superior arteriovenous anastomosis, we returned to the popliteal region, and after sectioning the vessels below the aneurysm, we also proceeded with ischaemia, and after ligating the central end of the artery (thus excluding the aneurysm) and the peripheral end of the vein to the subaneurysmal arteriovenous anastomosis, following the same technique, but with greater difficulties due to the sclerosis of the arterial wall, which produced the tearing of the first angular point.

Once this anastomosis had been performed, it could be observed that the aneurysmal tumour was not pulsating. Now the lower ischaemic forceps were released, and when the patient turned and released the forceps of the upper anastomosis and abandoned the compression of the femoral anastomosis, it could be observed that the current rushed with energy through the upper anastomosis above which a very thin bleeding emerged (a small puncture accidentally made in the artery above the anastomosis with the tip of the scalpel), which is coagulated with a stitch of suture. The popliteal vein changed its color to arterial red, pulsed vigorously along its entire length and even transmitted the current via the external saphenous vein, which pulsed in its turn. The popliteal artery below the anastomosis also pulsed clearly, although with less energy than the popliteal vein applied to the aneurysmal sac. The pedicle and posterior tibial arteries, without pulsation during the operative procedure, now began to pulsate clearly but weakly. The immediate patency of both anastomoses and the persistence of circulation to the leg and foot was thus demonstrated. The color of the limb changed from cyanotic to pink after the ischaemic forceps were released.

The 3 is a drawing taken from life by the illustrious Professor of Artistic Anatomy, Mr. Parada Santín, to whom I would like to reiterate my gratitude, and represents the definitive layout of the double arteriovenous anastomosis.

The operation was completed by suturing the two incisions and placing the dressing, fixing the limb with slight flexion of the knee…

This procedure is the first venous graft in history, used to bypass a diseased artery, in this case an popliteal aneurysm. A year after Goyanes, in 1909, Erich Lexer performed the first complete reconstruction using an internal saphenous vein to restore vascular continuity after the removal of an aneurysm in the axillary artery.

Goyanes' contributions were later taken up by Rudolph Matas of New Orleans in his famous paper on aneurysms presented at the International Congress of Medicine in London in 1913. In it, Matas presented and defended his methods of endoaneurysmorrhaphy, devoting extensive comments to the *'ideal method' of Goyanes and Lexer.*

J. Goyanes played a pivotal role in the advancement of surgical aneurysm therapy, being the pioneer and first clinical implementer of the 'ideal method' of treatment. Lexer continued his work with the use of the internal saphenous vein, and together they made this procedure universally known and adopted as the *'Goyanes-Lexer method.'* These interventions constitute a fundamental milestone in the development of modern vascular surgery.

Other contributions by Goyanes to the treatment of aneurysms include aneurysm resection followed by direct end-to-end anastomosis of the two ends (1908), aneurysm resection with repair by lateral arterial suture (1909), and the sectioning of a traumatic arteriovenous fistula in 1923, repaired with lateral sutures."

Throughout his career as a surgeon, Goyanes made numerous additional contributions, including venous surgery. He developed lateral venous sutures and proposed an innovative treatment for inferior vena cava wounds in 1911, using a temporary hemostasis clamp with 5 cm rubber-coated branches. This instrument, designed and manufactured by M. Collins in Paris, proved highly useful for controlling lateral hemorrhages in large-caliber veins, becoming a clear precursor to today's protected vascular clamps.

Goyanes also documented a resection of the subclavian vein followed by end-to-end anastomosis during en bloc excision of a recurrent breast carcinoma. With this case, he contributed with new data to the world literature on the resection of large veins infiltrated by cancer, making a significant contribution to the development of venous vascular surgery and radical oncological surgery.

Another of his outstanding contributions was his 1911 study on portal hypertension caused by liver cirrhosis, in which he proposed the inferior mesenteric-caval shunt (Fig. 8.6).

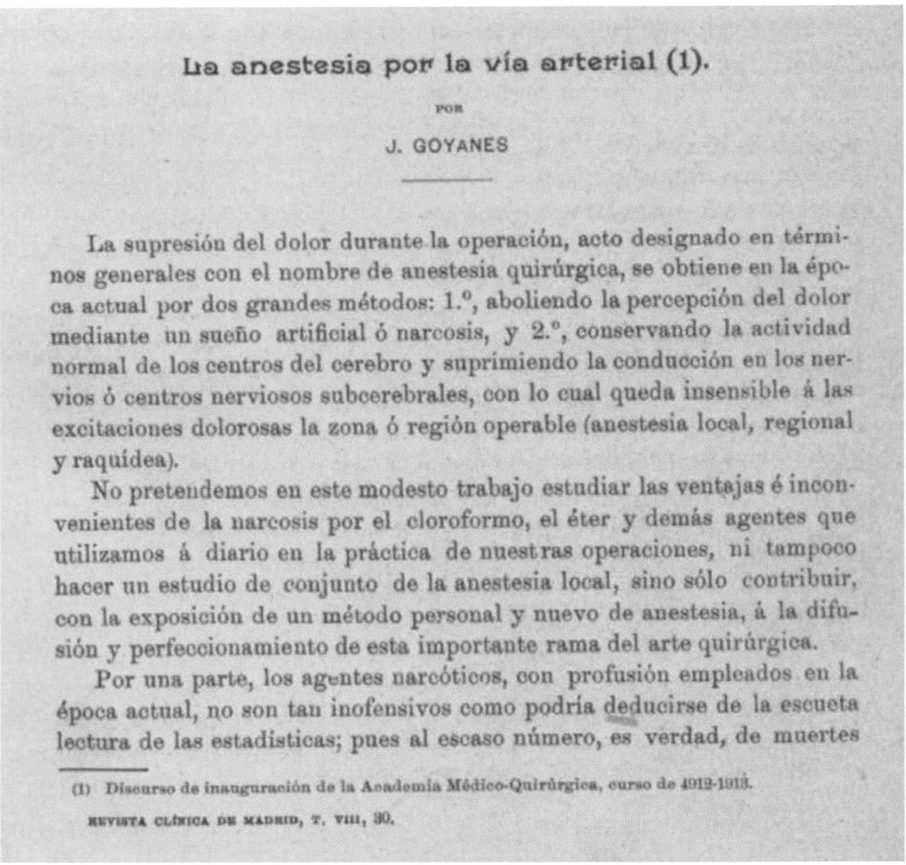

La anestesia por la vía arterial (1).

POR

J. GOYANES

La supresión del dolor durante la operación, acto designado en términos generales con el nombre de anestesia quirúrgica, se obtiene en la época actual por dos grandes métodos: 1.°, aboliendo la percepción del dolor mediante un sueño artificial ó narcosis, y 2.°, conservando la actividad normal de los centros del cerebro y suprimiendo la conducción en los nervios ó centros nerviosos subcerebrales, con lo cual queda insensible á las excitaciones dolorosas la zona ó región operable (anestesia local, regional y raquídea).

No pretendemos en este modesto trabajo estudiar las ventajas é inconvenientes de la narcosis por el cloroformo, el éter y demás agentes que utilizamos á diario en la práctica de nuestras operaciones, ni tampoco hacer un estudio de conjunto de la anestesia local, sino sólo contribuir, con la exposición de un método personal y nuevo de anestesia, á la difusión y perfeccionamiento de esta importante rama del arte quirúrgica.

Por una parte, los agentes narcóticos, con profusión empleados en la época actual, no son tan inofensivos como podría deducirse de la escueta lectura de las estadísticas; pues al escaso número, es verdad, de muertes

(1) Discurso de inauguración de la Academia Médico-Quirúrgica, curso de 1912-1913.

REVISTA CLÍNICA DE MADRID, T. VIII, 30.

Fig. 8.6 Inaugural conference of the course, 1912–1913, on arterial anaesthesia at the Academia Médico Quirúrgica Madrid

Intra-arterial anesthesia is a Goyanes contribution to the field of regional anesthesia, introduced by him after proving that arterial punctures could be performed without major complications. He began his studies in 1908 with animal experimentation and published his results in the following years.

Moreover, he also developed arterial anesthesia in limb surgery, a procedure that, in many cases, replaced spinal anesthesia. For this, he used cocaine solutions and their derivatives, designing extremely thin steel cannulas with a cross-sectioned end to avoid damaging the vascular endothelium [13].

In 1913, Goyanes described percutaneous arterial puncture, eliminating the need to expose the arterial vessel, as had been done up until that point. Regarding this procedure, he stated: '*It could be achieved, by the percutaneous procedure, to make the uncovering and separation of the vessel superfluous by penetrating from the outside with the needle through the skin.*' He then added: '*Our studies of arterial surgery and the practice of anesthesia by this route convinced us that arterial punctures with fine needles are harmless to these vessels; they do not cause thrombosis, do not generate aneurysms, and allow the circulation to persist normally.*'

In 1914, he began applying this technique to administer regional chemotherapy to tuberculosis patients.

Years later, in 1958, O. Creech would employ a similar procedure for regional perfusion with chemotherapeutic agents in the treatment of cancer.

In 1918, Goyanes described the clinical applications of catheterization using a distal balloon catheter, which proved useful in the aorta and common iliac during major pelvic surgery. Thanks to his pioneering research on arterial and venous catheterization, his publications are among the first to document these now routine methods. However, the medical community recognizes Bleichroeder (1912) as the originator of arterial and venous catheterization, and Forssmann (1929) as the pioneer of cardiac catheterization and angiocardiography (1931).

Goyanes also devised various surgical instruments, like specific clamps for aortic surgery, He also designed a wooden and glass box for thoracic interventions that allowed pressure to be raised, with which he operated on various pulmonary processes, anticipating the specialization in pulmonary surgery.

He was also renowned for his interventions in thyroid surgery, having addressed this subject in his doctoral thesis. In 1918, he published a study on goitre and endemic cretinism in the upper valleys of the Tormes and Alberche rivers in *El Siglo Médico*. In 1922, he traveled through Las Hurdes with Gregorio Marañón and Bardají as part of an official commission, accompanying King Alfonso XIII. As a result of this trip, he co-wrote the report "*El problema de Las Hurdes es un problema sanitario" (The problem of Las Hurdes is a public health problem.)*, which was published in *La Medicina Íbera* in 1922.

Oncology was also one of his areas of interest. In his laboratory, he studied the etiology and diagnosis of tumors, promoting extensive interventions in oncological surgery. He was one of the first to advocate the soft-ray mammography, a technique later consolidated in Uruguay with Leborgne and in the United States with Gerhon Cohen.

José Goyanes was member of the Royal Academy of Medicine (1918), president of the Spanish Medical-Surgical Academy (1911–1912), and founding director of the journal *Archivos Españoles de Oncología* and the *Boletín de la Liga Española contra el Cáncer.* He also chaired the Spanish Association of Surgeons.

Legacy

José Goyanes Capdevila stands as one of the most distinguished figures in the history of Spanish surgery, whose contributions transcended various fields, from vascular surgery to the study of surgical oncology, and even to the history of medicine itself.

Hos groundbreaking work in performing the first femoropopliteal vein grafting in the history opened a path in vascular surgery that has been followed to the present day. He also conducted experimental and clinical studies on a multitude of venous and arterial vascular topics such as vascular sutures, the substitution of arteries for veins, arterial anesthesia, arterial puncture and vascular catheterization. His oncology practice performing the first recorded interventions performing cancer resection with vascular reconstructions are pioneering of today's practices.

Goyanes' influence was not limited to his surgical innovations; he was also a keen intellectual, delving into classical languages and analyzing the works of renowned figures such as Michael Servetus and the literary critiques of doctors in the works of Quevedo.

His example is extraordinary for his vocation, passion and teaching.

His legacy as a doctor, researcher, and intellectual remains a pillar of inspiration in the fields of medicine, surgery, and beyond, influencing generations of medical professionals.

He has been recognized by the surgical world for his pioneering contributions to vascular surgery [14–16].

References

1. Criado E, Girón F. José Goyanes Capdevila, unsung pioneer of vascular surgery. Ann Vasc Surg. 2006;20:422–5.
2. Barros JL. Investigaciones sobre los trabajos del Dr. José Goyanes Capdevila. Cir Ginecol Urol. 1965;19:1–26.
3. Gilsanz F, Guasch E, Navarro-Suay R. José Goyanes Capdevila (1876–1964). Pionero de la cirugía vascular e introductor de la analgesia regional intraarterial. An Real Acad Doct Esp. 2024;9:59–80.
4. Die-Goyanes A, Die-Trill J. José Goyanes. Cirujano y humanista. Cir Esp. 2008;83:8–11.
5. Vaquero C, del Río L, San Norberto E, Brizuela JA. José Goyanes Capdevila (1876–1964). Pionero de la Cirugía Vascular Española. Ann Real Acad Med Cir Valladolid. 2017;54:71–82.
6. Libro-Homenaje Goyanes. Ed. Gaceta Medica Española. Madrid; 1930.
7. Die y Mas J. José Goyanes Capdevila. In Memoriam. Rev Esp Onc. 1964;11:11–20.
8. Jaboulay M, Briau E. Recherches expérimentales sur la suture et la greffe artérielle. Lyon Med. 1896;81:97–9.
9. Ochsner J. The complex life of Rudolph Matas. J Vasc Surg. 2001;34:387–92.
10. San Martin y Satrustegui A. Cirugia del aparato circulatorio, discurso leido en la sesion inaugural de la Real Academia de Medicina de Madrid Enrique Teodoro. 1902; 1–72.
11. Carrel A. Les anastomoses vasculaires et leur technique operatoire. Union Medical du Canada. 1904;33:521–7.
12. Goyanes J. Nuevos trabajos de cirugía vascular. Sustitución plástica de las arteria por las venas o arterioplastia venosa, aplicada, como nuevo metodo, al tratamiento de los aneurismas. Siglo Med. 1906;53:546–9; 561–564.
13. Lancina Martín JA. José Goyanes Capdevila: La aportación española a la anestesia regional por vía intraarterial [Internet]. Doctor Alberto Lancina Martín. Urología e Historia de la Medicina. 2015 [citado el]. https://drlancina.blogspot.com/2015/01/jose-goyanes-capdevila-la-aportacion.html.
14. Friedman SG. A history of vascular surgery. Blackwell Publishing; 2005.
15. Rickard RF, Hudson DA. A history of vascular and microvascular surgery. Ann Plast Surg. 2013;73:465–72.
16. Barker WF. A century's worth of arterial sutures. Ann Vasc Surg. 1988;2:85–91.

9

Fidel Pagés Miravé: Discovery of Epidural Anaesthesia (Metameric Anesthesia)—War Surgery in the RIF (Morocco)

Miguel A. Cuesta

2020 marked the centenary of the discovery of lumbar epidural anesthesia, an innovation by the Spanish surgeon Fidel Pagés Miravé. His name should be remembered not only for his skill as a surgeon but also for having developed a technique that revolutionized regional anesthesia (Fig. 9.1).

However, his international recognition has lagged far behind the worldwide success of his technique, widely used in obstetrics and pain management. Pagés's 1921 publication was the result of his profound experience in spinal or intradural anesthesia—administration of the anesthetic into the cerebrospinal fluid—and his vast anatomical, physiological, and pharmacological knowledge. Furthermore, he was well versed in the studies of pioneers in intradural and sacral epidural anesthesia. The clarity and precision of his publication, in which he describes his discovery with ambition and pride, remain an exemplary model for how to present an innovation in the field of anesthesia and surgery.

However, like so many other discoveries made in Spain, this breakthrough has remained forgotten for years, both in its country of origin and around the world, despite the fact that epidural anesthesia has become an essential procedure in operating rooms around the world for more than nine decades.

M. A. Cuesta (✉)
Department of Surgery, Amsterdam University Medical Centre (UMC), Amsterdam, The Netherlands

M. A. Cuesta, F. Mateo Vallejo (eds.), *Spain's Journey in Medicine*,
https://doi.org/10.1007/978-3-032-12221-6_9

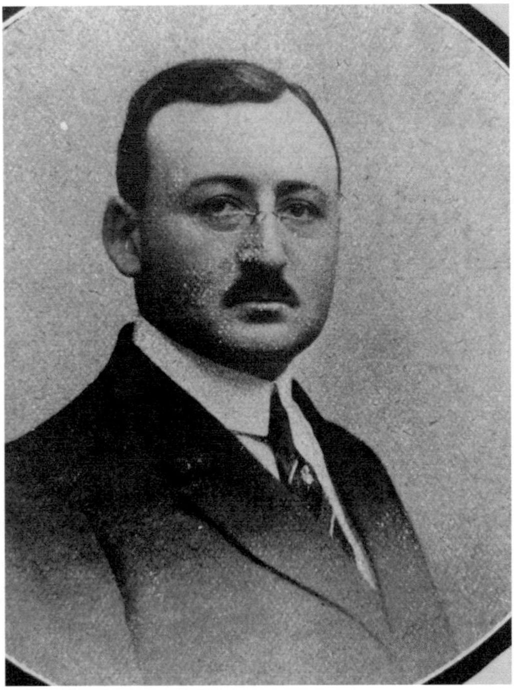

Fig. 9.1 Fidel Pagés Miravé

In 1965, Faulconer and Kays, in their classic work *Foundations of Anaesthesiology*, wrote about him: "*There is hardly any information about the life of this important Spanish surgeon,*" even noting that they did not know the date and place of his birth [1].

Fidel Pagés Miravé was born in Huesca on January 26, 1886, son of Juan Pagés, a Catalan merchant, and Concepción Miravé Sesé. Only child, he was orphaned at an early age. He completed his secondary education at Huesca, where he earned his bachelor's degree in June 1901. He subsequently entered the Faculty of Medicine at the University of Zaragoza as a scholarship student, where he discovered his calling for surgery under the tutelage of Ricardo Lozano Monzón, a prestigious surgeon of the time, renowned for his ability to operate in all cavities of the human body. On July 17, 1908, he obtained his degree in Medicine with Extraordinary Award and entered the Military Health Academy in Madrid at the end of September.

The RIF war, in what was then the Spanish Protectorate of Morocco, was experiencing intense fighting at that time, especially after the Disaster of Barranco del Lobo, which occurred on July 27, 1909, near Melilla. In that battle, Spanish troops suffered a serious defeat at the hands of Rifian fighters, with a high number of casualties.

Given the magnitude of the losses, in early August, Fidel Pagés was sent to the Military Hospital in Melilla, where he demonstrated his extraordinary skill as a surgeon, organizing an efficiently caring for the large number of wounded soldiers. His service at the front continued, with some interruptions, until June 1911, during which he performed various duties at different posts within the war zone.

In recognition of his merits in treating the wounded, he was awarded the First Class Cross of Military Merit, a distinction reserved for those who excelled in acts of bravery and service on the battlefield (Fig. 9.2).

Upon his return to the Peninsula, already holding the rank of Medical Captain in the Military Health Corps, Fidel Pagés underwent a series of successive postings across various Spanish cities between 1911 and 1913. In June 1913, he earned his Doctor of Medicine degree from the Central University of Madrid, presenting his dissertation titled "*Pathogenesis of Bradycardias*", which received a distinction.

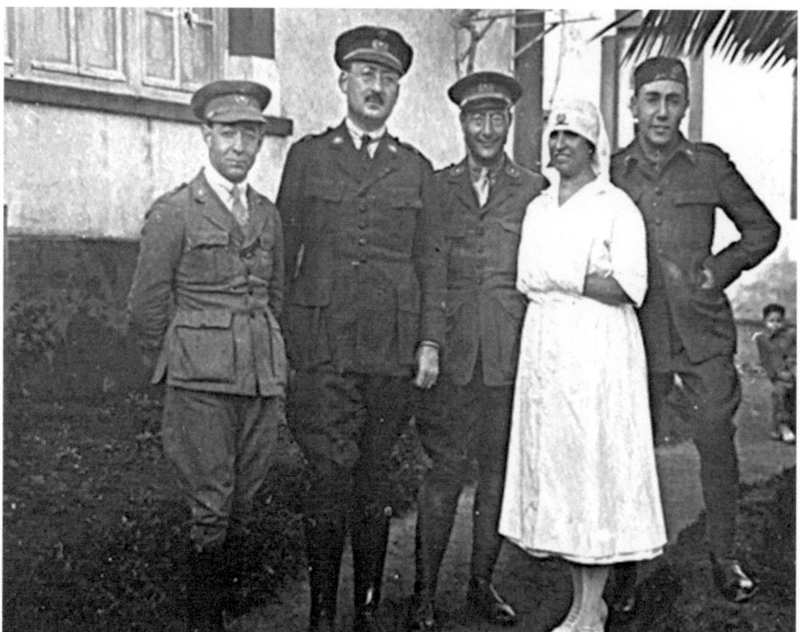

Fig. 9.2 Fidel Pagés in a break. Melilla 1920s

On August 13, 1913, he married Berta Concepción Bergemann y Quirós in Madrid, the daughter of Wilhelm Bergemann, a German citizen who had settled in the Spanish capital. Together they had five children (Fig. 9.3).

It was not until 1916 that he settled in Madrid and was assigned to the General Staff of the Army.

His brilliant career led him to get the first available post as a surgeon at the Hospital Provincial de Beneficencia in Madrid, as well as the position of family doctor for the Royal Patrimony of the Royal Family. His reputation as a surgeon—both for his technical skill and his humane treatment of patients—opened many doors for him within the country's surgical circles.

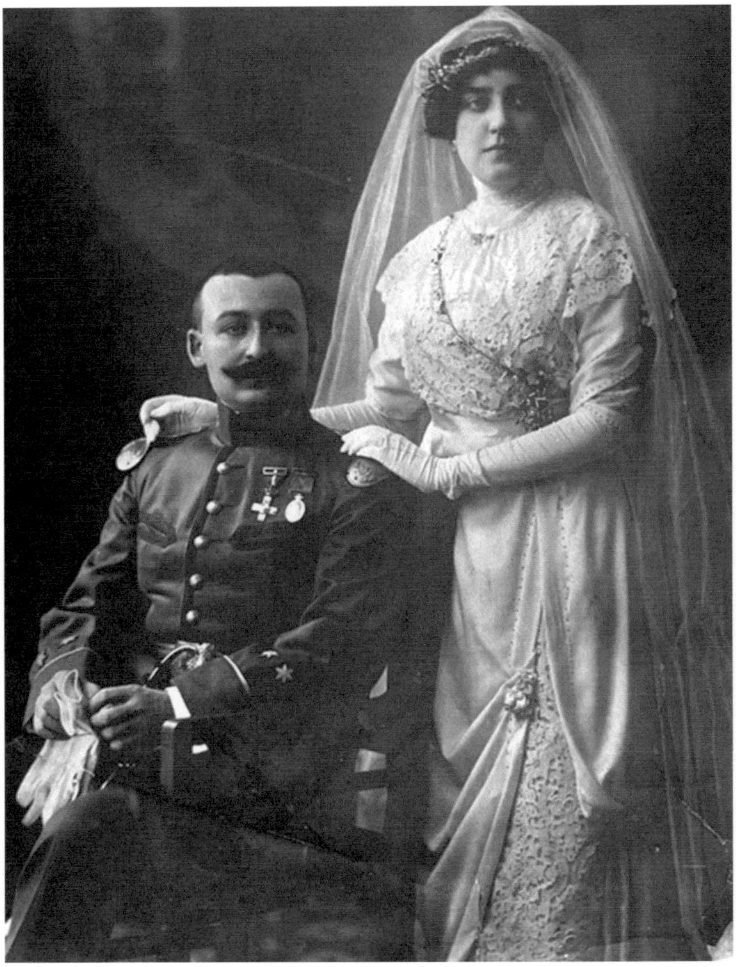

Fig. 9.3 Wedding photo of Fidel Pagés with Berta Concepción Bergemann y Quirós

In 1917, during the third year of the First World War, in which Spain remained neutral, Pagés was commissioned by Royal Order to travel to Vienna as a delegate of the Spanish ambassador. His mission was to inspect prison camps within the Austro-Hungarian Empire as a medical expert. In addition to his growing prestige as a surgeon, he was likely chosen for this task due to his fluency in French and German.

He arrived in Vienna in April and, beyond his inspection duties, between July and August he was attached as a surgeon to the Vienna Military Hospital, where he assisted in numerous surgical operations alongside the eminent Viennese surgeon Richard Werner. Having fallen ill, he returned to Madrid in September.

Upon his return, he took part in the reorganization of the Army, devising a plan to modernize the military medical units. His service record described him as a '*surgeon of merit, particularly for his outstanding intelligence and dedication to duty*,' which earned him promotion to Medical Captain at the age of 31.

In 1919, he developed a classification system for wounds and injuries based on triage, aimed at its application in military campaigns. An excellent communicator of his work, he dedicated himself to spreading surgical advances through specialized publications. That same year, he was appointed editor of the *Revista de Sanidad Militar*, and, with Tomás Rodríguez de Mata and Isidro Sánchez Covisa, he founded the *Revista Española de Cirugía*, the forerunner of today's *Cirugía Española*, the official journal of the Spanish Association of Surgeons (AEC).

All of his surgical contributions, from 1911 until his death, were published in these two journals (Fig. 9.4).

His work in Madrid, at the General Hospital, earned him widespread fame among the young surgeons who came there to train, both for his teaching skills to doctors and nurses and for his surgical innovations. He combined this role with his work at the Emergency Department in Carabanchel Hospital and with his practical surgery classes at the Hospital Clínico de San Carlos.

In July 1921, following the military disasters of Annual and Monte Arruit during the RIF War—where Rifian troops under the command of Abd el-Krim inflicted more than 18,000 casualties on Spanish forces led by General Silvestre—he was once again assigned to the Military Hospital in Melilla (Fig. 9.5).

His prestige as an organizer and surgeon led to his appointment as head of Field Surgical Team No. 1 at the Doecker Military Hospital. There, with the collaboration of his team—including his direct assistant Bernardo Areces Matilla, the anesthetist Fortunato García Gómez, and doctors Francisco

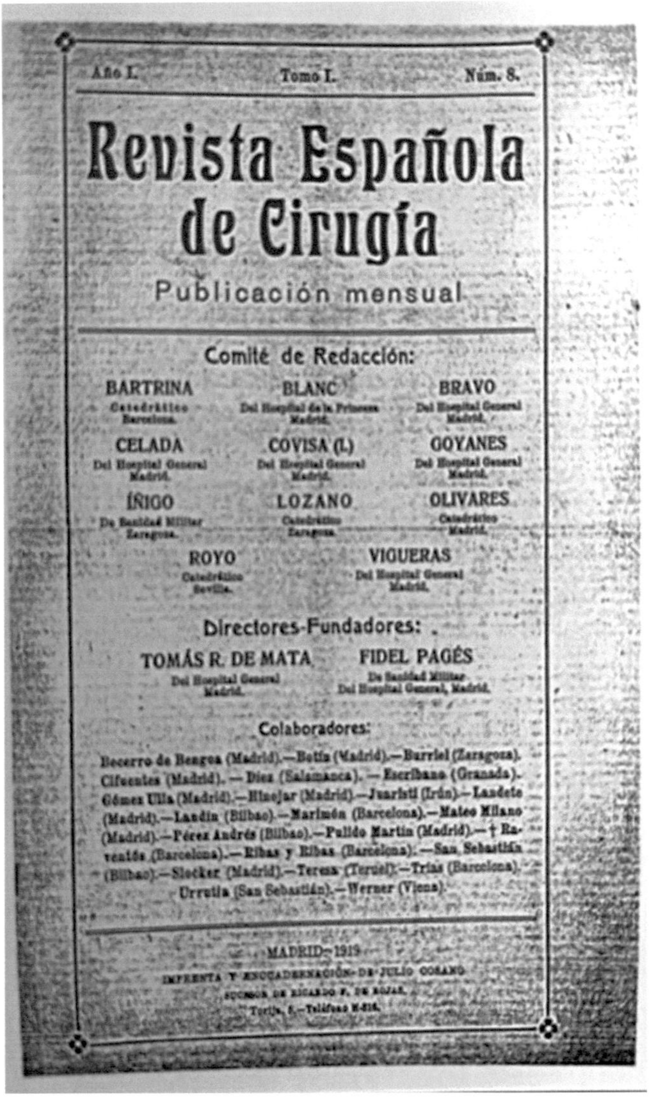

Año I. Tomo I. Núm. 8.

Revista Española de Cirugía

Publicación mensual

Comité de Redacción:

BARTRINA — Catedrático, Barcelona.
BLANC — Del Hospital de la Princesa, Madrid.
BRAVO — Del Hospital General, Madrid.
CELADA — Del Hospital General, Madrid.
COVISA (L.) — Del Hospital General, Madrid.
GOYANES — Del Hospital General, Madrid.
ÍÑIGO — De Sanidad Militar, Zaragoza.
LOZANO — Catedrático, Zaragoza.
OLIVARES — Catedrático, Madrid.
ROYO — Catedrático, Sevilla.
VIGUERAS — Del Hospital General, Madrid.

Directores-Fundadores:

TOMÁS R. DE MATA — Del Hospital General, Madrid.
FIDEL PAGÉS — De Sanidad Militar, Del Hospital General, Madrid.

Colaboradores:

Becerro de Bengoa (Madrid).—Botín (Madrid).—Barriel (Zaragoza). Cifuentes (Madrid). — Díez (Salamanca). — Escribano (Granada). Gómez Ulla (Madrid).—Hinojar (Madrid).—Juarbiti (Irún).—Landete (Madrid).—Landín (Bilbao).—Mariméa (Barcelona).—Mateo Milano (Madrid).—Pérez Andrés (Bilbao).—Pulido Martín (Madrid).—† Raventós (Barcelona).—Ribas y Ribas (Barcelona).—San Sebastián (Bilbao).—Slocker (Madrid).—Teresa (Teruel).—Trías (Barcelona). Urrutia (San Sebastián).—Werner (Viena).

MADRID—1919

Fig. 9.4 Cover of the Revista Española de Cirugía

Luque Beltrán, and Luis Marina Aguirre—he achieved outstanding results. According to the records, he obtained a survival rate of 70% among patients undergoing laparotomy for abdominal war wounds, an exceptional outcome for the time.

During the fighting in September at Tisza, Atlaten, Segangan, and Taxuda, the surgical team spent entire days in the operating theatre, performing countless triage and emergency operations. Their service record highlights "the most

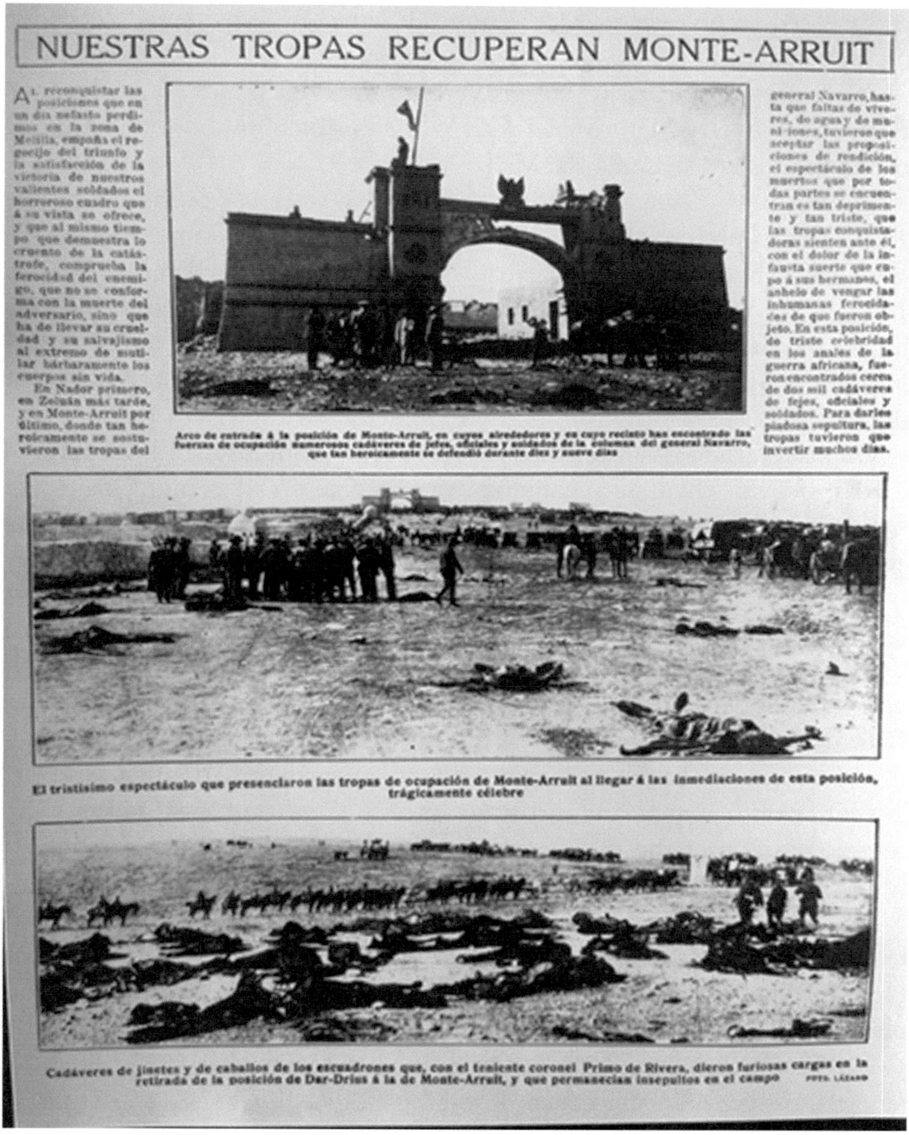

NUESTRAS TROPAS RECUPERAN MONTE-ARRUIT

Al reconquistar las posiciones que en un día nefasto perdimos en la zona de Melilla, empaña el regocijo del triunfo y la satisfacción de la victoria de nuestros valientes soldados el horroroso cuadro que á su vista se ofrece, y que al mismo tiempo que demuestra lo cruento de la catástrofe, comprueba la ferocidad del enemigo, que no se conforma con la muerte del adversario, sino que ha de llevar su crueldad y su salvajismo al extremo de mutilar bárbaramente los cuerpos sin vida.

En Nador primero, en Zeluán más tarde, y en Monte-Arruit por último, donde tan heroicamente se sostuvieron las tropas del general Navarro, hasta que faltas de víveres, de agua y de municiones, tuvieron que aceptar las proposiciones de rendición, el espectáculo de los muertos que por todas partes se encuentran es tan deprimente y tan triste, que las tropas conquistadoras sienten ante él, con el dolor de la infausta suerte que cupo á sus hermanos, el anhelo de vengar las inhumanas ferocidades de que fueron objeto. En esta posición, de triste celebridad en los anales de la guerra africana, fueron encontrados cerca de dos mil cadáveres de jefes, oficiales y soldados. Para darles piadosa sepultura, las tropas tuvieron que invertir muchos días.

Arco de entrada á la posición de Monte-Arruit, en cuyos alrededores y en cuyo recinto han encontrado las fuerzas de ocupación numerosos cadáveres de jefes, oficiales y soldados de la columna del general Navarro, que tan heroicamente se defendió durante diez y nueve días

El tristísimo espectáculo que presenciaron las tropas de ocupación de Monte-Arruit al llegar á las inmediaciones de esta posición, trágicamente célebre

Cadáveres de jinetes y de caballos de los escuadrones que, con el teniente coronel Primo de Rivera, dieron furiosas cargas en la retirada de la posición de Dar-Drius á la de Monte-Arruit, y que permanecían insepultos en el campo FOTO. LÁZARO

Fig. 9.5 News about the war in the Rif. Reconquest of the siege in Monte-Arruit

brilliant success" of their efforts, with special mention of "the extraordinary work carried out in response to the enormous number of wounded hospitalized."

The success of his interventions, later documented in several scientific articles, was attributed to three key factors: his organized teamwork, his outstanding professional skills, and his firm conviction that, following meticulous triage based on his experience, the survival of the seriously injured depended on immediate and precise surgical intervention.

In recognition of his work, he received important awards, including the First Class Military Merit Medal with White Distinction, the Gold Medal of the Spanish Red Cross and the Medal of Africa.

In December of the same year, he returned to work in Madrid. In August 1922, he was promoted to Medical Commander and appointed head of the Emergency Department at Carabanchel Hospital. A year later, in August 1923, he traveled with his family to the Cestona Spa in Guipúzcoa, and during his stay, he took the opportunity to attend the inauguration of the operating theatre at the Military Hospital in San Sebastián, where he would later perform his last surgery.

On his return to Madrid, while traveling by car with his family, the vehicle, driven by his chauffeur, collided with a tree in the municipality of Quintanapalla, in the province of Burgos (Fig. 9.6). Dr. Pagés died in the accident, while one of his daughters and the chauffeur were seriously injured [2, 3].

His body was transferred to Madrid, and his burial at the Sacramental Cemetery of San José y San Lorenzo drew a large crowd. This cemetery, originally intended for the artists, writers and scientists of the time, is located on Calle de la Verdad, in the Comillas district of Carabanchel.

The entire press at the time reported on the tragedy, describing it as a great loss for Spanish surgery and medicine. At only 37 years of age, Dr. Pagés was regarded as one of the most promising surgical figures of his time, with a bright future still ahead of him.

His close friendship with Queen Mother Doña Cristina gave rise to heartfelt tributes at the Hospital Militar del Buen Suceso in Madrid and at the Hospital Militar de San Sebastián, where just a day before his death, he had performed his last surgical intervention.

The *Revista de Sanidad Militar*, in its issue of 15 October 1923 (Fig. 9.7), reported the moving farewell words of his colleague, Dr. M. Gómez Ulla:

Tribute to a hero of science.

Pagés Has Died

These words will fill with sadness the hundreds of wounded he was able to rescue from the clutches of death. In the ranks of Military Health, among the list of Spanish surgeons, fate has claimed a casualty, leaving a void that is very difficult, if not impossible, to fill at this time. It is with deep sorrow that we learn of the

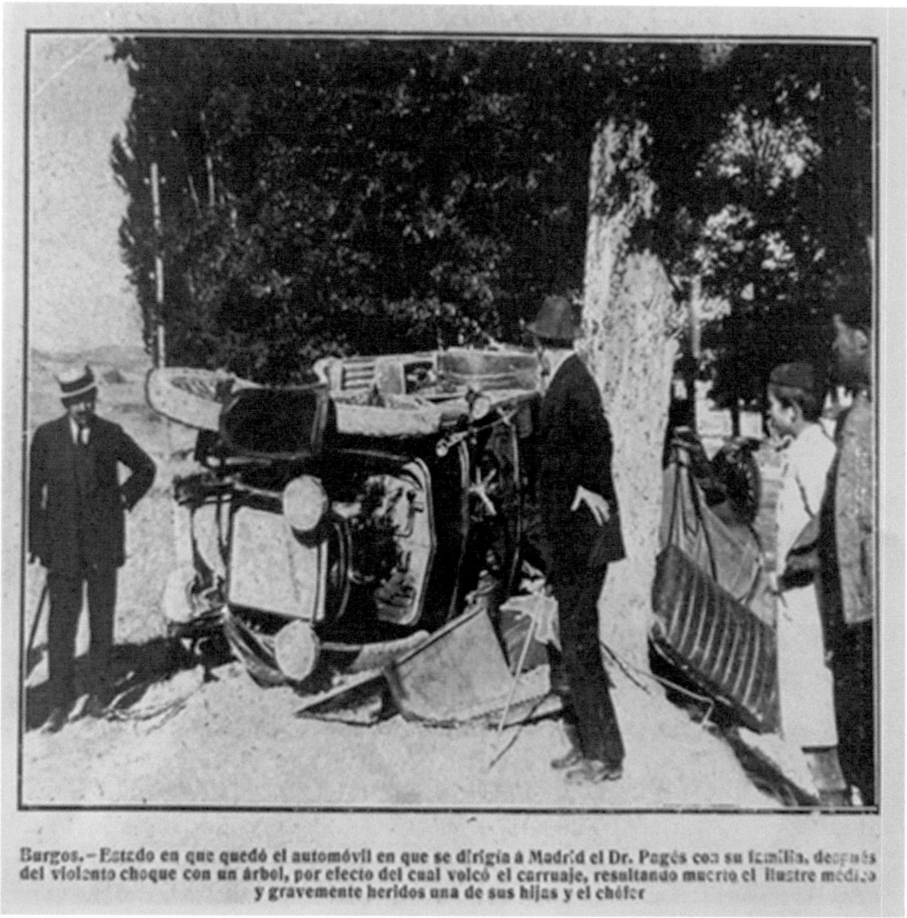
Burgos.—Estado en que quedó el automóvil en que se dirigía á Madrid el Dr. Pagés con su familia, después del violento choque con un árbol, por efecto del cual volcó el carruaje, resultando muerto el ilustre médico y gravemente heridos una de sus hijas y el chófer

Fig. 9.6 News of the fatal car accident

definitive departure of the great friend, the valiant military man, the wise surgeon, the eminent and skilled operator, the good, simple, and modest man—that great young man who, just two years ago, arrived here at the head of his team to contest with Death for the wounded who fell in the bloody battles of the time.

To highlight his prestige and the respect he inspired, Commander Francisco Franco mentions Pagés in "*Diario de una Bandera*":

> *The night is sad in Ambar; Major Fontanes is in a very serious condition, and everyone knows what an abdomen wound means with the hospital so far away. Dr. Pagés is all the wounded man's concern; he could save him. In the Legion, admiration is*

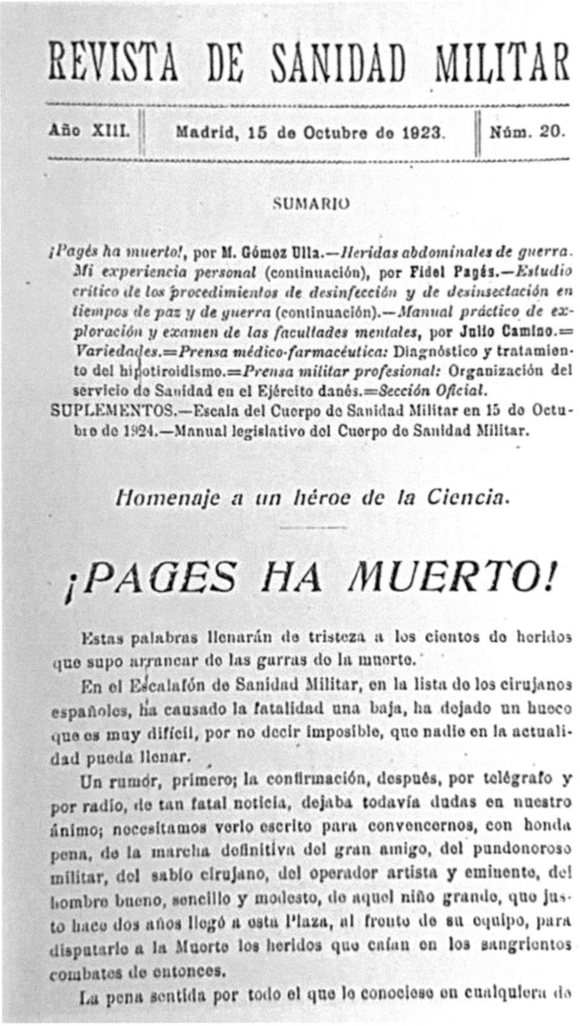

REVISTA DE SANIDAD MILITAR

Año XIII. | Madrid, 15 de Octubre de 1923. | Núm. 20.

SUMARIO

¡Pagés ha muerto!, por **M. Gómez Ulla.**—*Heridas abdominales de guerra. Mi experiencia personal* (continuación), por **Fidel Pagés.**—*Estudio crítico de los procedimientos de desinfección y de desinsectación en tiempos de paz y de guerra* (continuación).—*Manual práctico de exploración y examen de las facultades mentales*, por **Julio Camino.**=*Variedades.*=*Prensa médico-farmacéutica:* Diagnóstico y tratamiento del hipotiroidismo.=*Prensa militar profesional:* Organización del servicio de Sanidad en el Ejército danés.=*Sección Oficial.*

SUPLEMENTOS.—Escala del Cuerpo de Sanidad Militar en 15 de Octubre de 1924.—Manual legislativo del Cuerpo de Sanidad Militar.

Homenaje a un héroe de la Ciencia.

¡PAGES HA MUERTO!

Estas palabras llenarán de tristeza a los cientos de heridos que supo arrancar de las garras de la muerte.

En el Escalafón de Sanidad Militar, en la lista de los cirujanos españoles, ha causado la fatalidad una baja, ha dejado un hueco que es muy difícil, por no decir imposible, que nadie en la actualidad pueda llenar.

Un rumór, primero; la confirmación, después, por telégrafo y por radio, de tan fatal noticia, dejaba todavía dudas en nuestro ánimo; necesitamos verlo escrito para convencernos, con honda pena, de la marcha definitiva del gran amigo, del pundonoroso militar, del sabio cirujano, del operador artista y eminente, del hombre bueno, sencillo y modesto, de aquel niño grande, que justo hace dos años llegó a esta Plaza, al frente de su equipo, para disputarle a la Muerte los heridos que caían en los sangrientos combates de entonces.

La pena sentida por todo el que le conociese en cualquiera de

Fig. 9.7 Pagés is dead ¡ *Revista de Sanidad Militar* (October, 15, 1923)

felt for this remarkable surgeon, who has saved so many legionnaires from certain death. This is why the brave commander of the 2nd Brigade thinks of Pagés. In the early morning of the 20th, the heroic commander died in the position. The Legion is in mourning, it has lost one of its best commanders and the soldiers are sad; their eyes do not cry because there are no tears left in their sockets, they have already seen so many officers and comrades fall! … (Diary of a flag, Chapter XVIII, page 181.)

Scientific Activity

Despite his short yet intense life, Pagés had time to publish numerous scientific works on various subjects, which can be grouped into three categories. The first, and most numerous, are his studies on military surgery and war wounds. The second focuses on his research into cancer, while the third covers his experiences in civilian surgery.

However, his most recognized work is the March 1921 paper in the *Revista de Sanidad Militar* and the *Revista Española de Cirugía*, where he presented his study entitled *'Anestesia Metamérica'*. In this article, Pagés describes how, in November 1920, while performing spinal anesthesia for the repair of an inguinal hernia, he had the idea of stopping the needle after passing through the yellow ligament, without puncturing the dura mater, thus remaining in the epidural space. He then decided to block the nerve roots outside the meningeal space, before they passed through the intervertebral foramina [4, 5].

Instead of using the stovaine he had prepared, he dissolved three tablets of Novocaine Braun with suprarenin in 25 cc of saline in a boiled capsule and proceeded to inject the solution immediately through the cannula inserted between the second and third lumbar vertebrae. As a result, anesthesia was produced in the infraumbilical region of the abdomen and the anteroexternal aspect of the lower limbs. Twenty minutes after the injection, he successfully performed the radical cure of the right inguinal hernia, with the patient experiencing not the slightest discomfort.

This first epidural anesthesia was performed by Dr. Pagés in the surgical area on the third floor of the Hospital General de Madrid, a building that currently houses the Reina Sofía National Art Center Museum (Figs. 9.8 and 9.9).

The approach was based on tactile feedback, explaining that there are two ways to access the epidural space. The first is to reach the intradural space and then slowly withdraw the needle until no more cerebrospinal fluid is aspirated. The second, which he considers 'positively more elegant,' is the direct puncture, stopping after crossing the yellow ligament. According to Pagés, the latter 'is not difficult, once a certain amount of practice has been acquired.'

For this procedure, he used a standard short-beveled, not very sharp, 0.8 mm (21 gauge) spinal anesthesia cannula. The Record syringe he employed was similar to the Rekordpritze, manufactured in Berlin since 1906 by Dewitt & Herz. Its main advantage was that it allowed for the slow introduction of the anesthetic solution, ensuring an even diffusion in the epidural space.

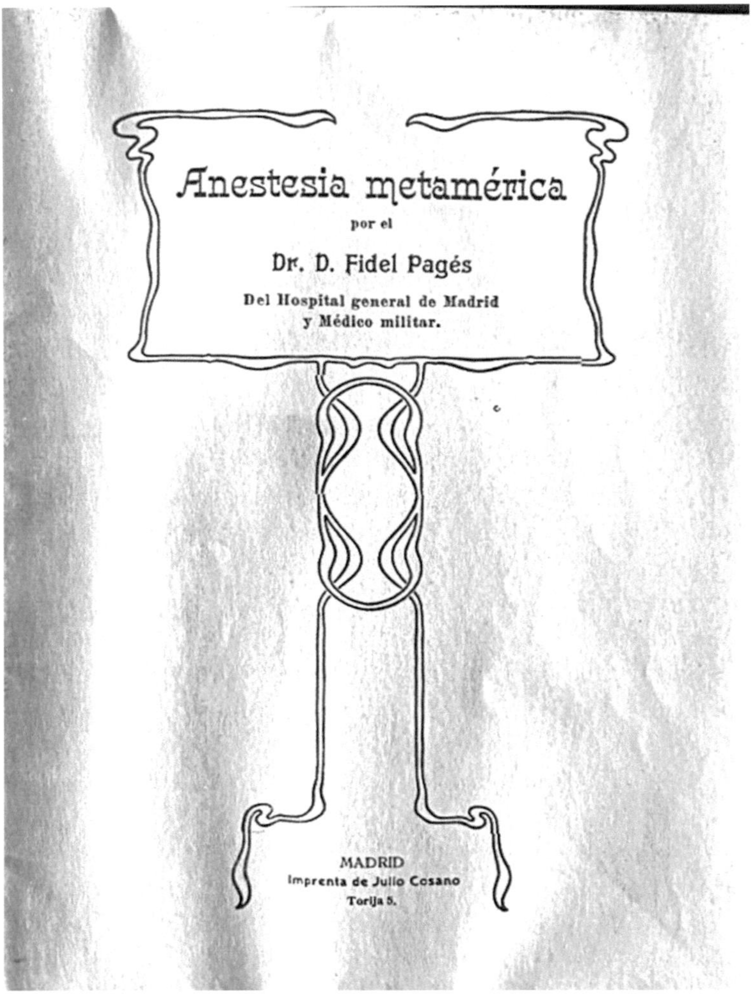

Fig. 9.8 Cover of the paper *Anestesia Metamérica*

Based on this experience, in his article, he analyzes the existing literature on regional anesthesia up to that point, particularly highlighting the French studies by F. Cathelin, P. Reclus, J.A. Sicard, and T. Tuffier on sacral epidural anesthesia. This technique involved injecting the anesthetic solution through the sacral hiatus, achieving sufficient anesthesia for procedures in the anal region and external genitalia, but proving inadequate for operations such as inguinal hernia repair.

Pagés also demonstrates a profound knowledge of German medical literature, referencing the work of M. Kappis, who, through injections of methylene blue, managed to color the epidural space by performing paravertebral

Nada diremos de la primera, por ser sobradamente conocida; pero en cuanto a la segunda, recordaremos que ya Sellheim, en 1905, consiguió insensibilizar la pared abdominal de un enfermo inyectando una solución anestésica alrededor de las raíces ner-

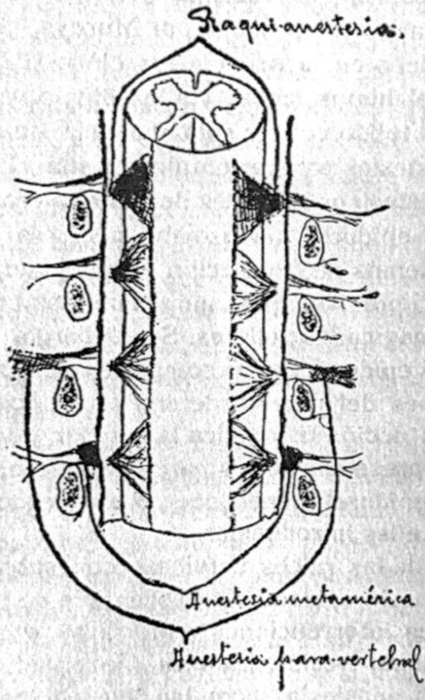

Fig. 1.ª—Esquema comparativo de las anestesias metamérica, paravertebral y aracnoidea.

viosas comprendidas desde la 8.ª a la 12.ª dorsal, a su salida del agujero de conjunción. El método paravertebral tiene por objeto bloquear la raíz inmediatamente de abandonar el raquis y antes de la división en sus dos ramas anterior y posterior, y de que haya cedido al simpático el ramicomunicante correspondiente (fig. 1).

Fig. 9.9 Comparative scheme: *anestesia metamérica, paravertebral and aracnoidea*

punctures. The injection of dye at the level of the first lumbar nerve, at its exit through the intervertebral foramen, allowed the distribution in the epidural space to be observed from the cervical spine to the sacrum. This technique of paravertebral extradural anesthesia had been published by several German authors in 1912.

Pagés' contribution represents a milestone in the history of anesthesia, marking the first successful access to the epidural space through a lumbar intervertebral route, achieving effective anesthesia for various surgical interventions depending on the height of the injection (Fig. 9.10). His work is a true descriptive masterpiece on how a scientific article should be structured, the result of an innovative experience. In it, he details the anatomy of the spinal canal, explains the different techniques of regional anesthesia—distinguishing between spinal anesthesia, epidural or metameric anesthesia, and paravertebral anesthesia—and illustrates them with very clear and simple diagrams. The drawings accompanying his publication "*Anestesia Metamérica*" were made by Antonio Fernández Victorio, Head of Studies at the Academia Especial de Sanidad Militar.

The article also describes in detail the technique, the instruments to be used, the recommended anesthetic solution, as well as the collateral phenomena accompanying metameric anesthesia, its possible failures, and complications.

"*Some patients presented nausea and vomiting along with blood pressure depression and were evaluated using the Pachón oscillometer. It is noted that 'an injection of ether or caffeine contributes to accelerate the evolution of this transient state*". Pagés states that epidural anesthesia should only be used in adults and contraindicates its use in children, as they "*interpret tactile sensations as painful*".

The advantages and disadvantages of this technique compared to other forms of anesthesia are discussed below. One of its disadvantages is the delayed onset of analgesia, which occurs approximately 20 min after injection, a longer latency time than with spinal anesthesia. This waiting time affects the efficiency of work in the operating room, where surgeons have limited time available due to the high workload. In this regard, it is clearly stated:

> *Therefore, given the intensity of work in our operating theatres, where it is common to operate on eight to ten patients in one session, the total time that the surgeon would have to spend on anesthesia would not be less than two hours, which is a great waste of time.*

To optimize the process, a practical solution is proposed: one patient is operated on while another is anesthetized, thus minimizing the loss of time.

Finally, the first 43 operations performed with this technique are described, including, in addition to inguinal and crural hernia surgeries, appendectomies, gastroenterostomies, gastric ulcer resections, adhesiolysis, cholecystectomies with exploration of the bile duct, drainage of pleurisy, amputations, and perineal surgery.

The results obtained are detailed below:

> "*Of the 43 anesthesia procedures performed, analgesia was complete in 40 cases. In two cases (one of pleurisy and one of shoulder dislocation), anesthesia failed, likely*

due to a technical error. In one patient, cervical root block was accompanied by alarming phenomena, which are described elsewhere. Nephropexy was performed in a patient whose neurotic temperament prevented the success of any anesthesia other than general anesthesia. However, a careful analysis led to the conclusion that the patient felt no pain, although she complained. It was enough to apply a mask with a few drops of ether to calm her completely". "*The results, being the first obtained with this technique, are considered sufficiently satisfactory to justify further research*".

The work, published in March 1921, is an example that any innovation in the development of humankind, whether in medicine or other fields, not only needs to be discovered but also communicated to the world for validation and adoption by the scientific community.

However, the lack of translation of the study into other languages, especially English, and the absence of its presentation at international congresses—then a rare occurrence—along with the short period between its publication, the intense life of its author, and his untimely death, limited the dissemination of the technique and its recognition with the name of its creator.

Therefore, it was the Italian surgeon Achille Mario Dogliotti (1897–1966) who, unaware—like the rest of the medical world at the time—of Fidel Pagés' discovery, described in 1931 epidural anesthesia via the lumbar spine, a technique that soon spread throughout Europe [6]. Dogliotti, professor of surgery in Modena, Catania, and later in Turin, was a great innovator in Italian surgery. His contributions included the development of one of the first heart-lung machines, the pioneering use of radiography for the biliary tract, and the organization of the first blood bank in Italy. He also lectured extensively, especially in England, where he spread his ideas, and became president of the International College of Surgeons.

From the discovery of epidural anesthesia by Pagés in November 1920 until its worldwide diffusion by Dogliotti in 1931, a ten-year period of obscurity elapsed. During this time, only a few advances were made, such as the reading of the paper "Anestesia metamérica" by the Argentine surgeon Alberto Gutiérrez and the timid attempts of Juan Robledo Sanz, anaesthsiologist in 1922. Gutiérrez, a surgeon and anesthesiologist at the Hospital Español in Buenos Aires, stood out for his anatomical studies and surgical innovations. Founder of the Revista Argentina de Anestesia y Analgesia, when he read Dogliotti's publication on epidural anesthesia, he remembered having studied Pagés' work years before. Therefore, in 1933, he vindicated Pagés' figure, publishing his experience with epidural anesthesia and his contribution to the approach to the epidural space via the hanging drop method.

His experience in dissecting cadavers allowed him to study in detail the anatomy of the spinal column, in particular the epidural and subarachnoid spaces, the arrangement of the nerve roots, and their relationship with the position of each vertebra. In his work, Gutiérrez stated that a surgeon intending to operate under regional or local anesthesia must have a thorough knowledge of topographical anatomy, be patient and calm, and manipulate the tissues with delicacy. Thanks to these qualities, he achieved excellent surgical results.

In May 1932, Gutiérrez presented his preliminary studies on metameric anesthesia in a clinical surgical class for medical students and colleagues [7]. During his presentation, he briefly reviewed previous reports by Pagés (1920) and Dogliotti (1931), explained the anatomy of the spine, and pointed out the differences between intradural and extradural injection of local anesthetics. After this presentation, most of his assistants and other colleagues in Buenos Aires began to apply the technique of epidural anesthesia.

Of the 12,000 surgeries he performed, 6000 were done under epidural or spinal anesthesia. A gynecologist from his team, Vicente Ruiz, published this experience in English, which allowed it to be read in the United States by Charles Odom from New Orleans. Odom visited Gutiérrez and Ruiz in Buenos Aires and contributed to the spread of the technique through his colleague Peter Graffagnino from Charity Hospital in Louisiana, who began performing the first caesarean sections with epidural anesthesia.

Dogliotti later became aware of Fidel Pagés' work on metameric or epidural anesthesia and publicly acknowledged him as the true initiator of the technique.

Works on War Experiences

His scientific output includes articles on war surgery and civil surgery [8].

His studies on war surgery are numerous. The study entitled "*Treatment of Diaphyseal Fractures of the Long Bones of the Extremities Caused by Firearm Projectiles*", published in the *Revista de Sanidad Militar* in 1914, received a special military mention.

His contributions to war surgery include works such as "*Traumatic Shock*," "*On the Existence of a Hypersonorous Paravertebral Space in Tension Pneumothorax*," "*Transcerebral Drainage*," and, above all, "*War Abdominal Wounds: My Personal Experience*" published in the *Revista Española de Cirugía* in two parts: the first in 1922 and the second, posthumously, in 1923. This latter study stands out for its description of 50 cases of open abdominal trauma due to gunshot wounds, treated by the author during the Melilla war campaign in 1921 [9].

In his analysis, he details the organization of a field hospital in wartime conditions and addresses doctrinal questions about the surgeon's approach to open abdominal wounds. Although the theoretical debate on emergency laparotomy had been considered settled since the First World War, there remained strong resistance from those who advocated surgical abstention. The author explains each case in detail, describing the surgical technique used, and is noted for his didactic clarity both in the surgical procedures and in preoperative preparation and postoperative care. He goes into great detail from the methodical exploration of the abdomen to the technical particularities for each type of lesion.

Finally, he compares his results, which reflect a 48% overall survival rate, breaking them down according to the type of injury, and contrasts them with data published in the world medical literature.

Work on Cancer

It is known that in 1913, he translated from German the work "*Tratamiento Incruento de los Tumores*" (Bloodless Treatment of Tumours), although no complete copy or reference has been found. His article "*Contribution to the Study of Plastic Surgery of the Cheek*", published in 1911, addresses the reconstruction of this area following injuries of various etiologies. In his analysis of maxillofacial reconstruction treatments, he emphasizes the importance of tracheal intubation, either blind or with the aid of Flagg's laryngoscope, to enable the use of the Meltzer-Auer technique, thus preventing asphyxia in patients undergoing highly hemorrhagic procedures.

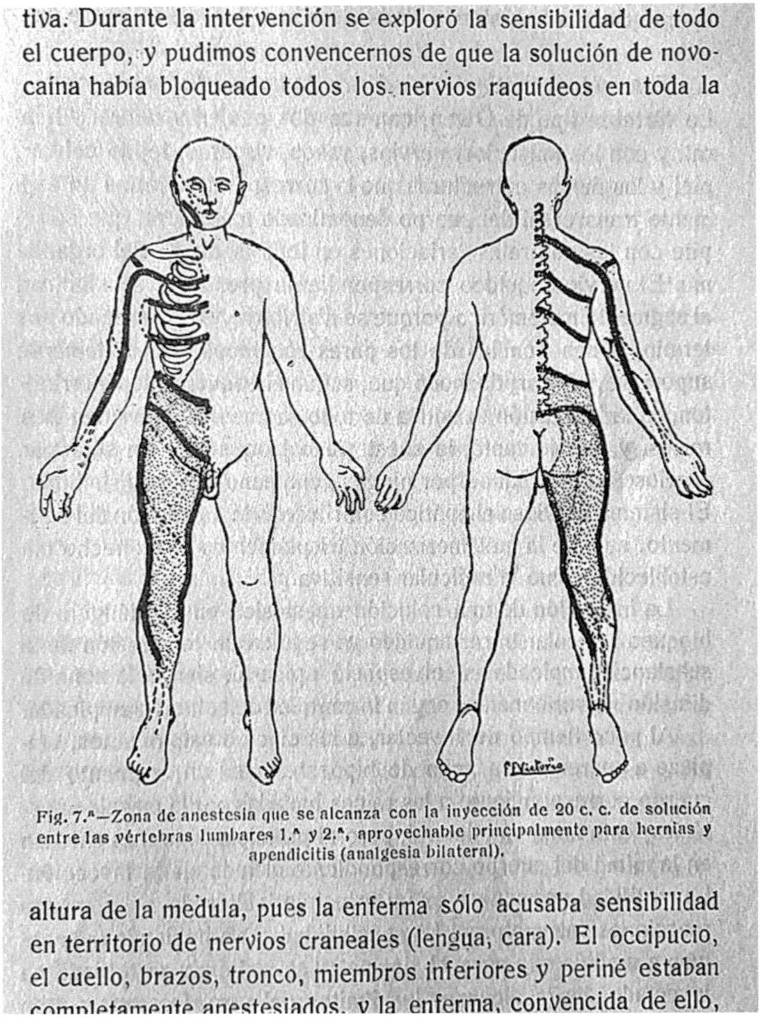

tiva. Durante la intervención se exploró la sensibilidad de todo el cuerpo, y pudimos convencernos de que la solución de novocaína había bloqueado todos los nervios raquídeos en toda la

Fig. 7.ª—Zona de anestesia que se alcanza con la inyección de 20 c. c. de solución entre las vértebras lumbares 1.ª y 2.ª, aprovechable principalmente para hernias y apendicitis (analgesia bilateral).

altura de la medula, pues la enferma sólo acusaba sensibilidad en territorio de nervios craneales (lengua, cara). El occipucio, el cuello, brazos, tronco, miembros inferiores y periné estaban completamente anestesiados, y la enferma, convencida de ello,

Fig. 9.10 Areas anaesthetised with the epidural anaesthesia (*anestesia metamérica)*

Works on General Surgery

He also published numerous studies on various surgical topics, including: the treatment of olecranon fractures, arteritis of the subclavian artery, diffuse infections of the hand, gastroenterostomy with an epiploic collar, and the use of fasciae in surgery. His final work, published posthumously, "*Surgical Aspects of Constipation*", provides a detailed description of this pathology, its methods of investigation, and the consequences of chronic constipation, considering it a state of general chronic intoxication of intestinal origin [12].

In this work, he discusses various causes of constipation, such as a mobile cecum or chronic appendicitis, which are treated by cecopexy or appendectomy; colonoptosis of the transverse colon, treated by Bier-style mesocolplication; and adhesions in the splenic flexure and descending colon, treated by Payr-style bypass between the transverse colon and the sigmoid colon. However, he also identifies a group of patients with severe essential constipation, in whom the causes described above are not found, thereby raising the need for surgical intervention.

The author discusses two possible procedures: the Senn and Salzer operation, which involves an anastomosis between the ileum and sigmoid, effectively functioning as a large bowel resection with the associated risks of preserving the colon in situ; and total colectomy with ileorectal anastomosis, a procedure he performed on three patients. He concludes that the best results are achieved with wide and early colectomies, emphasizing that partial colon resections are less effective than total colectomies. Furthermore, he addresses the challenges of colon surgery and outlines the principles of successful anastomosis.

This work is one of the few significant contributions to the study of constipation and colectomies in the medical literature, following Arbuthnot Lane's pioneering 1908 study on colectomy as a treatment for intractable constipation. Through this research, we gain insight into a surgeon who is both meticulous and dedicated to the comprehensive resolution of the problems he investigates.

Legacy

In Fidel Pagés' time, ether or chloroform anesthesia was administered by nurses, nuns, medical staff, or medical students. However, Pagés, with his profound understanding of spinal anatomy and anesthetic techniques, was uniquely positioned to make his groundbreaking discovery. His knowledge, coupled with the pressing need for pain-free surgery, provided him with the ideal conditions to innovate. His ambition to solve complex problems, organize information, and connecting concepts to innovate.

Pagés documented his findings in great detail, though he did not succeed in widely disseminating them to the international medical community. Today, it is our responsibility to ensure that his work receives the recognition it deserves. Pagés worked under challenging conditions in an unstable environment—during the years between 1909 and 1923, he practiced in six different locations. Nevertheless, his innovation and meticulous descriptions of surgical procedures continue to serve as a reference for future generations.

The legacy of Fidel Pagés offers many valuable lessons. He provides a window into the life of a Spanish military and civilian surgeon, a figure who remains relatively unrecognized in his homeland, though his recognition is steadily increasing, particularly among anesthesiologists. Pagés is the discoverer of a method of anesthesia that is now a routine part of surgical practice worldwide [10–12].

It is worth noting that, in 1955, the Asociación de Anestesiólogos de Barcelona published Pagés' full article in its journal, *Hypnos.* Additionally, the Fidel Pagés Military Hospital in Melilla and a classroom named after him at the Escuela de Sanidad Militar in Madrid bear his name. However, few in these institutions are fully aware of who Pagés was or the lasting impact of his legacy. His name lives on in streets, health centers, and his biography, available on Wikipedia in both Spanish and English.

References

1. Faulconer A, Keys TE. Foundations of anesthesiology. Springfield: C. C. Thomas; 1965.
2. De Lange JJ, Cuesta MA, Cuesta de Pedro A. Fidel Pagés Miravé (1886–1923). The Pioneer of lumbar epidural Anaesthesia. Anaesthesia. 1994;49:429–31.
3. de la Mata Pagés R. Fidel Pagés: discoverer of epidural anaesthesia. Dendra Médica. J Humanit. 2010;9:104–9.
4. Pagés F. Metameric anaesthesia. Rev Esp Cir. 1921;3:281–306.
5. López Álvarez S, Casas Reza P, del Río Fernández S. History of epidural anaesthesia: Fidel Pagés Miravé. 2021;MPJ.1:45–50.
6. Dogliotti AM. Research and clinical observations on spinal anesthesia: with special reference to the peridural technique. Curr Res Anaesth Analg. 1933;12:59–65.
7. Gutierrez A. Epidural metameric anaesthesia. Bol Asoc Med Bahia Blanca. 1933;16:791–3.
8. Velázquez Rivera, I (2011). Aproximación a la obra científica del Comandante médico Fidel Pagés Miravé. Sanidad Militar. 2011;67- suppl.1.
9. Pagés F. War wounds of the abdomen. My personal experience. Rev Esp Cir. 1922;10–12:419–77.
10. Chinn G, Gray AT, Larson MD. Overcoming obstacles: the legacy of Fidel Pagés, founder of the epidural, 100 years after his passing. Anaesth Analg. 2025;138:475–9.
11. Senovilla M One hundred years WITHOUT PAIN. Revista Española de Defensa. 2020.
12. Pagés F. Aspecto quirúrgico del estreñimiento. Rev.Esp.Cir. 1923; 8:363-382.

10

Santiago Ramón y Cajal and the Spanish Neurological School

Fernando de Castro Soubriet

Santiago Ramón y Cajal (1852–1934) holds a prominent place in the history of science. Widely regarded as the father of modern neuroscience, his groundbreaking work revolutionized our understanding of the nervous system and laid the foundation for the development of this discipline, pushing the boundaries of knowledge fifty to a hundred years ahead of his time (Fig. 10.1).

F. de Castro Soubriet (✉)
Myelin Dynamics & Repair Lab, Madrid, Spain

Centro de Neurociencias, Cajal-CSIC (former Instituto Cajal), Madrid, Spain

M. A. Cuesta, F. Mateo Vallejo (eds.), *Spain's Journey in Medicine*,
https://doi.org/10.1007/978-3-032-12221-6_10

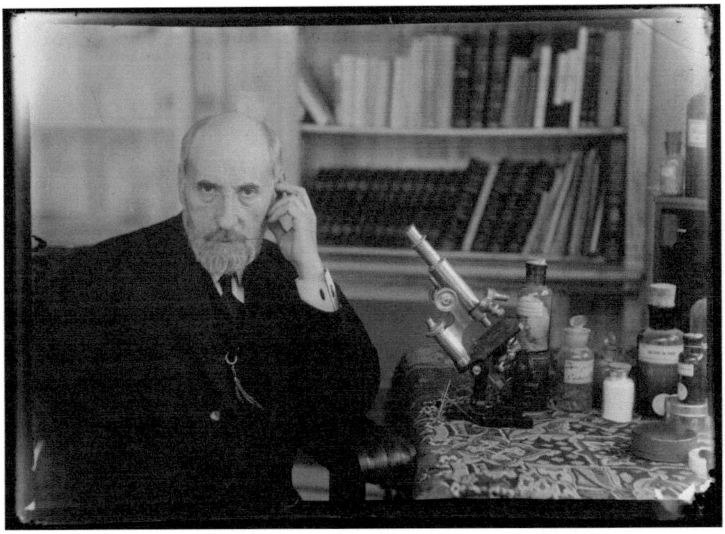

Fig. 10.1 Santiago Ramón y Cajal. (Legado Cajal, MNCN, Madrid)

Early Years and Education

Born on May 1, 1852, in Petilla de Aragón (Navarre), Ramón y Cajal showed an insatiable curiosity about the natural world from a young age. His father, a barber-surgeon and rural healer, was a man of determination who earned a medical degree in 1862 and eventually became a university professor in Zaragoza. He also played a crucial role in steering his son toward a career in medicine.

After earning his medical degree in Zaragoza in 1873, Cajal joined the army as a medical officer, serving in the Third Carlist War (mainly in the Lérida and Pyrenees fronts) and later in Cuba (1974–75) during the Ten Years' War in the province of Camaguey. While in the Cuban jungle, he contracted a severe case of malaria and was repatriated to Spain in June 1875, in critical condition. Perhaps the most valuable outcome of that harsh experience was that it allowed him to save enough money to purchase his first microscope, microtome, chemical reagents and dyes, making his first laboratory.

Thanks to his naturally strong constitution, the support of his family, and the healthy climate of the Pyrenees, Cajal was fully recovered. He then took the opportunity to begin studying anatomy in Zaragoza as an assistant to his father, Justo Ramón Casasús. In 1877, he went on to earn his doctorate at the Central University of Madrid.

Histology was at that time a compulsory subject for the doctoral degree, and it captivated Cajal—especially under the guidance of Aureliano Maestre de San Juan (1828–1890), a pioneer of the discipline in Spain. Maestre de San

Juan supervised Cajal's doctoral thesis, titled "Pathogenesis of Inflammation", with which he earned his doctorate on June 26, 1877. This work can be considered the true starting point of Santiago Ramón y Cajal's scientific career.

After several years in Zaragoza, where he served as Director of the Anatomical Museums at the Faculty of Medicine, and during which—already married to Silveria Fañanás García (1879–1930)—he deepened his knowledge of the chemical foundations of photography (even creating a small-scale industry for producing photographic plates) and obtained the chair of Descriptive Anatomy at the University of Valencia in 1883 (Fig. 10.2).

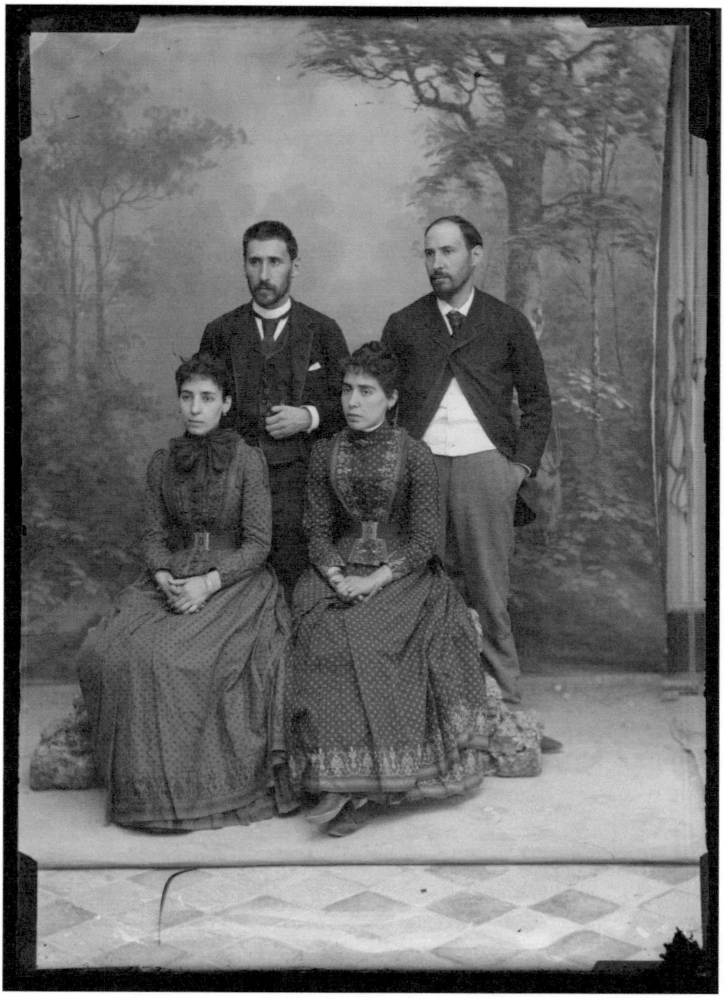

Fig. 10.2 Santiago Ramón y Cajal with his two sisters (Pabla and Jorja) and brother Pedro. (Legado Cajal, MNCN, Madrid)

From those joyful years in Valencia, one notable episode was Cajal's involvement in the 1885 cholera epidemic. In recognition of his work, the Zaragoza Provincial Council gifted him his first high-quality microscope—a Zeiss monocular—which would prove fundamental in his research on the nervous system.

During a trip to Madrid as part of an academic examination board, Cajal was introduced to the Golgi staining technique by the neuropsychiatrist Luis Simarro Lacabra (1851–1922). Cajal was instantly captivated by the striking, intricate shapes of nervous system cells stained with silver chromate. There was no turning back. Determined to master this histological method—known in Italian as the "reazione nera"—Cajal revived a technique that had been largely forgotten since Camillo Golgi (1843–1926) first published it in 1873 (Fig. 10.3).

Many of the most highly regarded histologists of the time had, over those fourteen years, abandoned Golgi's technique due to its inconsistency. For many, it could not even be considered a true scientific "method" because of the erratic and inconsistent images it produced. But Cajal, captivated and undeterred, drew on his deep understanding of chemistry—particularly photographic chemistry—to adapt and improve the technique, making it more reliable and systematic.

He refined the fixation process and introduced a second phase of silver impregnation, which helped reduce the unpredictability of Golgi's reazione nera (we never know which or how many cells will be stained in a given histological section). Most importantly, these adjustments significantly enhanced the staining of nerve cells themselves, allowing their structures and connections to be observed with far greater clarity—an improvement that would prove crucial to Cajal's later discoveries.

Golgi's method works by depositing silver salts onto fixed, emulsified tissue in such a way that it "draws" the outline of a cell and the intricate arborization of its extensions—much like how silver salts in classical photography are oxidized by light and deposited onto an emulsion. It's no coincidence, then, that Golgi's technique has also been called the "photographic method."

Cajal also discovered that the silver impregnation stopped precisely where the myelin sheaths began to encase the axons. This insight led him to apply the Golgi method to tissue from very young animals, including embryos, in which myelination had not yet occurred. In doing so, he succeeded in staining entire axons—from the soma (cell body) to their synaptic targets. This adaptation, known as the ontogenetic or embryological method, enabled Cajal to make some of his most fundamental and revealing discoveries about the structure and function of the nervous system.

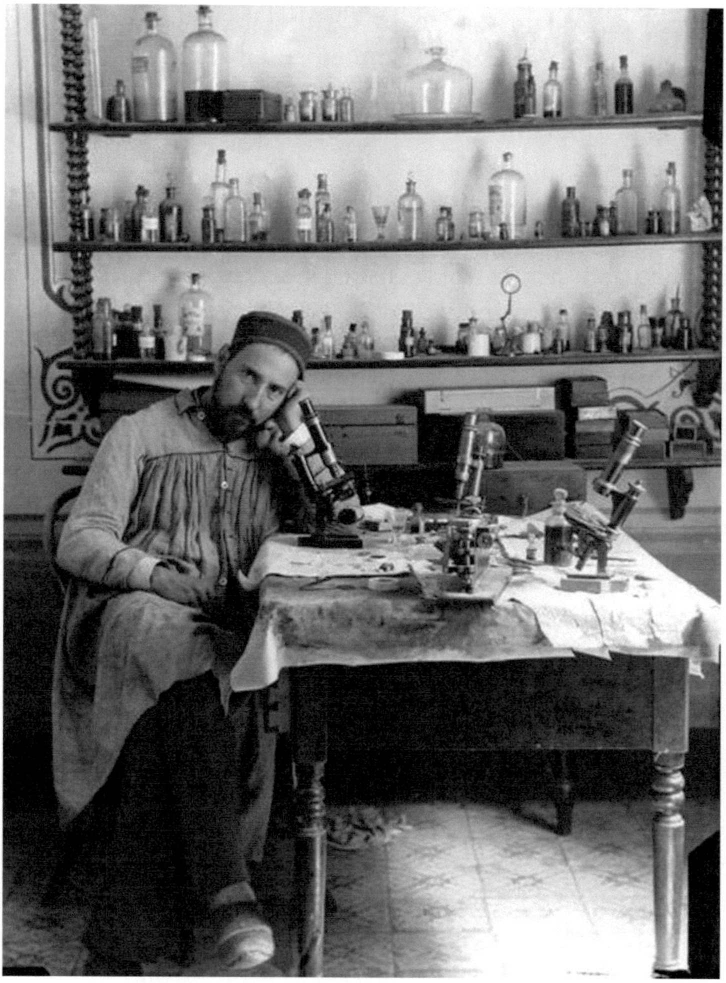

Fig. 10.3 Cajal in Valencia (1884–1887). Self-portrait taken in the Laboratory in his own home during his time in Valencia. Note his right hiding the shutter release cable of the camera. (Legado Cajal, MNCN, Madrid)

"My Peak Year, My Year of Fortune": Cajal Revolutionises Science with Neuronal Theory

On December 12, 1887, Cajal assumed the position of Professor of Histology, Histochemistry, and Pathological Anatomy at the University of Barcelona, whose Faculty of Medicine was housed in the building that now serves as the headquarters of the *Reial Acadèmia de Medicina de Catalunya*. From the moment of his arrival in Barcelona, Cajal systematically applied the new staining method to the nervous systems of various vertebrate species.

A torrent of groundbreaking findings began to emerge almost immediately from the modest laboratory he had set up in his own home. "My excessive scientific productivity in 1888 compels me to publish a micrographic journal," Cajal wrote. And indeed, he did everything himself—and funded it: conducting the experiments, hand-drawing the illustrations that summarized his key findings and "constructed" entire sequences on a single plane to reveal the relationships between individual nerve cells, editing and publishing the *Revista Trimestral Micrográfica*, and even handling its postal distribution.

From his very first article—focused on the structure of the cerebellar cortex—Cajal made a fundamental observation: the individuality of nerve cells (Fig. 10.4).

> ... *the collateral and terminal ramifications of all axon-cylinder* [what we know today as axon] *terminate in the grey substance, not by means of a diffuse network, as Gerlach and Golgi defended with the majority of neurologists, but by means of free arborizations), arranged in a variety of forms (pericellular baskets or nests, climbing branches, etc.). These ramifications are intimately applied to the body and dendrites of the nerve cells, establishing a contact or articulation between the receptor protoplasm and the last axonal branchlets (ramuncles)* [what we have known since 1897, thanks to Charles S. Sherrington, as synapses] [1].

This discovery—along with subsequent findings in the retina and spinal cord—brought light to the field of nervous system histology, which at the time was overshadowed by the prevailing dominance of the so-called reticularists. Nearly all leading specialists explained the nervous system as a continuous network of cellular extensions or, at least, of the neurofibrils of the cytoskeleton. This Reticular Theory had been formulated by the German anatomist Joseph von Gerlach (1820–1896) in 1871.

In each new issue of his journal, Cajal expanded his observations to more neural structures, repeatedly refuting the core tenets of reticularism. In doing so, he provided empirical support to the few scientists—only A. Forel, W. His, and a young, little-known neurohistologist named Fridtjof Nansen—who believed that the Cell Theory should apply to the brain just as it had been accepted for other organs since the mid-nineteenth century, thanks to the pioneering work of Matthias Schleiden, Theodor Schwann, and Rudolf Virchow.

But in the context of nineteenth-century Spain—a country then mired in political and scientific decline—Cajal's groundbreaking work emerged from a

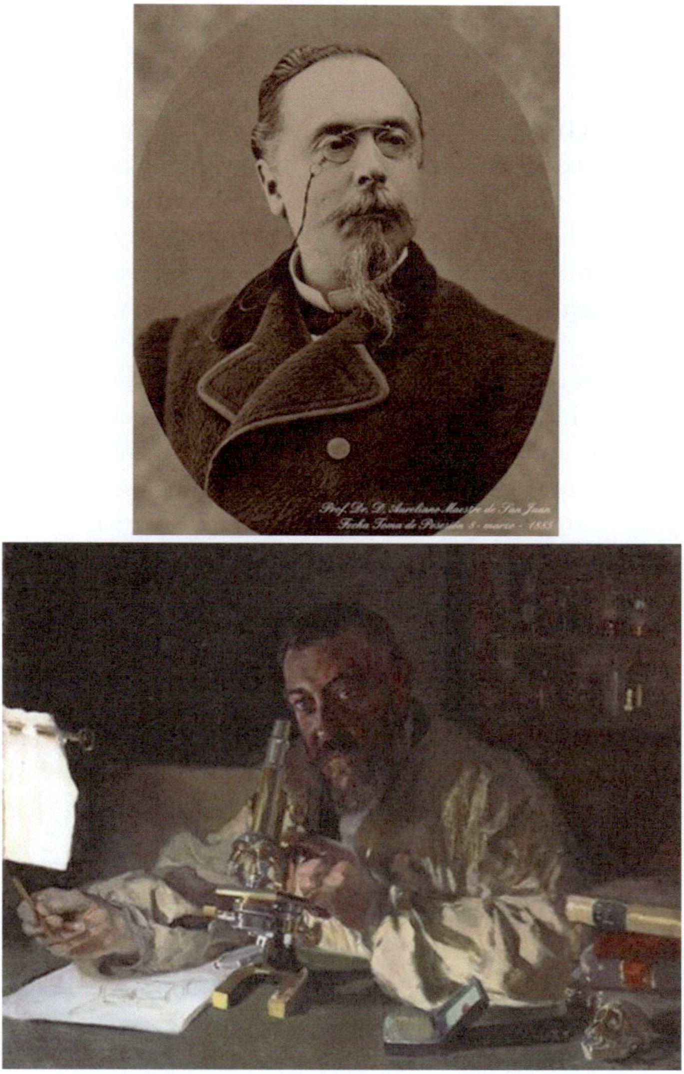

Fig. 10.4 The two teachers Cajal in Histology. Top: Aureliano Maestre de San Juan, introducer of the Histology in Spain. Below: Luis Simarro Lacabra who taught Cajal the method of Golgi (Portrayed by Sorolla in his Laboratory in Madrid) (With permission of the Collection of Images of the Real Academia de Medicine)

provincial university and was published in Spanish, a language with little relevance to the scientific vanguard of the time. Despite his tireless efforts, bold intuition, and the revolutionary nature of his findings, what real impact could his discoveries have had at that moment? In all honesty, very little.

The decisive breakthrough came at the renowned Congress of the German Anatomical Society, held in Berlin in 1889. There, the virtually unknown Cajal managed to impress the most influential histologist of the time, August Kölliker (1828–1904), who was astonished by the level of detail revealed in the remarkable histological preparations Cajal had brought from Spain—a country then considered as remote scientifically as it was geographically. "*I have discovered you, and I want to make my discovery known in Germany,*" exclaimed the astonished Kölliker—a promise he fulfilled with determination starting at that very meeting, held at Humboldt University in Berlin.

Another convert during that pivotal autumn of 1889 was the Swedish anatomist Gustav Retzius (1842–1919)—yet another providential advocate.

It is also worth noting that, from 1890 onward, Cajal's younger brother, Pedro Ramón y Cajal (1854–1950), began publishing his own research after returning from a long and perilous stay in Uruguay that had nearly cost him his life on several occasions. A graduate in Medicine from the University of Zaragoza, Pedro applied the Golgi-Cajal method to the nervous systems of amphibians, reptiles, and birds. He would go on to become, alongside Domingo Sánchez, one of the most important comparative neurohistologists of the Spanish Neurological School (Fig. 10.5).

In just four years (1888–1892), working from his modest home laboratory—located successively on Riera Alta, Carrer del Notariat, Bruch, and Consell de Cent streets—and publishing almost exclusively in Spanish, Cajal laid the foundational principles of modern neuroscience:

(a) **The individuality of nerve cells** (neurons are structurally and functionally independent units of the nervous system; 1888).
(b) **Axons terminate freely and form synapses** (contiguity space in which one neuron communicates with another; 1888);
(c) **The Law of Dynamic Polarization of Neurons** (nerve impulses travel in a defined direction within neurons—from dendrites and soma, the entry point, to the axon, the exit point—directions that Cajal was the first to illustrate using arrows; 1889–1891, with significant contributions from his brother Pedro Ramón y Cajal and some collaboration with Belgian histologist Arthur van Gehuchten.
(d) **The description of dendritic spines** (1888) and **axonal growth cones** (1889), microscopic structures essential for the formation of synaptic connections and for understanding the broader implications of the Neuron Doctrine introduced in these earlier postulates; and

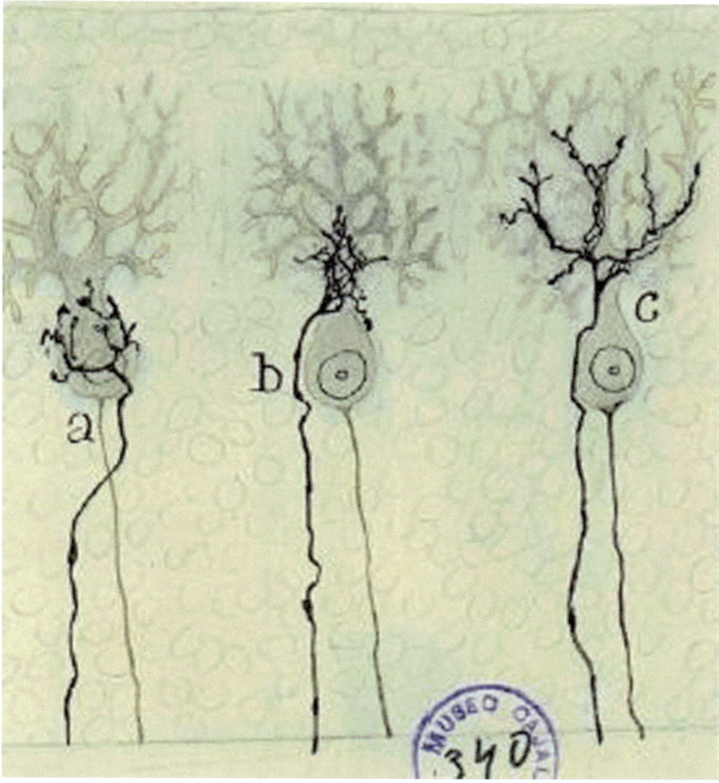

Fig. 10.5 Cajal shows this illustration of three neurons showing dendritic trees and free axons endings in the CNS. Original drawing of Cajal (1888) illustrating variants of climbing fibers forming synapses on Purkinje Cells in the cerebellar cortex. (Legado Cajal, MNCN, Madrid)

(e) **The Chemotropic Hypothesis** (axon growth cones are guided to their targets by chemical attractants and repellents; 1890–1892), a concept that took nearly a century to gain broad acceptance, finally validated with the discovery of chemotactic molecules by Marc Tessier-Lavigne and Corey Goodman (The molecular biology of axon guidance, Science 1996) (Figs. 10.6 and 10.7).

With these discoveries, Cajal not only challenged the dominant scientific paradigms of his time—he fundamentally revolutionized the study of the nervous system and opened previously unimaginable doors for understanding how the human brain works. Eric Kandel, Nobel Laureate in Physiology or Medicine (2000), summed it up succinctly and powerfully: "*Cajal taught us how to think about the brain.*"

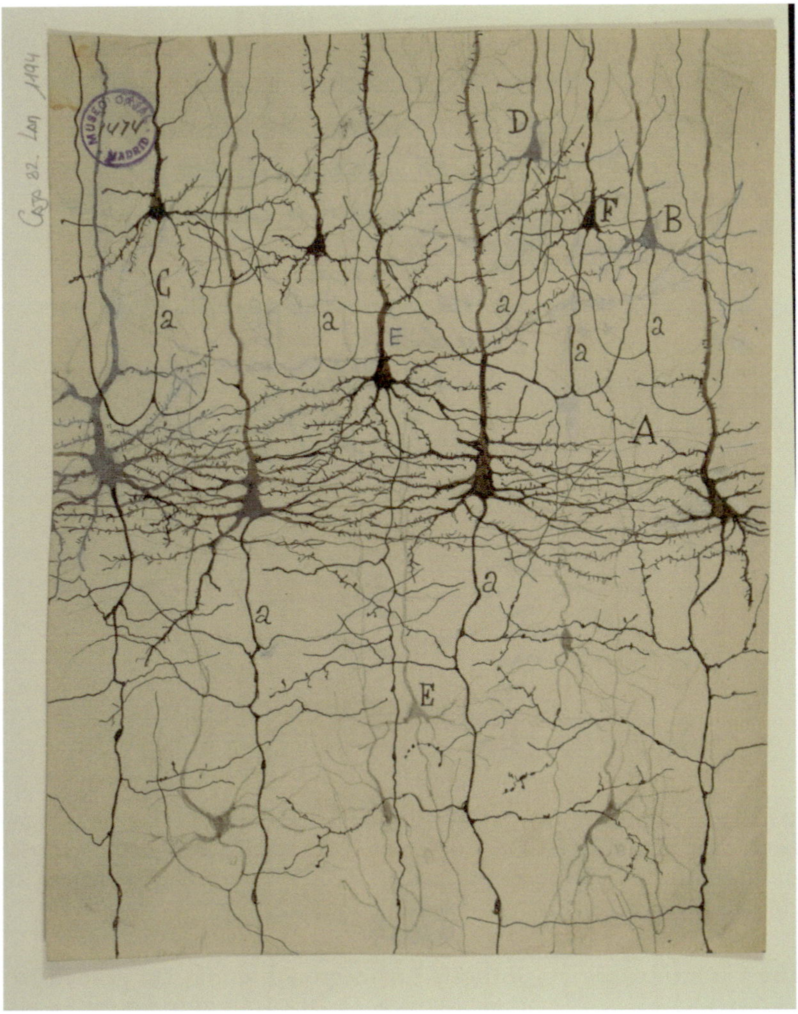

Fig. 10.6 Original drawing of Cajal, zones 5, 6, and 7 of the cat's visual cortex, showing the interconnection of neurons, displaying a complex network. (Legado Cajal, MNCN, Madrid)

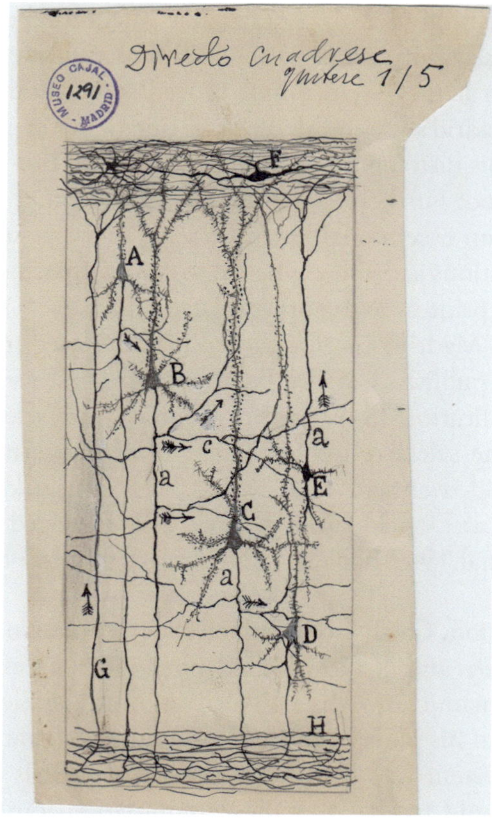

Fig. 10.7 Original drawing of Cajal (1891), illustrating with arrows the orientation followed by nerve impulses, the essence of the Law of Dynamic Polarization of Neurons (Legado Cajal, MNCN, Madrid)

Cajal, Professor in Madrid: The Major International Honors

In early 1892, Cajal was appointed to the Central University of Madrid, where he had got the chair of Embryology, Histology, and Pathological Anatomy. This was the highest academic post available in Spain at the time—at the country's most prestigious university, the only one authorized to confer doctoral degrees, and offering the best academic salaries. He would work in Madrid until his retirement in 1922, and he remained there until his death on October 17, 1934.

In Madrid, Cajal found a highly favorable intellectual climate—not only within the university but also in various cultural and scientific circles. And some details, even if they seem minor proved significant: for instance, the high quality of Madrid's water, thanks to its organoleptic properties, allowed him to optimize his histological techniques, including but not limited to the Golgi-Cajal method. Furthermore, the *Tipografía Artística* printing house in Madrid provided an exceptional level of fidelity and craftsmanship in reproducing the illustrations accompanying his work—surpassing, for decades, the quality offered by printers in major world capitals.

While based in Madrid, Cajal authored his renowned monograph on the vertebrate retina, published in the Belgian journal *La Cellule* (1893). In a lesser-known publication in 1895, he proposed that the learning process occurs through the selective reinforcement of certain synapses—a concept that, since the mid-twentieth century, has been widely known as *Hebbian learning*, though, as Donald Hebb himself acknowledged in the first paragraph of his seminal 1949 book, it should more properly be called *Cajalian learning*.

During this period, Cajal also described the phenomenon we now refer to as *neuronal plasticity*, and in 1897, he redefined in its definitive form his Law of Functional, Dynamic, or Axipetal Polarization of the Electrical Activity of Neurons. He began his pioneering studies on the degeneration and regeneration of nervous system—all before the cascade of awards and international recognition he would receive over the coming years from Italy, the United Kingdom, France, the United States, and, eventually, even from Spain itself—a country notoriously slow to honor its greatest figures, especially in the realm of science.

Among the many distinctions Cajal received, particular mention must be made of his invitation to deliver the Croonian Lecture at the Royal Society in London, honorary doctorates from the Universities of Cambridge (UK), Clark and Boston (USA), the Moscow International Prize (1890), the Helmholtz Medal (1905), and, most notably, the Nobel Prize in Physiology or Medicine (1906). He shared this last award with Camillo Golgi, despite their fundamentally opposing interpretations of nervous system organization. Remarkably, Cajal had been nominated for the Nobel every year since its inception in 1901.

During this prolific period, Cajal consolidated the majority of his discoveries in what is now considered one of the most influential scientific works of all time: *Textura del Sistema Nervioso del Hombre y los Vertebrados* (1899–1904). To facilitate international readership, it was later translated into French as *Histologie du Système Nerveux de l'Homme et des Vertébrés* (1909–1911), (Texture of the nervous system of man and vertebrates) [2–8].

It is particularly prescient in his inaugural speech on his entry as member to the Spanish Real Academia de Ciencias Exactas, Fisicas y Naturales (Royal Academy of Exact, Physical and Natural Sciences) in 1897, later published as Reglas y consejos para la investigación científica, (*Rules and Advice for Scientific Research)*, Cajal articulated a vision that, while largely overlooked at the time, it is becoming more and more important and relevant to contemporary science:

> The purest glory of a master lies not in forming disciples who merely follow him, but in shaping scholars who will surpass him. [...] To create entirely new minds, unique organs—if possible—in the machine of progress. To manufacture docile and interchangeable organs shows that the teacher has cared more for himself than for his country and for Science [9].

Until that point, Cajal had worked in solitude, from his home laboratory, aided only—though always from a distance—by his beloved brother Pedro. Despite the undeniable success he achieved through this solitary effort, now with truly global resonance, Cajal never lost sight of his duty to his country, nor of the urgent need to establish a first-rate scientific school in Spain. With the funds from the Moscow International Prize, he took the significant step of launching a new journal, the *Trabajos del Laboratorio de Investigaciones Biológicas* (1901), designed to replace—and publish more regularly than—his cherished *Revista Trimestral Micrográfica*.

More importantly, this award, sent from afar, symbolized the first cornerstone upon which Cajal would realize his vision: the foundation of what we now recognize as the Spanish Neurological School, or more simply, the Cajal School [10–12] (Fig. 10.8).

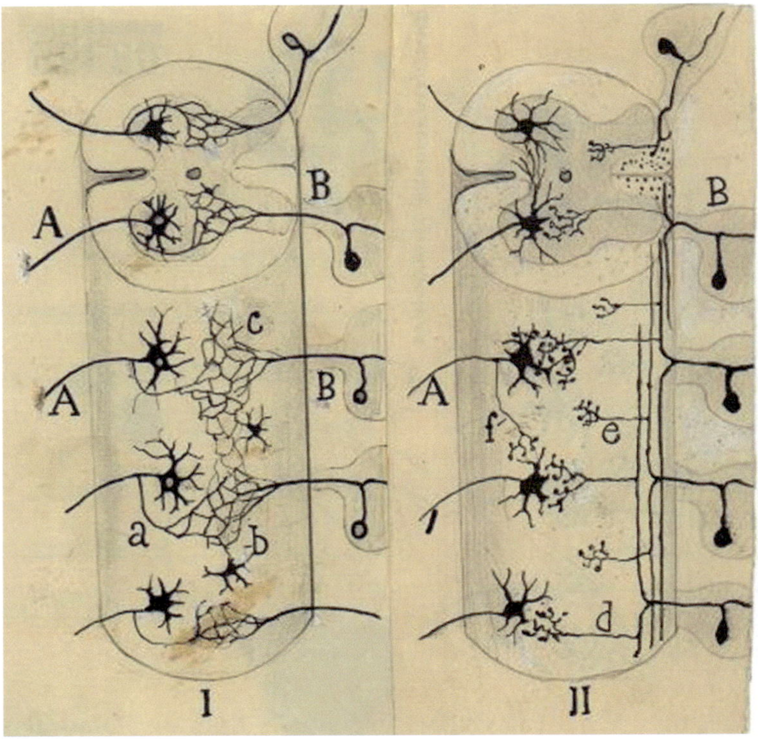

Fig. 10.8 The reticularism and the neuronism, Illustrated by Cajal (1917). On the left, schemes of afferent and efferents of the spinal cord according to the reticularists: the neurons form plexuses and there are no individual cells but a syncytium. On the right the same according to the neuronists: the neurons are individual cells connecting with others by the synapsis and the dendrites and axons are individual ending freely. (Original drawing of the Legado Cajal, MNCN, Madrid)

The Biological Research Laboratory and the Creation of His School

The young King Alfonso XIII and the political authorities of the time quickly (by our national standards) echoed the recognition coming from the capital of Tsarist Russia and decided to provide a modern, well-equipped laboratory, funded by the national budget, so that Cajal could continue his monumental task. In 1901, the Biological Research Laboratory (first known as Laboratorio de Investigaciones Biológicas which later became officially known as the Cajal Institute in 1920) opened its doors in the left wing of what is now the National Museum of Anthropology, opposite the Atocha railway station. And soon, at last, came the first permanent staff: some technical staff and, above all, Jorge Francisco Tello (1880–1958), an Aragonese who had studied Medicine at the Central University and with whom, senso stricto, the Cajal's School began in 1902. Tello remained with the Master until the retirement and subsequent death of Don Santiago (see below). Shortly afterward, Domingo Sánchez (1860–1947), a naturalist from Salamanca, repatriated from the Philippines where he worked as a zoological collector for the Museum of Natural History, before enlisting in the militia to fight against the North American Army that invaded that Spanish province in 1898, parallel to the invasion of the also Spanish Cuba and Puerto Rico. Therefore, between 1902 and 1904, Cajal already had true collaborators to achieve the titanic goal of unraveling the structure of the nervous system: we can already speak of what would later become known as the Spanish Neurohistological (or Neurological) School, more colloquially referred to as the School of Cajal or, in the style of the time, the School of Madrid. Because Cajal and his most brilliant disciples would turn the Spanish capital into a pilgrimage site for decades for anyone from anywhere in the world who wanted to learn about the nervous system, even after Cajal's death: only the outbreak of the Spanish Civil War would nip this center of knowledge in the bud.

Also as a consequence of the Moscow International Prize, Cajal presided over the 14th International Congress of Medicine, which was held in Madrid in April 1903. At the congress, Cajal presented his work on the organization of the optic thalamus, while the other star of the event, the Russian Ivan Pavlov (1849–1936), presented, for the first time, his theory of conditioned reflexes—a discovery that transformed physiology and psychology, and for which he was awarded the Nobel Prize in Physiology or Medicine the following year (1904). It is widely believed that the prominence of neurological topics at this Madrid congress marked the definitive rise of the neurosciences as a field of major global interest. With the Helmholtz Medal and the Nobel Prize, Cajal's prestige soared even higher, and he recommended to the government the creation of the Junta para la Ampliación de Estudios (JAE) (Board for the extension of studies), an organization he himself would preside over from its creation in 1907 until his death in 1934. The JAE would not only become a fundamental instrument for organizing and funding the Spanish Neurological School, but it would also evolve into a highly efficient and agile institution to promote all scientific and technological knowledge, as well as all areas of human creativity. This led to significant progress in Spain in these areas, contributing to the long-awaited modernization of Spanish science, culture, and, by extension, society as a whole.

Although overshadowed by his extensive research work, Tello is the author of pioneering studies on neurofibrils and the neurohistogenesis of the cerebral cortex. He described important structures in muscle fibers and went further than Cajal in his understanding of the regeneration of the central nervous system with his peripheral nerve implants, which are well-known today. Shortly afterward, the Franco-Belgian histologist Jules Havet (1866–1948), who would collaborate with Cajal and Domingo Sánchez until after the First World War before going on to develop an important academic and administrative career at the Université Catholique de Louvain (Belgium), made his first visit to Cajal's laboratory. The great neuropathologist from Bilbao, Nicolás Achúcarro (1880–1918), also settled in Madrid after his travels through Europe and North America in 1910. The following year, the British-Australian doctor Laura Forster (1854–1917) came from Oxford to learn neurohistological techniques and work on axon regeneration in the spinal cords of birds, replicating Cajal and Tello's experiments in mammals, and so on (Fig. 10.9).

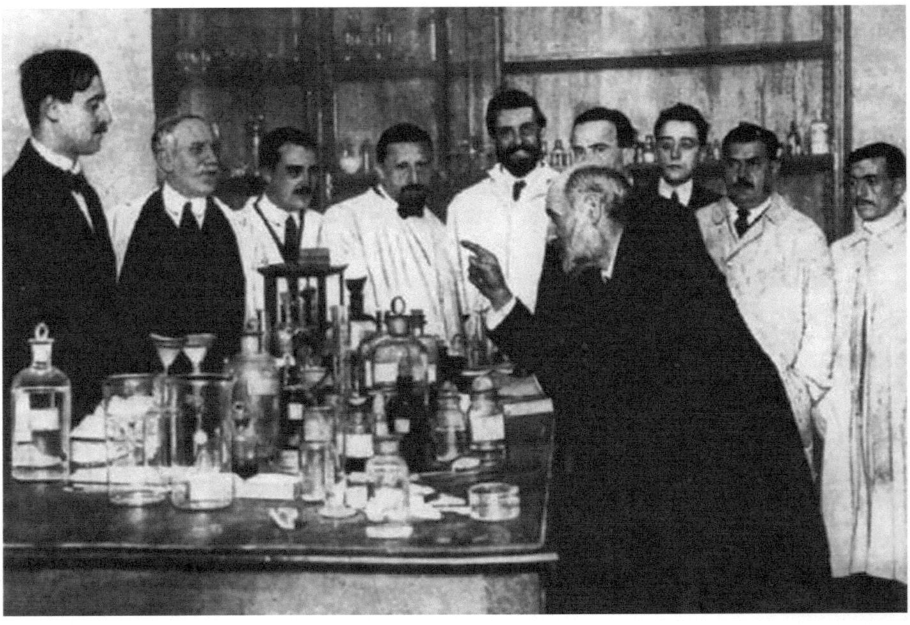

Fig. 10.9 Cajal forms School in Madrid. Photo taken in the Laboratorio de Investigaciones Biológicas, and published in 1915 by La Esfera. In the foreground, Cajal, finger raised, at the table piled with chemical reagents. In the second line, from left to right: Gonzalo R. Lafora, Domingo Sánchez, Julián Sanz-Ibáñez, Miguel Gayarre, Nicolás Achúcarro, the Brothers Sacristán (Luis Miguel and Juan de Dios), the Lab's caretaker and one of the Lab's waiters

The neurological knowledge generated by Cajal initially focused on exhaustively describing the structure of the nervous system in vertebrates (Pedro Ramón y Cajal, Tello, Río-Hortega, de Castro) and invertebrates (notably, Domingo Sánchez), as well as its normal development. With the incorporation of Achúcarro and his direct disciple, Pío del Río-Hortega (1882–1945), the Spanish Neurological School fully embraced the study of glial cells (Río-Hortega discovered two of the three fundamental types of glial cells: microglia and oligodendroglia) and neuropathology. In fact, del Río-Hortega tackled the first histogenetic classification of nervous system tumors in the second half of the 1920s, a classification that would later be adopted by the WHO when it was founded 50 years later. The School also explored purely neuropsychiatric aspects with the inclusion of Gonzalo Rodríguez Lafora (1886–1971) and José Mª Villaverde (1888–1936).

Nicolás Achúcarro's personality, his scientific expertise, and his linguistic abilities made him the natural successor to Cajal once *El Maestro* was forced to step back. However, Achúcarro died prematurely at just 38 years of age, and his death was mourned by the most prominent figures of Spanish intellectual life at the time, including Cajal, del Río-Hortega, poet Juan Ramón Jiménez, and philosopher José Ortega y Gasset. As the greatest visitors of Madrid as a world center for brain research, we should also mention the American Wilder Penfield (neuropathologist and neurosurgeon par excellence of the twentieth century, who headed the Montreal Neurological Institute) and Howard Florey (Australian pharmacologist, awarded the Nobel Prize in Physiology or Medicine in 1945 for his discovery of penicillin, but trained in histological techniques in Madrid around 1929).

Finally, the physiology that Cajal, a genius, had intuited and pointed out with his famous arrows was further developed by the last two "senior" disciples, the youngest and closest to Cajal in the last decade of his life: Fernando de Castro (1896–1967) and Rafael Lorente de Nó (1902–1990). Although trained as histologists in the sympathetic and auditory systems, respectively, it was they who introduced physiological methods (experimental neurosurgery, electrophysiology, etc.) and a fully physiological orientation of the School. We dedicate a chapter specifically to Fernando de Castro in this book (see Chapter XIII) (Figs. 10.10 and 10.11).

The young specialist in histology and the organization of the auditory system, Lorente de Nó, completed his studies on the vestibular system with Robert Bárány (Nobel Prize in Physiology or Medicine in 1914) in Sweden. After a brief stay at the Casa de Salud de Valdecilla as an otorhinolaryngologist and researcher, he accepted an invitation in 1931 to settle in the United States: first, in St. Louis, Missouri, and later, in 1936, at Rockefeller University

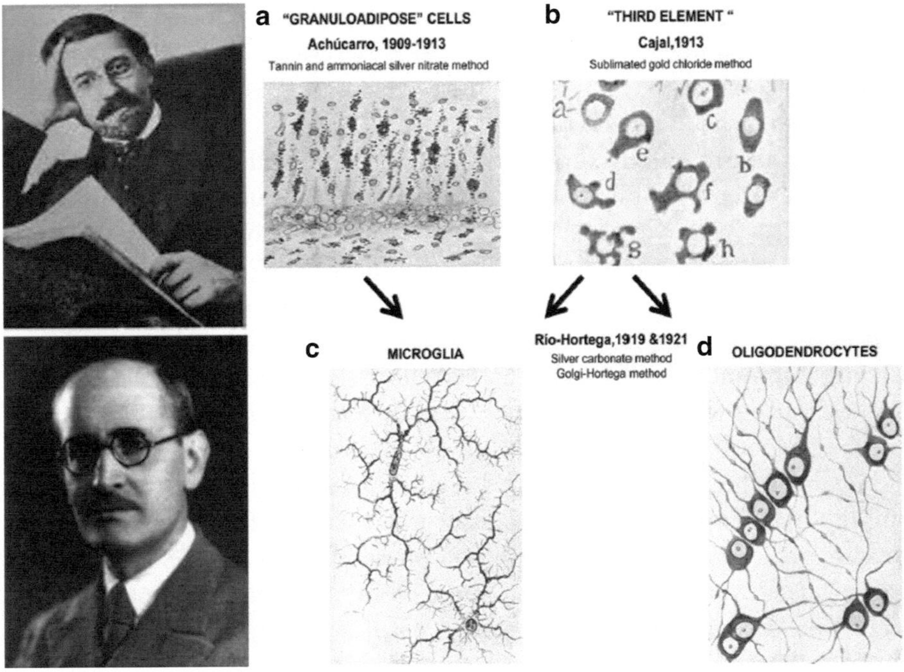

Fig. 10.10 Anatomical diagram showing the historical development of neuroglial cell identification. Achúcarro, Río-Hortega and the discovery of the oligodendroglia and the microglia. On the top left: Nicolás Achúcarro (ca. 1916; original photo in the Scientific Archive Fernando de Castro –Madrid)- and below, Pío del Río-Hortega (Permission of the Collection of Images of RANM). On the right summary-sequence of the Discovery of the two types of glial cells, as true components of the third element of the CNS as described by Cajal, (adapted from Tremblay, et al., 2015). (Original drawing, Fernando de Castro, (Madrid)

in New York. After retiring in 1972, he moved to UCLA. Lorente de Nó dominated the world of neurophysiology in the 1940s and 1950s, years during which he was a perennial candidate for the Nobel Prize. His descriptions of the first recurrent circuits in the nervous system were fundamental to the birth of cybernetics. In the shadow of the Manhattan Project and the first atomic bombs, the contributions of Norbert Wiener, Julian Bigelow, Warren McCulloch, Walter Pitts, Arturo Rosenblueth, and Lorente de Nó formed the group known as The Cybernetics, which was crucial for the development of the so-called "von Neumann architecture," the foundation for modern computers [13].

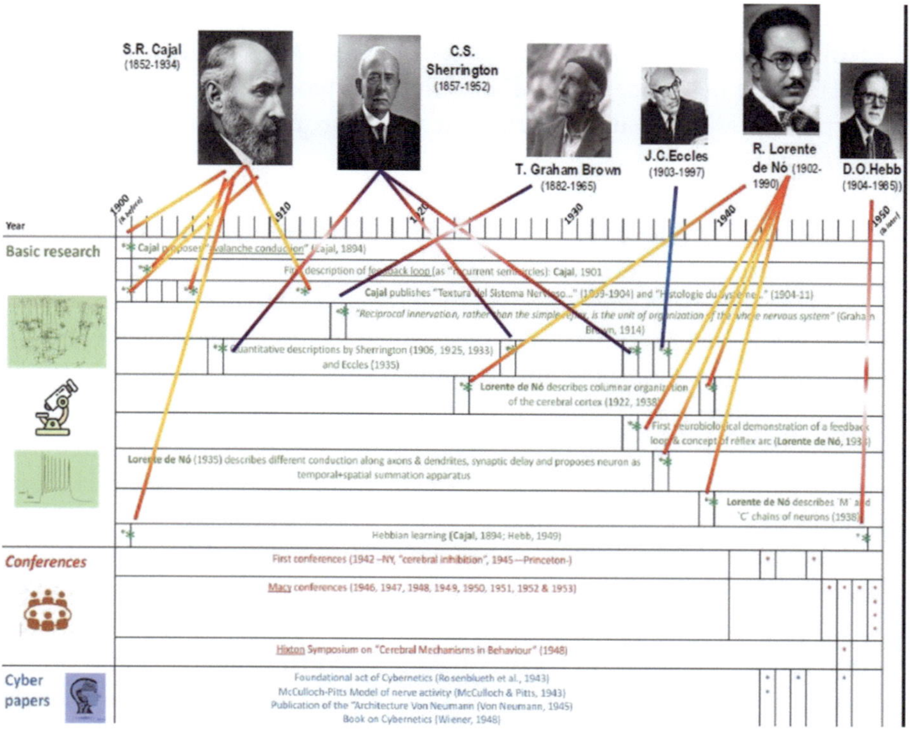

Fig. 10.11 Timeline flow chart of the neuroscientific discoveries that paved the way for the birth of Cybernetics from 1850 to 1950. The chart includes images of notable scientists with lines connecting them to their contributions, Cajal contributions were very early (1888–1914) and passed on mainly by his direct disciple Rafael Lorente de Nó, who also made relevant discoveries in this respect in the 1930s. (Adapted from: Espinosa-Sánchez et al., 2025)

Global Impact of Cajal's Discoveries and His School, beyond Neuroscience

All these direct disciples of Cajal contributed significantly to confirming the Master's findings, each focusing their studies on the orientations or structures that most interested them, freely, but always involved in the scientific battle that the reticularists were determined to maintain until the arrival of the electron microscope in the 1950s. The list of discoveries generated in or from Madrid up until the ill-fated summer of 1936, the Civil War, is impossible to include here, but we will highlight two key points as general characteristics:

A. Practically all the major discoveries made by Cajal, and his direct disciples remain valid today, even with the enormous technological advances. This is a rare feat in science, where discoveries are almost always transient truths, surpassed by others made with better tools or more accurate and intelligent methods.
B. In barely three decades of relative institutional and financial stability, despite wars, global crises, pandemics, and changes in political regimes in Spain, three of Cajal's direct disciples came close to winning a second, third, or fourth Nobel Prize in Physiology or Medicine before Severo Ochoa received his in 1959. The history of Spanish science would have to be rewritten in a radically different way if the Nobel had been awarded to del Río-Hortega in 1929 or 1937, de Castro in 1938, or Lorente de Nó in 1949, 1950, 1952, or 1953...! The list would be even longer if we included some of Cajal's indirect disciples, such as the aforementioned Howard Florey (1898–1968, who shared the 1945 Nobel Prize "for the discovery of penicillin and its curative effect on various infectious diseases"), Wilder S. Penfield (1891–1976), Rita Levi-Montalcini (1909–2012, Nobel Prize in 1986 "for her discovery of growth factors"), who always emphasized not only Cajal's scientific influence but also the fundamental role Cajal and de Castro played in the release of the great Italian histologist Giuseppe Levi from Mussolini's regime. Levi, nominated for the Nobel Prize and mentor to three prize-winning scientists—Salvatore Luria, Renato Dulbecco, and Levi-Montalcini herself)—credited Cajal and de Castro with being pivotal to his freedom. Additionally, the recent Nobel Prize winners John Hopfield and Geoffrey Hinton (Nobel Prize in Physics 2024), and David Baker, Demis Hassabis, and John M. Jumper (Nobel Prize in Chemistry 2024) have openly acknowledged that without neuromorphic models of neural networks and artificial intelligence, they would not have been able to make their major discoveries.

Another fundamental pillar of modern neuroscience, Charles Sherrington, winner of the Nobel Prize in Physiology or Medicine in 1932, described it in an unmatched way in 1935, in the obituary he published in the *Bulletin of the Royal Society* upon Cajal's death:

> "It is no exaggeration to say that he [Cajal], together with his disciples, especially Achúcarro [sic], Río-Hortega [sic], and de Castro, opened a new era of knowledge." [...] "It was an early ambition for him to create a Spanish school of science. No one, never, has done such great research on a more individual basis as he [Cajal] did in his early days. But as the years went by, if ever a scientist created a school, it was Cajal—a school of colleagues and disciples" [14].

Cajal created a school, and then almost every one of his direct disciples did so in turn, most notably del Río-Hortega, who was able to establish his own school in his laboratory at the Residencia de Estudiantes, as well as at the Instituto Nacional del Cáncer (National Cancer Institute). Outside Madrid, he also founded schools in Oxford and Buenos Aires. If Cajal directly founded modern neuroscience, he and his Spanish disciples transformed neurology, psychiatry, neurophysiology, and were fundamental to the birth of cybernetics, neural networks, artificial intelligence, and modern neuro-oncology. For all these reasons, UNESCO decided in October 2017 to include the "Archives of Santiago Ramón y Cajal and the Spanish School of Neurohistology" in the Memory of the World Register as part of the World Heritage (Collection ID: 2016-31).

> *These archives* [those of Santiago Ramón y Cajal, his brother Pedro Ramón y Cajal, Pío del Río-Hortega, Fernando de Castro and Rafael Lorente de Nó] *are essential for studying the history of the discoveries and theories that lead to our current understanding of the human brain in its double aspect of anatomical composition (individual cells) and physiological properties (formation of circuits and propagation of the nervous impulse).*

To date, the group of scientists thus distinguished by UNESCO is truly select: Copernicus, Linnaeus, Newton, Darwin, Pasteur, Tesla... and Cajal and his School. In fact, the School is considered exceptional by UNESCO. It is rare for the personality of such great geniuses to be compatible with the formation of brilliant disciples who grow and develop without their scientific roots mutually drying up. Cajal knew how to do it, and so did the aforementioned members of the Spanish Neurological School.

He was also an extraordinary writer on a variety of topics, such as his books about his life, old age and its difficulties, conversation with people in a café, and his advice to young people with a desire to research and innovate. These are all of them, true gems to read translated in to English! [15–18].

Legacy

Santiago Ramón y Cajal was not only a brilliant scientific pioneer; he was also a visionary with a deep faith in the transformative power of knowledge. His legacy, which includes the creation of an unparalleled scientific school in biomedicine, reminds us that investing in science and innovation is an urgent necessity for any society that aspires to development and true progress.

However, much remains to be done to preserve this legacy within the Spanish context and to make it known to future generations and the world.

As Cajal himself pointed out: "If we are disdained, we end up being disdained." That is why it is not only fair but also necessary that the promised Cajal Museum and School be brought to life—NOW!

The Royal Decree for the foundation of the Cajal Museum was enacted iin June 2024. It is still pending to give it a definitive installation and form, content and budget to be approved to put it into action in order to make the not so-distant examples of Cajal and his School our own so that they can serve as inspiration and continuity for the new generations. As scientists and as civil society, it is our responsibility to respect and not disdain each other. Today's elites, today's students, our entire society, must make it their own to support the Spanish R&D (research and development) system as a fundamental source of present and future wealth and well-being. This is especially important in the current circumstances, in a complex world that has already understood this and is rapidly demanding new scientific and technical knowledge at an accelerated pace.

References

1. Shepherd GM. Foundations of the neuron doctrine (history of neuroscience). New York: Oxford University Press; 1991.
2. Cajal SR. On the nerve fibres of the molecular layer of the cerebellum. Q J Normal Pathol Histol. 1888;1:33–49.
3. Cajal SR. Textura del Sistema Nervioso del Hombre y los Vertebrados. 3 volumes. Madrid: Imprenta y Librería de Nicolás Moya; 1899–1904.
4. Cajal SR. Histologie du Système Nerveux de l'homme et des Vertébrés. 2 volumes. Paris: Maloine; 1909–1911.
5. Cajal SR. Histology of the nervous system (2 vol), Translated by N. and L.W. Swanson. OUP, USA; 1995.
6. Cajal SR. Degeneration and regeneration of the nervous system. Oxford University Press; 1991.
7. Cajal SR. Studies on the cerebral cortex. Chicago Year Book Publisher; 1955.
8. Cajal S.R. New ideas on the structure of the nervous system. Cambridge, MA, MIT Press, 1990.
9. Cajal SR. Advice to a young investigator, Translated by N and L.W. Swanson. MIT Press; 1999.
10. de Castro, F. Cajal and the Spanish Neurological School. 180 pages. Madrid: Ed. Univ. Complutense.1981.
11. de Castro F. Cajal and the Spanish Neurological School: neuroscience would have been a different story without them. Front Cell Neurosci. 2019;13:187.

12. de Castro F, Merchán MA, editors. The major discoveries of Cajal and his disciples: consolidated milestones for the neuroscience of the XXIst century. 163 pages. Laussane: Frontiers Media; 2017.
13. Espinosa-Sanchez JM, Gomez-Marin A, de Castro F. The importance of Cajal's and Lorente de Nó's neuroscience to the birth of cybernetics. Neuroscientist. 2023;31:14–30.
14. Sherrington CS. Santiago Ramon y Cajal, 1852–1934. Obit Notices Fellows R Soc. 1935;1:424–41.
15. Cajal SR. Recollections of my life. (translated by E. Horne Craigie) Forword by W. Maxwell Cowan: Wellcome Collection. MIT Press; 1989.
16. Cajal, S.R. Aging and old age. Arno Press, 1934.
17. Cajal SR. Café chats. With B. Ehrlich. N Engl Rev. 1990;33:168–82. Middlebury College Publications.
18. y Cajal SR, Triarhou LC, editors. Cajal Beyond the Brain: Don Santiago contemplates the mind and education. Createspace Independent Publishing Platform; 2015.

11

Joaquín Albarrán y Domínguez: Universal Figure in Urology

Miguel A. Cuesta and Julio Virseda Rodriguez

Joaquín Albarrán y Domínguez was born on May 9, 1860, in Sagua La Grande, a prosperous city in the province of Villa Clara, located on the northern coast of Spanish Cuba. In those years, Sagua La Grande was distinguished by its dynamism and progress, remaining relatively untouched by the successive attempts at independence that shook the island. It was also an important center of political and literary innovation [1, 2] (Fig. 11.1).

The son of Dr. Pedro Pablo Albarrán, a native of Jerez de la Frontera, Cádiz, and María Micaela Domínguez de Lima, an aristocrat born in Matanzas, Joaquín was the fifth of six children. Albarrán's childhood was marked by the early loss of his parents, leaving him orphaned at the age of four. His godfather and tutor, Dr. Joaquín Fábregas, a renowned Spanish surgeon and family friend from Barcelona, undertook his education.

In 1869, Fábregas sent Joaquín and his older brother, Pedro Pablo, to Havana to pursue their baccalaureate studies with the Jesuits at Colegio de

M. A. Cuesta (✉)
Department of Surgery, Amsterdam University Medical Centre (UMC), Amsterdam, The Netherlands

J. V. Rodriguez
Department of Urology, Hospital of Albacete, Albacete, Spain

M. A. Cuesta, F. Mateo Vallejo (eds.), *Spain's Journey in Medicine*,
https://doi.org/10.1007/978-3-032-12221-6_11

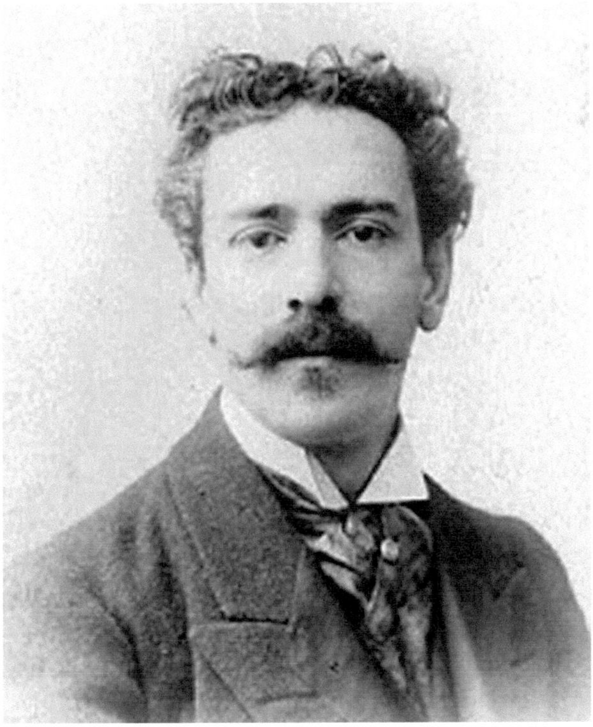

Fig. 11.1 Joaquín Albarrán

Belén. Shortly afterward, in 1872, amid growing instability caused by the island's insurrection, their tutor decided to transfer them to Barcelona to complete their academic education. The violence of those years in Cuba undoubtedly influenced this decision.

Joaquín completed high school at the age of thirteen and, determined to pursue medical studies, graduated with honors from the Faculty of Medicine in Barcelona in 1877, at the age of seventeen! His academic brilliance did not go unnoticed: surgeon Antonio Morales, Professor of Anatomical Topography and Operations, recognized him as his most outstanding disciple.

That same year, after a short stay in his hometown, he moved to Madrid to study for his doctorate, studying disciplines such as the History of Medicine, Clinical Analysis and Histology. During this period, the professor of Histology, Aureliano Maestre de San Juan, introduced him to Santiago Ramón y Cajal, who was studying one year ahead of him. A friendship marked by mutual admiration arose between the two, based on their passion for histology and their shared memories of Cuba, where Santiago Ramón y Cajal had done his military service years earlier.

Driven by his interest in physiology, Albarrán frequented the Experimental Physiology Laboratory directed by Professor Juan Magaz. The influence of these distinguished scholars proved crucial in his acquisition of knowledge that he would later apply in his medical research and treatises. In September 1878, he presented his doctoral thesis, entitled "*Contagio de la Tisis*" (Contagiousness of Tuberculosis), for which he earned his doctorate from the Faculty of Medicine in Madrid and was awarded the institution's gold medal.

The Ten Years' War (1868–1878), which pitted Cuban insurgents against forces loyal to Spain, had left the island in a state of great instability, making it difficult for the Albarrán brothers to return. Following the advice of the Fábregas family, and like other Cuban exiles, Joaquín found Paris an exceptional opportunity to continue his medical training.

Determined to enter the prestigious Faculty of Medicine at the Sorbonne, he applied for admission with the support of the Rector of the University of Madrid, who attested to his outstanding academic record through the Spanish Embassy in Paris.

From February 1879 to July 1881, in order to validate his Spanish degree, he completed five semesters of study in Histology (Prof. Louis Latteux), Histopathology (Prof. Louis Antoine Ranvier), Physiology (Prof. Charles Malassez), Bacteriology (Prof. Louis Pasteur), and Clinical Medicine (Prof. Edouard Brissaud). The training he received laid the foundation for the scientific contributions he would make throughout his career, integrating anatomical-histological knowledge, pathophysiology, bacteriology, clinical medicine, and experimental research.

At the end of this period, in 1884, he was given the opportunity to work as an extern doctor at the Paris Hospitals—initially as a histologist and microbiologist under Louis Pasteur—and a year later, he became a resident in Medicine and Surgery.

Joaquín Albarrán always regarded the anatomist Louis-Antoine Ranvier (1835–1922) and the urologist Jean Casimir Félix Guyon (1831–1920) as the key influences in his medical career.

For four years, he studied under renowned professors such as U. Trélat, J. Grancher, J. F. A. Le Dentu, and above all, J. C. Félix Guyon. It was at Necker Hospital—under Guyon's direction and widely considered the birthplace of modern urology—that Albarrán discovered a holistic approach to medicine, combining clinical practice, research, teaching, and direct patient care. This experience profoundly marked him. His dedication and talent did not go unnoticed by his mentor, who came to regard him as his most brilliant disciple.

Thanks to his strong background in histology and his deep knowledge of bacteriology and physiology, Albarrán wrote his doctoral thesis, "*Étude sur le Rein des Urinaires*" (Study of the Urinary Kidney), in 1888, during his fourth year of residency [3]. The work, which included four plates with fourteen illustrations and nine graphs, was presented in February 1889 before an examining board chaired by Professor Félix Guyon at the Faculty of Medicine of the Sorbonne. Among the jury members was the surgeon Paul Reclus, noted not only for his medical expertise but also for his connections to the anarchist movement in France. His brother, Élisée Reclus, was an influential thinker, a founder of French anarchism, and the author of "*The Conscience of the Earth*", a seminal work in social geography.

This second doctoral thesis by Albarrán would become a fundamental reference in the study of the kidney and in the field of urology, firmly establishing his reputation within the medical community(Fig. 11.2).

Professor Félix Guyon, Albarrán's mentor, played a pivotal role in the consolidation of urology as a medical specialty—an achievement as significant as that of the German urologist Max Nitze, the inventor of the cystoscope. As head of the urology department at Necker Hospital, Guyon trained specialists from around the world, making a substantial contribution to the discipline's development (Fig. 11.3).

His principal contributions centered on the study and treatment of genitourinary diseases, along with surgical advancements in bladder and prostate pathologies. Under his guidance, Joaquín Albarrán emerged as the most influential figure in urology at the turn of the twentieth century.

Urinary tract infections were considered extremely serious diseases, primarily due to the risk of sepsis. Although the bacterium *Escherichia coli* had not yet been identified by that name, Albarrán described its presence and its role in urinary infections, referring to it as the "*pyogenic bacillus.*" This microorganism played a central role in kidney infections, bacteriaemia, renal failure, sepsis, and frequently, patient mortality.

Albarrán also investigated, both experimentally and clinically, the pathways of renal infection, distinguishing between upward and downward hematogenous spread. Furthermore, he identified and analyzed the clinical, evolutionary, and histopathological differences between pyogenic bacilli and pyogenic streptococci infections. His doctoral thesis is regarded as a landmark work in the field of urology.

In 1891, Joaquín Albarrán married Paulina Ferri, with whom he had two children. After being widowed, he remarried in 1899 to Carmen Sanjurjo Ramírez de Arellano, with whom he had two more children.

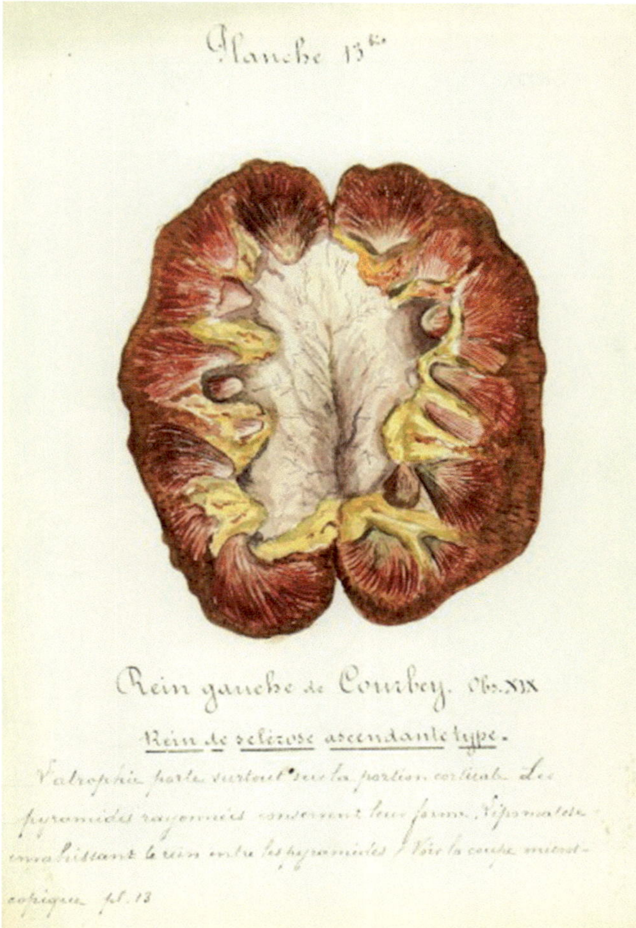

Fig. 11.2 Drawing of a tuberculous kidney in his doctoral thesis

In 1892, he got the position of Assistant Professor of Surgery through a competitive examination. That same year, his book "*Les tumeurs de la vessie*" (*Tumors of the Bladder*), written with a profound mastery of the anatomoclinical approach of the new urology, earned him the prestigious Godard Prize, awarded by the Institut-Académie des Sciences de Paris [4].

Two years later, he was appointed Surgeon of the Paris Hospitals. With a strong scientific orientation, he advocated in 1896 for the use of nephrectomy in the early treatment of renal tuberculosis, presenting his findings the following year alongside other studies on renal pathology.

His scientific work contributed to clarifying the physiology and pathology of the urinary system. This, along with his innovations and improvements in

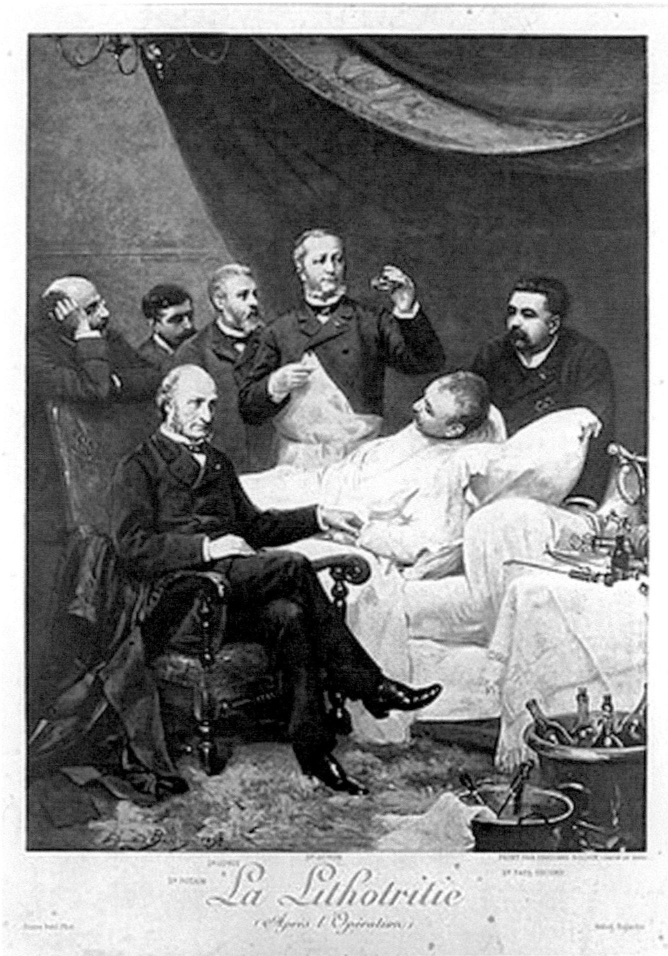

Fig. 11.3 Prof. Felix Guyon performing lithotripsy

instrumental techniques, significantly advanced the field of urology in his time.

Among his contributions to medical instrumentation was the so-called *Albarrán's nail* (or *Albarrán's lever*), presented to the Paris Academy of Medicine in 1897. This cystoscope, based on Nitze's original model, enabled catheterization of both ureters all the way to the kidneys, thereby facilitating the diagnosis and treatment of renal diseases. For this invention, Albarrán was awarded the prestigious Barbier Prize by the Faculty of Medicine (Fig. 11.4).

In addition, he designed a thermoforming sterilizer for disinfecting instruments and catheters, which operated by combusting metal vapors in contact

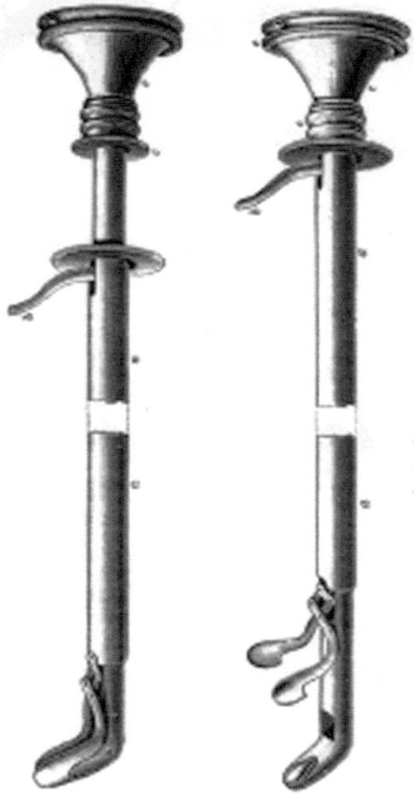

Fig. 11.4 Albarrán cystoscope with the famous fingernail for catheterizing both ureters

with a platinum sponge to release formaldehyde. He also developed various metal catheters, syringes, and urethral retractors.

In 1903, he published his treatise "*Les tumeurs du rein*" (*Kidney Tumors*), a work of considerable significance enriched by numerous personal observations [5]. His anatomoclinical approach was also evident in earlier studies on renal adenomas and epitheliomas (1897), as well as in his research on renal cancer (1900). He is likewise credited with pioneering investigations into the adenomatous nature of what was then referred to as prostatic hypertrophy. In April 1903 he participated in the 14th International Congress of Medicine held in Madrid, congress where Ramón y Cajal and Pavlov presented their new discoveries.

Albarrán also proved able to incorporate radiological techniques into the diagnosis of kidney stones and renal diseases.

But Albarrán did not stop there; he also succeeded in incorporating pathophysiological principles into the specialty. This led him to develop an original and highly effective method for assessing renal function. He presented it in a 1905 publication that has since become a classic in urological literature: "*Exploration des fonctions rénales*" (*Exploration of Renal Function*) [6] (Fig. 11.5).

This marked the inception of the first systematic assessment of renal functional capacity. The so-called "polyuria test," which Albarrán successfully

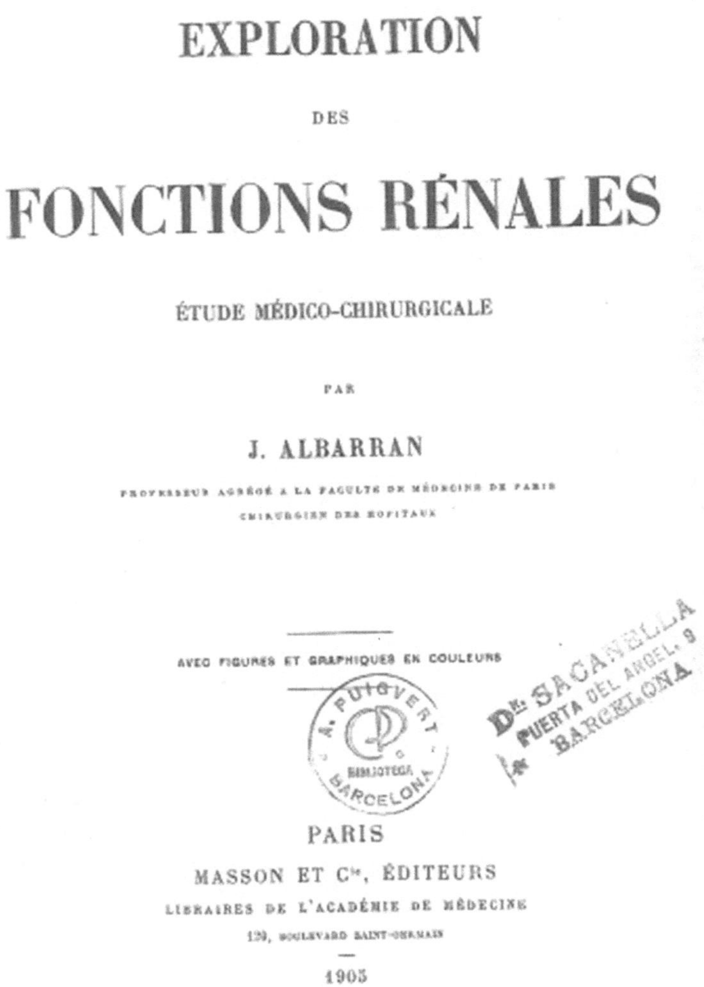

EXPLORATION

DES

FONCTIONS RÉNALES

ÉTUDE MÉDICO-CHIRURGICALE

PAR

J. ALBARRAN

PROFESSEUR AGRÉGÉ A LA FACULTÉ DE MÉDECINE DE PARIS

CHIRURGIEN DES HOPITAUX

AVEC FIGURES ET GRAPHIQUES EN COULEURS

PARIS

MASSON ET Cie, ÉDITEURS

LIBRAIRES DE L'ACADÉMIE DE MÉDECINE

120, BOULEVARD SAINT-GERMAIN

1905

Fig. 11.5 Cover of the book: Exploration of renal function.1905

introduced, enabled the evaluation and comparison of each kidney's function before and after the ingestion of a specific volume of water, thereby facilitating the study of individual renal production of urine.

In 1906, at the age of 46, Albarrán succeeded his mentor, Félix Guyon, in two significant roles: as Director of the Department of Urology at Necker Hospital and as Professor of Urology at the University of Paris (Sorbonne), positions he attained through competitive examination. In his inaugural lecture, titled "*Clinique des maladies des voies urinaires*" (*Clinic of Urinary Tract Diseases*), he emphasized that a specialist in urinary system disorders must possess both comprehensive medical knowledge and surgical expertise, thereby defining urology as a medical-surgical specialty (Fig. 11.6).

In 1908, he inaugurated the First International Congress of Urology in Paris. A year later, his health suffered a major setback due to severe pulmonary tuberculosis, which prevented him from working and led him to travel to spas and clinics across Europe in search of a recovery that never came. His most

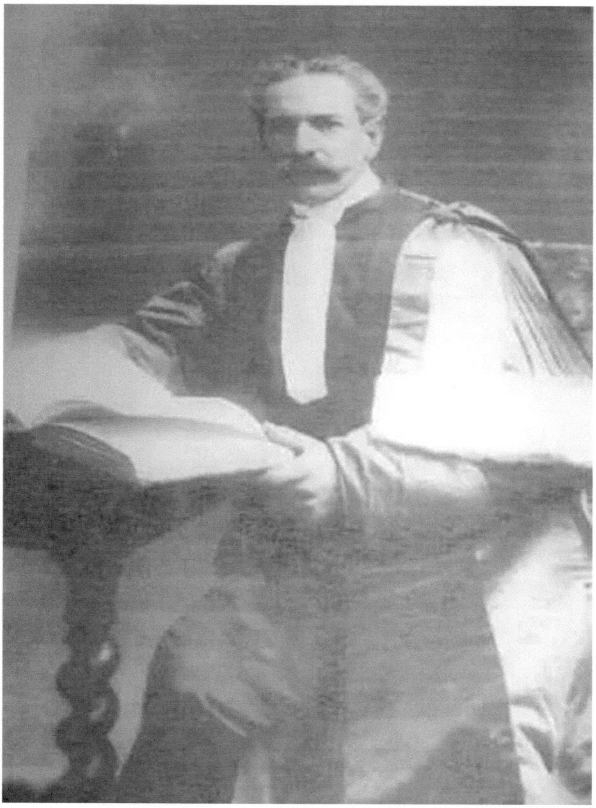

Fig. 11.6 J. Albarrán in professor's gown of the University of the Sorbonne in Paris

important masterpiece was published in 1909 under the title "*Médecine opératoire des voies urinaires*" *(Operative Medicine of the Urinary Tract)*, which was considered the best treatise on surgical urology for many years [7]. In this extensive work, Albarrán reaffirmed his vision of operative medicine, grounded in both normal and pathological anatomy and physiology (Fig. 11.7).

Joaquín Albarrán was the first surgeon in France to perform a perineal prostatectomy for prostate carcinoma. In addition, his design of the "*Albarrán nail*" for catheterization of the ureters with many applications established him as a pioneer in endourology.

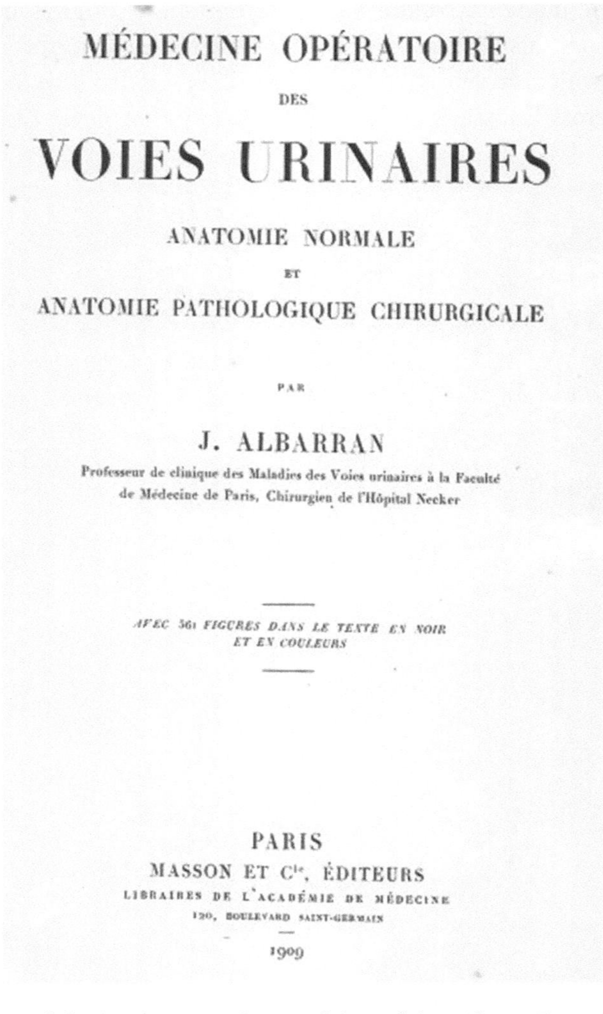

MÉDECINE OPÉRATOIRE

DES

VOIES URINAIRES

ANATOMIE NORMALE

ET

ANATOMIE PATHOLOGIQUE CHIRURGICALE

PAR

J. ALBARRAN

Professeur de clinique des Maladies des Voies urinaires à la Faculté
de Médecine de Paris, Chirurgien de l'Hôpital Necker

AVEC 561 FIGURES DANS LE TEXTE EN NOIR
ET EN COULEURS

PARIS
MASSON ET Cie, ÉDITEURS
LIBRAIRES DE L'ACADÉMIE DE MÉDECINE
120, BOULEVARD SAINT-GERMAIN

1909

Fig. 11.7 Cover of the book: Operative Medicine of the Urinary Tract. 1909

He was not only a prolific writer and scientist but also an innovator in urology. He introduced the concept of tube nephrostomy and the need for proximal urinary decompression in cases of anuria caused by obstructive stones, prior to performing surgery for stone removal. He was also the first to use urine cytology for diagnosing endothelial tumors. His work revolutionized the knowledge of renal pathophysiology, thanks to experimental evidence that allowed him to establish the laws of renal function.

Albarrán also described the so-called Albarrán glands of the prostate, submucosal glands located in the subcervical prostatic region, and Albarrán-Ormond syndrome, an inflammatory retroperitoneal fibrosis of unknown etiology that causes ureteral obstruction. Additionally, he identified the Albarrán sign, characterized by ureteral hemorrhage when serum is injected into the renal pelvis to distend it, which may indicate the presence of urothelial cancer in the kidney.

Other contributions included:

"*The Albarrán test*" involves assessing the degree of kidney tissue loss by measuring the volume and concentration of urine excreted.
"*Albarrán disease*" refers to an E. coli infection.
The "*Albarrán operation*" involves the resection of the dilated renal pelvis.
The "*Albarrán urethrotome*" is an instrument used to cut through a urethral stricture with a flexible guide.

He was awarded the Godard Prize of the French Medical Academy on three occasions (1884, 1893, and 1903), the Tremblay Prize from the Paris Academy of Medicine (1897, 1899, and 1904), and the Oulmont Prize, also from the same Academy, in 1889. He also received the Gold Medal in Surgery of the Hospitals, awarded in Paris in 1887.

He was a distinguished member of several prestigious scientific institutions, including the Anatomical Society of Paris (1888), the Royal Academy of Medical, Physical, and Natural Sciences of Havana (1890), and the Paris Society of Surgery (1899). He received the French Legion of Honor and was nominated for the Nobel Prize a few months after his death in 1912.

Joaquín Albarrán died in Arcachon, near Bordeaux, on January 17, 1912, from pulmonary tuberculosis at the age of only 51. It is said that he accidentally injured and infected himself with the scalpel he was using to dissect a tuberculous kidney, which likely aggravated his lung condition. His bust is preserved at the Necker Hospital, and his remains are buried in the Neuilly-sur-Seine cemetery in Paris. In Cuba he has another funerary monument in Havana (Fig. 11.8).

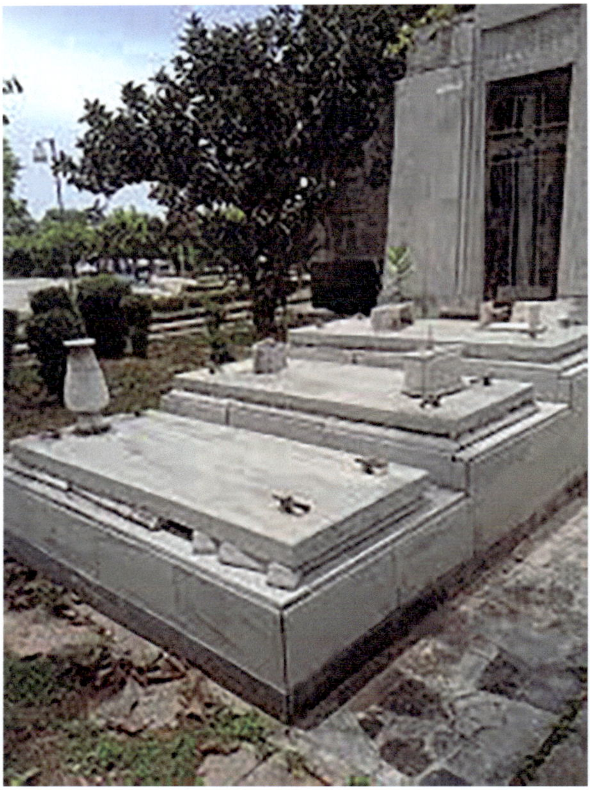

Fig. 11.8 Funerary monument of the Prof. J Albarrán in Havana

Maurice Heitz-Boyer wrote his epitaph in the *Journal de Urologie* on February 15, 1912:

> *The vibrant voice of the master is now silent. Never again will we see in those unforgettable eyes the luminous radiance of his intelligence. Yet, the work he accomplished, though perhaps not as grand as his ambition dreamed, is already so magnificent that it has added a new prestige to the Necker school. Guyon, Albarrán: master and disciple. Their two inseparable names dominate the imperishable work they created, this fiery center of urological science in the world, to which doctors from all countries are drawn. It is not appropriate to say a final farewell to the departed: every day, in each of our works, in each step of our scientific life, we will find the trace of his passing, his living thought, the memory of his guiding image.*

Legacy

Joaquín Albarrán is one of the most significant figures in urology of all time, universally recognized for his contributions. His research on bladder tumors, prostatic hypertrophy, renal function, urinary sepsis, and anatomopathological studies, as presented in his books, marked a milestone that continues to impress today for its scientific rigor and the brilliance of its exposition. In particular, his work *Operative Medicine of the Urinary Tract,* has been considered the best urological treatise written until recent times.

In 1906, at the age of 46, he was appointed head of the Urology Department at Necker Hospital and professor of Urology at the Sorbonne University. Exceptionally intelligent, erudite, and polyglot—fluent in five languages—he was a tireless worker and a thoughtful thinker. He was a regular presence at urology congresses, and his vision for the development of the specialty established him as a world authority on urinary system surgery.

In addition to his important scientific contributions, he also excelled in the design of urological instruments, such as the *cystoscope "fingernail,"* of Albarrán which, with minor modifications, is currently used to facilitate ureteral catheterization. His surgical talent, combined with his innovative capacity, made him one of the most influential personalities in the history of urology.

His Significance for Urology in Spain

In January 1911, the Spanish Society of Urology was formed, and due to Albarrán's close ties with Spanish urology, he was appointed honorary president of the society in recognition of "*his contributions to the development of our specialty and the training of numerous Spanish compatriots in the late 19th and early 20th centuries.*" Those who knew him personally passed on to younger urologists not only his teachings, but also various aspects of a personality that was as complete as it was fascinating.

Prominent Spanish urologists, including Vicente Company, José María Bartrina, Antonio Morales Pérez, and Leonardo de la Peña, traveled to Paris to perfect their skills under his guidance. He remained a close friend of de la Peña until his death. In 1900, he traveled to Spain to give a lecture at the Instituto Rubio in Madrid on the "*Diagnosis of Kidney Tumors,*" where he highlighted the role of this institution as a pioneer of surgical specialization in Spain.

Albarrán maintained deep ties with Spain, both familial and academic, having completed part of his training in Barcelona and Madrid. He was always admired by the urological community for his important scientific studies, surgical innovations, and the high quality of his treatises, as well as for being a pioneer in endourology [8–10].

Throughout his life, he kept a vivid memory of his native Cuba and maintained a special connection with Spain, a country he visited frequently. He kept a home in Barcelona for many years and never lost his Spanish accent.

In 1890, during a trip to Cuba and a visit to his city, he wrote:

If the vagaries of life have made me adopt the great French nation as my homeland, I never forget that I am Cuban and will always strive to make myself worthy of the land of my birth.

Beyond the field of urology, he established connections with eminent physicians such as Otto Zuckerkandl, Theodor Billroth, and Johann Mikulicz. Outside of medicine, he frequented the literary circles of George Sand, Frédéric Chopin, and Antonín Dvořák. He met Gustave Flaubert, whose *Madame Bovary* set the literary tone of the time, and the Cuban poet José María Heredia, one of the most avant-garde figures of the nineteenth century. He was also captivated by the splendor of Impressionism in Paris, admiring the works of Claude Monet, Pierre-Auguste Renoir, and Edgar Degas.

However, although Spanish-Cuban in origin and culture, his urological legacy belongs entirely to the history of French medicine, establishing him as one of the creators of the specialty of urology.

His biographer, Professor Cathelin, wrote of him:

He was great by the heart, as well as by the spirit... He was certainly the clearest, most lucid, most insightful, and most understanding mind I have ever known.

References

1. Casey RG, Thornhill JS. Joaquín Maria Albarrán y Dominguez: microbiologist, histologist and urologist – a lifetime from orphan in Cuba to Nobel nominee. Int J Urol. 2006;13:1159–61.
2. Angulo Cuesta J, Fernández Arias M. Joaquín Albarrán y los caminos de la Urología. Published by the AEU (Spanish Association of Urology); 2020.
3. Albarrán J. Étude sur le Rein des Urinaires, doctoral thesis. Paris: G. Steinhell; 1889.

4. Albarrán J. "Les tumeurs de la Vessie", Masson et Cie, Paris, 1892.
5. Albarrán J. Les tumeurs du Rein. Paris: Masson et Cie; 1903.
6. Albarrán J. Exploration des fontions rénales, Masson et Cie, Paris, 1905.
7. Albarrán J. Medicine operatoire des Voies Urinaires. Paris: Masson et Cie; 1909.
8. Laín Entralgo P. Homenaje al Profesor J Albarrán. Arch Esp Uro. 1962;15:200–6.
9. Puigvert Gorro A. Joaquín Albarrán (Barcelona-Madrid) (1872–1878). Actas Urol Esp. 1979;3:245–8.
10. Fernández Arias M. Joaquín Albarrán. Vida y pasión científica de un médico genial. Ed. Científico-Técnica, Habana, 2012.

12

Pío del Río Hortega: Discoverer of the Oligodendroglia and Microglia and the First Histogenic Classification of Central Nervous System

Carlos Vaquero Puerta

During the first third of the twentieth century, neurohistology in Spain were marked by a number of eminent scientists dedicated particularly to the study of the nervous system. These scientists framed a brilliant period in the history of Spanish science, with notable figures including Santiago Ramón y Cajal, del Rio Hortega, Federico Olóriz, Jorge Francisco Tello, and Nicolás Achúcarro, among others (Fig. 12.1).

In particular, Santiago Ramón y Cajal, awarded the Nobel Prize in 1906, and Pío del Río Hortega are two of the most prominent names in this context. The biography of Pío del Río Hortega is fascinating, and his contributions to the understanding of the Central Nervous System are especially significant. His work focused on the study of glial cells, thereby complementing Cajal's contributions related to neurons. The interplay between their research has been fundamental to a comprehensive understanding of the nervous system.

Pío del Río Hortega was born on May 7, 1882, in Portillo, Valladolid, into a wealthy family involved in the management of agricultural estates. He was the fourth of seven children born to Juan del Río Sanz and Dolores Hortega Guerra.

C. V. Puerta (✉)
University of Valladolid, Valladolid, Spain

M. A. Cuesta, F. Mateo Vallejo (eds.), *Spain's Journey in Medicine*,
https://doi.org/10.1007/978-3-032-12221-6_12

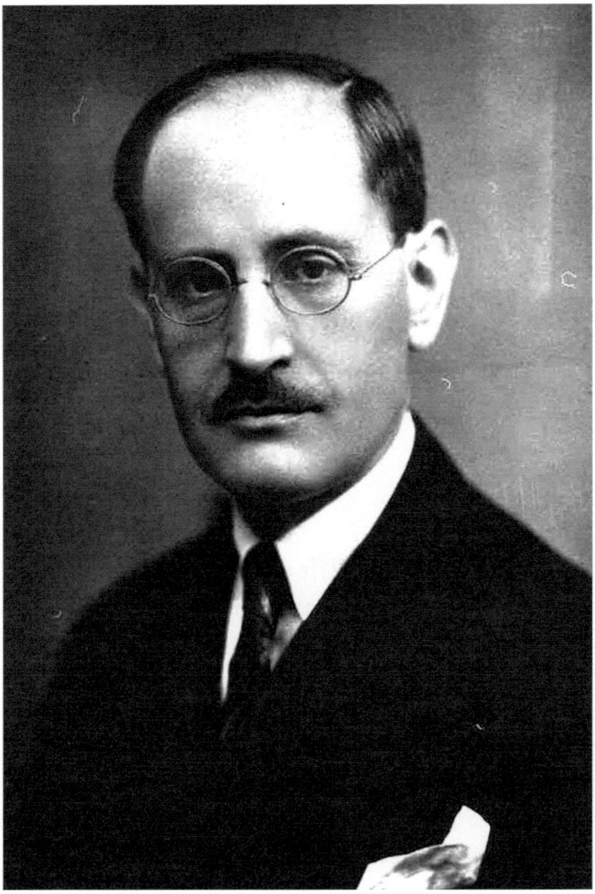

Fig. 12.1 Pio del Rio Hortega. (Archives of the University of Valladolid)

During his childhood, he attended the local school and in 1892, the family moved to Valladolid to ensure their children could pursue formal education in the provincial capital. Pío enrolled at the local Institute to complete his baccalaureate, which he finished in 1898. During the last three years of this study, he also studied Fine Arts, with a particular focus on drawing.

In 1900, he began his medical studies at the Faculty of Medicine in Valladolid, where he obtained his degree in June 1905.

From his early years as a student, he showed a marked interest in anatomy, which led him to obtain the position of alumno interno (intern student) in the Department of Anatomy, under the guidance of Leonardo de la Peña, who directed the anatomical work.

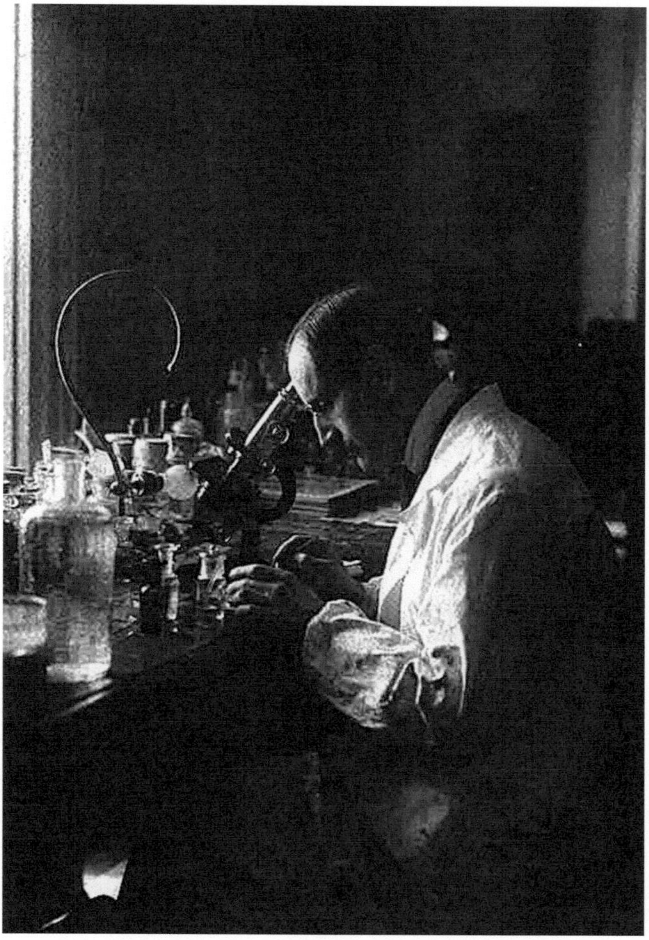

Fig. 12.2 Del Rio Hortega working with the microscope. (Archives of the University of Valladolid)

Likewise, his interest in histology led him to work alongside Leopoldo López García, who appointed him as honorary assistant student when he joined the Histology Laboratory in the fourth year of his study. To support his son's passion for histology, his father gave him a Zulauf optical microscope, which enabled him to study the histology of different tissues and organs of the human body (Fig. 12.2).

During his university years, he developed a close friendship with two fellow students: Ramón López Prieto, with whom he worked as an intern in the Department of Anatomy, and Tomás Gutiérrez Perrin, who shared his interest in Histology. Despite his dedication and extensive work in the laboratory, located on the top floor of the Faculty building, his academic record was not particularly outstanding—possibly due to his strong focus on practical work rather than theoretical studies.

After completing his degree, he decided to travel to Madrid with his friend Tomás Gutiérrez in the hope of meeting Santiago Ramón y Cajal, the recent Nobel Prize laureate, whom they greatly admired. However, their first attempt to join his research group was unsuccessful.

As an alternative, he decided to practice medicine as a general practitioner, which he did in Valladolid from 1907 to 1910. During this time, he also worked on his doctoral thesis under the supervision of his professor, Leopoldo López García. He defended his thesis, titled "*Etiología y anatomía patológica de los tumores del encéfalo*" (*Etiology and Pathological Anatomy of Brain Tumors*), at the Central University of Madrid in 1909, earning the degree of Doctor with the highest distinction.

In 1911, he decided to return to the Faculty of Medicine in Valladolid when he was appointed as Assistant Professor in the Department of Normal and Pathological Histology, again under the guidance of López García. During this time, he showed a stronger inclination toward research than teaching.

In 1912, Pío del Río Hortega made several trips to Madrid in an effort to work with the Cajal's School. He eventually succeeded in joining the Laboratorio de Investigaciones Biológicas (Biological Research Laboratory) at the San Carlos Faculty of Medicine, where he worked alongside Jorge Francisco Tello, Cajal's right-hand man. However, the experience turned out to be disappointing, as he did not receive the recognition or support, he had hoped for, this led him to look for another type of work.

He succeeded in joining the Laboratory of Histopathology of the Nervous System, directed by Nicolás Achúcarro. Unlike his previous experience, he was warmly welcomed there, forming a friendship with Achúcarro and gaining valuable training and experience across various practical fields. Among his colleagues were Miguel Gayarre y Espinal, José Miguel Sacristán y Gutiérrez, Luis Calandre Ibáñez, Luis Fortún Alcalá, Miguel Prados, and Gonzalo Rodríguez Lafora.

In 1913, he got a scholarship by the Junta para Ampliación de Estudios to continue training abroad, as a result, he moved to Paris, where he worked until 1914, first at the Pathology Laboratories of Boucicaut Hospital, under the direction of Maurice Letulle, and after at the Histology Laboratory of the Faculty of Medicine, led by Auguste Prenant.

He then moved to Berlin to work at the Institut für Infektionskrankheiten (Institute of Infectious Diseases), where he collaborated with Joseph Koch in the fields of bacteriology and experimental cancer research. However, his stay in Berlin was cut short by the outbreak of World War I, forcing him to return to Spain in 1915.

To complete his fellowship, he spent a period in London working with J.A. Murray at the Imperial Cancer Research Foundation, concluding his training at Middlesex Hospital under the supervision of W.S. Lazarus Barlow.

Upon returning to Spain, he resumed his position at the Laboratorio de Histopatología del Sistema Nervioso, where he worked alongside Nicolás Achúcarro until his death from Hodgkin's disease in 1918. After his death, Pio del Rio Hortega, together with Miguel Gayarre y Espinal, assumed leadership of the Laboratory. In recognition of his scientific contributions, he was awarded the first Achúcarro Prize in 1919.

During this period, he was also appointed Secretary of the Spanish Society of Biology under the presidency of Ramón y Cajal, replacing Jorge F. Tello. This role involved significant administrative responsibilities, particularly regarding the management of the Society's Journal, but it also brought him into closer contact with Ramón y Cajal.

In 1920, the Laboratory continued to share the building on Calle Infanta Isabel with Ramón y Cajal's own laboratory. However, due to professional rivalries, personal tensions and intrigues, a serious disagreement arose between the two. This culminated in a letter from Cajal dated October 9, 1919, and a subsequent confrontation of both at the laboratory, during which Cajal reportedly directed personal insults—including homophobic remarks—at del Rio Hortega and expelled him from the Laboratory.

As a result, del Río Hortega decided to relocate his laboratory to the Residencia de Estudiantes, which, at his request, was renamed as the Laboratorio de Histología Normal y Patológica. There, he made significant contributions to the field of neurohistology, which greatly enhanced his reputation, attracting numerous national and international professionals to his laboratory (Figs. 12.3 and 12.4). The laboratory continued to operate under his direction until 1937, when he was succeeded by his disciple, Manuel López Enríquez.

Pío del Río Hortega continued his work in the laboratory alongside his disciples and a large group of visiting researchers, producing numerous scientific contributions that were published in various national and international journals. These works earned him significant international recognition,

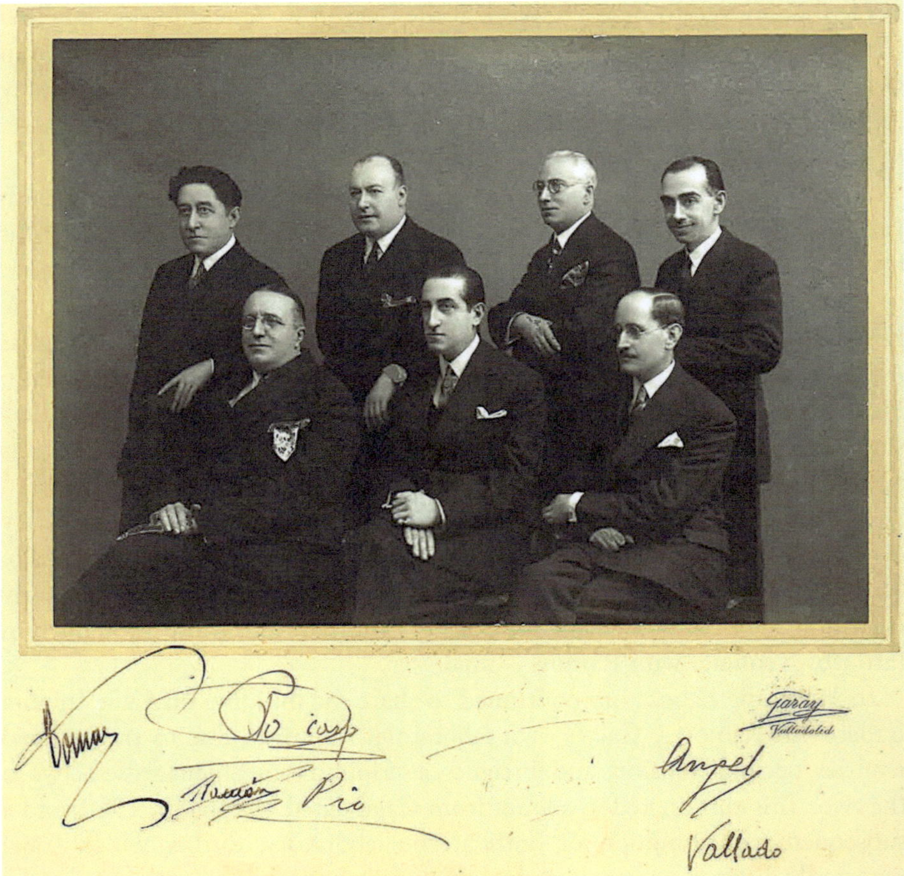

Fig. 12.3 Del Rio Hortega with other colleagues: Andrés Torre Ruiz, Policarpo Mingote, Valentín García Perrin, Ramon López Prieto, Tomás García Perrin, and Angel López Pérez. Valladolid, April 2, 1924. (Archives of the University of Valladolid)

establishing him as a leading figure in several areas of neurohistology and oncology.

In 1928, upon the recommendation of his director, José Goyanes Capdevila, he was appointed Head of the Laboratorio de Cancerlogía Experimental at the Instituto Nacional del Cáncer, which at the time was known as the 'Príncipe de Asturias' Institute. Later, in 1931, he was appointed Director of the Institute, following the dismissal of Prof. Goyanes by the Republican government—possibly for political reasons—after being accused of the disappearance of some radium needles as an excuse (Fig. 12.5).

Following the proclamation of the Second Spanish Republic on April 14, 1931, del Río Hortega was appointed to several political and cultural positions such as member of the Ministry of Education's Cultural Relations Board,

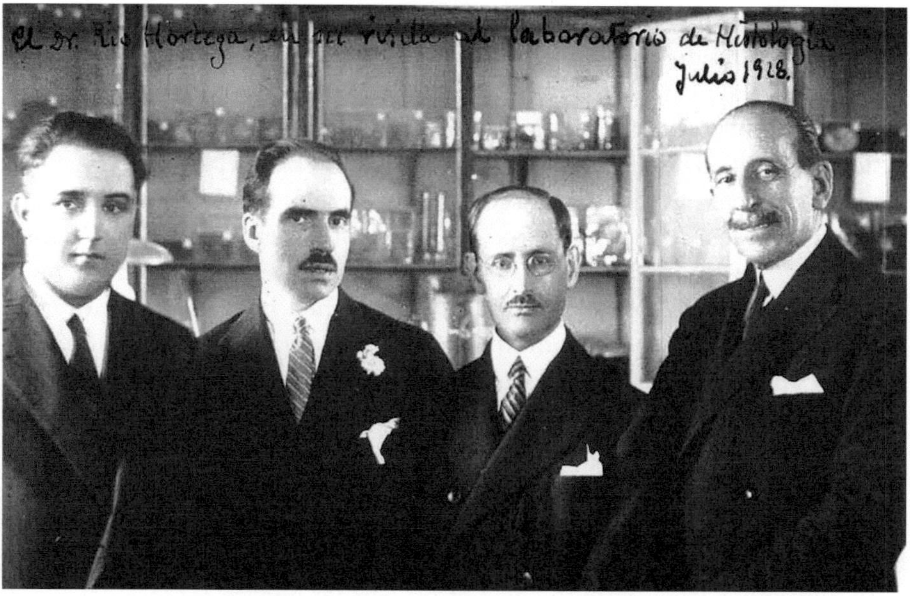

Fig. 12.4 Photo taken during the visit to the University of Santiago de Compostela in 1928. (Archives of the University of Valladolid)

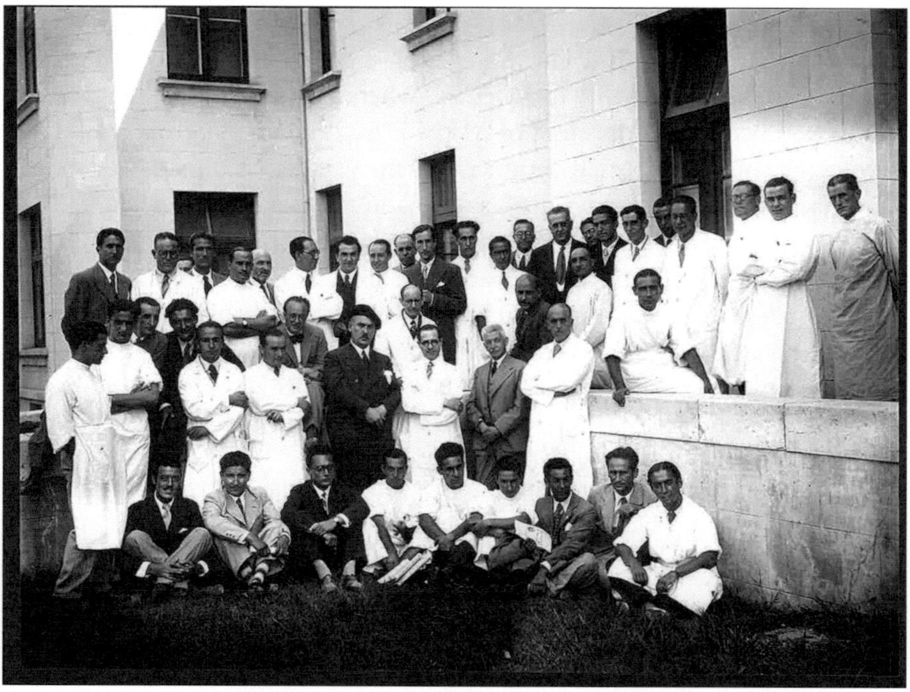

Fig. 12.5 Pío del Rio Hortega at the Oncology Institute of Madrid in August 1933. (Archive of the University of Valladolid)

with other prominent scientists, advisor of the National Health Board in 1933 by the President of the Republic and in 1934, he assumed the position of advisor for the Ministry of Culture.

In 1934, following the death of Santiago Ramón y Cajal, his seat at the Academia Nacional de Medicina became vacant. Pío del Río Hortega was widely considered the natural successor; however, he had to compete for the position with José María Villaverde, who was ultimately elected by the academy members. This decision was regarded as unjust by some other academics, including Gonzalo Rodríguez Lafora, who resigned from the institution in protest. As a gesture of recognition, a tribute was organized for both, del Rio Hortega and Rodríguez Lafora. During this time, he also signed a manifesto in support of the Republican government, alongside other intellectuals.

On July 18, 1936, the Spanish Civil War broke out. In September, he traveled to Brussels to attend the International Cancer Congress, remaining there until early November. Upon returning to Spain, he carried radioactive material on behalf of the Republican government for the Cancer Institute.

In November 1936, with the help of his partner Nicolás Gómez del Moral and his niece Ascensión Amo del Río, del Rio Hortega managed to save from destruction caused by the bombardments his numerous histological preparations, working materials, and radioactive material that he had brought from Brussels.

In the same month of 1936, he received an order from the Minister of Health, Federica Montseny, to Valencia, where the Republican government had moved because of the siege of Madrid. Accompanied by his family and Nicolás, he could work briefly in the Laboratory at the Faculty of Medicine in Valencia, collaborating with Luis Urtubey and Alcover Campos.

In January 1937, he decided to go into exile in Paris with his family, where he joined the Neurosurgical Department of Clovis Vincent at the Pitié Hospital to move on November 1937 to Oxford, with his family, to work with neurosurgeon Hugh Cairns, who offered him a position as a neuropathologist with the possibility to start a laboratory. Del Rio Hortega remained at the Nuffield Institute at the Radcliffe Infirmary until 1940, when London was hit by the first bombing raids of World War II.

In the same year, he traveled to Argentina, arriving on August 28, after being invited by the Spanish Cultural Institution to give a course in Buenos Aires deciding to stay in the city. Initially, he worked with the neurosurgeon, Manuel Balado, in the Laboratorio de Histología Patológica at the Santa Lucía Hospital, and then the Spanish Cultural Institution in Argentina, chaired by Rafael Vehils, offered him the opportunity to establish an Histological and Histopathological Research Laboratory in a room of the Spanish Patriotic

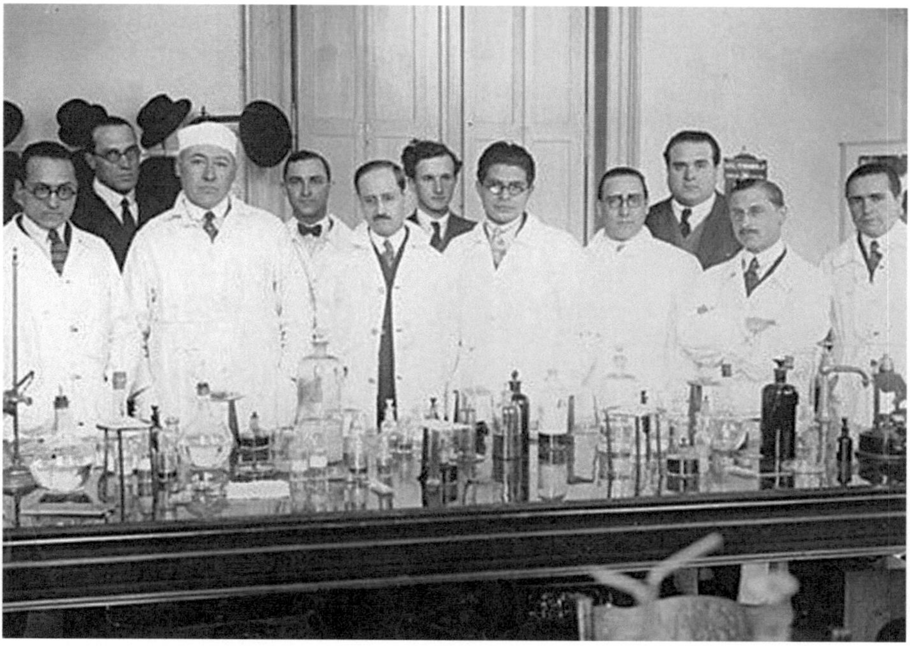

Fig. 12.6 Pio del Rio Hortega during the Histology Course taught in Buenos Aires

Association, which was inaugurated in 1941. The Laboratory was named 'Laboratorio Ramón y Cajal.' (Fig. 12.6).

During his time in Argentina, he was joined by new disciples, including Moisés Polak, José Manuel Prado, Washington Bruño, Pardiñas, David Celener, León Zimman, Aranovitch, Manuel Ojea, and Amanda Pellegrino de Iraldi (Fig. 12.7).

Del Río Hortega died of cancer in Buenos Aires on June 1, 1945, at the age of 63, after being admitted to the Avelino Gutiérrez Sanatorium in January 1945. His body was embalmed.

After his death, his brothers moved his belongings and personal archive to his hometown of Portillo, where they were stored in the Pharmacy, owned by his brother Julián, until being transferred to the family home in Valladolid in 1969. In 1986, his body was repatriated to Spain and buried in the Pantheon of Illustrious Men in the city of Valladolid.

Regarding his personal and family life, his partner was the businessman Nicolás Gómez del Moral, who stood by him for 25 years, accompanying him from the time of his disagreement with Ramón y Cajal until his death [1–5].

Politically, Don Pío del Río Hortega appeared to be a member of Lerroux's Republican Party, a political group with an anti-clerical, liberal, and initially

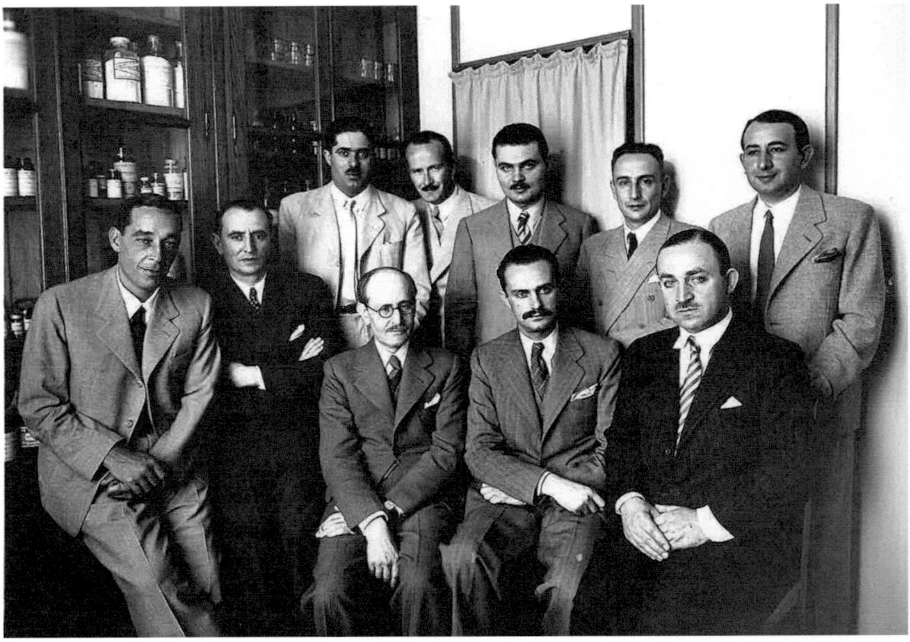

Fig. 12.7 Del Rio Hortega with his disciples in Argentina, 1940: Sverdlik, Pardiñas, Celener, Doutat, Zimman, Aranovich, Polack, Ojea, and Prado. (Archives of the University of Valladolid)

left-wing profile. He was one of the co-founders, on 11 February 1933, of the Association of Friends of the Soviet Union during the time of Stalin, along with other scientists and intellectuals. He also signed a manifesto in support of the Soviet Union, which likely influenced his future identification as a man of the left. In his will, he expressed his wish to be buried in the robe of an honorary doctorate from Oxford, with the Republican insignia (Fig. 12.8).

On the international stage, many scientists visited his laboratory to gain knowledge, assess his techniques, offer their collaboration, or simply receive training. Among those who visited were Wilder Graves Penfield, Bernardo Alberto Houssay, Lewis H. Weed, Lawrence S. Kubie, Bernard Alpers, Lewis Stevenson, Charles Scott Sherrington, Knud Krabbe, Percival Bailey, Harvey Cushing, Giuseppe Levi, Adolf Meyer, and Charles Harrison Frazier, among others.

It is also important to point out that del Río Hortega maintained relations with the intellectuals of his time in Spain, interacting with personalities such as Gregorio Marañón, Juan Negrín, Ramón Pérez de Ayala, Alejandro Lerroux, José Ortega y Gasset, Victorio Macho, among many others.

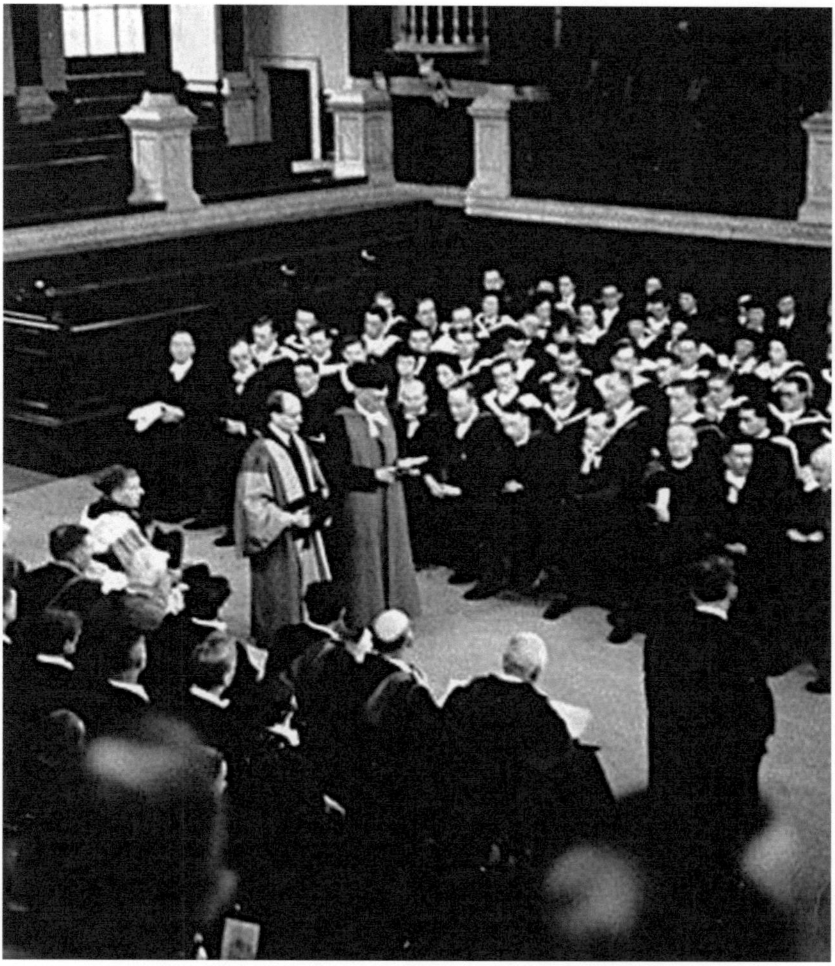

Fig. 12.8 Ceremony of appointing Pio del Río Hortega as an honorary doctor in sciences by the University of Oxford. February 25, 1939. (Archives of the University of Valladolid)

He was nominated for the Nobel Prize in Physiology and Medicine in 1929, when he was a member of the Junta de Ampliación de Estudios e Investigaciones Científicas in Madrid and in 1937, in the midst of the Civil War. On both occasions, according to the Swedish Academy, his nomination was due to his contributions to microglia and oligodendroglia, although the prize was not awarded, apparently because much of his work was written in Spanish.

Contributions

Pío del Río Hortega's contributions to scientific knowledge are numerous, particularly in the field of the structural and functional understanding of the central nervous system. His most significant contribution was undoubtedly the discovery and description of the Third Element of the CNS, the neuroglia, specifically oligodendroglia and microglia.

Glial cells or neuroglia perform very important auxiliary functions in the nervous system, complementing neurons, forming an interneuronal matrix, supporting and nourishing neurons. There is a central glia in the central nervous system formed by oligodendroglia and microglia and a peripheral glia formed by Schwann cells (Fig. 12.9).

In 1918, Don Pío developed an innovative histological staining technique known as the ammoniacal silver carbonate method, a procedure that proved crucial in histological research and essential to his contributions, particularly regarding certain cellular components of the nervous system. He also made significant modifications to other histological methods and techniques to enhance their efficiency, as demonstrated in his work with Achúcarro's tannin and silver technique, for which he developed four different variants.

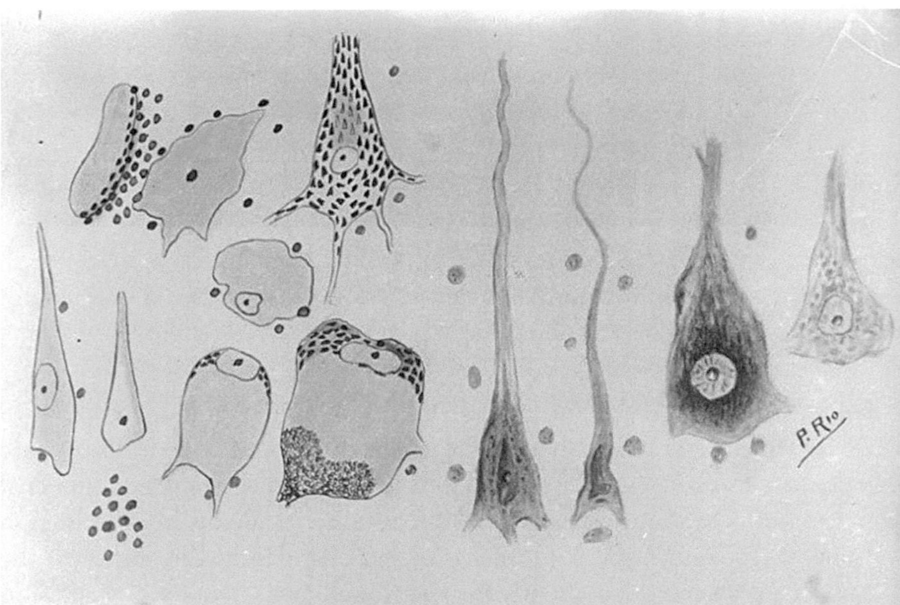

Fig. 12.9 Drawing of nerve elements signed by Pio del Rio Hortega

These innovations not only advanced the understanding of neuroanatomy but also laid the groundwork for future research in neuroscience, establishing del Río Hortega as a pivotal figure in the histopathology of the nervous system.

Through his research, he discovered two distinct types of cells in the neuroglia: microglia—later called *Hortega cells*—which are of mesodermal origin and serve as the brain's immune cells, acting as macrophages that respond to pathogens and provide the main active immune defense in the central nervous system (CNS); and **oligodendroglia**, which are of ectodermal origin and are responsible for forming and maintaining the myelin sheath around axons [6–13].

Another of his significant contributions was the demonstration that Schwann cells of peripheral nerves also belong to the oligodendroglia category. Other research topics included the pineal gland, whose lobes contain fibrous neuroglia and the centrosomes, the cell organelles involved in cell division.

During his time in Argentina, he continued his work on the cells that surround neurons in sensory ganglia and the autonomic nervous system, identifying these cells as oligodendroglia.

Although he initially showed little interest in undergraduate teaching, he was deeply engaged in instructing in the laboratory, imparting his knowledge at the microscope—an uncommon practice among many researchers. He also organized several courses on histological techniques, where he taught tissue processing, staining methods, and, of course, the histological structures, including his innovative contributions to them.

Additionally, he worked in the field of pathological anatomy, concentrating on the study of various brain tumors, which was the focus of his doctoral thesis, with a particular emphasis on gliomas. These contributions solidified his legacy in neuroscience and histopathology [14].

Further Reading (from Boullerne A.I. and Feinstein D.L. [13])

1. Cajal S. R. (1913. a). Un nuevo proceder para la impregnación de la neuroglia [A new procedure for the impregnation of neuroglia]. Boletín de la Sociedad Española de Biologia, 2, 104–108. Cajal succeeded in being the first to stain both fibrous and protoplasmic astrocytes with unequaled selectivity while neurons remained pale, using a gold and mercury chloride-sublimate technique.
2. Cajal S. R. (1913. b). Contribución al conocimiento de la neuroglia del cerebro humano [Contribution to the knowledge of the neuroglia of the human brain]. Trabajos del Laboratorio de Investigaciones Biológicas de la

Universidad de Madrid, 11, 255–315. Cajal famously designated neuroglia cells he could barely visualize, despite his staining artistry and genius, as the "third element."

3. Río-Hortega P. D. (1919). El "tercer elemento" de los centros nerviosos [The "third element" of the nerve centers]. Boletín de la Sociedad Española de Biología, 9, 68–166. I. La microglía en estado normal (pp. 68–82) II. Intervención de la microglía en los procesos patológicos (pp. 91–103) III. Naturaleza probable de la microglía (pp. 108–120) IV. Poder fagocitario y movilidad de la microglía (pp. 154–166) These four installments (I to IV) published back to back in the same journal issue formally introduced microglia to the world. Microglial cells had been formerly described i.e. by Alzheimer in the late nineteenth century, but until the 1919 Río-Hortega series, microglia were just strange amoeboid cells. Río-Hortega devised a staining which showed microglia in all their activation states from resting ramified to phagocytosing amoeboid, thereby establishing a new cell type and showing its versatility.
4. Río-Hortega P. D. (1921). Estudios sobre la neurologia. La glía de escasas radiaciones (oligodendroglía) [Studies on neurology. Low-radiation glia (oligodendroglia)]. Boletín de la Real Sociedad Española de Historia Natural, 21, 63–92. This article introduced the oligodendrocyte as a new cell type. This report antagonized Cajal more than the newly described microglial cell, because Cajal was now famous world-wide and had already received the Nobel Prize. Despite his staining genius, Cajal failed in visualizing oligodendrocytes which he dubbed the" third element" or "apolar elements" since he could never see their processes. Cajal finally acknowledged the existence of oligodendrocytes a mere 5 years before his death in a personal letter to Pío, but never in a scientific publication.
5. Río-Hortega P. D. (1928). Tercera aportación al conocimiento morfológico e interpretación funcional de la oligodendroglia [Third contribution to the morphological knowledge and functional interpretation of oligodendroglia]. Memorias de la Real Sociedad Española de Historia Natural, 14, 5–122. The sum of a monumental amount of work on oligodendrocytes of which we are still rediscovering. Essentially everything Pío discovered about oligodendrocytes is contained in this book of 120 pages. The classification into four cardinal types depending upon the orientation and size of myelinated axons is still used to this day.
6. Río-Hortega P. D. (1932). *Microglia in cytology and cellular pathology of the nervous system* (W. Penfield, Ed., pp. 480–534). Hoeber. The first account of microglia in English. For a while microglia were called "Rio-Hortega's cells".

7. Río-Hortega P. D. (1993). Art and artifice in the science of histology. (Originally published in Spanish in 1933, translated by W.C Gibson) Histopathology, 22, 515–525. Philosophical thoughts of Río-Hortega on the relationship between histology, drawing, and art; which revealed him as a true artist. Río-Hortega could draw with both hands and was the author of all of his drawings (like Cajal), in contrast to others who had artists draw their cells (such as Ranvier).
8. Río-Hortega Bereciartu J. D. (2020). Pío del Río-Hortega: The revolution of Glia Anatomical Record, 303, 1232–1241. A personal account by the grandnephew of Río-Hortega, detailing his complicated relationship with Cajal and the special WWII political upheaval in Spain that forced his exile to Argentina. This short biography also details the unsuccessful attempt made for the discoverer of microglia to receive the Nobel Prize.
9. Tremblay M. E., Lecours C., Samson L., Sánchez-Zafra V., Sierra A. (2015). From the Cajal alumni Achúcarro and Río-Hortega to the rediscovery of never-resting microglia. Frontiers in Neuroanatomy, 9, 1–10. An interesting historical account describing the context in which microglial cells were discovered, crediting Achúcarro and not Cajal, as commonly assumed. Río-Hortega never trained with Cajal but mastered histological staining with another forgotten genius of the time: Achúcarro.

References

1. Aguirre de Viani C, Jiménez Carmena JJ. Pío del Río Hortega, Valladolid, Junta de Castilla y León Consejería de Cultura y Turismo. Villalar Collection. 1991.
2. Campos A. del Río-Hortega. The forging of a histologist (I). An RANM. 2018;135:222–9.
3. Gil Sanz Rodríguez F. Pio Del Rio Hortega (1882–1945). Arch Fac Med (Valladolid). 2020;2:6–12.
4. González Calvo V. A well-deserved tribute to Don Pío del Río Hortega. Anal Real Acad Med Cir Vall. 1971;9:70–3.
5. Houssay BA. Speech at the burial of Dr. Pío del Río Hortega, Anales de la Academia Nacional de Medicina de Buenos Aires. 1945;28:306–10.
6. Del Rio Hortega P. The microglia. Lancet. 1939;233:1023–6.
7. Masson P. L'ouvre scientifique de Pío del Rio Hortega. J Hotel Dieu. 1945;6:405–16.
8. Ortíz Picón JM. La obra neuro-histológica del doctor Pío del Río Hortega. Arch Neurobiol. 1971;34:39–70.

9. Río Hortega J. On the discoveries of microglia and oligodendroglia: Pío del Río-Hortega and his relationship with Achucarro and Cajal (1914–1934). Neurosci Hist. 2013;1:176–90.
10. Sierra A, de Castro F, Del Rio-Hortega J, et al. The "Big-Bang" for modern glial biology: translation and comments on Pío del Río-Hortega 1919 series of papers on microglia. Glia. 2016;64:1801–40.
11. Vera Sempere F. The scientific production of Pío del Río Hortega (1882–1945) and the laboratory of the Residencia de Estudiantes. Neurosci Hist. 2022;10:126–44.
12. Del Río Hortega Bericiartu J. Pío del Río Hortega: the revolution of glia. Anat Rec (Hoboken). 2020;303:1232–41.
13. Boullerne AI, Feinstein DL. History of neuroscience I. Pío del Río Hortega (1882–1945): the discoverer of Microglía and Oligodendroglía. ASN Neuro. 8open access. 2020;12(I)
14. Penfield WG. The Spanish School of Anatomy: homage to Cajal and del Rio-Hortega from a grateful pupil. https://HOA/Penfield-Wilder-La-Escuela-Española-de-Anatomia-pdf.

13

Fernando de Castro: Disciple of Cajal, Key Figure of the Spanish Neurological School and His Transcendent Discovery of Arterial Chemoreceptors in the Carotid Body

Fernando de Castro Soubriet

Fernando de Castro Rodríguez (Madrid, February 25, 1896–Madrid, April 15, 1967) was one of the youngest and most brilliant disciples of Santiago Ramón y Cajal. A native of Madrid, born on Calle del Arenal, he developed an interest in scientific research—particularly neurohistology—early on during his medical studies at the Central University of Madrid (1913–1920) (Fig. 13.1).

In June 1920, he earned his degree with distinction, and in 1922 he defended his doctoral thesis titled "*Study of the Sensory Ganglia of Humans in Normal and Pathological Conditions*", a work that was awarded the Nicolás Rodríguez Prize.

That same year, he was also recognized with the Abaytúa Prize, awarded by the Spanish Royal National Academy of Medicine.

Like many others, he was drawn by the magnetism of Santiago Ramón y Cajal's towering figure. However, he did not initially obtain a position at the Biological Research Laboratory. After receiving the Helmholtz Medal in 1905

F. de Castro Soubriet (✉)
Myelin Dynamics & Repair Lab, Centro de Neurociencias Cajal–CSIC (former Instituto Cajal), Madrid, Spain

M. A. Cuesta, F. Mateo Vallejo (eds.), *Spain's Journey in Medicine*,
https://doi.org/10.1007/978-3-032-12221-6_13

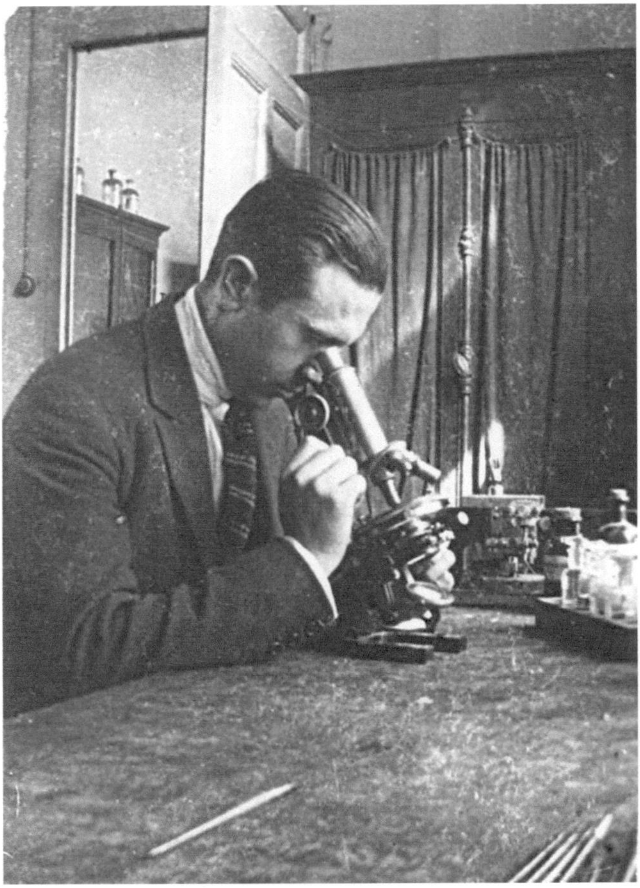

Fig. 13.1 Fernando de Castro using a monocular microscope in the laboratory of the Faculty of Medicine at the Central University (Madrid), 1922

and the Nobel Prize in Physiology or Medicine in 1906, Cajal Laboratory was full of doctors and students eager to work alongside him.

The young de Castro was recruited by Nicolás Achúcarro (1880–1918), a Bilbao native, to join his own laboratory—the Laboratory of Histopathology of the Nervous System—established by the *Junta para Ampliación de Estudios* on the floor directly above Cajal's lab in the mansion at 13 Paseo de Atocha. Achúcarro was a brilliant scientist who had trained with some of the most prominent neuropathologists in Europe and had distinguished himself in the United States, where he came recommended by Alois Alzheimer to set up a modern neuropathology service (Fig. 13.2).

Still quite young, Achúcarro returned to Spain, and his groundbreaking research on glial cells—combined with his charismatic personality—quickly

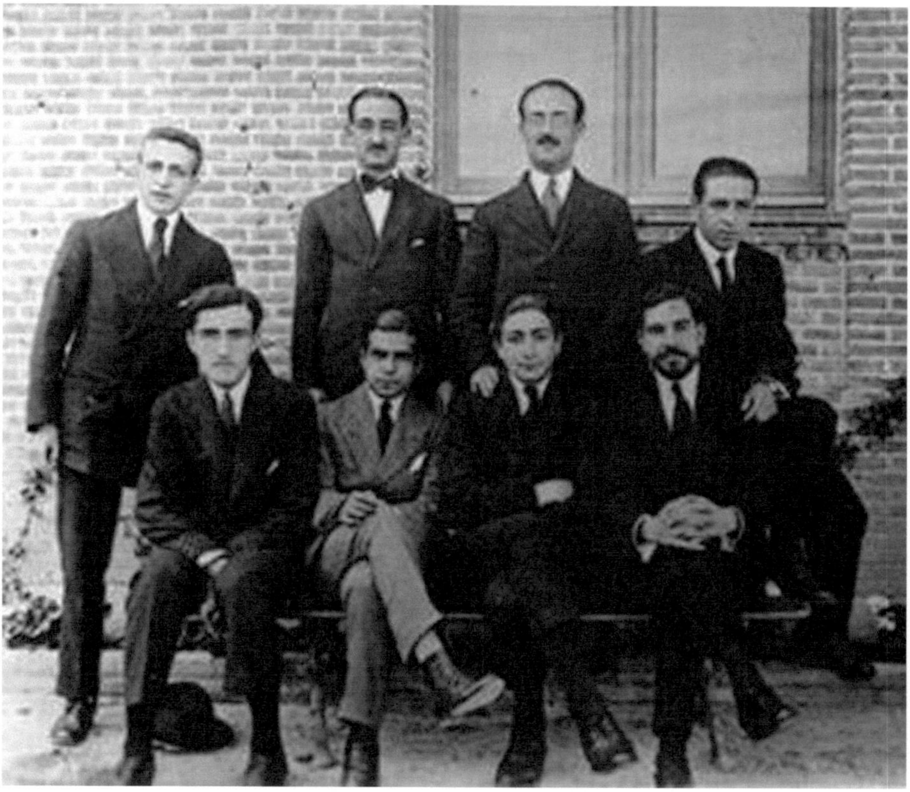

Fig. 13.2 Nicolás Achúcarro (seated, right) with some of his students at the Residencia de Estudiantes (ca. 1916). Standing, second from the left, are Pío del Río-Hortega, Luis Calandre, and Fernando de Castro (seated, behind Achúcarro), Sebastián Raz, J.M

made it clear that he, and no one else, should be the natural successor to lead the Cajal School when El Maestro eventually chose (or was perhaps compelled...) to step aside.

Achúcarro also had a remarkable talent for mentoring: under his guidance, major figures in neuroscience such as Pío del Río-Hortega and Fernando de Castro entered the field. He also influenced leading neuropsychiatrists like Miguel Gayarre Espinal, and José Miguel Sacristán; the anatomopathologist Luis Ruiz de Arcaute; and the renowned cardiologist Luis Calandre Ibáñez.

Achúcarro co-authored research articles with all of them—except for Río-Hortega and de Castro, the youngest members of this so-called "Achúcarro School."

De Castro's work in Achúcarro's laboratory soon bore fruit, resulting in noteworthy publications on the histogenesis of neuroglia in the olfactory bulb and cerebral cortex. These studies, highly valued by de Castro himself, were intended to form the foundation of an ambitious project conceived by Nicolás Achúcarro during his time in Germany: the study of the glioarchitecture of the entire central nervous system.

However, Achúcarro fell seriously ill at a young age, left the laboratory in 1916, and passed away in 1918. As his health declined, Fernando de Castro continued to meet with him weekly, both at his home and later in a sanatorium in the Sierra de Guadarrama, to discuss scientific matters. When Achúcarro relocated to Neguri (Vizcaya) for what would be the final stage of his life, Santiago Ramón y Cajal—who had taken notice of de Castro's promising output and, above all, his great skill with the diverse histological techniques employed in the Biological Research Laboratory—recruited him to join his own lab.

Cajal appointed Pío del Río-Hortega to take over leadership of Achúcarro's former laboratory, while Fernando de Castro would continue to work closely with Cajal until his death. In fact, it could be said that de Castro would not stop working with Cajal until the latter's death and could hardly be considered to have left the Cajal institute—the official name given to the Biological Research Laboratory in 1920—remaining associated with it until his own death in 1967.

De Castro was, along with Francisco Tello and Domingo Sánchez, one of Cajal's longest-serving collaborators (18 years), and also one of the most brilliant—second only to Pío del Río-Hortega and on par with the younger Rafael Lorente de No. [1]

Unravelling the Structure and Organisation of Sensory Ganglia

The nervous system is traditionally divided into the central nervous system (CNS)—comprising all nervous tissue enclosed within the bony structures of the skull and spine—and the peripheral nervous system (PNS), which includes the nerves and ganglia located outside the CNS.

Historically, many neurohistologists attempted to resolve the morphological and functional complexities of the PNS, a particularly demanding challenge both technically and logistically.

The debate between the "neuronists" and the "reticularists" was especially intense in the context of the PNS. A key example of this controversy was the dispute over the embryological origin of Cajal's interstitial cells in the intestine—considered fibroblastic by the reticularists, but of neural origin according to Cajal and the neuronists.

At the time, the scientific community was actively discussing the nature of axonal collaterals that innervate the ganglia, as well as the atypical forms that some of these structures displayed. The complexity of the issue, coupled with the fierce opposition of the reticularists, prompted Cajal to make a decisive move: he entrusted his young disciple, Fernando de Castro, with the delicate task of definitively clarifying the organization of the peripheral ganglia.

After completing his medical studies, Fernando de Castro began investigating the structure of the sensory ganglia, which today are recognized as part of the sympathetic and parasympathetic nervous systems.

He applied the silver staining methods developed by his mentors, Cajal and Achúcarro, to tissue samples from various species—both in normal conditions and in pathological states—thereby corroborating and refining several conclusions previously drawn by Cajal and the Romanian neurologist Georges Marinesco. For example, he confirmed that monopolar neurons—those with a single process emerging from the soma—are the most common cell type in normal sensory ganglia, though bipolar neurons—with two extensions emerging from the soma, typically a dendrite and an axon extending in opposite directions—can also be present.

More significantly, de Castro reorganized and definitively simplified the classification of neuronal cell types in normal sensory ganglia, refining the complex schema initially proposed by the Russian histologist Alexander Dogiel (1852–1922). Through elegant experimental work, he also resolved the debate over the ectodermal origin of satellite cells in ganglia, proposing the concept of a "neuro-neuroglial symbiosis"—an interaction between neurons and glial cells [2, 3]

Furthermore, in contrast to the trophic hypothesis proposed by Cajal and others regarding the spherical swellings observed in intraganglionic fibers after axotomy, Fernando de Castro supported the regenerative function suggested by G. Marinesco and J. Minea through in vitro studies. Castro's interest in nerve regeneration went further, as during the 1930s, he conducted complex experimental studies on reinnervation and cross-anastomosis between PNS motor fibers and sensory ganglia to demonstrate the nature of chemoreceptors in the carotid body. These conclusions were widely and universally accepted, as evidenced by the fact that the neurosurgeon and neuropathologist Wilder S. Penfield invited Fernando de Castro to write a chapter on the structure of sensory ganglia; and, as we will see later about the sympathetic ganglia in his renowned treatise on the nervous system, "*Cytology and Cellular Pathology of the Nervous System*", published a decade later.

However, the remarkable study on the cytoarchitecture of sensory ganglia not only earned de Castro the highest academic distinction but also the greatest recognition of his technical expertise. Santiago Ramón y Cajal decided that Fernando de Castro should supervise the technical training of new staff at the Institute but also the work of visiting researchers from various Spanish and international institutions. He held this position until 1932. Among these researchers were prominent figures in the history of biomedicine, such as Howard Florey (Nobel Prize in Physiology or Medicine, 1945), Hungarian neurologist Deszo Miskolczy, Uruguayan neuroscientist and educator Clemente Estable, American zoologist Edward Horne-Craigie, Portuguese scientist Celestino Da Costa, Belgian physiopharmacologist André Dewulf, and Ukrainian (then Soviet) researcher Oleksandr Chernyakhivsky. As a sign of his trust in the young de Castro's expertise in neurohistological techniques, Cajal assigned him the task of compiling all the protocols for the neurohistological techniques used and developed at the Laboratory of Biological Research (which became the Cajal Institute in 1920) over several decades, with the intention of publishing them. This resulted in the 1933 publication of what is perhaps the first textbook exclusively focused on neurohistological procedures (Cajal and de Castro, 1933), which, despite numerous attempts, was only published in English translation in 2016 [4, 5] (Fig. 13.3).

Conquering the Sympathetic and Parasympathetic Systems

Since the reticularists—led by Golgi—persistently defended the idea that the nervous system formed a continuous network (no longer composed of neuronal extensions, but of neurofibrils which, they claimed, extended from one neuron to another), they were reluctant to accept the theories proposed by Cajal and the so-called neuronists. The neuronists asserted that the nervous system was made up of individual cells—neurons—connected to one another via synapses. In response to this controversy, Fernando de Castro chose to directly investigate the histological structure of the autonomic ganglia.

In vertebrates, the autonomic nervous system—also called the vegetative nervous system—helps control the internal organs and keeps the body's internal environment stable. It works closely with the somatic nervous system, which controls voluntary movements. The autonomic system has groups of nerve cells called ganglia, which can be either sensory or motor. The motor ganglia are divided into two types: sympathetic ganglia (near the spine) and

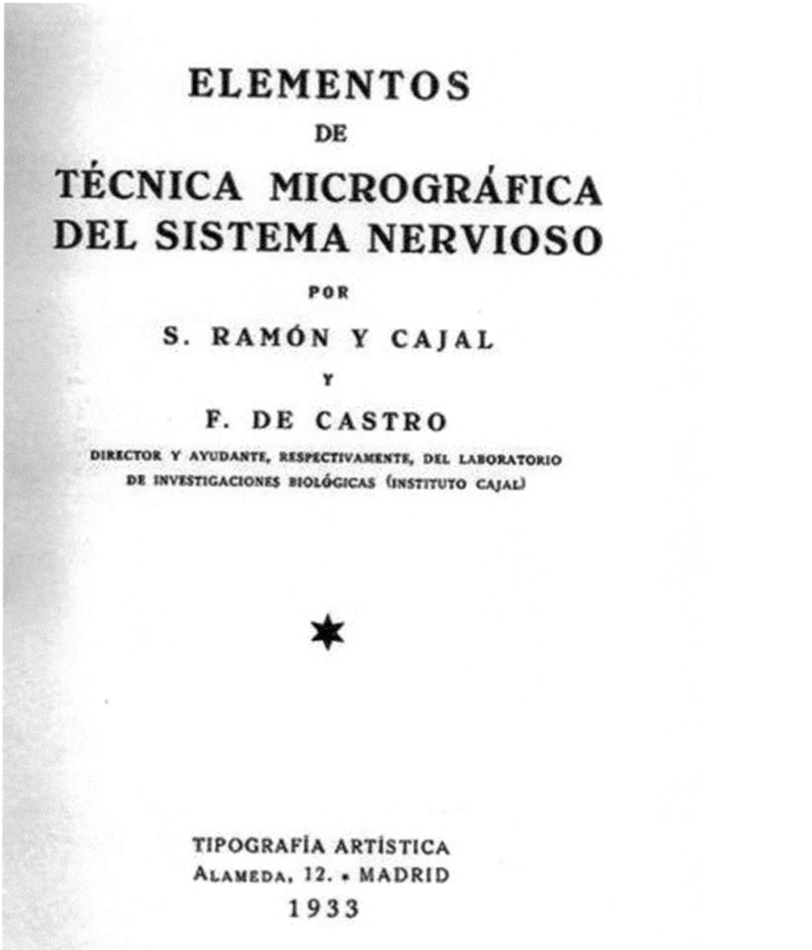

ELEMENTOS
DE
TÉCNICA MICROGRÁFICA
DEL SISTEMA NERVIOSO
POR
S. RAMÓN Y CAJAL
Y
F. DE CASTRO
DIRECTOR Y AYUDANTE, RESPECTIVAMENTE, DEL LABORATORIO
DE INVESTIGACIONES BIOLÓGICAS (INSTITUTO CAJAL)

TIPOGRAFÍA ARTÍSTICA
ALAMEDA, 12. • MADRID
1933

Fig. 13.3 Elements of the micrographic technique of the Nervous System. (S. Ramón y Cajal and Fernando de Castro, 1933)

parasympathetic ganglia (closer to the abdominal organs). This system also includes two partly independent parts: the cardiac system, which helps control the heart, and the enteric system, which manages the digestive organs.

Between 1923 and 1951, Fernando de Castro focused on studying the intercellular connections in the sympathetic ganglia, using various mammalian species as models [6] (Fig. 13.4).

After thoroughly reviewing the work of his predecessors in this field—including Dogiel, Cajal, von Lenhossék, Marinescu, Nageotte, Schaeffer, Bielschowsky, and Giuseppe Levi, among the most notable—Fernando de Castro confirmed that the spiral connections arranged around Paul Ehrlich's

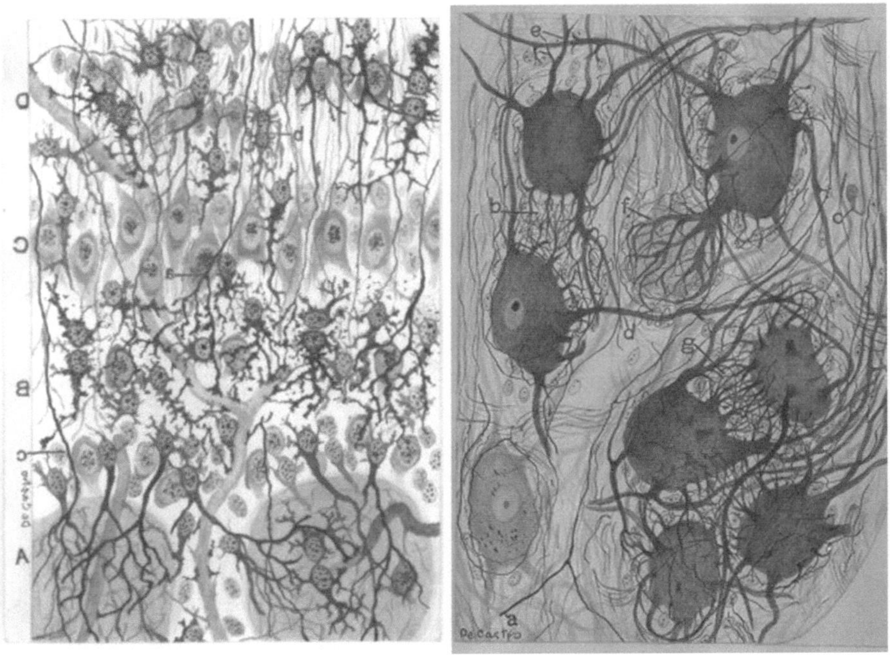

Fig. 13.4 Two drawings: (a) astrocytes. Original drawing by Fernando de Castro in pencil, India ink, and ink wash, illustrating various aspects of astrocyte genesis in the olfactory bulb of an eight-day-old cat, stained using Cajal's gold sublimation method, published as Figure 1 in: de Castro, F. (1920). Some observations on the histogenesis of neuroglia in the olfactory bulb. Trab. Lab. Invest. Biol. (b) Illustrates neurons of a lumbar sympathetic ganglion (and their connections). (F. de Castro Scientific Archive, Madrid)

so-called "*pericellular nests*," previously observed in amphibians, are also present in mammals. With this finding, he demonstrated that these pericellular nest structures were the most common form of connection of preganglionic afferent fibers in the sympathetic ganglia, later referred to as "*receptive plaques*."

Nearly a decade later, both De Castro and the Russian scientist Boris I. Lavrentyev (1892–1944), along with other researchers, provided evidence of synapses at the terminal boutons of these preganglionic fibers (see Ros and de Castro, 2020, for a historical overview). In 1932, De Castro described with great clarity that each sympathetic ganglion contains three types of neurons—large, medium, and small—have neurites that intertwine and appear to be distributed randomly [6]. This observation provided a histological basis for interpreting previous electrophysiological recordings by S. W. Ranson and P. R. Billingsley (1918), which had suggested that each type of preganglionic fiber formed synapsis exclusively with a specific type of ganglion cell.

Between 1914 and 1935, Henry Dale and Otto Loewi demonstrated the existence of chemical neurotransmission and identified the first neurotransmitters of the sympathetic nervous system—work that earned them the Nobel Prize in Physiology or Medicine in 1936

Following this line of research, Fernando de Castro focused on the nature of synapses within the myenteric ganglia—clusters of neurons located in the myenteric plexus, a network of nerves embedded in the intestinal wall. This study, disrupted by the Spanish Civil War, was completed under difficult conditions with the help of his doctoral student at the time, María Luisa Herreros [7, 8].

In the course of this work, Fernando de Castro also described the presence of "synaptic boutons close to astrocytes"—an observation whose functional significance would not be understood until several decades later, with the development of the concept of "*tripartite synapses*" [9]. This finding is now recognized undoubtedly one of the first and most striking milestones in what is known today as the "*glial cell revolution*," a rapidly growing field of neuroscience.

Some of De Castro's other contributions to the anatomy and physiology of the peripheral nervous system (PNS) remain relevant to this day. Among them is his description of the "*glial veil*" surrounding ganglionic neurons—a sort of "*neuronal atmosphere*" that protects axons once they have lost their myelin sheaths.

Throughout these decades of meticulous and elegant research on the cytoarchitecture of sympathetic and parasympathetic autonomic motor ganglia, De Castro placed particular emphasis on synaptology—the study of synapses and neuronal connections that enable communication. This focus on synaptic structure and function became a hallmark of his scientific career.

Fernando de Castro thus laid the definitive anatomical and histological foundations of the sympathetic nervous system. By the mid-1920s, despite his young age, he had established himself as one of the world's foremost experts in the field, alongside Boris I. Lavrentyev—a Russian histologist internationally known for his morpho-functional experiments on interneuronal synapses and the interoceptive and neurotrophic functions of sympathetic ganglia in the PNS.

Interoception is the understanding of your body's internal senses. It is a learned skill that you develop as you grow (that your heart is beating or that you are hungry or that you need to pee).

Neurotrophic relate to the influence of nerves on the nutrition of tissue.

Working from opposite ends of Europe, De Castro and Lavrentyev advanced the understanding of the sympathetic system well beyond that of their mentors, Cajal and Dogiel [6, 10].

De Castro remained committed to this line of research until the end of his career, which was thereafter devoted almost entirely to the study of various structures of the peripheral nervous system. Among his notable contributions was his detailed study of the innervation of the pancreas—still considered one of the most thorough descriptions of pancreatic innervation to date. This work was published in a commemorative volume honoring Cajal upon his retirement, to which all of Cajal's students and many international colleagues contributed.

De Castro also investigated the innervation of the intestine, but his most groundbreaking and widely recognized contribution to the history of science was the discovery and conceptualization of the first arterial chemoreceptors. A comprehensive overview of all these research lines can be found in Ros and de Castro [10].

Carotid Innervation and the First Description Arterial Chemoreceptors

Two papers published in French between 1926 and 1928 by Fernando de Castro in the Trav. Lab. Rech. Biol: "Sur la structure et l'innervation du sinus carotidien de l'homme et des mammiferes. Nouveaux faits sur l'innervation et la function du glomus caroticum" caused a stir in the biomedical community of the time. In them, he described the existence of chemoreceptors capable of detecting changes in the composition of arterial blood—clearly distinct from baroreceptors—each located in entirely different regions of the cardio-aortic area (Fig. 13.5).

He was the one who demonstrated that the dilatation at the bifurcation of the common carotid artery—known today as the carotid sinus—is not an artifact caused by tissue fixation or processing, but a genuine anatomical feature present in all mammalian species. He showed that two types of sensory receptors are concentrated in this region: baroreceptors, which detect changes in blood pressure and are embedded in the vascular wall, and chemoreceptors—first described and characterized by him—which are located in a small, highly vascularized structure known as the glomus caroticum or carotid body.

De Castro was the first to study these structures in detail and to consider their physiological functions. He was also the first to describe it and propose

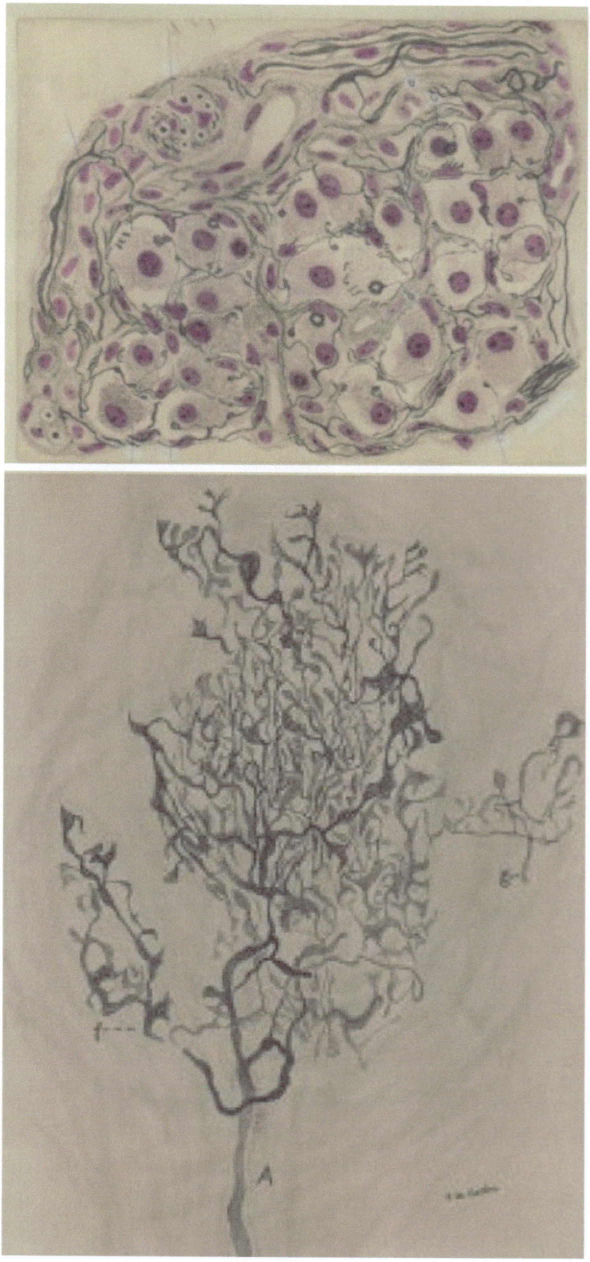

Fig. 13.5 Two drawings (**a**) Polychrome illustration of the carotid body stained with cresyl violet to show the chemoreceptor cells (de Castro, 1926) (**b**) Termination of a baroreceptor in the human carotid sinus, graphite and India ink drawing (de Castro, 1928). (F. de Castro Scientific Archive, Madrid)

that it was responsible for detecting qualitative changes in blood composition, with functional implications for the activity of other organs.

Using methylene blue staining techniques, he determined that this area was innervated almost exclusively by the first branch of the glossopharyngeal nerve after it exits the skull. He named this branch the intercarotid nerve—formerly known as Hering's nerve.

De Castro himself stated: *"In our opinion, the glomus represents an organ with multiple sensory receptors, equipped with specialized receptor cells, similar to those found in other sensory organs [...] We hypothesize that the glomus caroticum serves as a sensory organ, the only one so far known to detect certain qualitative variations in blood composition. This function, possibly mediated by reflex action, would influence the functional activity of other organs"* [11, 12].

De Castro made three key contributions:

1. He was the first to demonstrate the existence of sensory endings sensitive to the blood pressure in the carotid sinus wall.
2. He showed that the *glomus caroticum* is a sensory organ that responds to changes in the chemical composition of the blood.
3. He established that the sensory afferents from the carotid sinus and the *glomus caroticum* are transmitted through a nerve, specifically the first branch of the glossopharyngeal nerve.

Unfortunately, for various reasons, De Castro was unable to maintain the momentum he had set for his research. However, the path he had paved allowed other research groups, particularly those led by H. E. Hering and Corneille Heymans, to further investigate cardiovascular reflexes.

De Castro's work completely reoriented this field of research and specifically that developed in Ghent by father Francois and son Corneille Heymans and their disciples known as the Ghent school of physio-pharmacology. While de Castro chose a laborious way to demonstrate the nature and functioning of his chemoreceptors by cross anastomoses between nerves of different natures, procedures that required deep knowledge of the processes of degeneration and regeneration of the nervous system, the Ghent school used simple and elegant experiments in parabiosis (experiments in biology whereby two different animals share a single blood circulation).

In 1929, De Castro was invited by C. Heymans to Ghent, an invitation that was repeated in 1932, to conduct experiments that provided Heymans with crucial insights into the mechanisms of the carotid sinus.

Various factors, including competitive exams for a Histology chair at the University of Seville, the writing and publication of "*Técnica Micrográfica del*

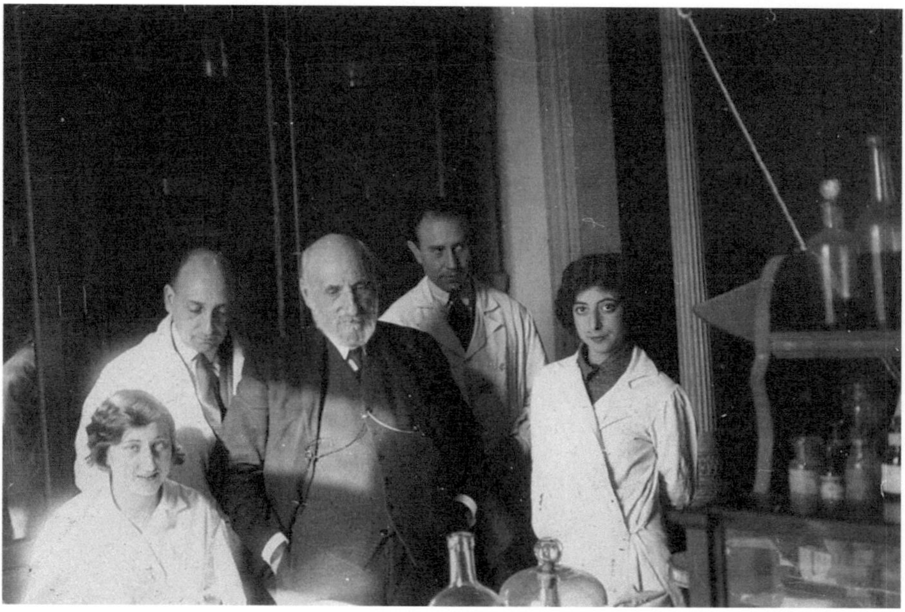

Fig. 13.6 Cajal and some of his disciples and collaborators at the first Cajal Institute (formerly Paseo de Atocha, 13), 1926. From left to right: Carmen Serra (laboratory worker), neuropsychiatrist José Mª Villaverde, Santiago Ramón y Cajal, Fernando de Castro, and Enriqueta "Kety" Lewy (librarian at the Institute)

Sistema Nervioso" [4], the death of Cajal, and the outbreak of the Spanish Civil War (1936–39), slowed down De Castro's research. Meanwhile, Corneille Heymans was awarded the Nobel Prize in Physiology or Medicine in 1938 *"for the discovery of the role of the sinus and aortic mechanisms in the regulation of respiration"*—an honor that de Castro undoubtedly deserved as well, a fact that caused him considerable frustration.

De Castro had actually been the discoverer of the functions of the *glomus caroticum,* and the recognition had gone to someone else [13] (Figs. 13.6, 13.7, and 13.8).

Although Pío del Río-Hortega was proposed by the University of Valencia for the Nobel Prize the previous year, Fernando de Castro was never nominated for the prize that year—an essential requirement for sharing it with the Belgian physio-pharmacologist. This situation was even discussed within the halls of the Karolinska Institute in Stockholm, which was responsible for awarding the prize. At the time, they were uncertain whether De Castro was still alive, as Madrid had been a battlefront since 1936, a city where almost everything had happened in those 2 years.

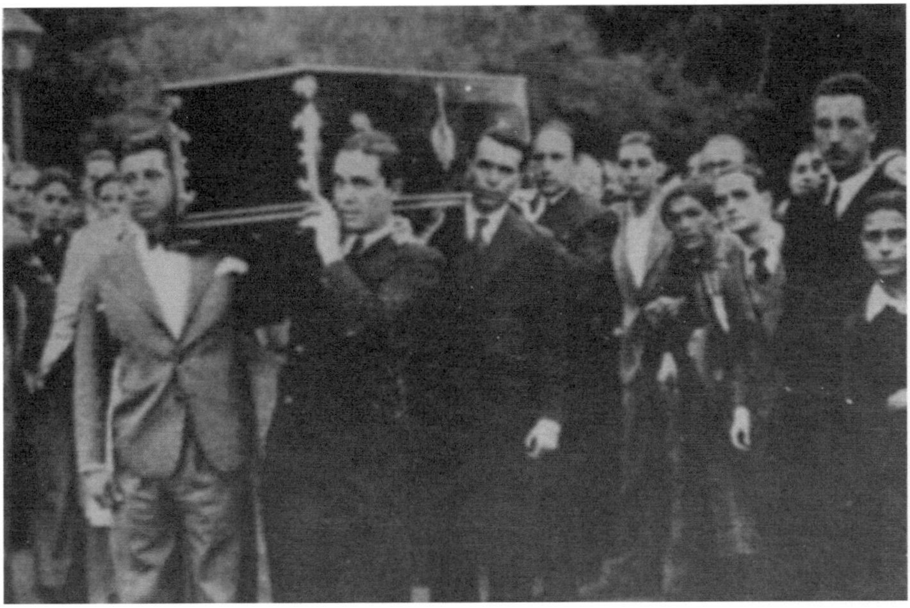

Fig. 13.7 Cajal's coffin is carried from left to right. Remartínez (an orderly at the Cajal Institute), Luis Calderón, Ramón Martínez (Tello's son-in-law), and Fernando de Castro. (F. de Castro Scientific Archive, Madrid)

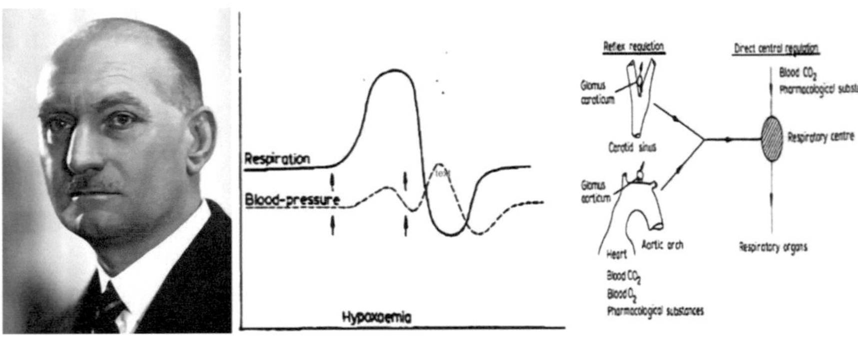

Fig. 13.8 Corneille Heymans and two diagrams from his Nobel Lecture showing the effect of hypoxemia on the respiration of a healthy dog (center) and a diagram showing the relationship between baroreceptors and chemoreceptors and cardiorespiratory reflexes. In the center, labeled G, a graph showing the relationship between respiration and blood pressure over time, with a focus on the effects of hypoxemia. On the right, labeled H a flow chart illustrating the regulation of respiration. It includes pathways from the carotid sinus and aortic arch to the respiratory center, influenced by blood CO2 levels and pharmacological substances. (adapted from Ros and de Castro, 2020). It was de Castro who guided this work, identifying and separating the distribution of these and other types of receptor neurons

The Spanish Civil War and the Irretrievable End of an Era

During the Spanish Civil War, Francisco Tello and Fernando de Castro—then, respectively, the Director and Deputy Director of the Cajal Institute—went there daily to protect it. At the end of the conflict, they handed over the Institute's belongings, equipment, and facilities to the new authorities, ensuring that they remained largely intact. However, both were tried and removed from their positions at the Central University and the Cajal Institute. Despite this, they continued their research under almost heroic conditions (Fig. 13.9).

Although Fernando de Castro was the most active researcher during those difficult years, Tello, Domingo Sánchez, and Pedro Ramón y Cajal (from Zaragoza) also continued to publish papers in the Institute's journal. However, the war had taken a significant toll on his scientific career, and with few resources or stable collaborators, Castro's output—focused on arterial chemoreceptors and the sympathetic system—never regained the level it had been at before the conflict.

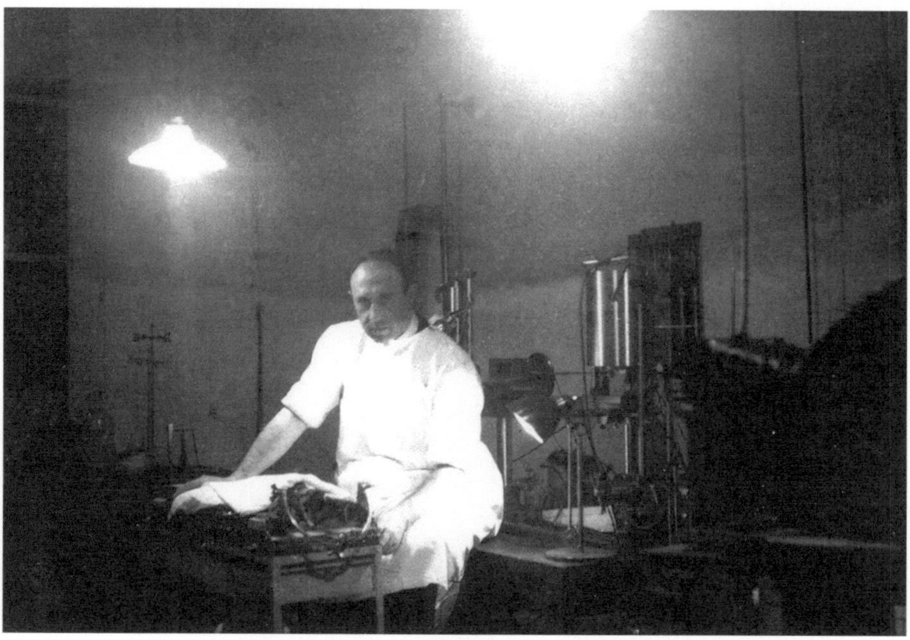

Fig. 13.9 1942. Fernando de Castro working at the postwar Cajal Institute (photograph by his friend and collaborator Dr. Miguel Calvo, 1942), operating on a cat. (F. de Castro Scientific Archive, Madrid)

Despite the lack of resources, in the early post-war period, the anatomopathologist Agustín Bullón and M. ª Luisa Herreros, among others, joined Castro's laboratory. His attempt to learn electrophysiological techniques at Rockefeller University in 1947, when the end of World War II allowed him to travel, with Professor Herbert S. Gasser, also failed to return his work to the pre-war pace. [1, 10].

With the departure of Lorente de Nó (who had been based in the USA from 1931 until his death in 1990), the exile and subsequent death of Pío del Río-Hortega in Buenos Aires in 1945, and the deaths of Domingo Sánchez in 1947, and Francisco Tello in 1958, Fernando de Castro ultimately became the leading figure of the Spanish Neurological School, the School of Cajal, in Madrid.

In 1952, De Castro took part in tributes to Cajal abroad for the centenary of his birth and, perhaps more significantly, became the undisputed architect of the tribute held in Madrid from November 14–20, 1952. This event brought an unprecedented number of Nobel laureates to the Spanish capital (Fig. 13.10).

Fernando de Castro also succeeded in persuading the Consejo Superior de Investigaciones Científicas (CSIC) to reprint Cajal's work, "*Histologie du Système Nerveux de l'Homme et des Vertébrés*", which had been out of print for decades. Despite the brief reprint, it quickly became unavailable again. The success of this well-deserved tribute was so significant that it encouraged the Franco dictatorship to promote scientific research in Spain. Among its consequences was the relocation of the Cajal Institute to new headquarters on Calle Velázquez, accompanied by a partial renovation of its equipment.

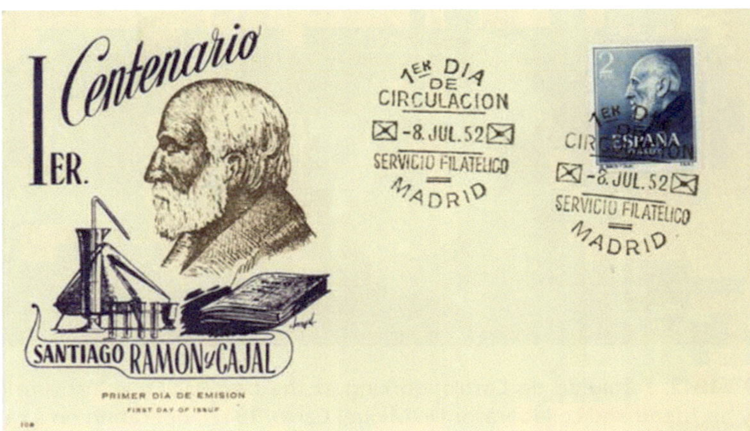

Fig. 13.10 Commemorative envelope featuring Cajal's first centenary, 8. Jul. 1952. Servicio Filatelico-Madrid

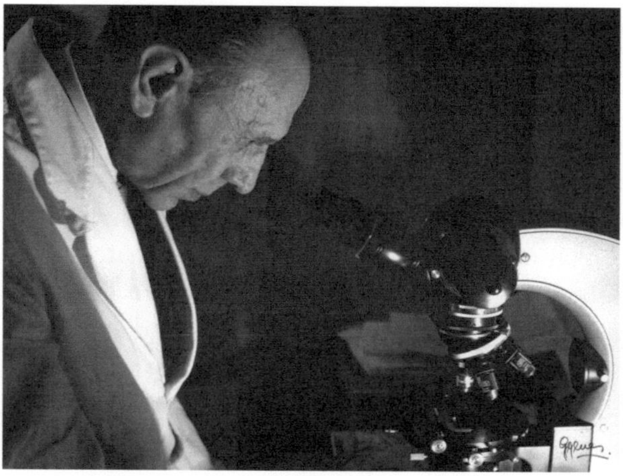

Fig. 13.11 Fernando de Castro looking through a microscope at the Cajal Institute (1966), Gyenes Photographer. (F. de Castro Scientific Archive, Madrid)

In the final years of his life, Fernando de Castro received numerous national and international honors and appointments. He led the official Spanish delegation at the Nobel Prize ceremony for Severo Ochoa in 1959 and was elected a member of the Accademia Nazionale dei Lincei in Italy, the Royal Academy of Exact, Physical, and Natural Sciences, and the Royal National Academy of Medicine in Madrid. However, he did not assume these latter two positions as he passed away before doing so.

He was also named Honorary Director of the Cajal Institute, although he never formally took up the post (Fig. 13.11).

In the final years of his career, Fernando de Castro mentored several outstanding disciples, including José Gómez Sánchez, the Chilean Juan de Dios Vial Correa, who would later become rector of the Pontificia Universidad Católica de Chile, and César Aguirre Viani. Among his most brilliant students, who went on to have significant scientific careers, were Constantino Sotelo, residing in Paris and Facundo Valverde.

Just before Fernando de Castro's retirement and his premature death from kidney cancer, the Dutch neuroscientist Hendrik van der Loos, known for his work on the structure of the cerebral cortex, stayed in his laboratory.

His last intern student at the Histology Department, Jaime Merchán Cifuentes, devoted his doctoral thesis to studying the scientific work of Fernando de Castro.

Epilogue

For all these reasons, the role of Fernando de Castro is considered fundamental in the development of neurohistology. He was one of Cajal's youngest direct disciples—chronologically, together with Rafael Lorente de Nó—and also one of those who achieved the most relevant scientific production, comparable only to that of Lorente de Nó himself (nominated for the Nobel Prize in Physiology or Medicine on four occasions, between 1948 and 1953) and to that of Pío del Río-Hortega (nominated in 1929 and 1937).

As has been pointed out, Fernando de Castro was the one who worked the longest with the Maestro: eighteen uninterrupted years after his time in Achúcarro's laboratory, where he stayed for another 2 years. He maintained, as a whole, a continuous and profound relationship with the different members of the Spanish Neurological School, as well as with numerous foreign researchers who passed through Cajal's laboratory.

Fernando de Castro also stood out for his loyalty to his Master and his spirit of camaraderie with all those with whom he worked. He was a faithful collaborator of Achúcarro until his death, a defender of the Cajal Institute alongside Jorge Francisco Tello during the Civil War—a time when both tirelessly and at great risk to their lives visited various Madrid "chekas" in an attempt to save José M. ª Villaverde from an execution that was ultimately carried out in Paracuellos del Jarama. He was friends with Domingo Sánchez and Pedro Ramón y Cajal, despite their generational differences, and maintained a close intellectual and personal relationship with Rafael Lorente de Nó, until an enigmatic distancing in the early 1950s. He was also a friend and later a supporter of Gonzalo Rodríguez Lafora upon his return from Mexican exile.

The only possible blemish in such an impeccable career was perhaps his involvement—along with Lorente de Nó—in the unjust criticisms published in 1923 against some discoveries of Pío del Río-Hortega, which he soon regretted, even publicly in 1946. Even this controversial episode cannot be fully understood without considering the strong sense of esprit d'école that permeated that time. The publication in question occurred during the height of a brief but painful personal rift between Cajal and Río-Hortega—a conflict largely fueled by third parties acting as instigators.

Fernando de Castro's commitment to honoring his mentor and preserving the legacy of the Spanish Neurological School was evident not only in his tireless work between 1939 and 1967 but also in his pioneering efforts as a chronicler of that extraordinary era. He was the first to write in depth about Cajal and the members of his school. These writings, originally dispersed across various publications, were compiled and published in 1981 by the Complutense University, thanks to the initiative of his only son, Fernando-Guillermo de Castro. [1, 14].

This work is essential for anyone seeking a deep understanding of Santiago Ramón y Cajal and the significance of his most distinguished disciples. As none other than Charles Sherrington—another giant of neuroscience and Nobel laureate in 1932—wrote in his obituary for Cajal, published by the Royal Society in early 1935 (see full reference in Chap. 10 of this book):

> It is no exaggeration to say that he [Cajal], together with his disciples—especially Achúcarro, Río-Hortega, and de Castro—opened a new era of knowledge [...] If ever a scientist created a school, it was Cajal; a school of colleagues and disciples.

Anyone wishing to write about Cajal must also remember his own words from *Rules and Advice for Scientific Investigation*:

> The purest glory of the master consists not in forming disciples who follow him, but in forming wise men who surpass him.

To attempt an account of Cajal's contributions without understanding the legacy of his school is to miss the essence of his work. And to truly grasp the depth of the Master's character and influence—especially in this regard—one must study in detail what Fernando de Castro wrote in *Cajal and the Spanish Neurological School*. It is rare to find such a powerful blend of personal insight, scientific understanding, admiration, and literary elegance as is found in those pages.

The *Fernando de Castro Scientific Archive* is a comprehensive collection of documents, drawings, histological preparations, photographs, and personal belongings—amounting to several tens of thousands of items. While the majority of the archive stems from Fernando de Castro's own life and scientific activity, a significant portion consists of materials he acquired personally (and, to a lesser extent, those obtained by his son, Fernando-Guillermo de Castro) in an effort to preserve everything related to Santiago Ramón y Cajal. This preservation was especially urgent given the risk that, for various and mainly unfortunate reasons, Cajal-related materials might fall into hands that neither valued nor cared for them.

After decades of dedicated effort, the *Fernando de Castro Scientific Archive* was officially registered in the *Census-Guide of Archives of Spain and Latin*

America (reference: ES. 28079.ACFC). Since October 2017, it has been part of *UNESCO's Memory of the World Programme*, included in the collective inscription of the archives of Santiago Ramón y Cajal, Pío del Río-Hortega, Fernando de Castro, Rafael Lorente de Nó, and Pedro Ramón y Cajal [15]. UNESCO recognized these archives as essential for understanding the history of the discoveries and theories that shaped our current knowledge of the human brain—both in terms of its anatomical structure (individual cells) and its physiological functions (circuit formation and nerve impulse transmission).

References

1. de Castro F. Cajal and the Spanish Neurological School. Madrid: 1981. Ed. Univ. Complutense. Madrid. Spain.
2. de Castro F. Study on the sensory ganglia of man in normal and pathological state. Typical and atypical cellular forms. Arch Neurobiol. 1922;3:256–318.
3. de Castro F. Sensory ganglions of the cranial and spinal nerves normal and pathological. In: Penfield W, editor. Cytology and cellular pathology of the nervous system, vol. 1. New York: Hoeber Publishers; 1932. p. 93–143.
4. Cajal SR, de Castro F. Técnica micrográfica del sistema nervioso. Madrid: Tipografía Artística; 1933.
5. Merchán M, De Felipe J, de Castro F, editors. Cajal and de Castro's neurohistological methods. Oxford University Press; 2016.
6. de Castro F. Sympathetic ganglia, normal and pathological. In: Penfield WD, Penfield W, editors. Cytology and cellular pathology of the nervous system, vol. I. New York: Hoeber Publishers; 1932. p. 317–9.
7. de Castro F. Sur la régénération fonctionnelle dans le sympathique (anastomoses croisées avec des nerfs de type iso et hétéromorphe). A special reference to the constitution of synapses. Trav Lab Rech Biol. 1937;31:271–345.
8. de Castro F, Herreros ML. Functional activity of the superior cervical ganglion in relation to the number and modality of its preganglionic fibres. Model of the synapse. Trab Cajal Res Inst Biol. 1945;37:287–342.
9. Perea G, Navarrete M, Araque A. Tripartite synapses: astrocytes, process and control synaptic information. Trends Neurosci. 2009;32:421–31.
10. Ros F, de Castro F. Fernando de Castro: Cajal's man on the peripheral nervous system. Anat Rec. 2020;303:1206–14.
11. de Castro F. Sur la structure et l'innervation de la glande inter-carotidienne (glomus caroticum) de l'homme et des mammifères, et sur un nouveau système d'innervation autonome du nerf glosopharyngien. Trav Lab Rech Biol. 1926;24:365–432.

12. de Castro F. Sur la structure et l'innervation du sinus carotidien de l'homme et des mammifères: nouveaux faits sur l'innervation et la fonction du glomus caroticum. Trav Lab Rech Biol. 1928;25:330–80.
13. Author's translation of the official information on https://www.nobelprize.org/prizes/medicine/1938/summary/.
14. de Castro F. Towards the sensory nature of the carotid body: Hering, de Castro and Heymans. Front Neuroanat. 2009;3:23–30. https://doi.org/10.3389/neuro.05.023.2009.
15. More information at: http://www.unesco.org/new/en/communication-and-information/memory-of-the-world/register/full-list-of-registered-heritage/registered-heritage-page-1/archives-of-santiago-ramon-y-cajal-and-the-spanish-neurohistological-school/.

14

Josep Trueta i Raspall: Surgeon, Researcher and Committed Citizen

Luis A. Fariña

"Trueta's work is vast, diverse and complex. But, at the same time, it is poorly known. Despite being an established figure in European medical history".

Felipe Cid, 1996.

"It is a scientific monstrosity to believe that "purity of blood" is maintained by the elimination of crossbreeding, when we know that the opposite is true".

Josep Trueta, 1978.

Josep Trueta, born in the Poblenou district of Barcelona in 1897, graduated from the Faculty of Medicine of Barcelona in 1921 and earned his doctorate from the University of Madrid in 1922. He was one of the most prominent, influential, and renowned European surgeons of his time [1–3] (Fig. 14.1).

Supported by his father, who was also a doctor in Barcelona, Trueta began his studies of Medicine in the University of Barcelona with teachers as Augusto Pi Sunyer in physiology, Jaume Ferran in microbiology and Joaquim Trias i Pujol as professor of surgical pathology; he was also intern in de department of internal medicine with prof. Francesc Ferrer Solervicens. In 1921 he began his surgical training in Barcelona, the same year he graduated, at the

L. A. Fariña (✉)
Department of Urology, Ribera Povisa Hospital in Vigo, Vigo, Spain

M. A. Cuesta, F. Mateo Vallejo (eds.), *Spain's Journey in Medicine*,
https://doi.org/10.1007/978-3-032-12221-6_14

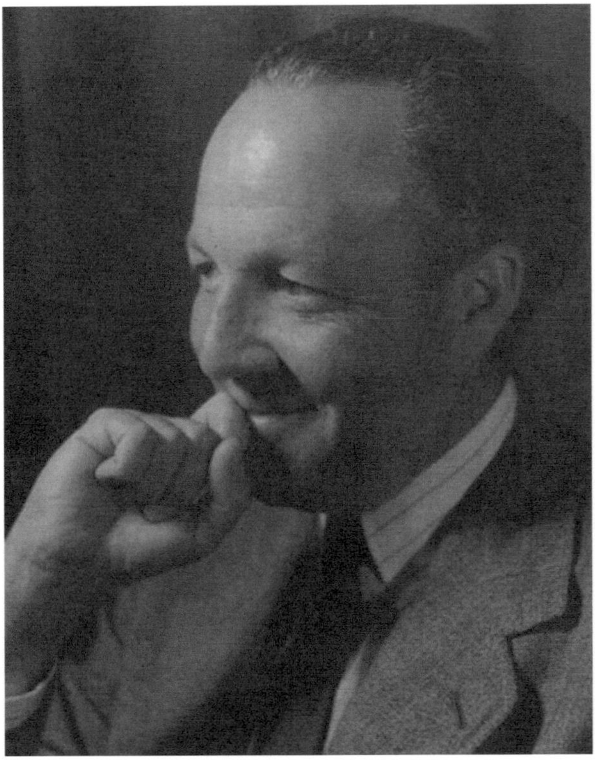

Fig. 14.1 Josep Trueta in 1944, when he was 47 years old and leading a traumatology and orthopedics team in Oxford (UK)

newly modernized Hospital de Santa Creu i Sant Pau, working as assistant to Dr. Manuel Corachán—one of the surgeons of the Catalan school at the beginning of the twentieth century, who left a significant mark on Spanish surgery.

With M. Corachán they visited the department of Lorenz Bohler in the AUVA-Hospital in Vienna, pioneer of the modern traumatology of accidents, where Francesc Gimeno Vidal studied. Both Trueta and Gimeno Vidal are considered the fathers of the new traumatology in Spain.

In 1935, after the death of Enric Ribas i Ribas professor at the Universitat Autònoma, when Trueta was to be his successor, the Civil War in Spain broke out.

Trueta Surgeon

In July 1936, coinciding with the military rebellion against the Republican government that led to the Spanish Civil War (1936–1939), Trueta took charge of one of the Surgical Units at the Hospital de Sant Pau in Barcelona, city where armed conflicts were taking place between forces loyal to the government and others supporting the coup d'état. A city that was the rearguard of several war fronts and where its population was a prolonged military target, including heavy aerial bombardments by Italian and German aircraft.

The large influx of wounded and the scarcity of resources prompted Trueta to extensively implement a novel method of deep surgical wound cleaning, combined with occlusive and immobilizing treatment using plaster casts for complex open fractures of the extremities. He had already gained experience in trauma management from working in industrial accidents [4, 5] (Fig. 14.2).

This approach was based in complicated open fractures in which combined early, thorough cleaning of the wound—removing foreign bodies, excision of wound edges, necrotic tissue and bruised tissue (P.L. Friedrich wound excision)—with careful sparing blood vessels and nerves, and as much of the bone

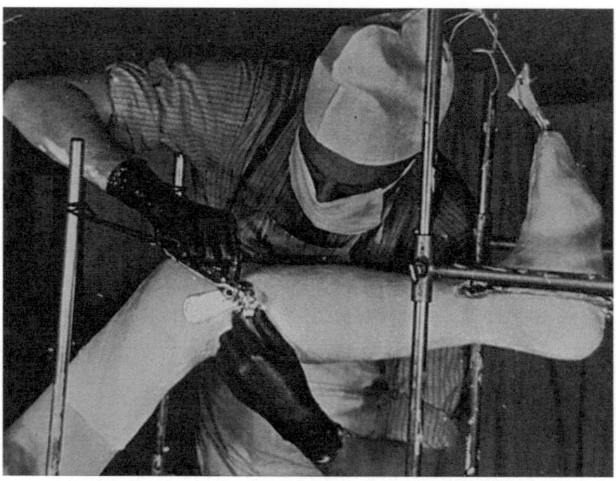

Fig. 14.2 Trueta operating, completing the cast on a wounded lower limb during the Spanish Civil War (1937)

and its fragments as possible. It also involved drainage and immobilization of the limb in extension with a plaster bandage. This treatment could be followed by transfer from the front or, if the patient was already in a well-equipped center, by periodic and prolonged dressings. Inspection of the wounds, weeks after, showed a clean wound with granulating tissue covering the bones fragments and fracture. This approach to treating complex wounds involving open complicated fractures, bone fragmentation, and contamination had precedents. Techniques for debriding complicated wounds and methods for the prolonged immobilization of war-related fractures—areas in which the Spanish surgeon Manuel Bastos gained significant experience during colonial wars and conflicts within the Iberian Peninsula—were already known, just as it was for treatment of chronic osteomyelitis. However, it was Trueta who systematized and widely disseminated this approach, beginning with a publication in Catalan in 1938, followed by several in English from 1939 onward. He referred to it as the "*closed method*". These works were shared and discussed internationally (Fig. 14.3).

Trueta and his collaborators demonstrated that the method significantly reduced cases of gangrene and the need for limb amputations in battlefield injuries—at a time when technical and human resources for evacuation and medical care were scarce, little was known about the microorganisms causing wound infections, and antibiotics had yet to be tested on humans. His method's broad dissemination through well-illustrated books and articles earned Trueta well-deserved recognition among both civilian and military surgeons worldwide.

Interesting is the lecture of the vascular surgeon Rudolph Matas, son of Catalonian parents, during the LII Congress of the Southern Surgical Association in 1939. He referred to his experiences in Catalan hospitals during the Spanish Civil War, speaking about the "Spanish or Catalan method" to treat the open complicated fractures. He told that after several weeks, when the plaster cast was removed, the wound had a foul smell as consequence of the pus and secretions accumulated, but once cleaned with sterile water, the wound showed a clean aspect covered with healthy granulation tissue. He ended his conference saying: "Not all cheese that smell bad, is bad".

In early 1939, with the Spanish Civil War nearing its end, Trueta went into an exile with his family. After a brief stay in France, he was invited by the British Health Service, which was eager to learn from his experience treating war wounds. He was authorized to practice surgery and began working at the Nuffield Orthopaedic Centre in Oxford, a hospital sponsored by automobile manufacturer William Morris, Lord Nuffield. In 1942, he was awarded an honorary Doctor of Orthopedics at the University of Oxford, and in 1947, he

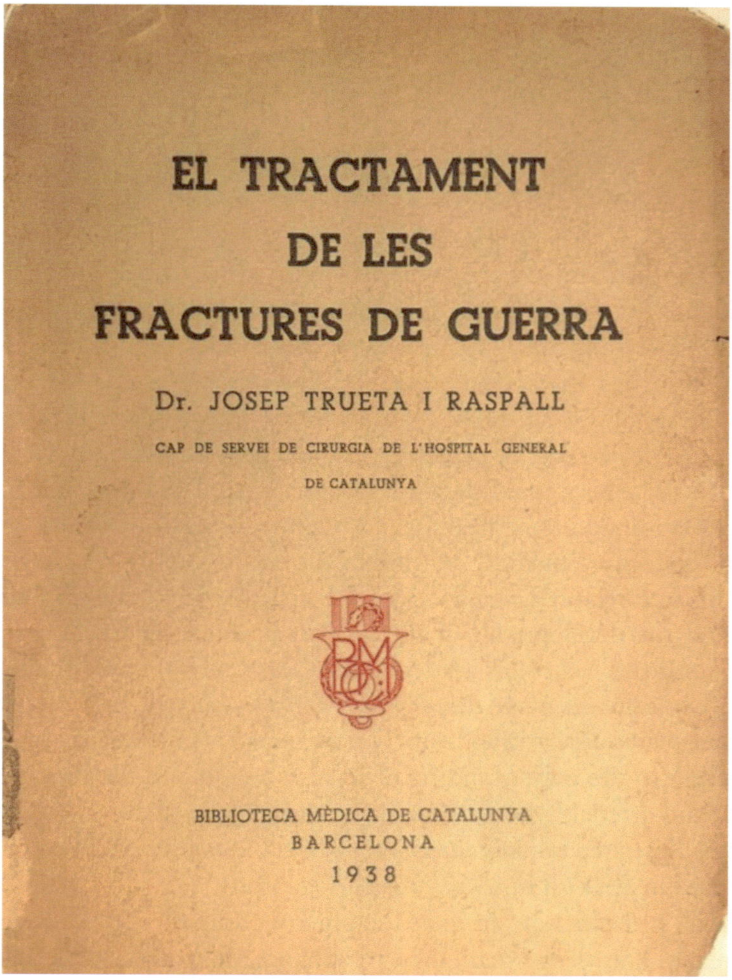

Fig. 14.3 Offprint from Trueta's first publication on the treatment of war fractures, in Catalan (1938)

became the university's first Professor of Orthopedics. There, he taught his knowledge of war surgery to medical students and nurses—expertise that was widely applied by many armies during the Second World War and in subsequent conflicts such as those in Korea and Vietnam.

His books "*The Principles and Practice of War Surgery: With Reference to the Biological Method of the Treatment of War Wounds and Fractures*" (1943) [6] and "*An Atlas of Traumatic Surgery: Illustrated Histories of Wounds of the Extremities*" (1949) [7] became widely recognized reference texts. From his early years as a surgeon in Barcelona, Trueta was a dedicated communicator and publicist. His numerous works on war wounds and bone diseases reveal a thoughtful and inquisitive clinician committed to understanding the scientific foundations of his practice.

Trueta Researcher

Also in Oxford, Trueta worked in the laboratory where the first clinical studies on penicillin—the world's first antibiotic—were conducted by the team led by H. W. Florey and E. B. Chain. Florey and Chain, along with Alexander Fleming, who had discovered penicillin in 1928, were awarded the Nobel Prize in Physiology or Medicine in 1945. Trueta was among the first to demonstrate the effectiveness of penicillin in treating osteomyelitis.

In Oxford, he also established a school of clinical research that produced significant studies on bone healing and pathology, many of which were published in the leading medical journals of the time. Later in his career, Trueta focused his research on osteogenesis and the relationship between the vascular system and the development of the human skeleton—a line of inquiry he pursued until the end of his academic life. This body of work culminated in his 1975 book *Studies of the Development and Decay of the Human Frame* [8].

Another major area arising from Trueta's research in severe trauma was his contribution to the understanding of renal function and the damage caused by shock and arterial hypertension. This work culminated in the publication of his well-illustrated book *Studies on the Renal Circulation*, released in English in 1947 and in Spanish in 1949 [9–11] (Fig. 14.4).

The book presents how an interdisciplinary group of researchers —in different areas of knowledge -radiology, physiology, and pathological anatomy—develop an original study of the causes of post-traumatic oliguria in war casualties. Based on their experience with the severely traumatized people from the Spanish Civil War, and on early studies of Crush Syndrome published in 1941, which had identified acute renal failure following extensive limb injuries, Trueta and his team were able to demonstrate specific changes in renal circulation. They observed a pattern of cortical ischemia—where blood flow in the outer region of the kidney was reduced or even halted—while medullary and juxtamedullary circulation was preserved or increased.

Initial experiments involved inducing localized trauma to the limbs of animals to observe the resulting renal ischemia and oliguria. Through a series of studies documented with original diagrams, angiographic images, and anatomical preparations, they showed that in various pathological conditions, the transit time of blood flow from the renal artery to the renal vein was reduced

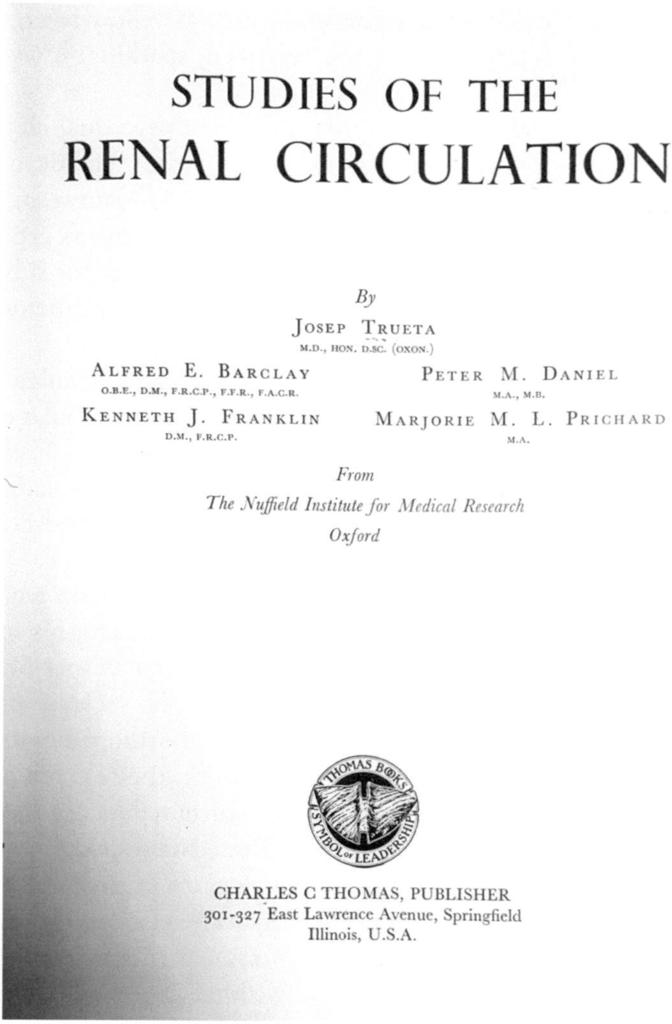

STUDIES OF THE
RENAL CIRCULATION

By

JOSEP TRUETA
M.D., HON. D.SC. (OXON.)

ALFRED E. BARCLAY
O.B.E., D.M., F.R.C.P., F.F.R., F.A.C.R.

PETER M. DANIEL
M.A., M.B.

KENNETH J. FRANKLIN
D.M., F.R.C.P.

MARJORIE M. L. PRICHARD
M.A.

From

The Nuffield Institute for Medical Research
Oxford

CHARLES C THOMAS, PUBLISHER
301-327 East Lawrence Avenue, Springfield
Illinois, U.S.A.

Fig. 14.4 Cover page of the English edition of "Studies of the Renal Circulation" Charles C. Thomas, Springfield, Illinois, U.S.A. (1947)

by one-third to one-half with occasionally reduced arterial caliber and, critically, a diversion of blood flow from the cortex to the medulla via the straight vessels—an effect that became temporarily known in scientific literature as ‘Trueta’s shunt.

Trueta and his collaborators proposed that the origin of renal ischemia lay in a reflex or centrally mediated stimulus of the vascular nerves, which triggered distant arterial spasm in various organs. They believed this spasm was responsible for the oliguria observed in combat-injured patients. At the same time, numerous other causes of renal anoxia—such as yellow fever, cholera, surgical bleeding, and sepsis—were being described, sparking intense scientific debate.

Trueta's experiments, and his description of the kidney's dual circulation, were validated by research in other European and North American centres and were reaffirmed in 1968, when cortical ischemia was again recognized as a central feature of oliguric acute renal failure. Although Trueta's explanation was not definitive, his work became a foundational reference for subsequent studies on acute renal failure caused by septic, traumatic, and hemorrhagic shock, transplant rejection, and other conditions.

Over the past fifty years, a vast body of knowledge has accumulated about renal disease, particularly regarding the pathogenesis of acute tubular necrosis. This condition, now understood as a common final pathway of diverse renal injuries—not only traumatic in origin—has been linked to early changes such as increased renal vascular resistance and decreased cortical blood flow, both of which contribute to the onset of the lesion.

All of Trueta's experimental work—particularly his research on renal circulation, for which he may one day be remembered as much as for his contributions to war surgery—stands as a model of research driven by specific clinical questions. What is especially remarkable is the breadth of his scientific inquiry, extending far beyond his primary role as a trauma and orthopedic surgeon.

Following the publication of this final major work, the research group at the Nuffield Institute in Oxford disbanded, and Trueta redirected his focus to the study of bone development and ageing. These interests culminated, as mentioned above, in his 1975 book *The Structure of the Human Body: Studies on Its Development and Decay*. For both his surgical practice and his scientific contributions, Trueta received numerous professional and academic honors across Europe and the Americas. In contrast, within Spain, he shared the fate of many exiles—deliberately overlooked and excluded from recognition.

Trueta, Humanist and Committed Citizen

Trueta was an intellectual and humanist with remarkably broad interests, which he expressed through memoirs, travel writings, studies on the history of surgery, and brief biographical essays on classical Catalan and Spanish scholars such as Ramon Llull and Luis Vives, as well as physicians like Arnau de Vilanova, Michael Servetus, Santiago Ramón y Cajal, and his mentor and predecessor in orthopedics at Oxford, the surgeon G. R. Girdlestone.

His unwavering commitment to freedom and solidarity with Spain's legitimate Republican government led him to accept the uncertainties of exile in

February 1939. He briefly participated in the first Catalan government in exile—the *Consell Nacional de Catalunya*, which represented Catalan interests in the United Kingdom and among the Allies—and in 1941 he authored "*The Spirit of Catalonia*" (published in English in 1946) a historical and cultural essay aimed at introducing Catalonia's identity to an English-speaking audience. The book was later translated into Catalan in 1950, where it was read clandestinely under Franco's regime, and only posthumously translated into Spanish in 1989 [12] (Fig. 14.5).

Dedicated "to the memory of Pau Casals, great artist and great Catalan," the book was intended as "an inventory of the Catalan contribution to the

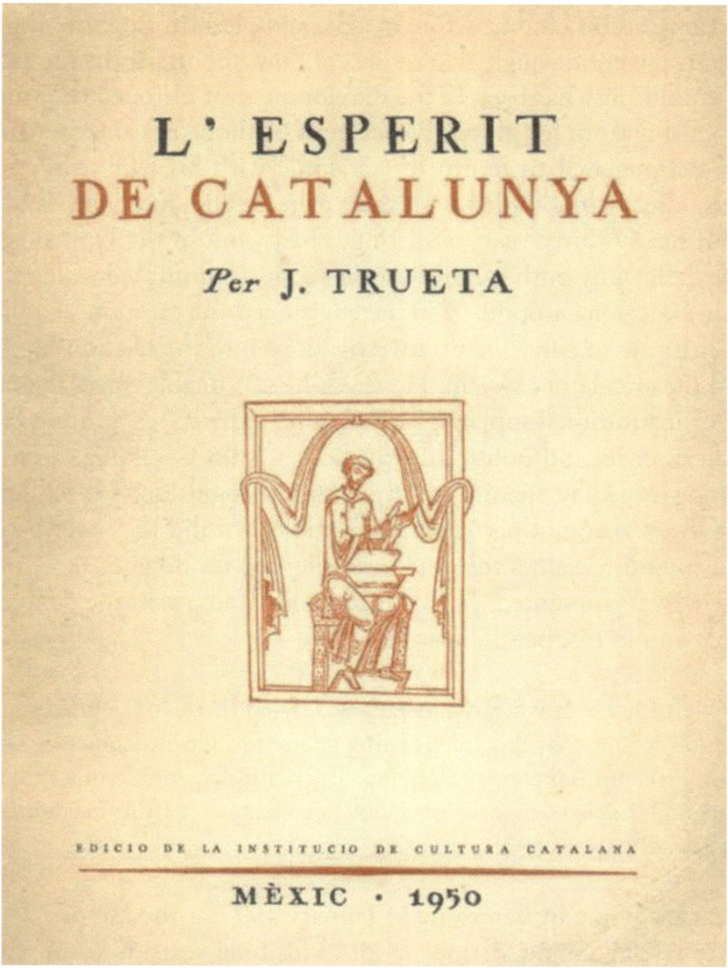

Fig. 14.5 First Catalan edition of the book "L'esperit de Catalunya", Mexico by the Institució de Cultura Catalana (1950), originally published in English

progress of Western Civilization". It offers Trueta's perspective on the history of Catalan institutions and culture, including scientific and medical achievements within the medieval kingdoms of Aragon and Catalonia. The work is supported by references drawn from his extensive readings in the London bookshop of Joan Gili, a prominent Catalan bookseller and publisher. Trueta himself acknowledged in later editions that *The Spirit of Catalonia* was not a conventional history book "as understood by professional historians," but rather "a clinical history written by an expert about the people to whom he belongs and for whom he writes".

Some conclusions seem controversial, when they invoke certain collective ideals or when they interpret certain conflicts, without considering how complex the history is, but Trueta had an in-depth knowledge of history, the arts and human relations, and he wrote in agile and pleasant English. The numerous editions it went through give an idea of how important the prestige of the Catalan community has been in the development of European culture.

After retiring from his post as Professor of Orthopedics at Oxford in 1965, Josep Trueta prepared to return to Catalonia with his wife, while his three daughters, already had settled with their own families in Spain. This marked the end of nearly thirty years of distinguished work in the United Kingdom and a life defined by both surgical excellence and committed exile.

Back in Barcelona around 1970, he envisioned the creation of a biological research institute to continue his investigations into the relationship between bone and the circulatory system. However, he was unable to get the necessary funding or institutional support. Although he received recognition from several medical, civic, and political institutions within Catalonia, he was never fully acknowledged by Spanish society at large recognition that was long overdue. The times were not particularly favorable, nor did they ever become so, as Trueta embodied values that had been silenced for decades.

In 1976 was appointed "Doctor Honoris Causa" of the University of Barcelona, and in his speech, he said:

> Having left Catalonia when democracy was dying there, it is a great source of satisfaction for me that this title is being granted to me as democracy is being reborn... Freedom is intrinsic to my life. This act today signifies my true return to my land, which I left because I did not want to see the freedom of my country dead!

He died at his home in Barcelona in January 1977 at the age of 79 [13] and was laid to rest in Santa Cristina d'Aro. In his final years, he wrote his memoirs, which were organized and edited by his daughter Amelia and published as "*Fragments d'una vida*" (1978) [14], with an English edition titled "*Trueta: Surgeon in War and Peace*" (1980). This moving and richly detailed account captures not only the extraordinary life of Josep Trueta but also the dramatic historical period he lived through, as hero of two wars (Spanish Civil and the

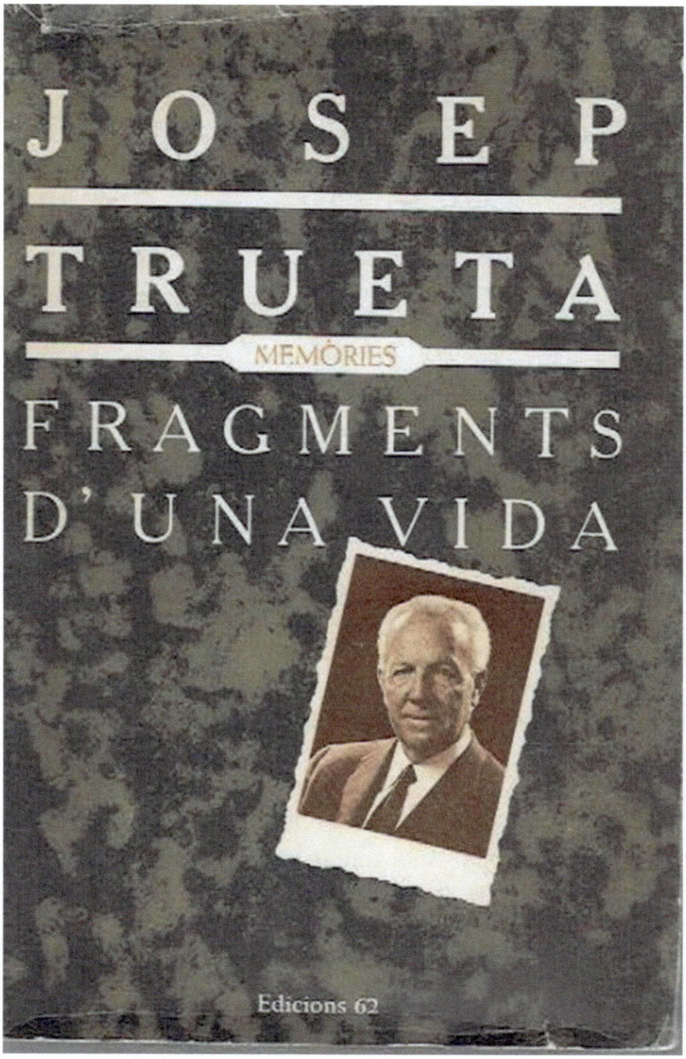

Fig. 14.6 Cover of the first edition of Trueta's memoirs "Fragments d'una vida", Editions 62, (1978)

world War II [15] as well as many of the pivotal medical and surgical advances of the twentieth century (Fig. 14.6).

References

1. AAVV. Josep Trueta (1897–1977). In homage. Fundació Barcelona, Col.legi Oficial de Metges de Barcelona; 1996.
2. Trueta. Angels Aymar. UK: Five Leaves Publications; 2010.
3. Cid F. Josep Trueta, esbós d'una obra médica i biológica. Barcelona: Tibidabo; 1991.
4. Moral Torres J. El "Método Español" en el Tratamiento de las heridas de guerra. (Técnica de Orr-Bastos-Trueta). In: Los Médicos y la Medicina en la Guerra Civil Española. Monografías Beecham; 1986. p. 157–66.
5. Cid F. La contribució científica catalana a la medicina y cirurgía de guerra (1936–1939). Fundació Uriach 1838, Barcelona 1996.
6. Trueta J. The principles and practice of war surgery: with reference to the biological method of the treatment of war wounds and fractures." Introduction by O.W. Wangensteen. St Louis: C.V. Mosby Co; 1943.
7. Trueta J. "An atlas of traumatic surgery: illustrated histories of wounds of the extremities" Oxford: Blackwell Scientific Publications. 1949.
8. Trueta J. Studies of the development and decay of the human frame. London: University of Oxford/William Heinemann Medical Books; 1975.
9. Trueta J, Barclay AE, Daniel PM, Franklin KJ, Prichard MML. Studies of the renal circulation. Blackwell Scientific Publications; 1947.
10. Epstein M, Eknoyan G. A forgotten chapter in the history of the renal circulation: the Josep Trueta and Homer Smith intellectual conflict. Am J Physiol Renal Physiol. 2015;309:F90–7.
11. Fariña LA. Studies on the kidney and the renal circulation by Josep Trueta I Raspall (1897–1977). Actas Urol Esp. 2008;32:276–80.
12. Trueta J. L'esperit de Catalunya. Barcelona: Edicions 62; 2003.
13. In Memoriam. J. Trueta. Bone & Joint. 1977;57 B: 243–45.
14. Trueta J. Fragments d'una vida. 1978. Edicions 62, Barcelona 1978.
15. Rodrigo A, Doctor Trueta. Anonymous hero of two wars. Barcelona: Plaza y Janés; 1977.

15

Carlos Jiménez Díaz: Basic Sciences Are Fundamental for Clinic Medicine

Miguel Ángel Piris Pinilla

Carlos Jiménez Díaz was born in Madrid in 1898, the second of four sons of Mariano Jiménez Hortés and Jacoba Díaz Benito. He came of age during the vibrant cultural and intellectual awakening of 1920s Spain and later endured the hardships of the Civil War and the postwar period (Fig. 15.1).

A gifted student from an early age, Carlos was drawn to medicine, inspired by the groundbreaking work of Santiago Ramón y Cajal, recipient of the Nobel Prize in 1906. He pursued his medical studies at the San Carlos Faculty of Medicine in Madrid, where he had the opportunity to attend lectures by some of the most renowned figures of the time: Ramón y Cajal, Teófilo Hernando Ortega in Therapeutics at the Hospital Clínico, and Juan de Azúa Suárez in Dermatology at the Hospital Provincial.

Despite this impressive academic environment, Carlos soon became disillusioned with the quality of instruction at the Faculty. Disappointed, he and several of his classmates chose to stop attending formal lectures, instead dedicating themselves to rigorous self-study. During this period of independent learning, he resided as an intern student at the Academic Hospital of San Carlos.

M. Á. Piris Pinilla (✉)
Department of Pathological Anatomy, Fundación Jiménez Díaz, Madrid, Spain

M. A. Cuesta, F. Mateo Vallejo (eds.), *Spain's Journey in Medicine*,
https://doi.org/10.1007/978-3-032-12221-6_15

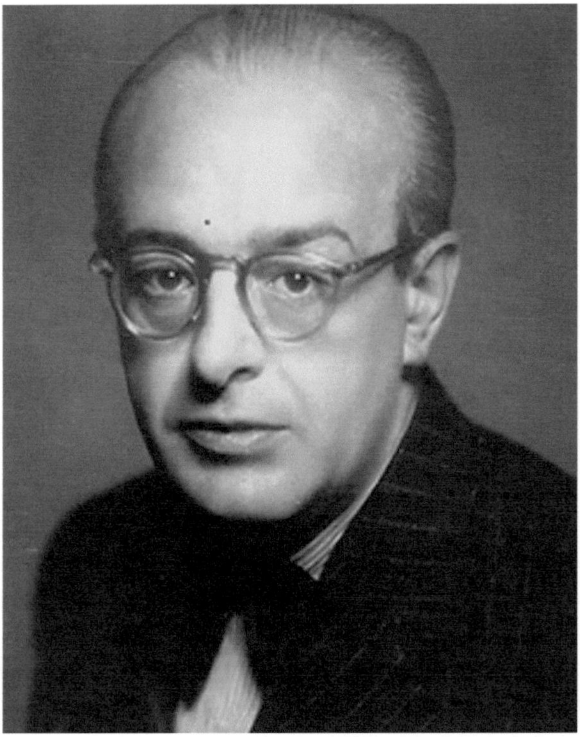

Fig. 15.1 Carlos Jiménez Diaz. (Permission of the Foundation C. Rábago, Madrid)

He completed his medical degree in 1921 and defended a doctoral thesis titled "*Factores esenciales de la dieta y el crecimiento*", ("*Essential Factors of Diet and Growth*"), an experimental study that earned him the University's Extraordinary Prize. His thesis director was Professor Fernando Enríquez de Salamanca, a prominent internist just 6 years his senior. The two would go on to share a complex relationship marked by both collaboration and rivalry throughout their professional lives.

With aspirations of an academic career, Carlos faced an early setback when, at just 22 years old, he was unsuccessful in his first attempt to get a professorship in Barcelona. The outcome sparked a public controversy involving notable figures such as Gregorio Marañón and Santiago Ramón y Cajal—then president of the examining board—who both intervened in the debate.

Soon after, Carlos was awarded a scholarship from the *Junta para Ampliación de Estudios*, which allowed him to continue his training in Germany. He studied clinical medicine in Berlin under prominent physicians such as Karl von Noorden and Adolf Strümpell, pathological anatomy with Otto Lubarsch, and internal medicine with Frederick Kraus. He later moved to Frankfurt to work with Paul Michaelis in biochemistry and Adolf Bickel in experimental medicine. This formative period abroad was pivotal to his development and proved decisive for the direction of his professional career.

At the age of 25, Carlos obtained his first professorship at the University of Seville. Just 3 years later, he secured a chair at the Faculty of Medicine in Madrid, firmly establishing his academic standing—competing with his former thesis advisor, Fernando Enríquez de Salamanca.

Once settled in Madrid, Carlos quickly recognized the limitations of the scientific environment in Spanish medicine. In response, he spearheaded the creation of the *Asociación Protectora de la Cátedra* (Association for the Protection of the Chair), which supported the Department he directed. A year later, in the early 1930s and with the support of Juan Negrín, physiologist and politician, he founded the Instituto de Investigaciones Clinicas y Médicas conceived as part of a broader reform of the new Faculty of Medicine. Within this institute, he developed departments dedicated to Pathological Anatomy, Biochemistry, Microbiology, and Nutrition and Hormones.

The banker Pablo Garnica played a very important role in the project development and remained a steadfast ally throughout Carlos's career.

In 1932, Carlos published *Asthma and Other Allergic Diseases*, a landmark work that marked a turning point in both his scientific and personal trajectory.

His career was abruptly disrupted by the outbreak of the Spanish Civil War. Forced to leave the country for a time, he spent several months in London, Rome, and Paris before returning to Spain under precarious circumstances. By then, the Institute he had helped to build had been completely destroyed by bombardments. In 1939, following his return to Madrid, he was summoned by the Regional Court of Political Responsibilities. Among the charges brought against him was his participation in a banquet honoring Gonzalo Rodríguez Lafora and Pío del Río Hortega—an event tied to the controversy surrounding Río Hortega's exclusion from the Royal Academy of Medicine. Despite these accusations, Carlos managed to survive the hostile postwar climate by forging strategic relationships with key figures within the Franco's regime, allowing him to continue his professional work.

In 1940, he founded the *Revista Clínica Española*, a medical journal that would become a significant platform for clinical research in Spain. He also resumed his scientific work at the temporary headquarters of the Instituto de Investigaciones Clinicas y Médicas. In 1945, he formally returned to his chair at the Faculty of Medicine.

During this period, Carlos strengthened his reputation as one of Spain's most esteemed physicians, alongside contemporaries like Gregorio Marañón.

He also initiated a new line of research exploring the therapeutic use of nitrogen mustards in the treatment of autoimmune diseases.

After years of negotiation, Carlos achieved a major milestone in 1953: the official recognition of his Institute, which was rebuilt on the site of the former Rubio Institute. This achievement was made possible through the political support of Francisco Franco and the then Minister of Education, Joaquín Ruiz Jiménez.

In 1955, the *Clínica de Nuestra Señora de la Concepción* was formally inaugurated. The facility opened with 200 beds, including 10 designated for private patients. Over time, the clinic underwent several expansions, ultimately evolving into the institution known today. Its structure and philosophy were directly inspired by the Mayo Clinic in Rochester, Minnesota—a model that Carlos personally visited and studied as a reference for his own vision of modern, integrated clinical care [1–3] (Fig. 15.2).

The *Aula Magna*, preserved almost entirely in its original form since its construction, served as the venue for the 1956 International Congress of Internal Medicine—the first time the prestigious event was held in Spain.

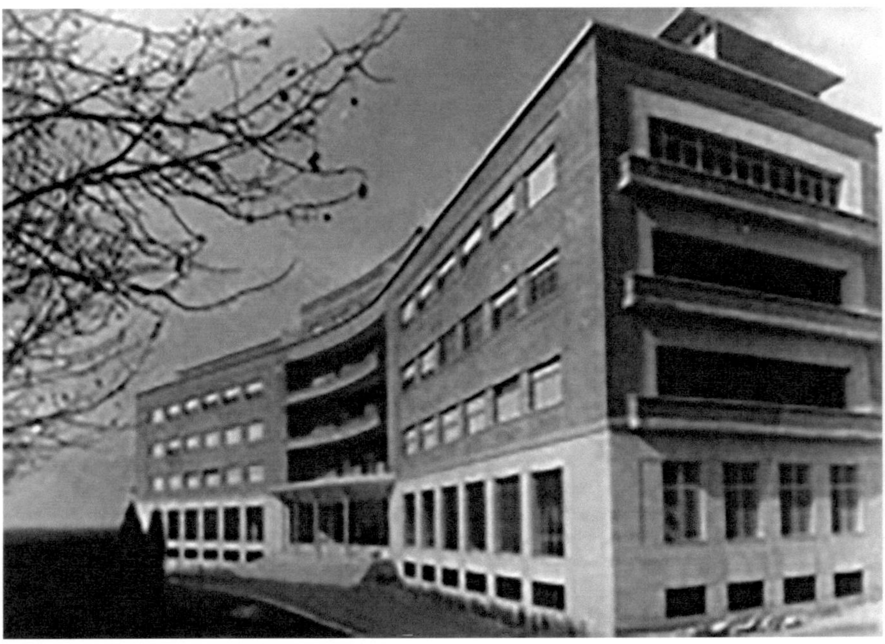

Fig. 15.2 "La Fundación Jiménez Diaz" in its early days. (Permission of Jimenez Casado)

Beginning with the 1955–1956 academic year, Carlos launched a structured residency training program for young physicians, initially offering twenty positions annually. Recognizing the growing dominance of English as the international language of science—gradually replacing German—he supported the creation of an English-language journal, the *Bulletin of the Institute for Medical Research, University of Madrid* (1948–1966), to complement the *Revista Clínica Española.* Both publications featured numerous articles authored by Jiménez Díaz and his collaborators, contributing to the dissemination of Spanish medical research at an international level.

In 1963, he founded the *Fundación Jiménez Díaz* to provide the *Clínica de Nuestra Señora de la Concepción* with a stable legal and financial structures. From that point forward, ensuring the sustainability of the Foundation became his foremost concern. One of his most significant accomplishments was obtaining official recognition of the Foundation as a healthcare provider within the Spanish Social Security system—a crucial step in ensuring its long-term future.

Carlos Jiménez Díaz passed away in 1967. Although he had survived both a myocardial infarction and a serious car accident—despite being hypertensive and a smoker—he succumbed to a second heart attack at his own clinic. His death came shortly after learning the devastating news that his wife and lifelong companion, Conchita de Rábago, had been diagnosed with pancreatic cancer.

Merits

Capable and brilliant, Carlos Jiménez Díaz distinguished himself through unwavering dedication during his years as a student and young physician. A true innovator, he critically examined the state of medical education and clinical practice in Spain, determined to break with tradition and prevent the system from continuing on with "business as usual."

He possessed a sharp, critical perspective on the realities of the university system, the healthcare sector, and the burdens of bureaucracy. Like Santiago Ramón y Cajal—whose influence loomed large in his thinking—Jiménez Díaz consistently proposed thoughtful reforms to improve these institutions. He shared intellectual and ethical affinities with reformist contemporaries such as Pedro Laín Entralgo and Gregorio Marañón and maintained close personal and professional ties with both. He also benefited from a longstanding friendship with Severo Ochoa and collaborated with Juan Negrín during the formative years of his career, before the civil war.

As a mentor and leader, Jiménez Díaz trained an entire generation of internists and hospital specialists, among them notable figures such as Luis Hernando and José María Segovia de Arana. Deeply influenced by his own training in Germany, he retained a strong international perspective throughout his career. He actively encouraged his collaborators to pursue advanced training abroad and, upon their return, entrusted them with genuine professional responsibility and autonomy—fostering a culture of excellence and innovation in Spanish medicine (Fig. 15.3).

Carlos Jiménez Díaz played a pivotal role in the development of numerous subspecialties within Internal Medicine and was a founding member of both the Spanish Society of Cardiology and the Spanish Society of Allergy. Despite these contributions to specialization, he remained a steadfast defender of the internist's role as the physician best equipped to understand the patient as a whole—beyond the fragmented lens of subspecialties disciplines.

A passionate advocate for the incorporation of emerging diagnostic technologies—in Radiology, Pathology, and Laboratory Medicine—he consistently emphasized their integration into a unified, patient-centered model of care, coordinated by the internist. This philosophy came to life in the renowned Clinicopathological Sessions held several times a year in the *Aula*

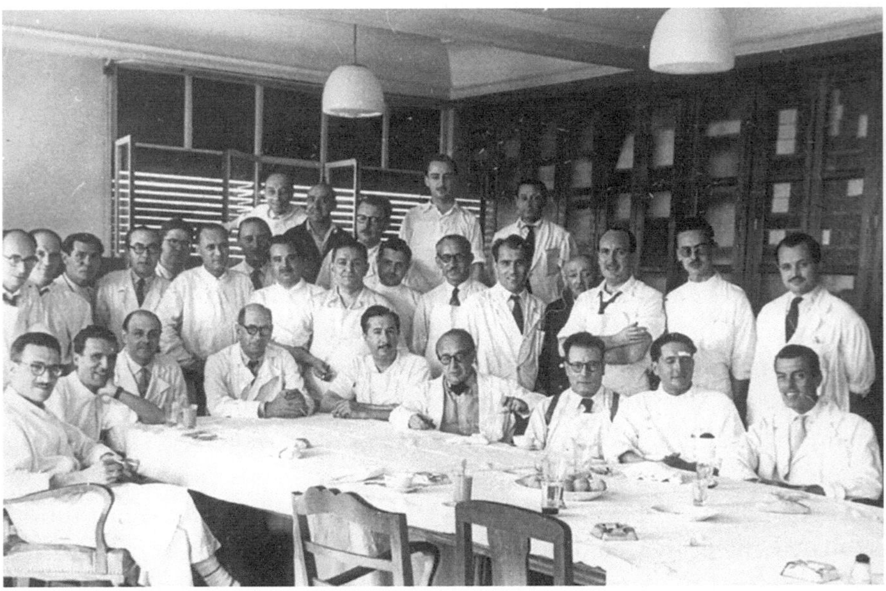

Con sus primeros colaboradores en la Clínica de la Concepción.

Fig. 15.3 Carlos Jiménez Díaz, with his first collaborators. (Permission of Jimenez Casado)

Magna of the Fundación Jiménez Díaz, where internists and other specialists rigorously presented and defended their diagnoses and clinical decisions. These sessions were inspired by the *Clinicopathological Conferences* of the Massachusetts General Hospital, regularly published in the *New England Journal of Medicine*.

Remaining faithful to the principles of his German training, Jiménez Díaz championed a model in which basic and experimental research was fully intertwined with clinical practice. Guided by this approach, he transformed the Fundación Jiménez Díaz into a pioneering institution—not only in postgraduate education, serving as a key reference in the development of Spain's MIR (Medical Residency) system—but also in academic teaching, where instruction was closely tied to real-world clinical care.

Throughout his life, he never wavered from his vision: the creation and consolidation of a Research Institute that would serve as the foundation for a scientific, innovative, and patient-centered form of medicine. That vision ultimately materialized in his Fundación Jiménez Díaz, an institution that remains a cornerstone of Spain's medical and academic landscape (Fig. 15.4).

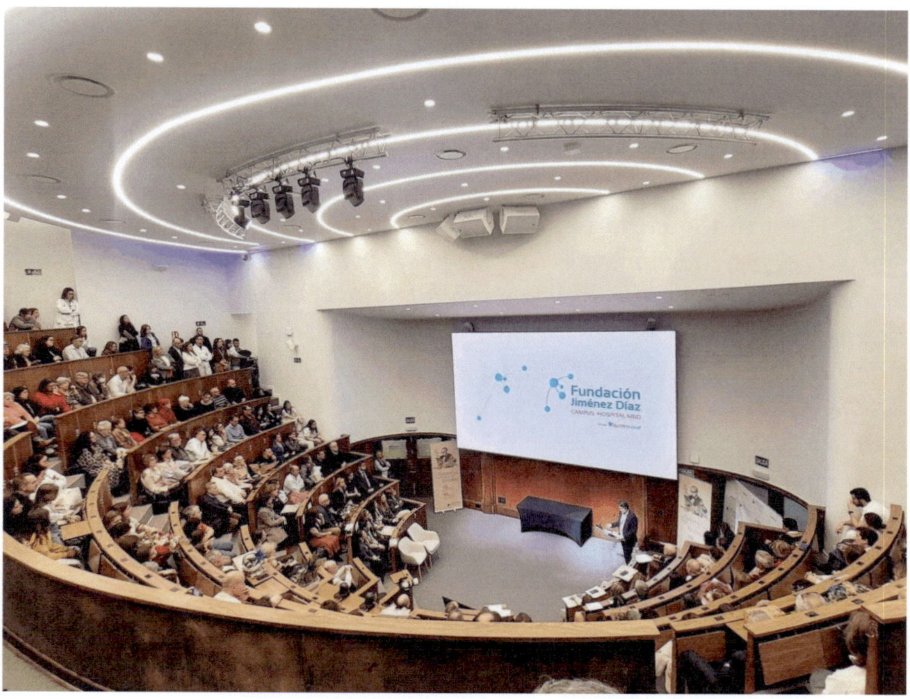

Fig. 15.4 Celebration of the 90th anniversary of the Fundación

Most Relevant Clinical Findings and Observations

Early in his career, Jiménez Díaz intuited that many diseases could stem from a dysregulated immune response—what would later be defined as autoimmune diseases. In 1951, he published a groundbreaking article in JAMA titled "Treatment of Rheumatoid Arthritis with Nitrogen Mustard: Preliminary Report," in which he described nine cases of rheumatoid arthritis treated with nitrogen mustard. This study opened a pioneering path in the immunomodulatory treatment of autoimmune disorders.

Alongside Francisco Vivanco, he studied the *latirism*, a toxic neurological condition, and identified Lathyrus or grasspea (*almorta* flour) as its primary causative agent. His research interests were broad and forward-looking: he explored the pathophysiological mechanisms of hypertension, particularly the secretory function of the arterial wall, and conducted studies on renal function in Addison's disease, analyzing the connections between adrenal activity and renal metabolism [4–12].

His precocious intellect and intense drive to innovate propelled him to break down scientific and institutional barriers. However, these same qualities occasionally led to tensions and disagreements with some of his collaborators, including Juan Rof Carballo and José Luis Arteta, among others.

Some Illustrative Sentences

1953, letter to the Head of State, Francisco Franco: *...These conditions (to promote original scientific work) (means, group and modest but sufficient economic situation) which we consider necessary, fail in such a way in our country that they determine the penury of our scientific production. Cajal, undoubtedly the most authentic scientific researcher Spain has ever had, was able to carry out his work in isolation and with meagre resources because he cultivated histology, which lends itself to this...*

...I must point out the absolute inadequacy of this teaching (of medicine) in our country. The teaching is, except for a small part of the students, those who work as interns in a Department, absolutely dogmatic and memoristic. ....

1954, The doctor exploring his patient:
The attitudes that should preside over the clinical examination:

1. *Interest in finding out why he suffers, what he (or she) has*
2. *Mental sincerity*

3. *Objectivity and firmness of data (... intuition is of no use unless it is based on firm and reliable facts).*
4. *Congruence contrast of the data obtained*
5. *Hierarchical ordering of the symptoms (...the artist or the clinician has to order things in a similar way, highlighting the essential from the accessory, using all that is revealed to complete the whole).*
6. *The diagnosed disease has to explain the symptoms.*

1960, Rio de la Plata Congress of Internal Medicine:
One of the fatal disadvantages of excessive specialization is the withdrawal of most of the valuable young people in all countries from the practice of medicine, turning to the specialties, …

1963, In the history of my Institute:
The version towards research is originally an uneasiness which springs from contemplation, first, and concern, next, for the unknown. This situation can originate in the sensitive person through various types of contact, but it is undoubtedly particularly strong when it arises at the bedside of the sick person; so often we do not explain what we see and we have the impression of a limited possibilities of suppressing the suffering, the progression of the illness and its fatal or disabling end.

Legacy in Spain

The contributions of Carlos Jiménez Díaz to Spanish medicine has been multiple and significant. Yet, his most enduring legacy lies in his unwavering commitment to scientific evidence and intellectual rigor in the practice of diagnosis and clinical care. A staunch advocate of continuing medical education, he aimed to elevate the overall standard of the medical profession and promote collaborative work among specialists [13–15].

His influence was instrumental in integrating basic medical and biological sciences into everyday clinical practice—an approach that helped Spanish medicine into a new era of modernity. Throughout his career, he thought and trained an entire generation of physicians and researchers who went on to enrich universities and hospitals not only across Spain but also throughout Latin America. These disciples, trained under his demanding yet inspiring guidance, embraced his rigorous methodology and patient-centered philosophy. They distinguished themselves by their commitment to evidence-based practice and their courage to challenge the boundaries of conventional medicine.

Among his most outstanding disciples were José Cruz Auñón, Manuel Díaz Rubio, Felipe Morán Miranda, Eduardo Ortiz de Landázuri, Vicente Gilsanz García, Eloy López García, Carlos de Oya Salgueiro, José María Segovia de Arana, Miguel Garrido Peralta, José Perianes Carro, Rafael Alcalá Santaella, Mariano Jiménez Casado, and Alfonso Merchante Iglesias.

Acknowledgements Fabiola Trivino Guiza, FJD librarian.

References

1. Historia de mi Instituto. History of my Institute. Madrid: Editorial Paz Montalvo; 1965.
2. Jiménez CM, Diaz DJ. Vida y Obra: la persecución de un sueño. Madrid: Fundación Conchita Rábago de Jiménez Díaz; 1993.
3. Cuervo A.M. LVI Commemorative Jiménez Diaz C. Lecture (27/5/2025). Madrid
4. Jiménez Díaz C, Sánchez Cuenca B. Right heart catheterisation. Arch Cardiol Hemat. 1930;2:1–4.
5. Jiménez Diaz C, Cruz Auñón J, Mascaró J. Renal pathology studies I communication. The aqueous diuresis tests. Ann Med Int. 1933;2:977–1006.
6. Jiménez Díaz C, de la Barreda P, de Molina AF, Machado B. Further studies on the neurochemical mechanism of arterial pressure regulation. Bull Inst Med Res Univ Madr. 1948;1:145–55.
7. Jiménez Díaz C, Castro-Mendoza H. The role of the kidney in fat metabolism. Bull Inst Med Res Univ Madr. 1948;1:1–5.
8. Jimenez Diaz C, Lopez Garcia E, Merchante A, Perianes J. Treatment of rheumatoid arthritis with nitrogen mustard; preliminary report. JAMA. 1951;147:1418–9.
9. Vivanco F, Jimenez DC. Further studies on the toxic effects of leguminous proteins (leguminism); lathyrism odoratus (odoratism). Bull Inst Med Res Univ Madr. 1951;4:1–13.
10. Jimenez Diaz C, Barreda P, Af M, Alcala R. Role of arterial wall secretion in the regulation of blood pressure. Circulation. 1954;9:903–7.
11. Jiménez Diaz CJ. Collagen and allergic diseases. Acta Med Scand Suppl. 1956;312:297–302.
12. Ales Reinlein JM, Jiménez Díaz C, Ortiz MF. Immunological Study of the antigenic composition of house and barn dust. Bull Inst Med Res Univ Madr. 1956;9:53–70.
13. La investigación científica y la enseñanza y orientación de la medicina, Madrid, Paz Montalvo, 1952.
14. Clinical examination methods and their evaluation: El médico explorando a su enfermo, Madrid, Editorial Paz Montalvo, 1954.
15. Tratado de la Práctica Médica, Madrid, Editorial Paz Montalvo, 1959 (1963, 1964).

16

Severo Ochoa y Albornoz: Discovering Enzymes and the Genetic Code and Founding the Spanish Society of Biochemistry

Inmaculada Yruela Guerrero

Severo Ochoa de Albornoz was born on 24 September 1905 in Luarca (Asturias). His father died of a heart attack when he was only 7 years old. In his memoir "*Visión y recuerdo de mi tierra*" (*A Vision and Memory of My Homeland*,) published in ABC on February 27, 1987, Ochoa reflects (Fig. 16.1):

> My earliest memories are from Asturias, specifically from Gijón and Luarca. In Gijón, during the winter I went to school; in Luarca I spent the summer [...] My life in the village made me an enthusiastic observer of Nature from a very young age [...]. During low tide I spent endless hours observing the enormous variety of animal and plant life that inhabited the countless pools formed as the sea receded into the hollows of the rocks. Perhaps that was the awakening of my future passion for biology.

In 1912, the family moved to Málaga due to his mother's delicate health. She suffered from chronic bronchitis, which worsened in the cold, damp Asturian winters. They lived in Málaga for 11 years, spending the school year there—from September to June—and returning to Asturias for the summer months.

I. Yruela Guerrero (✉)
Senior Research Scientist. Experimental Station Aula Dei (EEAD), Spanish Research Council (CSIC), Zaragoza, Spain

M. A. Cuesta, F. Mateo Vallejo (eds.), *Spain's Journey in Medicine*,
https://doi.org/10.1007/978-3-032-12221-6_16

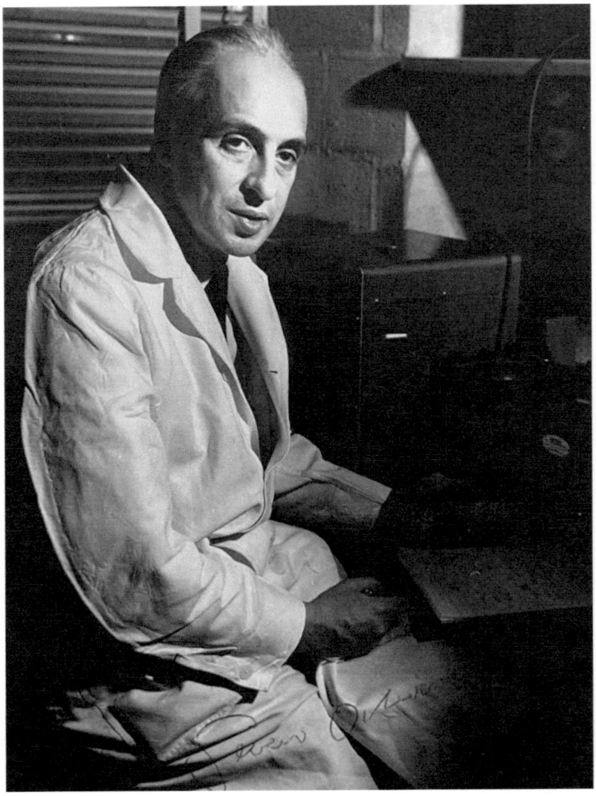

Fig. 16.1 Severo Ochoa y Albornoz

During those summers, young Severo would use one of the outbuildings of their farmhouse as a laboratory, where he examined the entrails of small animals he had caught with other village boys. He also recalls in *A Vision and Memory of My Homeland*:

> *As the years went by, my memory returns to Villar, where I had saturated my senses with "Nature" and where my mind began to mature, and my spirit was moulded by reading and the spirit. It was there during the holidays that, already intensely interested in biology, I spent long hours to the study of physics, chemistry, physiology and biochemistry. There I began to read original research papers in a French journal, the "Journal de Physiologie et Pathologie Génerale" to which I had subscribed in my second year of medicine.*

In Malaga he assisted the first years of primary education at the Sagrado Corazón de Jesús school (Jesuits), and the second years of secondary education (baccalaureate), between 1915 and 1921, at the General and Technical

Institute, which was known for having some of the best teachers in the city. Two of his teachers at this Institute had an enormous influence on his intellectual development: Eduardo García Rodeja, a physics and chemistry teacher, and Luis Muñoz Cobo, a natural history teacher. In particular, García Rodeja made him fall in love with biology, as he himself recounts in his autobiography "*The pursuit of a hobby*" (*Annual Review of Biochemistry*, 1980):

> *It was in the last years of secondary school that I began to feel enormously attracted to the natural sciences. It was largely due, I am sure, to the stimulating teaching of a brilliant young chemistry teacher, Eduardo García Rodeja. For a while I thought about studying engineering, but on the one hand I had little talent for mathematics and on the other I realized that what really interested me was biology. For this reason I enrolled in the Faculty of Medicine in 1923 [...].* [1–3]

This period of his education was interrupted by the 1918 influenza pandemic (so-called Spanish flu), which forced the closure of schools across Spain. The pandemic claimed more than two-hundred thousand lives in the country, and Ochoa himself was among those affected. He contracted the flu, which developed into severe pneumonia and posed a serious threat to his health. However, after several months of convalescence, he eventually recovered. In 1922, he earned his bachelor's degree. This phase of his education had an undeniably profound impact on him, and on more than one occasion he stated that it was in the classroom where he discovered his scientific vocation.

During his time in Málaga, Ochoa cultivated many hobbies that would stay with him throughout his life. He practiced horseback riding, had a passion for automobiles, and maintained a deep interest in music—despite never learning to play an instrument. He was also an avid reader of novels by Jules Verne, Emilio Salgari, and Arthur Conan Doyle.

Another of his great passions was the figure of Santiago Ramón y Cajal, whom he deeply admired. Determined to follow in Cajal's footsteps, he moved to Madrid to study medicine—not with the goal of becoming a practicing physician but driven by a scientific calling. He was accompanied on this journey by his inseparable friend José María García Valdecasas, whom he had met at the Institute. However, Ochoa never had the chance to meet Cajal at the Faculty of Medicine at the Central University of Madrid, as Cajal retired before Ochoa began his studies.

During his medical studies (Fig. 16.2) Ochoa came under the influence of several professors, most notably Juan Negrín, who invited him and García Valdecasas to join the Physiology Laboratory he directed, located at the

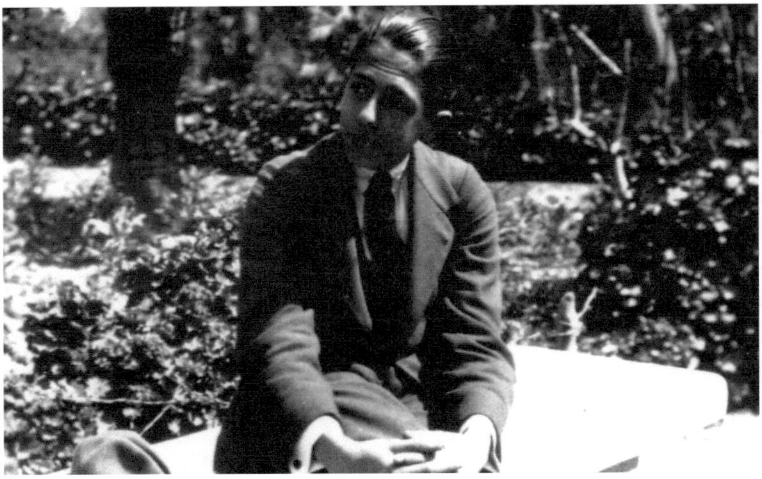

Fig. 16.2 Severo Ochoa as a student

Residencia de Estudiantes in Madrid. Ochoa later wrote in his "*Memories and Longings*" (*ABC*, November 26, 1983).

> *My first contact with the Residencia was when, back in 1924, Don Juan Negrín invited me and inseparable companion José María García Valdecasas to work in the Physiology Laboratory of the Residencia de Estudiantes, which he directed. The Residencia housed several biological research and teaching laboratories on the first floor and in the basement of its third pavilion. These included the world-renowned Normal Histology and Pathology Laboratory, directed by Don Pío del Río Ortega, the Physiology Laboratory, directed by Don Juan Negrín, and two essentially teaching laboratories, one for Biology, directed by the distinguished cardiologist Don Luis Calandre, and the other for Microbiology, directed by Don Paulino Suárez. It was not easy to join the Residence. Being a "resident" was a highly sought-after privilege and I had to wait several years to become one.*

Ochoa joined Negrín's laboratory during his second year of medical school—a step that proved decisive in shaping his scientific training. It was Juan Negrín who introduced him to the fields of physiology and biochemistry. During the 1926–1927 academic year, Negrín proposed that he isolate creatinine from urine, a byproduct of creatine hydrolysis released during muscle contraction. At the time, creatinine levels in blood and urine were measured using Jaffe's colorimetric method. The new detection method developed by Ochoa and his close friend García Valdecasas was published in the *Boletín de la Sociedad Española de Biología in* 1927.

The findings of this study contradicted the theory of Noël Paton, a professor of physiology in Glasgow. In his fourth year of medical school, Ochoa wrote a letter to Paton, who accepted him for a research stay in his laboratory that lasted several months. There, Ochoa demonstrated that Paton's method was flawed and confirmed that there was no increase in creatinine during muscle contraction in frogs. He also made an unexpected discovery: guanidine caused contraction of melanophores in frog skin, making it turn pale.

Guanidine is a nitrogen-rich organic compound found in nature in plants and animals.

This finding was published in the *Proceedings of the Royal Society in* 1928, marking Ochoa's first scientific paper in an international journal.

A year later, in collaboration with García Valdecasas, he published a method for determining creatinine in muscle tissue in the *Journal of Biological Chemistry*. Together, they continued to investigate the role of creatine and creatinine in muscle contraction.

Although his introduction to research was in the field of physiology, Ochoa increasingly recognized the need for a new scientific discipline: biochemistry. In 1927, he collaborated on the writing of the book "*Elementos de Bioquímica*" *(Elements of Biochemestry)*, at the invitation of Professor J. Hernández Guerra. The book was published by Editorial España, a publishing house founded by Juan Negrín. It went through several editions and was possibly the first biochemistry textbook written in Spanish.

Another formative experience was his time at Otto Meyerhof's laboratory at the Kaiser Wilhelm Institute in Berlin. Meyerhof had been awarded the Nobel Prize in Physiology or Medicine in 1922, alongside Archibald Vivian Hill.

Ochoa's doctoral training under the supervision of Juan Negrín, carried out at the Residencia de Estudiantes in Madrid and lasting until 1931, was of great scientific and personal significance in his life. During this period, he attended lectures by renowned scientists such as Marie Curie and Albert Einstein. He also lived among influential cultural figures including Federico García Lorca, Salvador Dalí, and Luis Buñuel.

In 1931, Severo Ochoa married Carmen García Cobián, who was also born in Asturias and whose family had long known the Ochoa family. He dedicated one of his writings to her—"*Carmen, retrato de una Mujer*" (Carmen portrait of a woman) (*ABC*, January 31, 1987)—in which he wrote (Fig. 16.3):

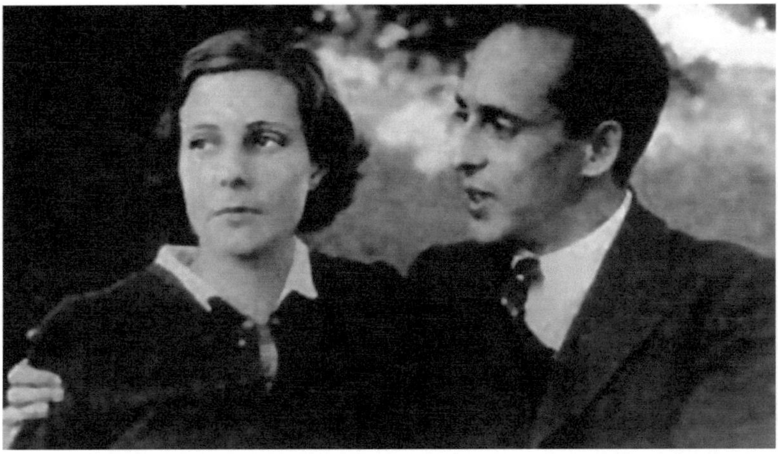

Fig. 16.3 Severo with his wife Carmen

> *Carmen knew very well the life that awaited her when she married me, a scientific quixote who had no other perspective than that of her illusions and hopes, and who could only contribute modestly to the support of our household. [...] I think I have said more than once that Carmen had a powerful influence on my life, although I undoubtedly had an influence on hers as well. Without Carmen my life could have been very different.*

In 1934, Ochoa defended his doctoral thesis, titled: "*Los hidratos de carbono en los fenómenos químicos y energéticos de la contracción muscular*" (*Carbohydrates in the Chemical and Energetic Phenomena of Muscular Contraction)* and was appointed assistant professor in Physiology at the Faculty of Medicine of the Central University of Madrid. However, Juan Negrín's gradual withdrawal from research to dedicate himself to political duties, along with Ochoa's discouraging experience during the competitive examination for the chair of Physiology at the University of Santiago de Compostela, left him with a sense of abandonment. These events led him to reconsider the direction of his scientific career.

In February 1935, he accepted an offer from Professor Carlos Jiménez Díaz to head the Physiology section of the newly established Institute of Clinical and Medical Research in Madrid. With this initiative, Jiménez Díaz aimed to bring together scientific research and clinical practice (see Chaps. 15 and 17). Despite taking on this new role, Ochoa did not abandon his postdoctoral training in leading European laboratories.

In 1936, the *Junta de Ampliación de Estudios* awarded him a grant to spend the summer at University College London, where he worked on muscle energy metabolism under the direction of Nobel laureate Archibald Vivian Hill. Upon returning to Spain, Ochoa found the political landscape dramatically altered—the Spanish Civil War had begun. He turned to Negrín, now serving as Minister of Finance, and requested help in relocating to a place more conducive to pursuing the kind of science he dreamed of.

A Race to the Nobel Prize

Severo Ochoa left Spain with his wife, Carmen, in 1936 following the outbreak of the Spanish Civil War, in pursuit of what he described as his "hobby"—a full-time dedication to a scientific career. As he recounts in his autobiography *The Pursuit of a Hobby* (*Annual Review of Biochemistry*, 1980), *"There was no possibility in Spain at that time, even without the war, of doing the kind of science I dreamed of doing."* [2].

He first moved to Heidelberg, joining the laboratory of Otto Meyerhof, with whom he had previously worked between 1929 and 1930 during the course of his doctoral research. However, the focus of Meyerhof's laboratory had since shifted—evolving from a physiology lab into one centered on the emerging field of biochemistry. This transition reflected the growing momentum of biochemistry as a discipline. In Meyerhof's lab, Ochoa was appointed a research assistant, and during this period he succeeded in isolating the coenzyme NAD from skeletal muscle.

Nicotinamide adenine dinucleotide (NAD) is a coenzyme that plays a crucial role in cellular metabolism. It is involved in many oxidation-reduction reactions, DNA repair and gene expression.

In August 1937, Ochoa was once again compelled to emigrate—this time due to increasing pressure from the Nazi regime, which made it untenable for Meyerhof and his team to continue their work in Germany. Ochoa relocated to the United Kingdom, where he held a six-month fellowship at the Marine Biological Laboratory in Plymouth. He later joined the Department of Biochemistry at the University of Oxford, working in the laboratory of Rudolph A. Peters under a grant from the Nuffield Foundation. There, he investigated the biological function of vitamin B1.

Given the worsening political climate in Europe with the onset of the Second World War, Ochoa made the decision in 1940 to emigrate to the United States, accompanied by his wife Carmen.

In the United States, Severo Ochoa initially worked with Carl and Gerty Cori at Washington University in St. Louis, focusing on the characterization of enzymes and phosphorylated compounds involved in carbohydrate metabolism. In 1942, he joined the New York University School of Medicine, first as associated researcher, supported by a Williams-Waterman Fund grant from the Research Corporation. In 1944, he was appointed Chair of the Department of Pharmacology in the same university.

Ochoa's work, in collaboration with other researchers, helped establish that oxidative processes are coupled with phosphorylation reactions—a fundamental mechanism by which ATP molecules are generated. These molecules store energy that serves as the universal energy currency for all cellular activities. As a result of these findings, the pathway became known as oxidative phosphorylation. Ochoa then undertook the formidable task of isolating the individual enzymes involved in this pathway from animal tissues and bacterial cultures, and of measuring their activity in vitro with precision—a significant challenge at the time.

Many of the discoveries he made from this period became foundational to modern biochemistry and are still featured in contemporary textbooks. His research also demonstrated that carbon dioxide fixation—the incorporation of CO_2 into organic molecules—is not exclusive to plant cells but occurs in animal cells as well.

Perhaps most notably, Ochoa identified several key enzymes of the citric acid cycle, including citrate synthase, citrate dehydrogenase, alpha-ketoglutarate dehydrogenase, succinyl coenzyme A synthetase, among others—discoveries that significantly deepened our understanding of cellular respiration and metabolism.

Ochoa quickly established himself as a distinguished enzymologist and became fully integrated into the scientific community of New York, gaining membership in the prestigious Enzyme Club. In 1943, he presented his first scientific paper on oxidative phosphorylation at a meeting of the Club, titled *"The Phosphate Bond in the Oxidation of Pyruvic Acid."*

In 1946, Ochoa was appointed Chair of the Department of Pharmacology at the New York University School of Medicine, a position he held until 1954. He later described those eight years as the most exciting and productive period of his career. His scientific achievements during this time garnered significant recognition. In 1951, the American Society of European Chemists and Pharmacists awarded him the inaugural Neuberg Medal, named after the eminent biochemist Carl Neuberg, acknowledging his exceptional contributions to the field of biochemistry.

In 1954, Ochoa became Chair of the Department of Biochemistry at New York University, position he held until his retirement.

His enzymology work focused on processes of oxidative phosphorylation, CO_2 fixation, and enzymes involved in the tricarboxylic acid (TCA) cycle (or Krebs cycle). Ochoa was a major contributor to elucidating the detailed steps of the TCA cycle. However, his work on oxidative phosphorylation led to what some biochemists believe to be his major contribution, RNA synthesis and the genetic code.

In 1954 Ochoa returned to the oxidative phosphorylation research and began looking for enzymes capable of converting ADP to ATP. Like most biochemistry labs at the time, the Ochoa lab now worked with radioisotopes, and Ochoa decided to approach the problem by looking for reactions that incorporated radioactively labeled phosphate.

Ochoa's enduring fascination with enzymes and metabolic pathways eventually led him to explore unexpectedly the nucleic acids. As he reflects in his autobiography "*The Pursuit of a Hobby*" [2]:

> *In 1954 it seemed to me that it was a good time to go back to oxidative phosphorylating. I thought that we should look for a group of enzymes capable of converting ADP to ATP and that this reaction should be followed by measuring the incorporation of radioactive phosphate into ATP. It also occurred to me that these enzymes might be found in extracts of Azotobacter vinelandii that oxidise carbohydrates and other compounds.*

He was working on this project with his postdoctoral researcher Marianne Grunberg-Manago, French biochemist of Russian origin (Fig. 16.4).

Unexpectedly, the experiments initially designed by Ochoa yielded surprising results. The enzyme they were studying it promoted the incorporation of radioactive phosphate into ADP to generate ATP, but also it was able of catalyzed the formation of long chains of adenylic acid (polyA), polynucleotides, closely resembling RNA (ribonucleic acid) polymers.

Adenylic acid is a nucleotide that forms a building block of RNA whereas PolyA refers to a sequence of many adenylic acid units linked together

Remarkably, the enzyme was also capable of forming polymers incorporating the rest of other nucleotides if added to the reaction. This marked the first time that nucleic acids had been synthesized *in vitro*—a groundbreaking achievement.

The discovery of the polynucleotide phosphorylase was published in both the *Journal of the American Chemical Society* and *Science* in 1955, generating significant international interest. In 1954 [4, 5].

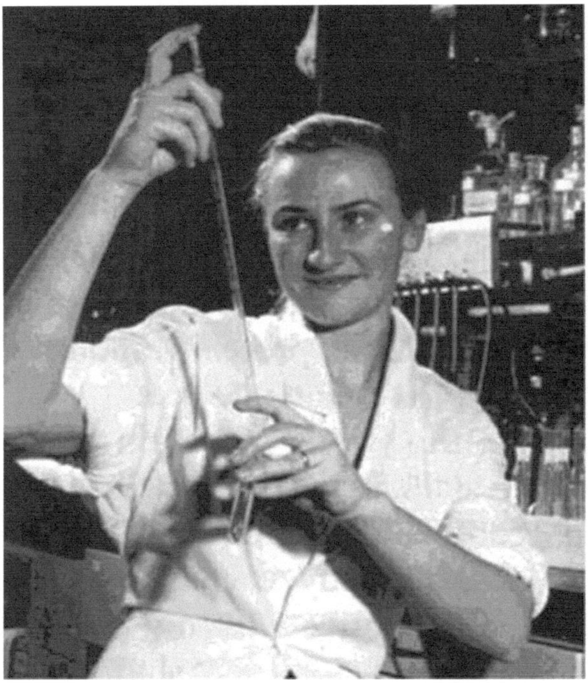

Fig. 16.4 Marianne Grunberg-Manago working in the laboratory

Severo Ochoa and Marianne Grunberg-Manago had discovered the first nucleic-acid-synthesizing enzyme, polynucleotide phosphorylase (PNPase). Initially, it was thought that the new enzyme was an RNA polymerase used by *E. coli* cells to make RNA chains from separate nucleotides. However, while the enzyme can link nucleotides together, the reaction is highly reversible and it later became clear that the enzyme usually catalyzes the breakdown of RNA, not its synthesis.

The discovery of PNPase happened shortly after James Watson and Francis Crick discovered the double helix structure of DNA in 1953.

Ochoa's name soon began to circulate as a potential Nobel Prize candidate. In 1956, he became a naturalized U.S. citizen.

Just 3 years later, in 1959, Severo Ochoa was awarded the Nobel Prize in Physiology or Medicine, an honor he shared with his former student and close collaborator, Arthur Kornberg, who had also worked in his laboratory.

The Nobel prize 1959 was awarded jointly to Severo Ochoa and Arthur Kornberg "for their discovery of the mechanisms in the biological synthesis of ribonucleic acid and deoxyribonucleic acid" [6] (Fig. 16.5 and 16.6).

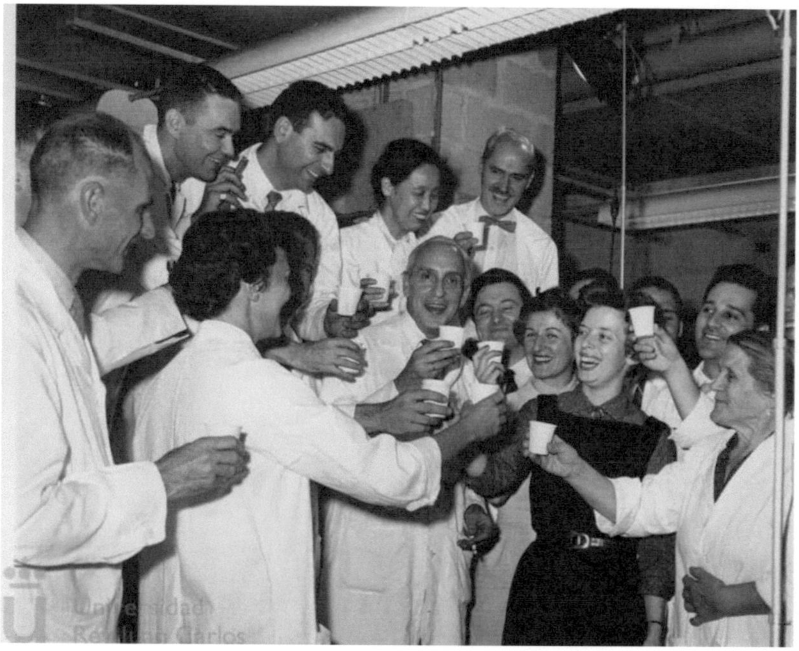

Fig. 16.5 The joy of being Severo Ochoa awarded the Nobel Prize

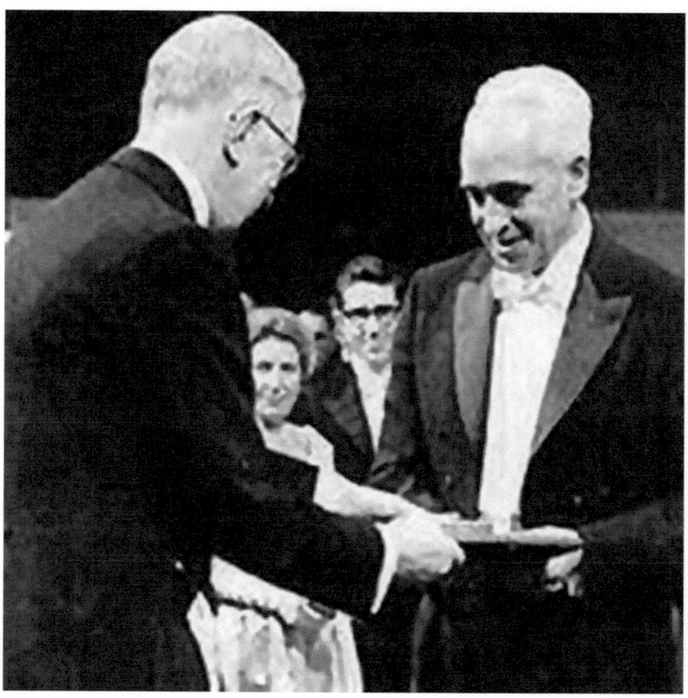

Fig. 16.6 Severo Ochoa receiving the Nobel Prize in 1959 from the King of Sweden Gustaf VI Adolf

In 1956, Arthur Kornberg's research group—by then based at Washington University in St. Louis, where he was a professor of microbiology—succeeded in isolating the long-sought DNA polymerase for the first time. This breakthrough enabled the synthesis of DNA strands *in vitro*, representing a major milestone in molecular biology. Ochoa's earlier discoveries had laid essential groundwork for this achievement and contributed significantly to the eventual deciphering of the genetic code. Throughout their careers, Ochoa and Kornberg remained close friends and collaborators, united by mutual respect and a shared passion for scientific discovery. He contributed to his recognition and respect paying tribute to S. Ochoa alongside many scientists and with his retirement and obituary [7, 8] (Fig. 16.5).

Severo Ochoa in the Run to Discover the Genetic Code

James Watson and Francis Crick discovered the double helix structure of DNA in 1953, rewarded with the Nobel Prize in 1962 (together with M. Wilkins). They announced that the structure of DNA, the molecule containing human genes, is a double helix. This discovery enabled a new understanding of heredity, how genes are passed down.

An organism's genotype resided in its DNA; protein was responsible for expressing the organism's phenotype. As the discipline of molecular biology began to evolve out of biochemistry, research focus shifted to understand the mechanisms driving those processes; a central problem of this research program was to understand the nature of the "genetic code." How was information contained in four DNA nucleotides converted into a functional sequence of twenty amino acids in a protein? Polynucleotide phosphorylase played an important role in answering that question.

In 1959 Marshall Nirenberg and coworkers at the National Institutes of Health (NIH) began experimental attempts to understand how DNA information was expressed as protein function.

In early 1961, Peter Lengyel and Joseph Speyer, in Ochoa's lab, started to work with cell-free protein synthesis systems. Their hypothesis was that synthetic polyribonucleotides, of known base composition, generated with polynucleotide phosphorylase would act as mRNA and incorporate amino acids into protein depending upon the polyribonucleotide base composition. The hypothesis was highly successful, and very shortly the Nirenberg and Ochoa labs were engaged in a tight, and highly competitive, race to solve the genetic code [9].

The use of polynucleotide phosphorylase was key for deciphering the genetic code since allowed the preparation of synthetic polynucleotides of different base composition with which, Severo Ochoa, in parallel with Marshall Nirenberg and J. Heinrich Matthaei, identified the nucleotide triplets that code for the twenty amino acids in the synthesis of proteins. Nirenberg and Matthaei's work along with contributions of Har Khorana, Severo Ochoa and Robert Holley led to the complete deciphering of the code over the next few years. According to Kornberg, Ochoa could have obtained a second Nobel Prize in 1968 shared with Holley, Khorana, and Nirenberg "for their interpretation of the genetic code and its function in protein synthesis."

Severo Ochoa's Legacy in Spain

The award of the Nobel Prize and the international recognition that followed they made Severo Ochoa a great influential figure, not only within the scientific community but also in broader political and institutional spheres. His international standing played a crucial role in shaping the early efforts to modernize and promote scientific research in Spain. Although by then a U.S. citizen, Ochoa remained deeply committed to supporting the development of Spanish science, particularly in the field of biomedicine. His residence in the United States never diminished his ties to his country of birth. On the contrary, he consistently supported and mentored initiatives aimed at fostering scientific progress in Spain.

Ochoa's leadership was instrumental in a number of foundational milestones: the organization of the first Biochemistry Congress in Spain in 1961; the creation of the Spanish Society of Biochemistry (SEB, now SEBBM) in 1963; the SEB's incorporation into the European Federation of Biochemical Societies (FEBS) that same year; the hosting of the 1969 FEBS Meeting in Madrid; and, most significantly, the establishment in 1975 of the Molecular Biology Research Center (Centro de Biología Molecular, CBM) that now bears his name—a joint initiative between the Universidad Autónoma de Madrid (UAM) and the Consejo Superior de Investigaciones Científicas (CSIC) (Spanish National Research Council).

A series of favorable circumstances helped make Ochoa's influence particularly effective. In January 1960, José María Albareda, Secretary General of the CSIC, invited Ochoa to serve as an honorary advisor to the Council and to lead the organization of the first National Biochemistry Congress [10]. Ochoa accepted, but under one condition: that the organization also include two distinguished Spanish scientists, Alberto Sols and Julio Rodríguez Villanueva—both of whom had trained in leading international laboratories. Sols had specialized in enzymology at the University of Washington under Carl and Gerty Cori, the Nobel Prize-winning duo in Physiology or Medicine in 1947 and Rodríguez Villanueva had worked in microbial biochemistry at Cambridge with Ernest Gale, a position he had secured through Ochoa's recommendation.

Thanks to their collaborative efforts, the first Spanish Biochemistry Congress was successfully held in Santander from July 19 to 22, 1961—marking a turning point in the institutionalization of biochemical research in Spain (Fig. 16.7).

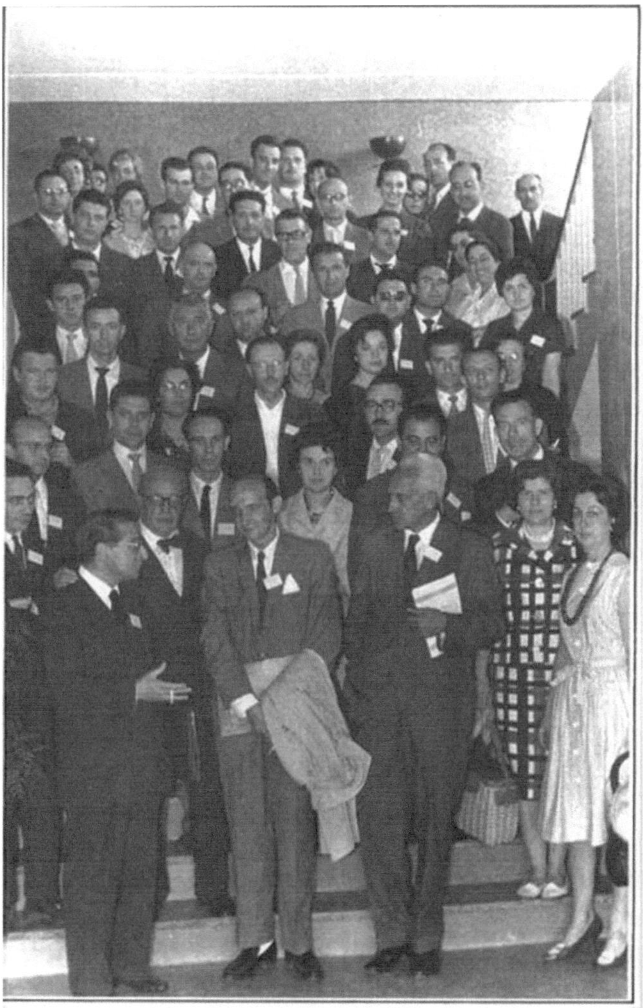

Fig. 16.7 First Spanish Biochemistry Congress. Santander, 1961

Two years later, on August 2, 1963, during the Second Meeting of Spanish Biochemists held in Santiago de Compostela, the Spanish Society of Biochemistry (SEB) was officially founded. The meeting was chaired by Severo Ochoa and received the explicit support of then-Minister Manuel Lora-Tamayo. At its inaugural assembly, the SEB unanimously conferred Honorary Membership upon Professors Carlos Jiménez-Díaz, Luis Federico Leloir (Argentinian biochemist, Nobel prize in 1970), Manuel Lora-Tamayo, and Severo Ochoa in recognition of their scientific leadership and contributions [8, 9].

The founders of the SEB laid the groundwork for biochemistry—and later, molecular biology—to develop into internationally competitive fields in Spain. Reflecting this evolution, the SEB formally changed its name in 1992 to the Spanish Society of Biochemistry and Molecular Biology (SEBBM). Today, the SEBBM boasts over 3,000 members and serves as the principal scientific body coordinating research and educational activities across the wide-ranging disciplines of biochemistry and molecular biology in Spain. In 2023, the Society proudly celebrated its 60th anniversary.

Another key milestone came in April 1969, when Spain hosted the Sixth Meeting of the European Federation of Biochemical Societies (FEBS), a landmark event that further solidified the country's integration into the European and international scientific community (Fig. 16.8).

The SEB became a constituent society of the FEBS in 1964, joining a network that then comprised 17 European countries. Despite the many political and social challenges Spain faced during that period, the FEBS Board of Directors, at its fourth meeting held in Oslo in 1967, approved the proposal for Spain to host the 1969 FEBS Meeting in Madrid.

The path to organizing the event was fraught with obstacles. The national and international political climate was tense. The reverberations of the student protests and political upheaval of spring 1968 in Paris and Prague cast serious doubts on the feasibility of holding such a high-profile scientific gathering in Spain. Strikes, student demonstrations, and university occupations erupted in major Spanish cities, creating widespread unrest. By January 24, 1969—just three months before the opening of the FEBS Meeting—the Spanish government declared a state of emergency. This escalation of tension heightened concerns within the international scientific community. Some FEBS member societies voiced strong reservations, even opposition, to the Congress taking place under such volatile conditions.

Nevertheless, after carefully assessing the situation, the FEBS Executive Committee confirmed its decision to proceed as planned. Against all odds, the Sixth FEBS Meeting was successfully held in Madrid in April 1969. It was a major scientific and organizational achievement, not only because of its academic impact but also due to the symbolic importance of international cooperation during difficult times.

Severo Ochoa played a key role as both a driving force and an emblematic figure behind the event, working from abroad alongside other prominent Spanish scientists such as Santiago Grisolía, Juan Oró, and Francisco Grande Covián [11] (Fig. 16.8).

The 1969 FEBS Meeting significantly raised the public profile of biochemistry in Spain and had the added benefit of bringing together nearly all of the country's biochemists—both established and emerging—at an event of major international scientific relevance. The congress not only marked a milestone in Spain's scientific integration with Europe but also served as a catalyst for collaboration and future research initiatives.

In a striking cultural crossover, the official poster for the Congress was designed by none other than Salvador Dalí. The renowned surrealist painter had been a longtime friend of Severo Ochoa, a bond that dated back to their early days as students at the *Residencia de Estudiantes* in Madrid.

The 1969 FEBS Meeting in Madrid attracted 2,200 participants from several continents, including eight Nobel laureates—Ernst Boris Chain, Carl Ferdinand Cori, Hans Adolf Krebs, Fritz Lipmann, Feodor Lynen, Severo Ochoa, Frederick Sanger, and Alex H. Theodor Theorell (Fig. 16.9)—as well as many leading scientists of the era [10].

On the day before the closing ceremony, a roundtable discussion was held on the teaching of biochemistry in Spain, attended by the Minister of Education, Villar Palasí. Topics included the role of biochemistry in medical education and the modernization of research training. Efforts were made to persuade Severo Ochoa to return to Spain to lead Centro de Biología Molecular (CBM) (Centre for Molecular Biology), though this vision would take many more years to materialize.

What was quickly achieved, following the 1969 FEBS Meeting, was the establishment of Autonomous Universities in Madrid, Barcelona, and Bilbao. This initiative aimed to ease student overcrowding and to encourage distinguished Spanish scientists working abroad—such as Severo Ochoa, Francisco Grande Covián, Nicolás Cabrera, and José Manuel Rodríguez Delgado—to return. However, these attempts were largely unsuccessful due to the many difficulties encountered. His encounters in Spain continued to be very frequent, especially with his friends Francisco Grande Covián and Santiago Grisolía (Fig. 16.10).

Ultimately, University autonomy ended up, Severo Ochoa did not return to Spain, and the plan to create a Centre for Molecular Biology remained stalled until 1973 [12].

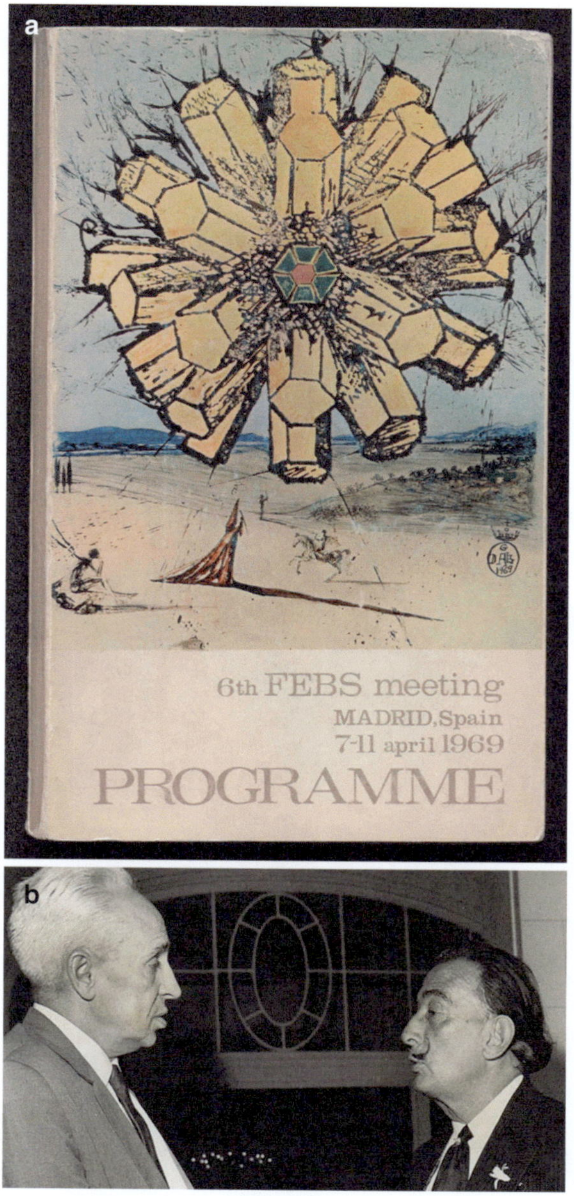

Fig. 16.8 (**a**) Poster made by Salvador Dalí for the Congress of the Federation of European Biochemical Societies (FEBS), held in Spain, April 1969. (**b**) Severo Ochoa with Salvador Dalí

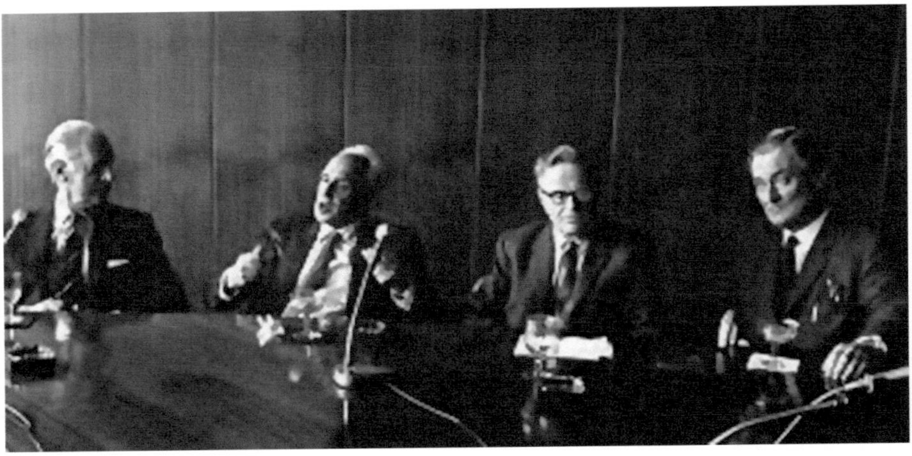

Fig. 16.9 Round table during the FEBS, Madrid 1969. From left to right: Carl Cori, Severo Ochoa, Hans Krebs and Hugo Theorell

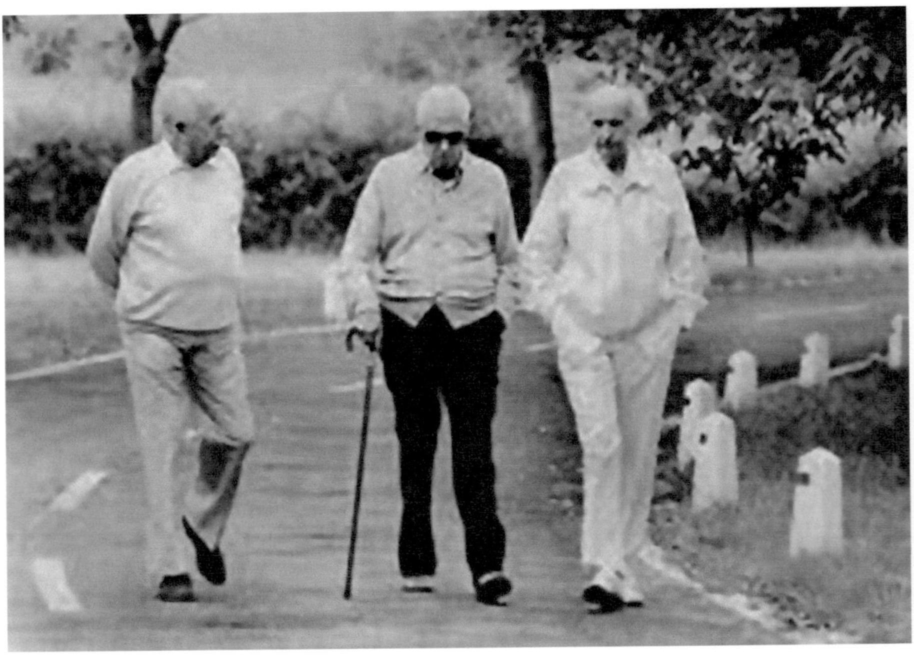

Fig. 16.10 Severo Ochoa with Francisco Grande Covián and Santiago Grisolía

The *Centro de Biología Molecular "Severo Ochoa"* (CBM Severo Ochoa) was finally inaugurated in September 1975 (Fig. 16.11).

Although the original plan envisioned that Ochoa would be the director of the centre—given his support and involvement in its planning—this never came to fruition. Ochoa abandoned the idea following the dismissal of Minister Villar Palasí. He did not return to Spain until his retirement from Roche Laboratories in 1982. Nevertheless, his legacy was a defining hallmark of the CBM from its beginnings.

Severo Ochoa often stated that "the CBM was my dream," a dream that was realized thanks to his support and guidance. From 1985 onward, the year he settled permanently in Spain, Ochoa played a prominent role in the scientific life of the CBM. There, he conducted research alongside his disciples César de Haro and José Manuel Sierra.

Over the years, the CBM 'Severo Ochoa' has evolved but continues to uphold the multidisciplinary and collaborative spirit that defined its early years. In 2008, the CBM, a joint centre with the Universidad Autónoma de Madrid, moved to a new building in Fuencarral-El Pardo, to expand its facilities. While primarily focused on basic research, it maintains strong collaborations with numerous academic institutions, hospitals, and biotech companies.

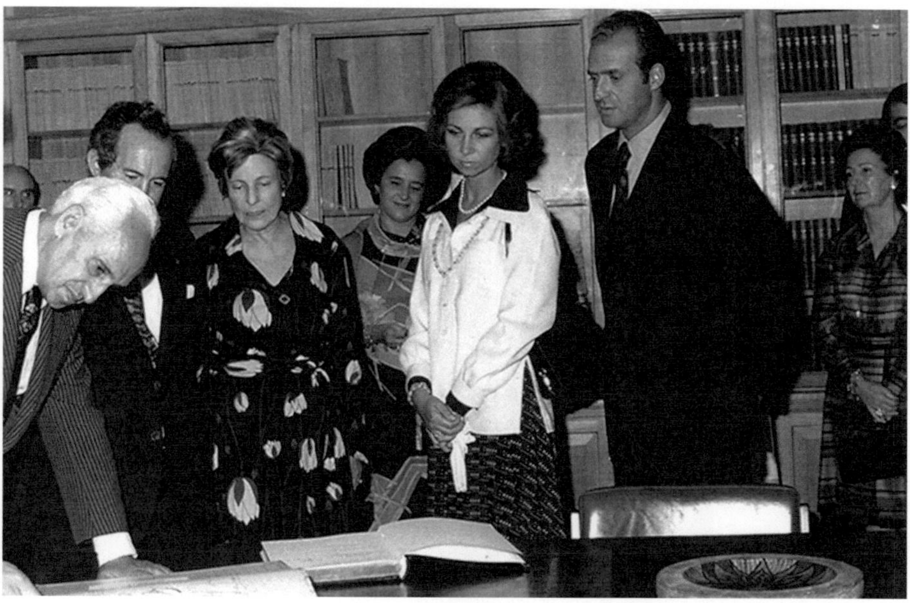

Fig. 16.11 The King and Queen of Spain Juan Carlos I and Sofia with Severo Ochoa at the inauguration of the Severo Ochoa Center for Molecular Biology (CBMSO) in September 1975

Following the example set by its founders, one of the CBM's key objectives remains the transfer of knowledge generated within the centre to clinical practice and industry.

Additionally, we must not overlook the disciples who trained with Ochoa in his New York laboratory. Among them were Margarita Salas and her husband, Eladio Viñuela. The newlywed couple arrived at Ochoa's lab in August 1964, where they benefited greatly from his mentorship. After 3 years, they returned to Spain and established their own laboratories.

Eladio Viñuela was one of the founding figures of the CBM, alongside Federico Mayor Zaragoza, Antonio García Bellido, and David Vázquez. He devoted much of his scientific career to the study of viruses. Margarita Salas focused on the bacteriophage Φ29, leading to the discovery of its DNA polymerase—the enzyme responsible for viral DNA replication—whose patent remains the most lucrative for the CSIC (see Chap. 30).

Today, Ochoa's legacy is also preserved through the foundation that bears both his and his wife's names. The Carmen y Severo Ochoa Foundation (FCySO) was established in 1994, following his will, after his passing on November 1, 1993. Its purpose is to honor his wife's name alongside his own and to uphold his passionate desire for Spain to one day join the ranks of scientifically advanced nations.

The Foundation's statutes, included in Ochoa's will, form his fundamental legacy. They define the Foundation's charitable nature and its commitment to awarding an annual prize for research in Molecular Biology to a scientist whose work has been conducted in Spain during the previous 5 years. To date, the quality of the awardees' research has been comparable to that of their European and American peers. The United States Postal Service issued a stamp in his honour in 2011 (Fig. 16.12).

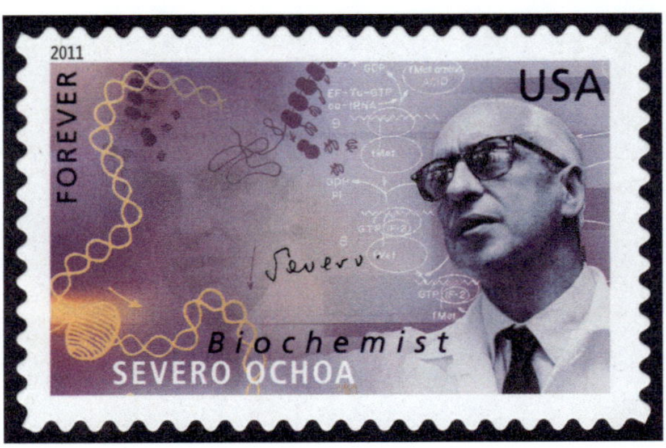

Fig. 16.12 US commemorative postage stamp honoring Severo Ochoa. 2011

References

1. Ochoa S. Escritos. Consejo Superior de Investigaciones Científicas, (Ed. Marino Gómez Santos) Madrid (1999).
2. Ochoa S. The pursuit of a hobby. Ann Rev Biochem. 1980;49:1–30.
3. Severo Ochoa: Un vida por la ciencia. Ed. José Manuel Sánchez Ron... [et al.], Geoplaneta and CSIC, Barcelona, 2024. pp. 1–225.
4. Grunberg-Manago M, Ortiz PJ, Ochoa S. Recollections on studies of polynucleotide phosphorylase: a commentary on 'Enzymic synthesis of polynucleotides. I. Polynucleotide phosphorylase of *Azobacter vinelandii*'. Biochim Biophys Acta. 1956;20:269–85.
5. Tan SY, Pettigrew K. Severo Ochoa (1905–1993). The man behind RNA. Singapore Med. 2018;59:3–4.
6. NobelPrize org. Severo Ochoa. Nobel Prize 1959.
7. Arthur Kornberg BL, Horecker LC, Oró J, editors. Reflections on biochemistry. In honour of Severo Ochoa. Oxford: Pergamon Press; 1976.
8. Kornberg A. Severo Ochoa (24 September 1905–1 November 1993). Proc Am Philos Soc. 1997;141:478–91.
9. Kresge N, Simoni RD, Hill RL. How Severo Ochoa determined the direction of the genetic code. J Biol Chem. 2006;281:16–17.12.
10. Santesmases MJ. Severo Ochoa and the biochemical sciences in Spain under Franco, 1959–1975. Isis. 2000;91:706–34. https://sebbm.es/revista/numeros/50-anos-del-congreso-febs-en-madrid-1969-2019/.
11. Documentary archive of the FEBS Meeting 1969 in open access on SIMURG: http://simurg.csic.es/browse?q=must,any,contains,P00209&limit=50&sort=-metadata.25_year.es.keyword&sort=-metadata.26_numero.es.keyword.
12. Santesmases MJ. Biomedical research and science policy in Spain, 1961–1975. Arbor. 2001:273–86.

17

Don Carlos and Don Severo: Double Partners for the Success of Spanish Biomedical Science

Damián García-Olmo

Spring 1935, Moncloa, Ciudad Universitaria de Madrid

Young Severo is driving the Ford his mother-in-law gave him to the San Carlos Hospital in Atocha. He needs to speak with his boss, Don Carlos Jiménez Díaz. He will inform him that he has just found out that the Faculty Board, in an extraordinary meeting, has withdrawn the budget assigned to his newly established Institute of Medical Research. The Institute had just begun its activities in the almost finished building of the new Faculty of Medicine.

It was an incident characteristic of Spanish university life—then and now. It was resolved through both academic and informal channels, without major consequences. Yet, this event undoubtedly marked the beginning of a deep friendship between the doctor and the scientist—two roles both men embodied, though in different ways.

D. García-Olmo (✉)
Universidad Autonoma de Madrid (UAM), Madrid, Spain

Department of Surgery, "Fundación Jiménez Díaz" University Hospital, Madrid, Spain

M. A. Cuesta, F. Mateo Vallejo (eds.), *Spain's Journey in Medicine*,
https://doi.org/10.1007/978-3-032-12221-6_17

Carlos, a brilliant clinician, always recognized the importance of combining scientific medicine with a deep understanding of fundamental mechanisms of basic science, in order to address the problems that arise daily in clinical practice.

Severo, a medical researcher—what we might now call a basic scientist—had already made the firm decision to dedicate himself entirely to scientific research, without the distractions of clinical work.

So when Don Carlos invited him to lead the Physiology Department at his newly founded Institute for Medical Research, Severo was more than happy to accept. More than 40 years later, in 1977, he would write: "*It would be difficult for me to express the great joy that this appointment caused me because for the first time it allowed me to realize my golden dream of dedicating my life entirely to scientific research, without limits, without hindrance, in a well-equipped laboratory, with technical assistance, with capable and enthusiastic collaborators; going to the laboratory in the morning and returning from it at night*" [1–3].

Why Did Don Carlos "Recruit" the Young Severo?

In 1935, Don Carlos was 37 years old and already a well-known and respected physician. At the time, he held the Chair of Internal Medicine at the Central University (today the Complutense University of Madrid), a position he had earned at just 28.

Five years earlier, in 1930, Don Carlos had been a member on the committee that evaluated the doctoral thesis of a 25-year-old physician from his faculty—Severo Ochoa—who left a strong impression on him. The thesis, titled "*Carbohydrates in the Chemical and Energetic Phenomena of Muscular Contraction,*" revealed to Don Carlos, thanks to his scientific intuition, that this was not a routine academic exercise designed to secure a university credential or post. It was, rather, a rigorous and meaningful piece of research, grounded in the scientific method.

From that moment, he began to take an interest in Severo's career. He remembered of his research stays in London with Sir Henry Dale and with Dudley, and he followed his progress. As soon as he had the opportunity, he invited Severo to head one of the departments of his newly founded Institute.

This decision had consequences. Severo's academic supervisor, Professor Juan Negrín—Chair of Physiology at the University and later President of the Second Spanish Republic—set a professional "trap" for him. In Severo's own words, recalled in his final days: "*The fact that Negrín forced me to take the exams and that I didn't pass them—something he must have been largely*

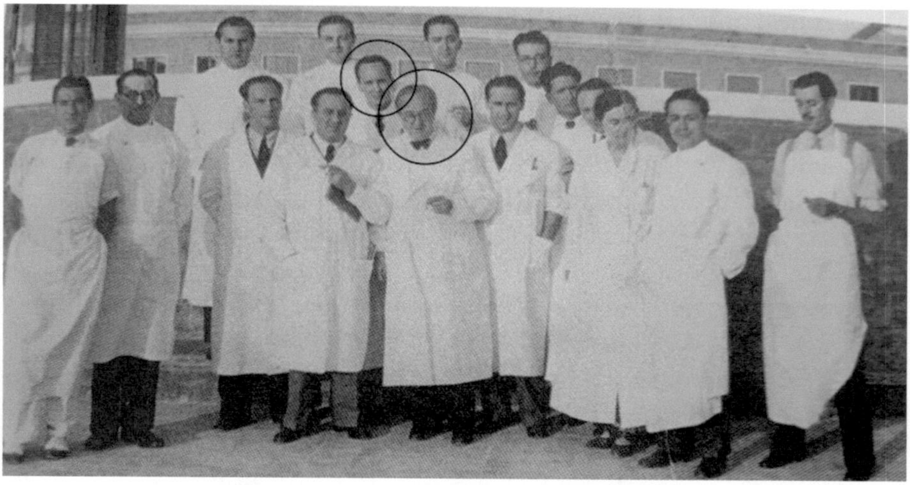

Fig. 17.1 Picture of 1935, possibly taken on February 13, on the roof of the new Faculty of Medicine in Madrid. Don Carlos (foregroun) with all the first founding group with Don Severo (background). (Permission Jimenez Casado)

responsible for—leads me to believe it was due to his displeasure at my association with Jiménez Díaz."

Don Carlos's decision to bring Severo Ochoa into his Institute clearly had consequences in the academic and political spheres—consequences that their opponents were going to exploit.

Even so, none of this prevented them from beginning their collaboration in 1935, a partnership marked by mutual respect and admiration [4, 5] (Fig. 17.1).

Much later, when Severo had become "Don Severo," he would recall:

> *We worked closely with Don Carlos, who—despite his many clinical and teaching duties—devoted two or more hours each day to the Institute and followed the course of our research very closely.*

But the golden days of the Institute were short-lived—less than a year of full activity. We all know what happened next. In the summer of 1936, the Spanish Civil War broke out. Don Carlos initially took a stand in defense of the Republic and tried to help however he could. He was assigned to the Hospital de Chamartín, a medical center organized by the Communist Party in the convent of the *Madres Reparadoras de Chamartín de la Rosa*, in northern Madrid. The building was relatively new and was named *Hospital Ada de la Fuente*, in memory of an activist who had died in the early fighting. It was not a proper field hospital, but rather a center for caring patients arriving from the front lines and conflict zones.

Don Carlos summoned his collaborators, and Severo came with his wife, Carmen García Cobián, whom he had married a year after completing his thesis and who had accompanied him throughout his travels and scientific work at the Institute. Conchita Rábago, Don Carlos's wife, also came to help and assist with the patients. From that moment, the bond between Conchita and Carmen was, without a doubt, one of the keys to the harmony between the two couples. Both men had been deeply in love with their wives from a young age. Neither couple had children.

Life in Madrid during those early days of the war was difficult for everyone—especially in a hospital that received both wounded soldiers from the front and victims of the purges in the rearguard. As the conflict worsens, Conchita suffered greatly, and Carlos began to feel disillusioned with the unfolding events in revolutionary Madrid. Carmen and Severo continued to help as much as they could in the hospital, but they too were upset by what they witnessed.

Eventually, both couples—each on their own but in parallel—began seeking a way to leave Spain. The decision to leave would be painful.

Don Carlos went to Paris and, after a tour through Europe, made the decision to return to Spain in the midst of the armed conflict (1936–39).

Like other intellectuals and scientists of his time—such as Gregorio Marañón and Teófilo Hernando—he changed his political stance and, during the war, managed to cross over to Nationalist Spain. There were many reasons behind this shift, but as Don Carlos himself explained, he considered himself a patriot and felt a duty to return and help rebuild Spain. Most importantly, Conchita needed the Spanish way of life; she could not adapt to living outside the country.

Don Severo also left for France and began his own journey—but he had no desire to return. He was captivated by the scientific world of the United States and Carmen adapted well to American life. Moreover, everything gave him the freedom to maintain his intellectual independence without any conditions or fear of reprisals. Although we must say that politics was never a dominant trait in his personality or in his public life.

Don Carlos, with his characteristic tenacity and intelligence, returned after the war to resume his work—rebuilding the Institute of Medical Research and later founding the Hospital Clínica de La Concepción. He missed Don Severo. But he knew he could not call on him. He understood that Severo would not return—his life had taken a different paths. He could not have pursued his life's work in the desolate, post-war Spain.

Even so, the friendship between the two couples endured. They continued to hold each other in high esteem and admiration. Though their lives had diverged greatly, the intense experiences they had shared in 1935 and 1936 created a powerful bond. They maintained a written correspondence—one that remained largely unspoken about, as it was politically inconvenient for Don Carlos during the darkest years of post-war political purges in Spain.

Don Carlos traveled to America to attend medical congresses, and his national prestige continued to grow. Meanwhile, Don Severo, working in New York, had already become a world-renowned scientist. In June 1954, Don Carlos visited Don Severo's laboratory. They called each other, they met, they enjoyed one another's company—but they no longer collaborated scientifically. Their professional paths had separated.

What's more, Don Carlos still had to be refined for his earlier Republican sympathies during the war, while Don Severo no longer needed it. He had changed his nationality and, since 1956, had been an American citizen.

In the autumn of 1959, Severo Ochoa was awarded the Nobel Prize in Physiology or Medicine. It was a milestone that went largely uncelebrated by official Spain at the time, yet it had a significant impact on the country's scientific community. The news appeared modestly on page 33 of the ABC newspaper on October 16, 1959.

Severo had fulfilled his dream—the dream first inspired by the writings of Don Santiago Ramón y Cajal during his early days at the Faculty of Medicine of the Central University of Madrid. His true friends—Don Carlos and his circle—were overjoyed.

The Spanish government may have tried to capitalize on Ochoa's international prestige, but he himself maintained an ambiguous stance toward the Franco's regime. He accepted official recognition without politically aligning himself with the dictatorship. This reflects the complex context in which Ochoa's achievement was received, and how Spain manages relationships with internationally acclaimed scientists.

Did Don Carlos and his entourage in any way influence the awarding of the Nobel Prize, and did the Spanish scientific community mobilize to support his nomination? These are two questions that have been asked repeatedly yet remain without a clear answer. What is certain is that Spain in 1959 was under a dictatorship, a political context that greatly affected the country's scientific development. Autarky, international isolation, and a lack of resources significantly limited the progress of Spanish science and, undoubtedly, its capacity for international influence. Many prominent Spanish scientists submitted nominations and spoke in support of him at conferences and forums, though likely with limited effectiveness. It could be said that Don Carlos, along with well-known figures from his university—such as Don José María Corral García, Professor of Physiology at the Faculty of Medicine of the University of Madrid—nominated him year after year for the Nobel Prize. However, these efforts may not have been decisive in the final decision.

When the Nobel Prize was awarded to Don Severo, the Government prepared an official delegation to represent Spain at the award ceremony in Stockholm. It was composed of Don Fernando de Castro, Professor of Histology and direct disciple of Cajal (see chap 13); Don Jesús García-Orcoyen, Professor of Gynecology; and Don José M. ª Corral himself—all from the University of Madrid. Everyone from the University of Don Carlos. However, Don Carlos, possibly the most prominent professor in the Spanish medical scene at the time, was not invited. The exact reasons are unknown, though we can speculate. What we do know is that he and Conchita prepared for the trip but, for reasons that have never been revealed, ultimately did not attend. On behalf of the Clínica de la Concepción, and thus Don Carlos, were doctors Sixto Obrador and Pedro Barreda.

All the testimonies of the time speak of Don Carlos's deep emotion and his strong sentimental bond with his great friend and companion in his adventures.

Later that year, Don Severo traveled to Madrid at the invitation of numerous institutions, and we know that his first stop was to visit the Maestro, Don Carlos. His first stop was at Clínica de la Concepción. It was a very emotional occasion, which was followed by scientific and festive gatherings that strengthened the professional and emotional ties between these two great figures. It is particularly interesting to look at the surviving photographs of the heifer bullfighting at the Hacienda Navalcaide in 1960 (Fig. 17.2).

Considering that it was less than 25 years after the events at Chamartín hospital, these images are striking and help us understand how deeply their friendship was sealed.

From then on, life brought them together on numerous occasions at scientific congresses and other events. When Don Carlos traveled to America, always accompanied by Conchita, he made every effort to see them, and they did the same. Their relationship with the recently founded Spanish Society of Biochemistry was especially moving; although somewhat distant from Don Carlos's daily work, it once again provided a great opportunity for them to meet and interact (Figs. 17.3 and 17.4).

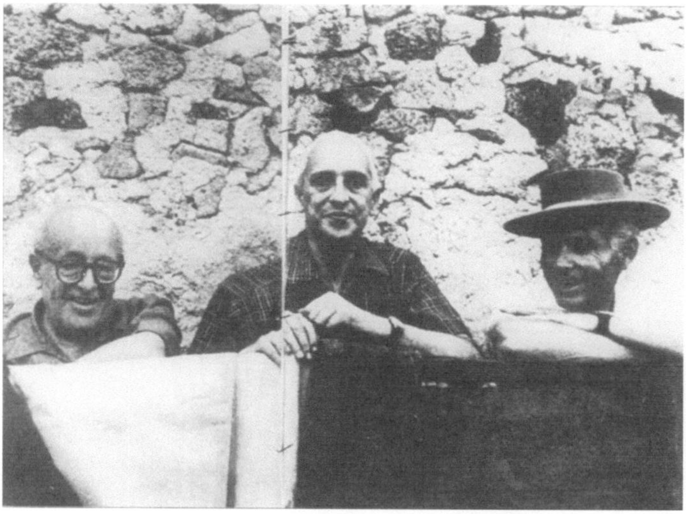

Fig. 17.2 Don Carlos and Don Severo in 1960 behind the barrier of the arena in Hacienda Navalcaide, together with the famous torero Domingo Ortega. (Permission Jimenez Casado)

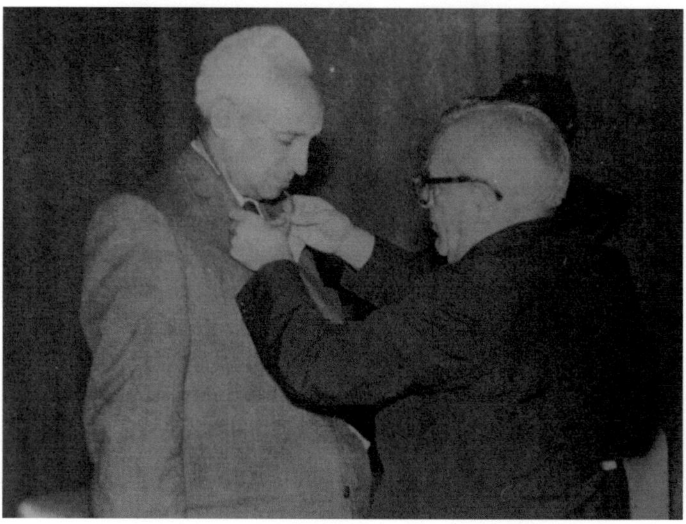

Fig. 17.3 Don Carlos imposing the Medal of the Spanish Society of Biochemistry to Don Severo Ochoa during the Congress of 1961. (Permission Jimenez Casado)

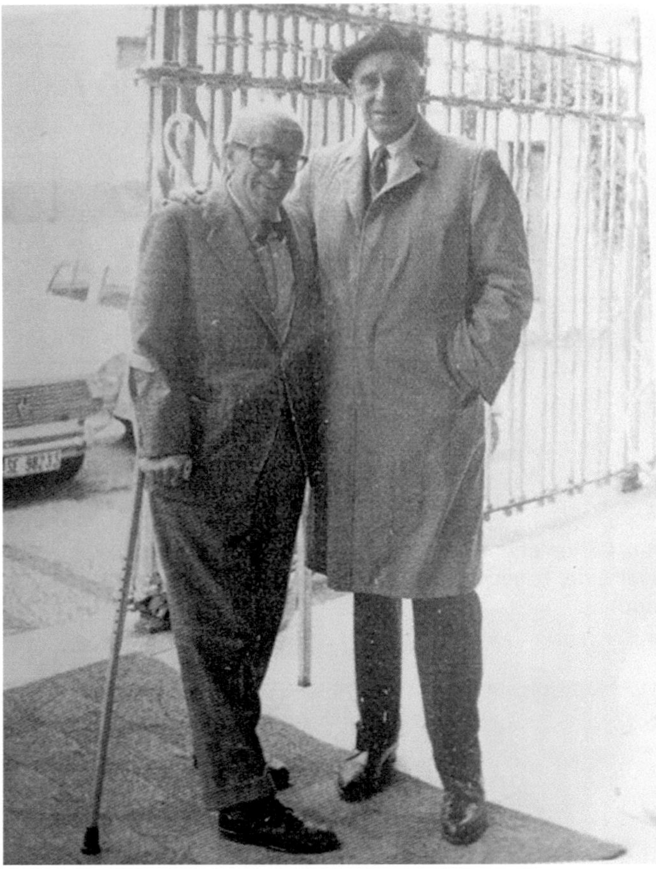

Fig. 17.4 Sevilla, 1967, during the National Biochemistry Congress. Don Carlos with a cane, after a serious traffic accident. It was the last time together. (Permission SEBBM)

In 1967, Don Carlos died suddenly at the doorstep of his practice, in what is now the Fundación Jiménez Díaz, at the age of 69, from a myocardial infarction. His death was undoubtedly hastened by the knowledge of his wife Conchita's serious and incurable illness, as she was at that time admitted to his clinic.

The funeral chapel was set up in "his" Aula Magna. Some accounts place Don Severo there on May 19th; however, direct testimonies indicate that he was unable to arrive from New York, although he would have wished to do so. He did send a condolence note which was read at the farewell ceremony. Shortly afterward, he wrote:

"The death of Don Carlos Jiménez Díaz was one of the most painful blows I have ever suffered in my life, as I was bound to him for years by bonds of deep affection. He was a man of great vision, who made it his mission to introduce the scientific spirit and method into Spanish medicine, and one of the few clinicians who, with his great intelligence and profound knowledge, appreciated the importance of the basic sciences in the practice of medicine". He then adds something premonitory that has survived to the present day: "Don Carlos survives in his work and in his school...".

The immediate creation of the Conchita Rábago Foundation served to preserve the values promoted by Don Carlos and his work. Along these lines, Santiago Grisolía—who had first been a disciple of Don Carlos and later of Don Severo (he can be seen between them in the photograph of the preparatory meeting for the Biochemistry Congress, Fig. 16.7 of Chap. 16)—proposed to Conchita Rábago the establishment of a la *Lección Conmemorativa* (Commemorative Lecture). The idea was that every year a prestigious scientist would give a lecture in memory of Don Carlos, helping to perpetuate his legacy. No one doubted that the first lecture should be delivered by Don Severo.

So, in May 1969, Don Severo Ochoa gave a lecture on biochemistry from the lectern in the Aula Magna, in the very place where Don Carlos had been laid to rest 2 years earlier—and just a few days after Conchita's death in her hospital. This symbolism did not escape anyone.

Deeply moved, Don Severo thus became indelibly linked to Don Carlos's legacy. He later became president of the *Board of Trustees of the Fundación Jiménez Díaz*. Beyond this formal role, there are testimonies of his ongoing support for the Fundación before the authorities, leveraging his prestige to prevent crises with the health system on several occasions.

Ten years after Don Carlos's died, Don Severo wrote: "*To conclude this review of the memory of Don Carlos Jiménez Diaz on the tenth anniversary of his death, I would like to reiterate that this model institution, this excellent postgraduate school, the Institute, everything in it today, is the work of a dreaming genius, the work of an iron will, the work of a man with a gigantic capacity for work. We all remember Don Carlos Jiménez Díaz with affection and will always remember him*".

On November 1, 1993, 26 years after the death of Don Carlos, Don Severo passed away at the Fundación Jiménez Díaz, where he had been admitted due to pneumonia—the very same center that had been his first stop in Spain for the celebration of his Nobel Prize [6]. Carmen's death, 4 years earlier, marked the beginning of his decline.

His funeral chapel was set up in the Aula Magna, the same place where Don Carlos was laid to rest and where Don Severo had given the first Memorial Lecture. In addition to the authorities of the time, dozens of students and young researchers paid their respects there.

So, we could say that something more than friendship united these two devoted doctors and scientists, who now rest beneath the same stones they helped lay for the rise of Spanish medical science [7].

And the story continues... at the Fundación Jiménez Díaz and in its Aula Magna!

References

1. Jiménez Casado M. Doctor Jiménez Díaz, vida y obra: la persecución de un sueño. [Madrid]: Fundación Conchita Rábago de Jiménez Díaz; 1993.
2. Gómez Santos M. La emoción de descubrir. Madrid: Editorial Pirámide; 1994.
3. Jiménez Casado M. History of the Fundación Jiménez Díaz. 1965–1995. Madrid: Editorial Ibáñez & Plaza Asociado; 1996.
4. Oliva Aldamiz H. Maestros y Dómines. Fundación Jiménez Díaz. Madrid: Editorial Ibáñez & Plaza Asociados; 1997.
5. Ochoa S. Jiménez Díaz y la Investigación. EL PAIS. 1977. https://elpais.com/diario/1977/05/22/cultura/233100003_850215.html?event_log=oklogin.
6. Argos L. Spanish science bids farewell to its Nobel Prize winner. EL PAIS. 1993. https://elpais.com/diario/1993/11/03/sociedad/752281206_850215.html.
7. De la Morena E. Confidencias personales. Jiménez Díaz Foundation. July 2024.

18

Francesc Duran Reynals: Beyond the Viral Theory of Cancer

Antoni Roca Rosell

Francesc Duran Reynals is remembered in the history of science as one of the early proponents of the viral theory of cancer, a concept he first advanced around 1927–1928 and later supported with experimental evidence in the 1940s. His theory sparked significant debate, as the international biomedical community was reluctant to accept that viruses—still poorly understood until the early 1940s—could be responsible for cancer, a disease traditionally considered non-contagious (Fig. 18.1).

Nevertheless, one seemingly "marginal" result of Duran Reynals' research soon earned him widespread recognition: the discovery in 1928 of the so-called "diffusion factor," also referred to as the "testicular factor" or "Duran Reynals factor." This substance, found in testicular tissue and snake venom, was shown to enhance the permeability of skin tissue. By 1936, this factor had been identified as hyaluronidase—an enzyme that breaks down hyaluronic acid, a key component of the skin's structural matrix.

Francesc Duran Reynals was born in Barcelona in 1899, the youngest of five siblings. Though the Duran Reynals family was relatively prominent in Catalan society, they had limited financial means. His parents, Manuel Duran i Duran and Agnès Reynals i Malloll, both passed away when he was still a child—his mother first, followed by his father, a draughtsman and illustrator,

A. Roca Rosell (✉)
Polytechnic University of Catalonia, Barcelona, Catalonia, Spain

M. A. Cuesta, F. Mateo Vallejo (eds.), *Spain's Journey in Medicine*,
https://doi.org/10.1007/978-3-032-12221-6_18

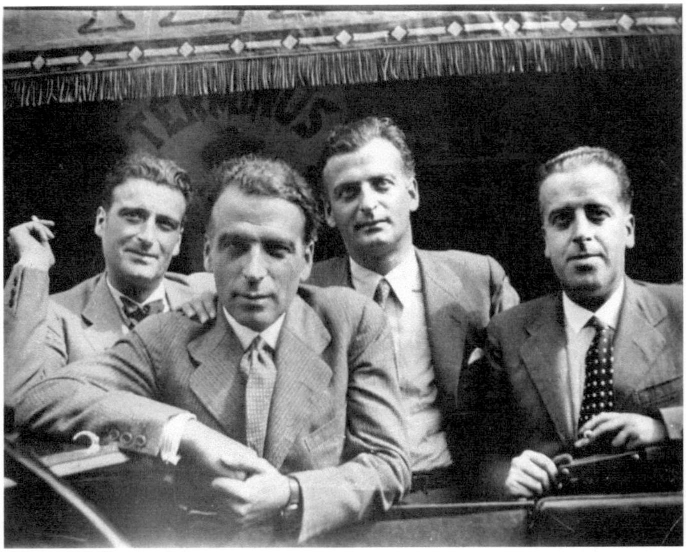

Fig. 18.1 The brothers Reynals in Barcelona, around 1930, probably in front of the "Términus" restaurant. (Photo: Courtesy of the Duran Reynals family)

in 1906. The siblings were left orphaned and were raised by their aunts, who became important guiding figures in their lives.

The eldest brother, Eudald (born 1891), was a writer and one of the first librarians of the Biblioteca de Catalunya, appointed in 1911. He died suddenly in Paris in 1917. Estanislau (1894–1950) became a lawyer and Catalanist politician; Raimon (1895–1966) was a distinguished architect; and Manuel (1896–1946), a chemical engineer, played a key role in the development of several companies in the chemical sector.

Francesc began studying at the Faculty of Medicine in Barcelona in 1916. That same year, he was admitted as assistant at the Municipal Microbiological Laboratory of Barcelona, then directed by Ramon Turró. From the first moment he quickly recognized the young student's talent. Duran Reynals simultaneous his academic work with laboratory research, although he gave priority to developing himself as an experimental researcher [1].

He focused his early investigations on immunology, one of the main lines of research led by Turró and his colleagues. In 1919, he presented his first

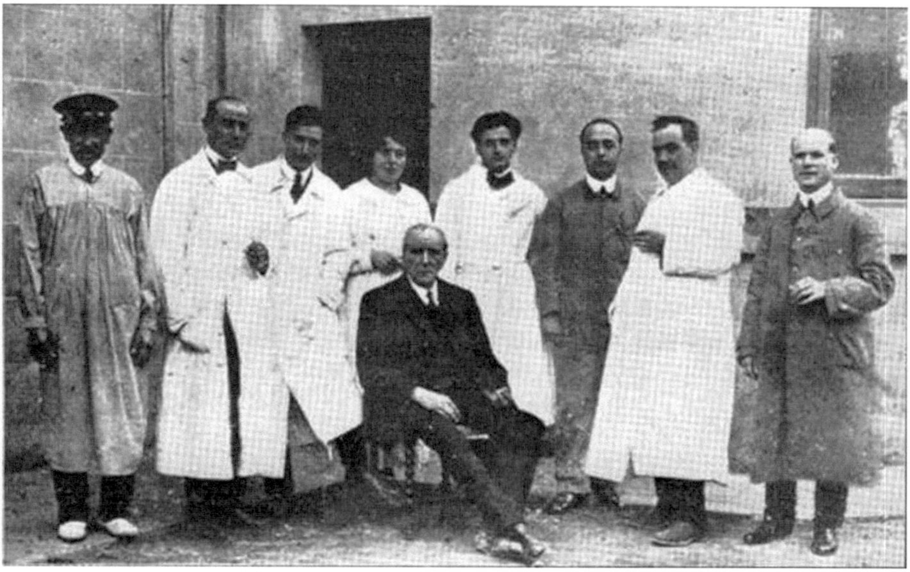

Fig. 18.2 At the Barcelona Municipal Laboratory: from left to right, a waiter, Dr. Puig de Valls, Pere Domingo, his wife, Ramon Turró (seated), Francesc Duran Reynals, Miquel A. Baltà, Pere González, and Mr. Inglada, curator of materials. (Photo: Barcelona Photographic Archive)

scientific study at the Laboratory's sessions, organized by the Societat de Biologia de Barcelona (the first branch of the Institut d'Estudis Catalans, founded in 1912). His work explored the transmission of anaphylaxis in pregnant mothers. Thanks to a collaboration agreement with the Société de Biologie de Paris, the note was also published in French in the bulletin of the French society [2] (Fig. 18.2).

Thereafter, Duran Reynals began a prolific career in experimental biology, working first at the Municipal Laboratory of Barcelona, which was equipped with state-of-the-art facilities and resources. In 1920, he was called up for military service, however, by paying a fee—a common practice at the time—he was assigned to the Military Health Command in Barcelona, this meant that he was able to continue his scientific studies and laboratory work during this period.

In November 1922, however, he was mobilized and sent to the Spanish Protectorate in North Africa to assist in the repatriation of wounded and ill soldiers following the Spanish military defeat known as the "Disaster of Annual." Duran Reynals endured what he later described as a harrowing, almost Dantesque experience due to the appalling conditions in the military concentration camps. He returned to Barcelona in May 1923, completing his medical degree in 1925.

Duran Reynals applied for a scholarship from the *Junta para Ampliación de Estudiose Investigaciones Científicas* (Board for the Extension of Studies and Scientific Research) to pursue further research at the Institut Pasteur in Paris. His aim was to deepen his investigations into anaphylaxis and pregnancy, as well as to explore the emerging field of bacteriophage viruses. In 1925, Duran Reynals' studies on bacteriophages were considered groundbreaking at the time. He even conducted clinical trials in Barcelona at the *Hospital de Infecciosos* (now *Hospital del Mar*) to explore the potential use of bacteriophages in treating typhus infections [3].

With the support of Ramon Turró, his application for a research fellowship was approved in September 1925, and by December of that year, he had likely settled in Paris.

There, he worked on bacteriophages with Eugène Wollman (1883–1943) and on anaphylaxis with Alexandre Besredka (1870–1940) and L. Rosenthal—renowned researchers with whom he collaborated productively, albeit briefly. He also worked with American bacteriologist Edna S. Harde at the Institut Pasteur on studies related to Rous sarcoma. His research on bacteriophages had introduced him to the emerging field of virology, and it seemed that Duran Reynals already suspected that the agent responsible for Rous sarcoma it could be a virus.

While in Paris, colleagues—including Edna Harde—introduced him to the work of Alexis Carrel, a French researcher based at the Rockefeller Institute in New York. Carrel, who had received the Nobel Prize in Physiology or Medicine in 1910, was a prominent advocate of the viral theory behind Rous sarcoma. Realizing that he would be unable to pursue this line of research further in Paris, Duran Reynals requested a transfer of his fellowship from the *Junta para Ampliación de' Estudios* to the Rockefeller Institute. He began his work there shortly after the summer of 1926 (Fig. 18.3).

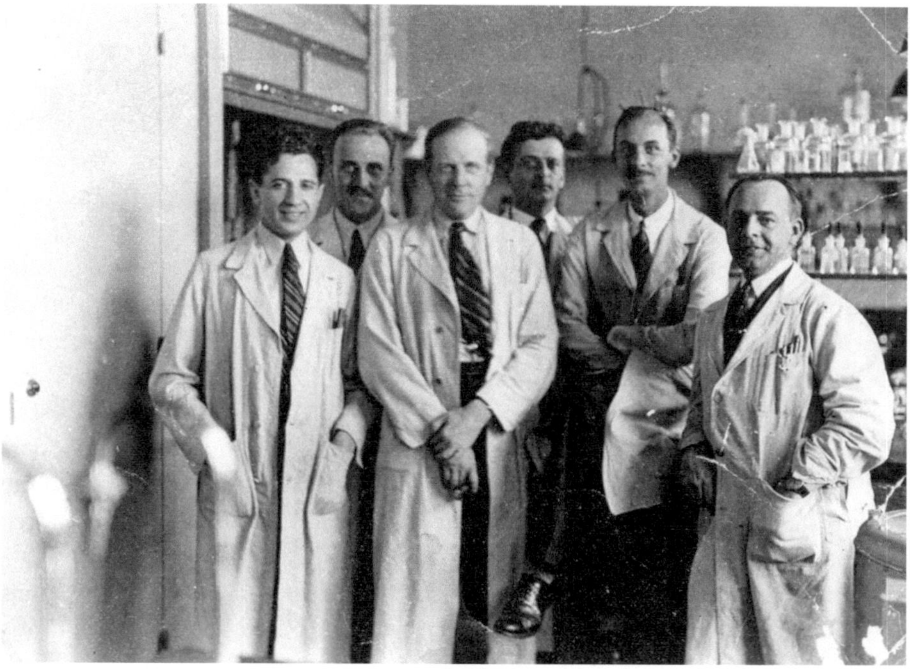

Fig. 18.3 At the Rockefeller Institute laboratory in New York. Albert Claude (first on the left), James Murphy is third, and Francesc Duran Reynals sticks out his head behind him. (Photo: Courtesy of the Duran Reynals family)

In the United States, First Stage

Upon arriving in New York, Duran Reynals quickly realized that he couldn't get along with Alexis Carrel and instead joined the laboratory led by James B. Murphy, where Francis Peyton Rous was also conducting research. However, the hypothesis Duran Reynals was developing—that Rous sarcoma was caused by a virus—was not well received by either Murphy or Rous. At the time, the international medical community firmly believed that cancer was not a contagious disease, and Duran Reynals' proposal challenged this deeply held conviction [4, 5].

Nevertheless, he was granted the freedom to pursue his research. One of his key lines of investigation into the nature of Rous sarcoma involved exploring the mechanisms by which microorganisms or viruses spread through tissues. In the course of this work, he identified a substance that facilitated such diffusion and named it "Factor T"—with "T" standing for "testicular." This substance soon came to be known as the "Duran Reynals Factor." He made this discovery in 1928, the same year his Spanish fellowship ended. However, possibly as a result of this significant finding, the Rockefeller Institute extended his contract [6].

Duran Reynals found this diffusion-promoting factor in testicular tissue, snake venom, and even spermatozoa. His research was not confined to New York—during the summers, he returned to Barcelona and continued working at the Municipal Laboratory, where he collaborated with former colleagues and close friends such as Jaume Sunyer Pi.

The Duran Reynals Factor attracted significant attention from researchers and was eventually identified in 1936 as a protein—specifically, the enzyme hyaluronidase, which breaks down the structure of hyaluronic acid, a key component of the skin's mesenchymal tissue [7, 8].

Although this work on the diffusion factor helped establish Duran Reynals as an internationally recognized scientist, it was only a secondary aspect of his broader research agenda, which focused on cancer and its possible viral origins. In that same year, 1928, he published a comprehensive study on prevailing theories of cancer in the journal *Ciència* of Barcelona. The following year, he contributed with two studies to the *Monografies Mèdiques*, published by Jaume Aiguader. Both publications were aimed at the Catalan medical and scientific community, with whom he remained closely engaged.

In addition, he delivered an extensive presentation on cancer prevention and treatment at the 1929 Congress of the Spanish Association for the Progress of Science, held in Barcelona.

By 1933, during the period of the Second Spanish Republic (1931–1936), he was proposed for a position as assistant professor at the Autonomous University of Barcelona—a role made possible by the university's newly gained autonomy. Around the same time, industrialist M. Roviralta, proprietor of Uralita (Spanish multinational enterprise dedicated to construction materials) expressed interest in establishing a private cancer research institute. Duran Reynals became involved in this initiative, ultimately choosing to prioritize it over a university appointment due to the growing political instability in Spain.

To build the research team for the new institute in Barcelona, Duran Reynals arranged for three young doctors to receive training in the United States at the Rockefeller Institute. In 1935, Jordi Folch-Pi traveled there to work with D. D. Van Slyke. At the beginning of 1936, Jordi Casals-Ariet joined Leslie Webster's laboratory, and Vincens Moragues Gonzalez trained under Leonor Michaelis [9].

In June 1936, Duran Reynals resigned from his position at the Rockefeller Institute to take part in launching the new center in Barcelona, which was to be named the *Institut Miquel Servet per a l'Estudi del Càncer i altres malalties d'etiologia desconeguda* (Miquel Servet Institute for the Study of Cancer and Other Diseases of Unknown Etiology).

However, as is well known, the Spanish Civil War broke out in July 1936, and the project was immediately cancelled. Duran Reynals suddenly found himself stranded in Barcelona but fortunately, his former colleagues and supervisors at the Rockefeller Institute quickly called him to return and being able to leave Spain, where he could continue his research in New York (Fig. 18.4).

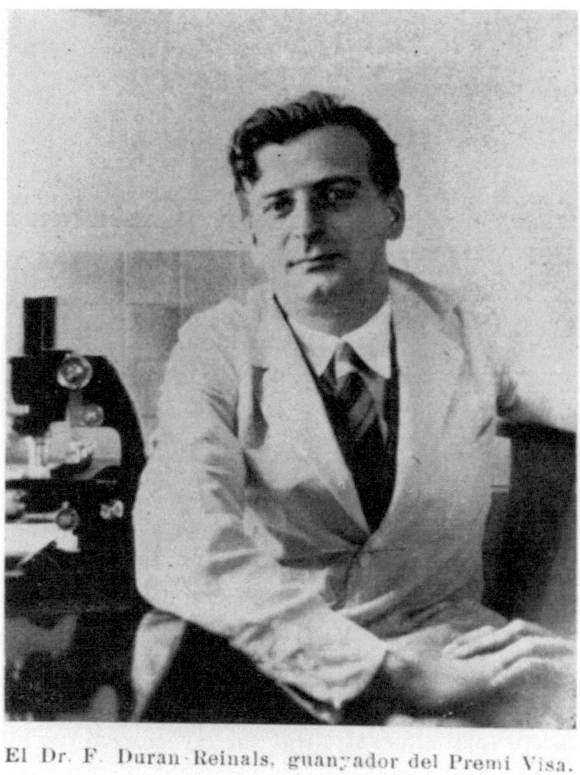

Fig. 18.4 Francesc Duran Reynals in 1935–1936, winner of the Visa Award from the Academy of Medicine and Surgery. (Photo appeared in La Medicina Catalana, January 15, 1936)

After the Unviability of the Barcelona Centre, Back to USA

The generosity extended to Duran Reynals during this period is also evident in the fact that, in 1938, James B. Murphy and Francis Peyton Rous facilitated his transfer to Yale University. There, he found abundant research facilities and a level of academic freedom that he may have lacked previously.

During the 1940s, he carried out a remarkable series of masterly experiments that provided compelling evidence that the agent responsible for Rous sarcoma was a "filterable" virus—meaning it could pass through filters that typically retain bacteria—and that it was not exclusive to chickens.

By 1942, after years of painstaking and complex research—particularly given the scientific limitations in understanding viruses at the time—Duran Reynals achieved what he considered the culmination of 15 years of work in experimental oncology. He had observed that the virus responsible for chicken sarcoma sometimes produced hemorrhagic lesions in the peritoneal cavity and internal organs, rather than forming tumors. This phenomenon occurred primarily in young individuals and had, in fact, already been noted by Rous and Murphy as early as 1912. For Duran Reynals, this observation confirmed a critical insight: a virus capable of causing cancer could also give rise to noncancerous disease manifestations [10, 11].

Could the reverse also be true—that is, that a virus that does not normally cause cancer eventually can induce it under certain conditions? This was the question that Duran Reynals pursued throughout his career. Through a highly complex experimental protocol, he succeeded in demonstrate that the virus responsible for hemorrhagic disease in young ducks will cause sarcoma in adult ducks. He had succeeded in disproving the apparent specificity of the sarcoma virus in chickens.

In doing so, he challenged the species and disease specificity of the Rous sarcoma virus, showing that through forced mutations, its behavior could be altered. These groundbreaking results were published in scientific papers in 1941 and 1942. It is important to note that, at the time, the first electron microscope images of viruses were just beginning to appear. Duran Reynals' experiments were able to set aside the limitation of knowing almost nothing about viruses except their small size (filterable with ceramic filters)—and little else.

Beginning in the 1940s, buoyed by his experimental findings, Duran Reynals launched an international effort to promote the viral theory of cancer. While his ideas were met with considerable skepticism, the strength of his scientific credentials and the rigor of his research led some members of the scientific community to reconsider their assumptions. He was frequently invited to speak at major international cancer congresses, where he continued to advocate for his theory—always grounded in experimental evidence [12–14].

It is no mere anecdote that F. Peyton Rous was awarded the Nobel Prize in Physiology or Medicine in 1966 for his "discovery of tumour-inducing viruses." In its official justification, the Nobel Foundation explicitly stated that, thanks to Rous—and in light of the new understanding of viruses—the relationship between viruses and cancer had become "a central area of modern cancer research."

However, in his Nobel Lecture, Rous referred to cancer-inducing viruses only indirectly, likening them to substances such as tar that can also trigger tumor formation, but he did not consider the cause-effect relationship between virus and cancer. Notably, he made no mention of Francesc Duran Reynals, who had died of cancer in New Haven in 1958.

Legacy

During his time in the United States, many Spanish researchers—primarily Catalans—looked to Duran Reynals for guidance and support in advancing their careers. Notably, among the researchers he had sent to the U.S. in connection with the unsuccessful Barcelona research center project, two—Jordi Casals-Ariet (1911–2004) and Jordi Folch-Pi (1911–1979)—went on to have highly distinguished scientific careers [6, 15, 16].

As mentioned earlier, Jordi Casals joined the Rockefeller Institute in 1936 to train in Leslie Webster's laboratory. When the unit he worked in moved to Yale in 1964, Casals was appointed professor at Yale University, where he remained until his retirement in 1981. Casals specialized in virology during this pioneering era, when experimental methods and resources were still in their infancy.

Thanks to the international reach of the Rockefeller Institute, Casals identified numerous viruses from around the world. He is best known for discovering the Lassa virus, named after the Nigerian town, where it was first identified. Primarly transmitted to humans with contact with items contaminated with rodent urine or feces. Person-to person transmission can also occur. This virus causes a hemorrhagic fever that nearly cost him his life. Casals became infected in the laboratory while testing for the virus, at a time when no treatment was known. To save him, doctors transfused him with blood from a nurse who had previously been infected and survived, which ultimately saved his life.

A man of experimental rigor, Casals revised the virus taxonomy system, which used capital letters for identification; his proposed system was soon adopted worldwide. Jordi Casals was also a dedicated supporter of Duran Reynals' legacy. His contribution to the volume *Virus and Cancer* (1971) stands as a testament to this.

In 1944, while at the Rockefeller Institute, Jordi Folch Pi was offered the opportunity to lead biological research at McLean Hospital, the psychiatric branch of Massachusetts General Hospital. His research focused on brain lipids and proteins, particularly their changes during development and diseases. There, he developed a highly original technique for identifying important brain lipids extracting brain lipids including phosphatidyl serine, mono, di and triphosphoinositides and myelin proteolipid, which quickly became a classic in neurochemical literature. The composition and changes in brain, are important particularly during development and of different neurological diseases. Folch Pi played a prominent role in both the American and International Neurochemistry communities, helping to promote the American Society for Neurochemistry—which awards a prize in his name—as well as the International Society for Neurochemistry.

Folch Pi passed away in 1979 and is regarded as a scientist of great renown. According to Google Scholar, his publications have amassed over 90,000 citations as of January 2025, his 1957 paper, "*A simple method for the isolation and purification of total lipids from animal tissues*," co-authored with M. Lees and G.H.S. Stanley and published in the *Journal of Biological Chemistry* (226: 497–509), has received over 80,000 citations.

In *Nature's* 2014 report on the top 10 most cited articles, was number 9 (at the time, with 45,000 citations). Finally, Folch Pi always acknowledged the great influence Duran Reynals had on him (Fig. 18.5).

Duran Reynals maintained his social and scientific influence. In 1980, the editors of the journal (*ciència*) prepared a monographic issue on cancer with the participation of very prominent Catalan researchers. Given that the journal wanted to link up with the journal that had appeared between 1926 and 1933, they proposed reprinting the article that Duran Reynals had published in 1928. The researchers initially received the proposal with skepticism. However, a few days later, they got enthusiastic about the freshness and relevance of Duran Reynals' insights on the importance of viruses. In fact, one of

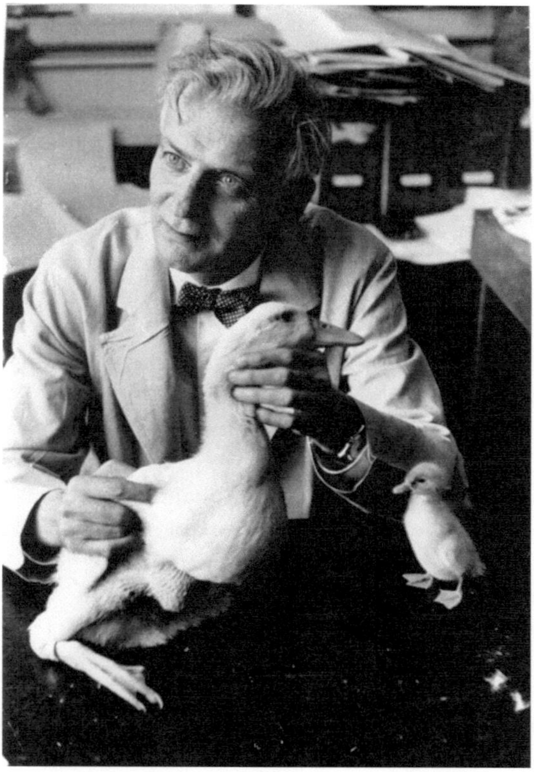

Fig. 18.5 Francesc Duran in his Yale laboratory, with an adult and a juvenile duck. (Photo by Ken Heyman, published in Life Magazine, January 1957)

them—Francesc-Xavier Bosch—played a key role in the development and epidemiological control of the papilloma vaccination at the Institut Català d' Oncologia, thanks to the identification of the virus responsible for causing and transmitting it.

While Duran Reynals' categorical assertion of the viral origin of cancer needs to be nuanced, today the international scientific community fully recognizes that certain cancers are virus-induced. Although he passed away in 1958, his work continues to be cited in research on diffusion factors as well as viruses and cancer.

Duran i Reynals remains a global pioneer in research into the origins of cancer.

References

1. Duran Reynals F. Galeria de Metges Catalans. https://www.galeriametges.cat/galeria-fitxa.php?icod=KD [the page contains a biography by Lluís Guerrero i Sala, photographs, bibliography, published work and links].
2. Duran Reynals F. Anaphylaxie et gestation. Comptes Rendus Hebdomadaires de Séances et Mémoires de la Société de Biologie. 1919;82:830–1.
3. Report to the Junta, París, June 14, 1926, Expediente Duran Reynals, Archivo de la Junta para Ampliación de Estudios; reproduced in Roca and Glick, Francesc Duran Reynals, pp. 174–5.
4. Rous FB, Murphy JB. On the causation by filterable agents of three distinct chicken tumors. J Exp Med. 1914;19:52–68.
5. Murphy JB. The possible role of viruses in the etiology of cancer. Third International Cancer Congress [Abstracts of papers, Atlantic City, 1939], p. 177.
6. Duran-Reynals F. The effect of extracts of certain organs from normal and immunized animals on the infecting power of vaccine virus. J Exp Med. 1929;50(3):327–40.
7. Duran-Reynals F. Tissue permeability and the spreading factors in infection – a contribution to the host: parasite problem. Bacteriol Rev. 1942;6:197–252.
8. Duran-Reynals F. Introduction, the ground substance of the mesenchyme and hyaluronidase. Ann New York Acad Sci. 1950;52:946–57.
9. Roca Rosell A. Francesc Duran Reynals i els seus col-laboradors als Estats Units. In: Lluís Garcia i Sevilla, Josep Carreras, Jacint Corbella, Antoni Roca Rosell i Oriol Casassas (coord.) Cicle de Conferències sobre les Ciències Experimentals i la Tecnologia a les Terres de Parla Catalana al Segle XX. 2009. 2: 99–109. Ciències biològiques, Barcelona, Institut d'Estudis Catalans.
10. Duran Reynals F. The reciprocal infection of ducks and chickens with tumor-inducing viruses. Cancer Res. 1942;2:343–69.
11. Duran Reynals F. Virus-Induced Tumors and the Virus Theory of Cancer. In: Homburger F, Fishman, editors. The physiopathology of cancer. New York: Hoeber; 1953. p. 298–337.
12. Duran Reynals F. Realities and Hypotheses of Viral Infection as a Cause of Cancer. Revue Canadienne de Biologie. 1956;14:411–28.
13. Glick TF, Roca-Rosell A, Duran Reynals F. (Barcelona 1899-New Haven 1958). Virus and cancer: a controversial theory. Contrib Sci. 1999;1:87–98.
14. Stanley WM, Oró J, Segura R. (eds.) Virus y cancer. Homenaje a F. Duran Reynals. V Congreso Nacional de la Sociedad Española de Bioquímica. Barcelona. 1971.
15. Hommage à Duran Reynals. Biol Méd. 1963;52:1–122.
16. Glick TF, Roca Rosell A. Francesc Duran i Reynals (1899–1958). La projecció internacional de la recerca biomèdica catalana. In: Camarasa JM, Roca Rosell A, editors. Ciència i tècnica als Països Catalans. A biographical approach. Barcelona: Fundació Catalana per a la Recerca; 1995. p. 1335–65.

19

Francisco Orts Llorca: The Anatomy and Development of Experimental Embryology

Jose Sanudo, Eva Maranillo Alcaide, and Arturo Prada Oliveira

Francisco Orts Llorca was born on June 10, 1905, in Tampico, Mexico, the son of Jaime Orts García de Presno and Margarita Llorca Orts. His birth in Mexico was due to his father's profession—he served as a pilot in the port of Tampico as part of his career in the Merchant Navy (Fig. 19.1).

At the age of three, Francisco and his mother returned to Spain, settling in Benidorm (Alicante) so that his mother, then expecting his sister, could give birth in her hometown. Shortly after, the family met again in Veracruz, Mexico. However, the outbreak of the Mexican Revolution in 1910 forced them to return once again to Benidorm when Francisco was just 5 years old. His father remained abroad for a time, relocating to New Orleans after securing a new position with a shipping company.

In pursuit of a proper education for their children, the family later moved to Valencia, where Francisco completed his secondary studies. It was during

J. Sanudo (✉)
Department of Anatomy and Embryology, Faculty of Medicine, Complutense University of Madrid, Madrid, Spain

E. Maranillo Alcaide
Professor of the Department of Anatomy and Embryology, Faculty of Medicine, Rovira i Virgili University, Reus, Tarragona, Spain

A. Prada Oliveira
Department of Anatomy, University of Cádiz, Cádiz, Spain

M. A. Cuesta, F. Mateo Vallejo (eds.), *Spain's Journey in Medicine*,
https://doi.org/10.1007/978-3-032-12221-6_19

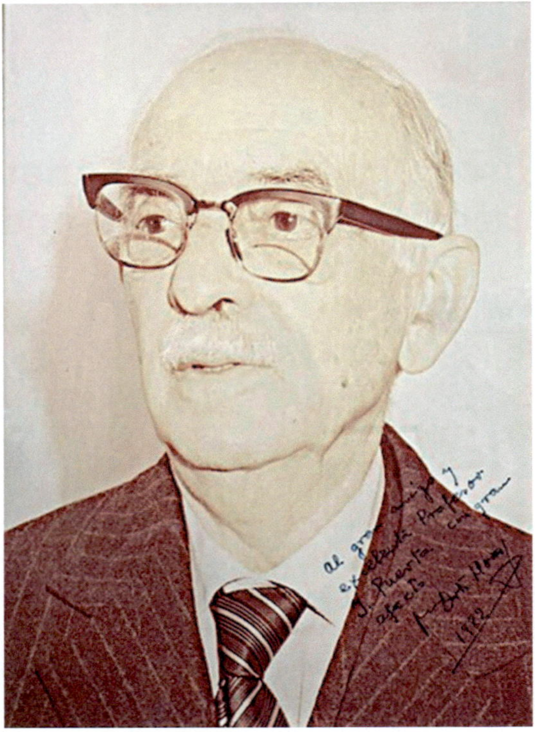

Fig. 19.1 Photograph by Professor Francisco Orts Llorca dedicated to his last disciple, Professor Javier Puerta Fonollá. 1982 (Permission Prof. F. Viejo)

these formative years—set against the backdrop of the First World War—that the Orts family came to be known for their liberal ideals and strong support for the Allied cause. This spirit is what he thought throughout his life, that of a liberal man.

Upon completing high school, Francisco Orts Llorca chose not to follow the family tradition of enlisting in the Merchant navy. His father dissuaded him by explaining the sacrifices that the sea demanded, and it was the figure of the doctor from Benidorm, a family friend, who inclined his vocation towards medicine, to his father's great joy. Reflecting on his early motivations, Orts would later write: *"As for my vocation, I can say that I have always been more interested in biology than in medicine. I am, therefore, more of a scientist than a doctor—more of a pragmatist, more of a laboratory man."* This perspective would remain a defining trait throughout his life.

In 1921, he enrolled at the University of Valencia in the Preparatory Course for Medicine, which covered topics such as Physics, Chemistry, Botany, and Zoology. Orts often emphasized the important role this course played in shaping his scientific mindset: *"...in that preparatory course I learned systematics, how to study, methodology, how to classify, how to organize, how to call each thing by its proper name—and not by an approximate one—and all of that had a profound effect on me."*

All of us devoted to the field of Morphology can wholeheartedly relate to these words, for we understand that such lessons form the very foundations upon which the disciplines of Anatomy and Embryology are built—fields in which Francisco Orts Llorca was, without question, a true master.

In 1922, Francisco Orts Llorca began his medical studies at the Faculty of Medicine in Valencia, graduating in 1928 with distinction in every subject and receiving the Extraordinary Prize for academic excellence. During these formative years, his vocation for anatomy was deeply shaped by Professor Jesús Bartrina, who taught Anatomy, and Dr. Navarro, his professor of Anatomical Technique. His dedication and talent in the field were quickly recognized; in his second year, he was awarded the Dr. Casanova Anatomy Prize, consisting of 500 pesetas and a diploma—an early acknowledgment of his remarkable possibilities [1–5].

As recalled by his nephew, Alfonso Puchades Orts, himself a Professor of Anatomy and Embryology at the University of Alicante, one anecdote perfectly illustrates the remarkable character and talent of the young Francisco Orts Llorca:

> *During a surgery class, the professor announced, 'You need to operate on an inguinal hernia. But of course, this is pure anatomy. Does anyone here actually know the inguinal canal?' Francisco immediately replied, 'I do!' The professor challenged him: 'Well then, explain it.' My uncle did so with such clarity and confidence that the professor stopped him midway and said, 'Very well—go down and operate.' Francisco went down to the table and performed the operation, with the professor himself acting as his assistant—utterly impressed by the student's knowledge and surgical skill.*

This marked the first of many surgical procedures Francisco Orts Llorca would later perform in Altea and Cádiz, once he had already become a Professor of Anatomy.

In 1928, upon completing his medical degree, he faced an important decision: whether to dedicate himself fully to surgery or to anatomy. To resolve this internal dilemma, he chose the most direct path—by immersing himself in both disciplines. With the financial support of his family, he moved to Paris, where he spent a full year refining his dual interests.

In the mornings, he trained in surgery under Armand Gosset, acquiring valuable hands-on experience in the operating room. In the afternoons, he worked in the anatomy laboratory of the renowned Henri Rouvière, where he began his formal initiation into the study of topographical anatomy. This dual exposure would profoundly shape his scientific identity and pave the way for his future contributions to anatomical science.

Topographical anatomy is the branch of anatomy that studies the arrangement of the structures of the human body in specific regions.

It was also in Paris that Francisco Orts Llorca first encountered what would become one of his lifelong scientific passions: the creation of a comprehensive collection of embryos and fetuses for the descriptive study of human development (Fig. 19.2).

This interest, born in the anatomy laboratory of Professor Rouvière, would accompany him throughout his career. Over the years, he established Embryology Collections at each of the universities where he worked—Valencia, Cádiz, and Madrid—laying the groundwork for generations of anatomical and embryological research.

And so, nowadays we have collections of human embryos and fetuses in several Spanish Universities. All these collections are collected in a small booklet sponsored by the Dean's Office of the Faculty of Medicine of the Complutense University (Fig. 19.3).

Impressed by his brilliance and tireless work capacity, Rouvière invited Orts Llorca to undertake a doctoral thesis on a subject that had, until then, received little academic attention: the lymphatic system of the lacrimal gland.

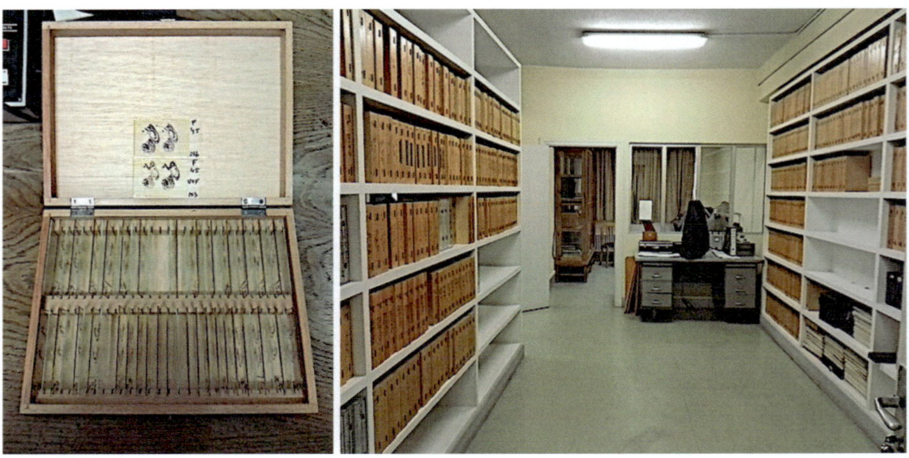

Fig. 19.2 Embryo Collection (Embryotheque) of the Department of Anatomy I (Professor Javier Puerta Fonollá) of the Faculty of Medicine of the Complutense University of Madrid. The box features a sagittal section of a 9-week-old fetus on the lid. On the right, the collection of human embryos and fetuses can be seen on the left, and the control chicken and quail embryos on the right

At the time, Rouvière was preparing his seminal book on the *Lymphatics of the human body* (published in 1932), and Orts' research proved to provide a significant contribution [6] (Fig. 19.4).

As a result, Figure 35 of Rouvière's book, featured Orts Llorca's detailed anatomical study of the lymphatics of the lacrimal gland, conjunctiva, and eyelids—a testament to the young academic's precision and skill. To carry out this meticulous work, Orts employed the lymphatic injection technique

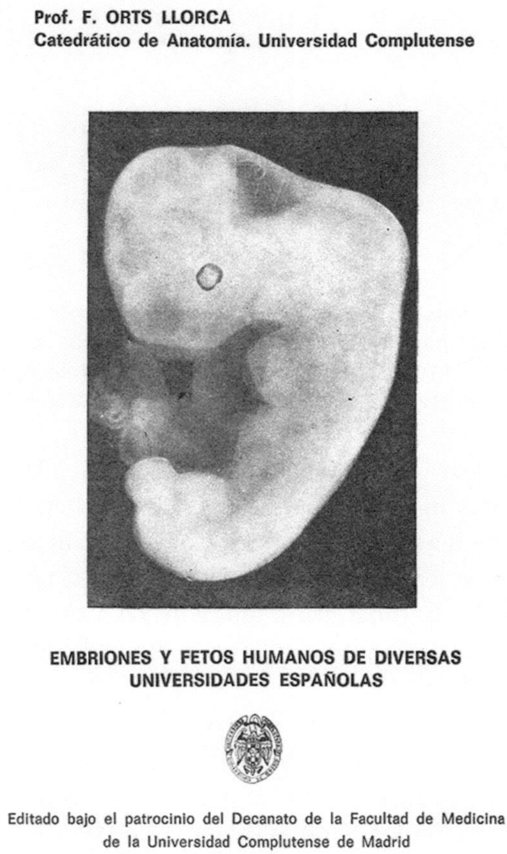

Fig. 19.3 Booklet published by the Faculty of Medicine of the Complutense University of Madrid. "Human Embryos and Fetuses from Various Spanish Universities." Professor F. Orts Llorca

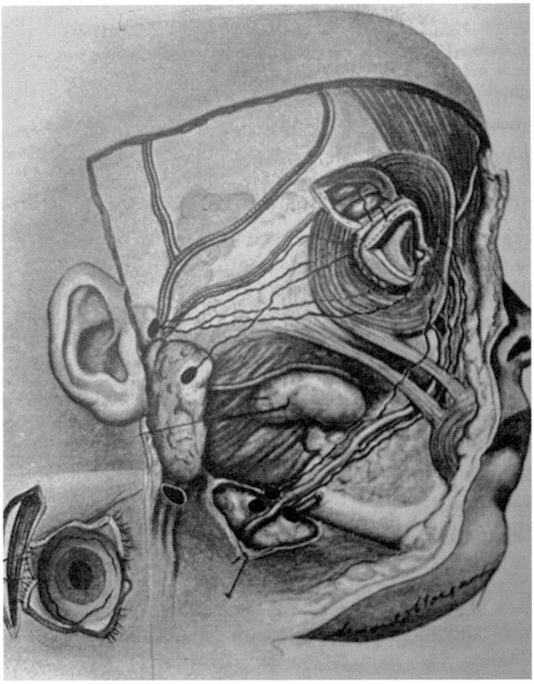

Fig. 19.4 Illustrative drawing of the study of the lymphatics of the lacrimal gland, conjunctiva, and eyelids, performed by Orts Llorca in Professor Rouvière's laboratory. It appeared as Figure 35 in Henri Rouvière's book "Anatomie des Lymphatiques de L'Homme" (Anatomy of the Lymphatics of Man). Masson: Paris, 1981

originally developed by Dimitrie Gerota (1867–1939), a method that allowed for exceptional clarity in visualizing the delicate lymphatic structures.

In his work he used a total of 12 specimens consisting of a sample of newborns, children up to 4 years old, and only one adult. His results show that the lymphatics of the lacrimal gland and adnexal areas drain mainly to the parotid lymph nodes, but also, and "anomalously", to the submandibular nodes.

Following this promising start, Professor Rouvière strongly encouraged Orts Llorca to devote himself fully to anatomy. To motivate him further, Rouvière proposed that he deliver a lecture to his class of over 600 students, choosing the submandibular gland as the topic. Before allowing him to present, however, Rouvière personally reviewed the lecture three times, ensuring it met his rigorous standards. The result was a success—the lecture was delivered to a packed auditorium and received with great acclaim.

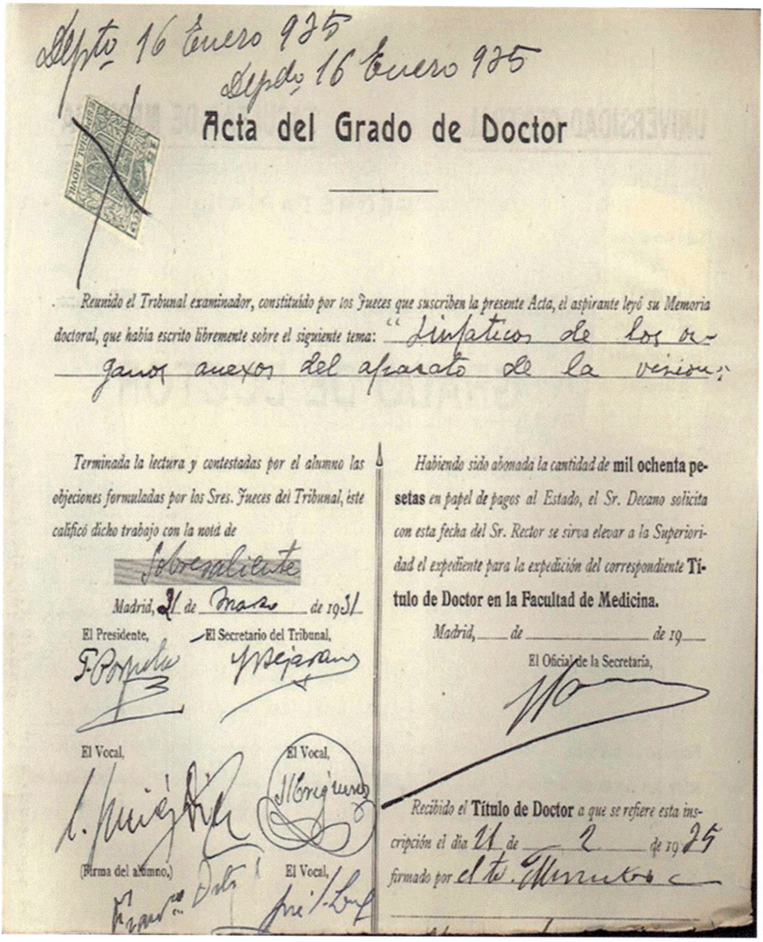

Acta del Grado de Doctor

Reunido el Tribunal examinador, constituído por los Jueces que suscriben la presente Acta, el aspirante leyó su Memoria doctoral, que había escrito libremente sobre el siguiente tema: "Linfáticos de los órganos anexos del aparato de la visión".

Terminada la lectura y contestadas por el alumno las objeciones formuladas por los Sres. Jueces del Tribunal, éste calificó dicho trabajo con la nota de Sobresaliente

Madrid, 21 de Marzo de 1931

El Presidente, El Secretario del Tribunal,

El Vocal, El Vocal,

(Firma del alumno.) El Vocal,

Habiendo sido abonada la cantidad de mil ochenta pesetas en papel de pagos al Estado, el Sr. Decano solicita con esta fecha del Sr. Rector se sirva elevar a la Superioridad el expediente para la expedición del correspondiente Título de Doctor en la Facultad de Medicina.

Madrid, __ de __ de 19__

El Oficial de la Secretaría,

Recibido el Título de Doctor a que se refiere esta inscripción el día 11 de 2 de 1935

Fig. 19.5 Certificate of Professor Orts Llorca's obtained for his doctoral thesis entitled "Lymphatics of the ancillary organs of the visual apparatus," on March 21, 1931, at the Central University of Madrid

At the same time, Orts Llorca presented the remarkable findings from his doctoral research at the Academy of Medicine in Paris, earning further recognition.

In 1931, he defended his doctoral thesis at the Central University of Madrid, receiving the highest distinction [7] (Fig. 19.5).

Between 1929 and 1931, in addition to his dissertation, he also published six other scientific works, marking an extraordinarily productive and formative period in his early academic career.

One study focused on the lymphatics of the orbital portion of the lacrimal gland, another on the lymphatics of the lacrimal sac and caruncle, and a third on the lymphatics of the conjunctiva. In addition to this series concerning the lacrimal gland and its associated structures, he also published a fourth work on the lymphatics of the abdominal wall, a fifth on the lymphatics of the cranial vault, and a sixth on the lymphatics of the sternum, clavicle, and vertebral bodies.

It is important to highlight that Orts was a cultured man with refined tastes, who enjoyed reading authors from the Generation of '98 and listening to the music of Bach. However, his time in Paris was not all work; he also participated in gatherings of Spaniards in Montparnasse, where, according to his own account, he met also Maurice Chevalier, Josephine Baker, Raquel Meller, and other notable figures.

With this scientific background on his CV, upon returning from Paris in 1930, he applied for a position as assistant professor in Descriptive Anatomy under Professor Ramón López Prieto at Valladolid University—a position he got through a competitive examination.

Descriptive anatomy is the branch of anatomy that studies the shape, size, position and relationships of the organs of the human body.

With a meager salary of 250 pesetas, he had to give private lessons to make ends meet. He spent 2 years in Valladolid, during which he presented his doctoral thesis at the Central University of Madrid and witnessed the proclamation of the II Spanish Republic on April 14, 1931. Around this time, he joined the Radical-Socialist Party, remaining a member from 1931 to 1934.

Radical-Socialist Party defended a social liberalism, strongly anticlerical with important influences from social democracy.

This is, as far as we know, previously unpublished information and offers a clear insight into the person and mindset of Orts Llorca. While he was always recognized for his prestige and significant research achievements, his personal career remained largely unknown, largely due to political affiliations that decisively impacted his academic future in the immediate post–Civil War period.

In 1932, he applied for a grant from the Junta de Ampliación de Estudios (JAE), then chaired by Ramón y Cajal, which was awarded to him to return to the laboratory of Henri Rouvière in Paris. There, he continued his studies on the lymphatic system and began research in descriptive embryology within Rouvière's collection.

That same year, he sat for the competitive examinations for a professorship in Barcelona, where he received only two votes—from Salvador Gil Vernet and Joaquín Trías Pujol. He made such a strong impression on the latter that he was appointed Professor of Anatomy at the Universitat Autònoma de Barcelona, a position he was ultimately unable to hold due to the turbulent political climate in Spain. According to Orts, "the root of these policies lay in the fact that ideological discord, rather than enriching our souls, came instead to harass and destroy them."

In 1933, he received a second grant from the Junta de Ampliación de Estudios, thanks to the support of Pedro Ara, who would become one of his strongest advocates and one of the teachers who most influenced his education. Ara recommended that he expand his knowledge of embryology by going to Vienna to study with Eduard Fischel, a leading expert of the time. During his stay, he met members of the Spanish community who would later play significant roles in his life, including Laín Entralgo and his future wife, Ana Bartis.

During this period, he published three articles in German journals, one of which described a human embryo with four pairs of somites.

Somites are bilaterally blocks of mesoderm that appear on either side of the neural tube in the embryo.

Having completed his training in Descriptive Embryology, he returned to Madrid, where Professor Ara, then Professor of Anatomy at the Central University, offered him a position as Assistant Professor—a post he held for about a year and a half.

On December 6, 1935, he won the chair of Anatomy in Cádiz through a competitive examination with the presidency of Pedro Ara y Pio del Rio Hortega. He immediately traveled to Vienna to bring his fiancée to Spain and marry her; they would live together for 58 years, unfortunately without children.

In 1935, supported by a grant from the Rockefeller Foundation, he went to Munich to work with the disciples of the recently awarded Nobel Prize in Medicine laureate, embryologist Hans Spemann, J. Holtfreter and W. Vogt. However, Holtfreter had emigrated to the United States that same year, so together with Walter Vogt, he took a two-month course in Experimental Embryology. This experience marked an important step in his training, shifting his focus from the study of static morphogenesis based on histological sections to gaining expertise in Experimental and Developmental Embryology techniques, and familiarizing himself with new concepts in Cell Biology.

The couple returned to Spain to assume his professorship in Cádiz in October 1935.

A few days before the outbreak of the Civil War in 1936, he received an invitation again from the Rockefeller Foundation to return to Munich to complete his studies in Experimental Embryology. However, this trip never materialized due to the turbulent situation in Spain. Orts himself reflected, *"If I had gone on that occasion, it is very likely that by now I would be teaching at an American university."*

When the Civil War broke out, he happened to be on holiday in Valencia. He and his wife then moved to Benidorm, which Orts described as an exemplary town with a cosmopolitan and tolerant population where there were no casualties.

Following the publication of a decree requiring all professors to affiliate with the nearest university, he joined the University of Valencia. There, he was assigned to the Provisional Hospital in Altea (Alicante) to treat wounded soldiers arriving from the front, serving as a medical lieutenant in the Health Department of the Guardia de Asalto (republican police).

On February 25, 1937, the Military Government in Burgos officially had dismissed him from the academic ranks, and when the war ended, he attempted to return to his position in Cádiz but was vetted from holding positions of responsibility during the war. His Dean, Enrique Muñoz—of whom he always spoke fondly—did not exempt him from teaching and research duties.

His dismissal was due to his membership in the Radical Socialist Party in Valladolid from 1931 to 1934. As a consequence, he began earning a salary of 1,400 pesetas—a sum entirely insufficient to support a married couple. He had to return to private practice, not to teach anatomy, but to work as a surgeon. He considered this a great sacrifice, as he had to give up the research he loved purely for financial reasons. Moreover, he disliked surgery for two reasons: first, because of the discomfort it caused him, and second, because he felt he was not healthy enough for it.

In 1952, the government urged him to ask for forgiveness, but Orts felt this was inappropriate, believing that the time for purification had passed. Fortunately, between 1948 and 1953, he also held his work as surgeon at the Hospital de Mora in Cádiz, with his salary rising to 28,000 pesetas in 1951. Despite those difficult years, his scientific output continued with numerous national and international publications and the supervision of many doctoral theses.

These were heroic times for Orts, during which he achieved so much with so little. He could only do this because he was a true leader who believed that *"continuous and self-sacrificing work would bring its reward."*

To learn more about the personal side of this great man, I recommend reading the letter he wrote to the last class of his students in Cadiz, which is included in the obituary dedicated to him by Professor López Rodríguez in the year of his death, 1993 [4, 8].

During the 15 years between the end of the war and his move to Madrid in 1954, he remained highly active. While his laboratory work was largely limited to creating a collection of sections of human embryos and fetuses for study, he devoted much of his time to writing his major work: Anatomia Humana (Human Anatomy), published in three volumes (Fig. 19.6).

His teaching reflects the spirit of this treatise, which is grounded in the principles of Functional Anatomy established by Hermann Braus (1868–1924), while also honoring the Descriptive Anatomy of Henri Rouvière (1875–1952).

Functional anatomy is the branch of anatomy that studies the relationship between the anatomical structure of organs and their origin, morphology and function.

The treatise on *Human Anatomy* was gradually published, but it fundamentally revolutionized the teaching of anatomy in twentieth-century Spain. Its significance lay in introducing international terminology in Latin and presenting anatomy through multiple paradigms: descriptive (following Vesalius and his followers, such as Rouvière), functional (Galen and his followers), cellular (Virchow and his followers), and evolutionary (C. Gegenbaur and his followers). According to Laín Entralgo, *"In Spain, it was Orts who had the*

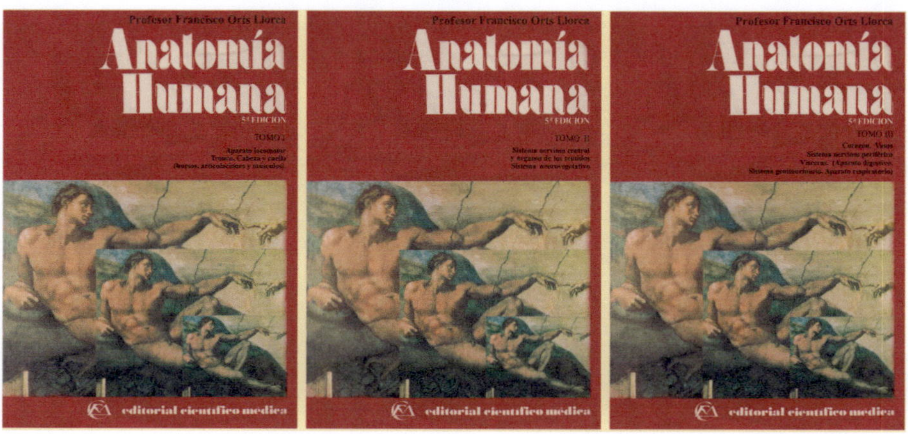

Fig. 19.6 Covers of the three volumes of Professor Orts Llorca's treatise on Human Anatomy. Volume I on the musculoskeletal system, Volume II on the central nervous system and Volume III on the peripheral nervous system, digestive and genito-urinary systems. In this case, its 5th edition

enormous merit of modernizing anatomy by introducing this important conceptual innovation—a true intellectual revolution."

The first volume of his comprehensive treatise on Human Anatomy is dedicated to the Locomotor System (1944), followed by a second volume focusing on the Central Nervous System. The series concludes with a third volume published in 1950, covering the Cardiovascular, Peripheral Nervous System, Digestive, GenitoUrinary and Respiratory, Systems. Of course, the sales of these volumes provided the authors with significant financial support, which was crucial in helping their modest salaries.

After spending 15 years in Cádiz—years he fondly recalls as the happiest of his life with his wife—he competed for a move to Madrid in 1954. His great friend, Professor Laín Entralgo, described this achievement as *"one of the few personal satisfactions during his tenure as Rector of the Complutense University, as he was able to contribute to this significant milestone for his institution."* However, a couple of years later, following the student revolt of February 1956, Professor

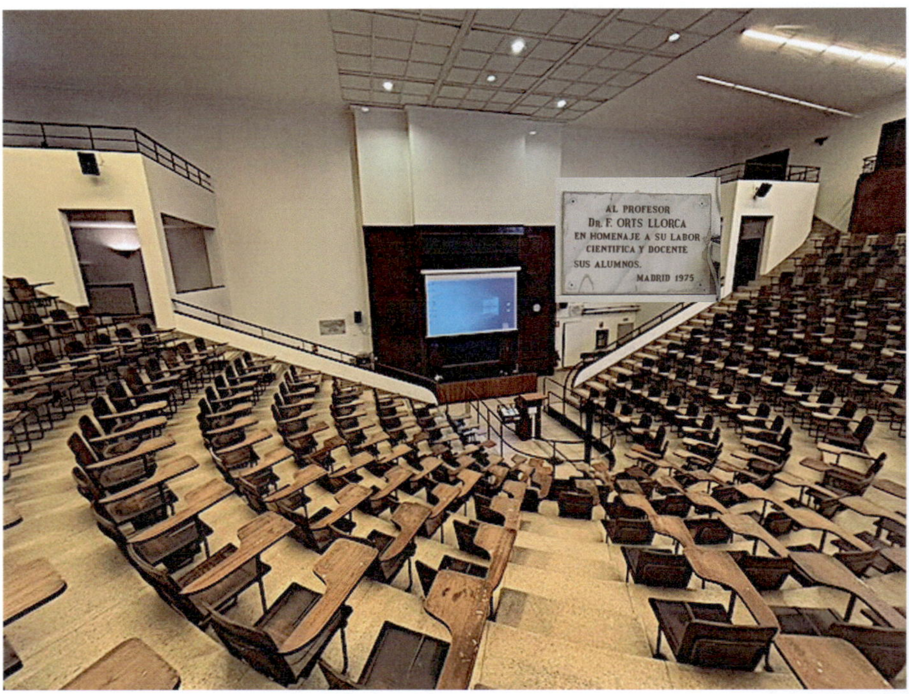

Fig. 19.7 Aula 2 of the Faculty of Medicine at the Complutense University of Madrid, where Professor Orts Llorca taught his classes. In this space is a commemorative plaque, paid for by his students in the year of his retirement, 1975, in recognition of his scientific and teaching work

Laín Entralgo was also dismissed from his position as Rector, as was the Minister of National Education, Joaquín Ruíz-Giménez.

Although he was appointed Director of the Hospital Clínico San Carlos, he continued his research tirelessly until his retirement at age 70 in 1975 (Fig. 19.7).

Yet, a man like him never truly stopped his academic pursuits. He continued researching alongside his pupils, visiting them regularly to monitor their progress and learn about their research lines. Orts dedicated himself to his scientific work until his death on April 21, 1993, in Madrid—not in his beloved hometown of Benidorm, which had honored him by dedicating an avenue to him in 1966.

Contributions

If we are to highlight his most significant contributions, they would be in the field of experimental embryology, particularly in two areas: the morphogenesis of the heart and the eye. Not forgetting is the pioneering work of one of his most talented disciples, Professor Murillo Ferrol, who later became Rector of the University of Zaragoza. Regarding his research on the morphogenesis of the eye, it is noteworthy that in his 1975 acceptance speech as a Full Member of the Royal National Academy of Medicine (RANM), he began with a quotation from a poem, reflecting his poetic sensibility and depth of thought.

> *We have had two hearts*
> *which merged into the midline*
> *into one - what a pity!*
> *And on the contrary, a single eye*
> *That was split in two.*
> *What luck! We have been Cyclops!*

Orts devoted himself to the morphogenesis of the eye in several works.

He observed that in the fourth week of gestation, the cleavage of the single eye sketch splits into two independent eye sketches (embryonic cyclopia). He also helped to explain that when one of these two sketches was excised, regeneration of the excised sketch occurred if it was grafted onto the coelom of a second embryo, not otherwise. No less valuable was his discovery of the influence of the vascular factor on the development of the eye: sectioning of the vitelline veins results in homolateral micro-ophthalmia.

However, although his work on teratogenesis and ocular morphogenesis is still often cited as important, his work in the field of cardiac morphogenesis remain very important as well.

His studies highlight that there are two prospective cardiac areas in the embryo's mesoderm, the left and right. The cells in these prospective regions exhibit affinity, meaning that when they are previously disaggregated using Moscona's method, they can recognize each other again and regroup if placed in a suitable medium, allowing the development of the heart. Cardiac differentiation, therefore, requires the inductive action of the underlying endoderm (or entoblast). Conversely, the ectoderm (or ectoblast), particularly in the cephalic region, induces a smaller heart and alters its normal curvature.

Finally, it is known that the venous-arterial vascular axis gives rise to a vascular plexus, which, through the specific selection of some channels and the obliteration of others, leads to the genesis of two cardiac tubes. These tubes eventually fuse at the midline to form a single heart. Experimentally, if this fusion is prevented using a nylon thread, two separate hearts can be formed.

For readers interested in the work of this Spanish academic who traveled beyond our borders and was visited by researchers from around the world, his scientific publications in national and international journals amount to a total of 163 papers.

All of them are referenced in a paper published in 2009 (Arechaga, Jiménez-Collado and Ruano Gil, 2009). In this work, all the articles are listed in chronological order.

On the other hand, to gain a deeper understanding of Orts Llorca's figure, we also recommend reading the chapter on the History of Embryology in the excellent book published by Raúl Velasco Morgado, titled Embriologia en la Periferia [9]. This work explores the Developmental Sciences in Spain during the Second Republic and Franco dictature.

Among the co-authors of the aforementioned works are his disciples, many of whom became professors in different universities: López Rodríguez (University of Cádiz); Genís Álvarez (University of Seville); Ruano Gil (University of Barcelona); Murillo Ferrol (University of Zaragoza, Rector); Jiménez Collado (Complutense University of Madrid); Puchades Orts (University of Alicante); Ribes Blanquer (University of Córdoba); Domènech Mateu (Autonomous University of Barcelona) and Puerta Fonollá (Complutense University of Madrid, Vice-Rector).

He was also a member of editorial boards of important journals in the field of anatomy and embryology, such as Acta Anatomica and Bulletin de L'Association des Anatomistes.

His activity was also projected outside our country. He was a visiting professor at many different universities: Washington, St. Louis (Missouri), Toledo (Ohio), California: Los Angeles and Stanford, Minnesota, Columbia and Rockefeller Center in New York, Cordoba (Argentina), Rio de Janeiro, Nacional de Mexico, Panama, and the Carnegie Foundation in Baltimore.

One of the attributes to highlight in his person is that of his kindness.

We could conclude the biography of Francisco Orts Llorca, by saying that he always complied with the assertion that *"the University is not only to transmit knowledge, but also to increase it"*, as he did throughout his life

References

1. Arechaga J, Jiménez Collado J, Ruano Gil D. A glance at Spanish embryology and teratology during the XX century through the academic life of Francisco Orts-Llorca (1905–1993). Int J Dev Biol. 2009;53:1165–77.
2. Díaz Rubio M. Spanish doctors in the 20th century. 2000. pp: 138–9. Madrid: D.L. ISBN: 84-921474-5-8.
3. Gómez-Santos M. Cinco Grandes de la Ciencia española: Severo Ochoa, Carlos Jiménez Díaz, Fernando de Castro, Francisco Grande Covián, Francisco Orts Llorca (Orts-Llorca, pp 158–182). Biblioteca Nueva: Madrid, 1968.
4. López Rodríguez A. Tribute in memory of Professor Francisco Orts Llorca (1905–1993). The teacher in Cadiz. 1993.
5. Méndez D. Orts Llorca, de la Anatomía a las raíces de la vida. Biograma n° 6. 1974;1:237–59.
6. Rouvière H. Anatomie des Lymphatiques de l'Homme. Paris: Masson; 1932.
7. Orts Llorca F. Lymphatics of the adnexal organs of the visual apparatus. Doctoral thesis, Central University. Madrid; 1931.
8. Laín Entralgo P. Necrology session in memory of his excellency Francisco Orts Llorca. Ann Sp R Nat Acad Med. 1993;110:528–34.
9. Velasco Morgado R. Embriología en la Periferia. The developmental sciences in the Spain of the Second Republic and Franco regime. Madrid: Consejo Superior de Investigaciones Científicas; 2016.

20

The ABC of Spanish Ophthalmology: Arruga, Barraquer And Castroviejo

Raquel Salazar Méndez and Sara Sánchez Canto

The specialty of ophthalmology began to take shape in Spain during the second half of the nineteenth century. Its founding figures—Francisco Delgado Jugo, Rafael Cervera, Luis Carreras Aragó, and Cayetano del Toro—received their training in leading European ophthalmology departments. Thanks to these pioneers and their disciples, the field entered a phase of consolidation, marked by the contributions of notable figures such as José Antonio Barraquer, Manuel Menacho, and Manuel Márquez.

It was in the subsequent generation that the three most internationally renowned Spanish ophthalmologists emerged: Hermenegildo Arruga, Ignasi Barraquer, and Ramón Castroviejo—collectively known as the "ABC of Spanish ophthalmology (Fig. 20.1)." Their groundbreaking work advanced the field across three distinct subspecialties, in which each became a global leader: Arruga in retinal detachment surgery, Barraquer in cataract surgery, and Castroviejo in corneal transplantation (keratoplasty) [1].

All three were the sons of ophthalmologists, began practicing the specialty at an early age, and completed advanced training abroad. In addition to their clinical excellence, they also contributed significantly to the development of ophthalmic surgical instruments—some of which remain in use to this day.

R. Salazar Méndez (✉) • S. Sánchez Canto
Ophthalmology DepartmentHospital, Universitario San Agustín, Avilés, Spain

M. A. Cuesta, F. Mateo Vallejo (eds.), *Spain's Journey in Medicine*,
https://doi.org/10.1007/978-3-032-12221-6_20

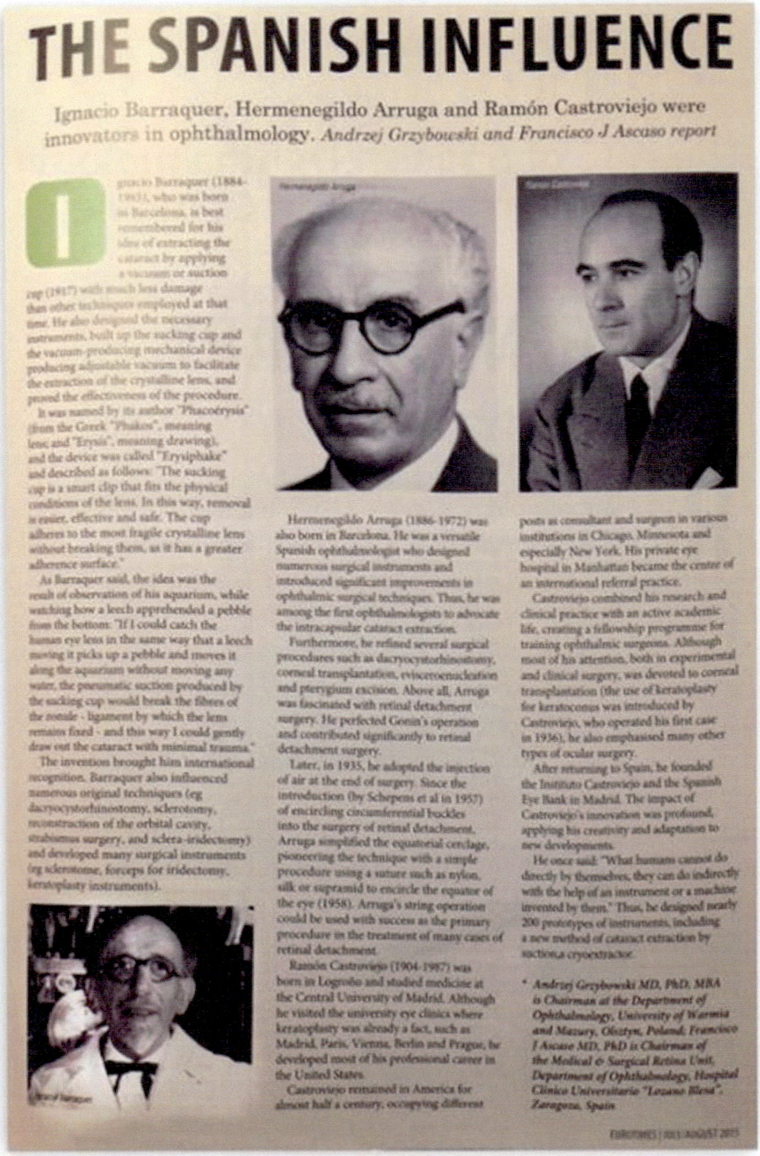

THE SPANISH INFLUENCE

Ignacio Barraquer, Hermenegildo Arruga and Ramón Castroviejo were innovators in ophthalmology. *Andrzej Grzybowski and Francisco J Ascaso report*

Ignacio Barraquer (1884-1965), who was born in Barcelona, is best remembered for his idea of extracting the cataract by applying a vacuum or suction cup (1917) with much less damage than other techniques employed at that time. He also designed the necessary instruments, built up the sucking cup and the vacuum-producing mechanical device producing adjustable vacuum to facilitate the extraction of the crystalline lens, and proved the effectiveness of the procedure.

It was named by its author "Phacoérysis" (from the Greek "Phakos", meaning lens and "Erysis", meaning drawing), and the device was called "Erysiphake" and described as follows: "The sucking cup is a smart clip that fits the physical conditions of the lens. In this way, removal is easier, effective and safe. The cup adheres to the most fragile crystalline lens without breaking them, as it has a greater adherence surface."

As Barraquer said, the idea was the result of observation of his aquarium, while watching how a leech apprehended a pebble from the bottom: "If I could catch the human eye lens in the same way that a leech moving it picks up a pebble and moves it along the aquarium without moving any water, the pneumatic suction produced by the sucking cup would break the fibres of the zonule - ligament by which the lens remains fixed - and this way I could gently draw out the cataract with minimal trauma."

The invention brought him international recognition. Barraquer also influenced numerous original techniques (eg dacryocystorhinostomy, sclerotomy, reconstruction of the orbital cavity, strabismus surgery, and sclera-iridectomy) and developed many surgical instruments (eg sclerotome, forceps for iridectomy, keratoplasty instruments).

Hermenegildo Arruga (1886-1972) was also born in Barcelona. He was a versatile Spanish ophthalmologist who designed numerous surgical instruments and introduced significant improvements in ophthalmic surgical techniques. Thus, he was among the first ophthalmologists to advocate the intracapsular cataract extraction.

Furthermore, he refined several surgical procedures such as dacryocystorhinostomy, corneal transplantation, evisceroenucleation and pterygium excision. Above all, Arruga was fascinated with retinal detachment surgery. He perfected Gonin's operation and contributed significantly to retinal detachment surgery.

Later, in 1935, he adopted the injection of air at the end of surgery. Since the introduction (by Schepens et al in 1957) of encircling circumferential buckles into the surgery of retinal detachment, Arruga simplified the equatorial cerclage, pioneering the technique with a simple procedure using a suture such as nylon, silk or supramid to encircle the equator of the eye (1958). Arruga's string operation could be used with success as the primary procedure in the treatment of many cases of retinal detachment.

Ramón Castroviejo (1904-1987) was born in Logroño and studied medicine at the Central University of Madrid. Although he visited the university eye clinics where keratoplasty was already a fact, such as Madrid, Paris, Vienna, Berlin and Prague, he developed most of his professional career in the United States.

Castroviejo remained in America for almost half a century, occupying different posts as consultant and surgeon in various institutions in Chicago, Minnesota and especially New York. His private eye hospital in Manhattan became the centre of an international referral practice.

Castroviejo combined his research and clinical practice with an active academic life, creating a fellowship programme for training ophthalmic surgeons. Although most of his attention, both in experimental and clinical surgery, was devoted to corneal transplantation (the use of keratoplasty for keratoconus was introduced by Castroviejo, who operated his first case in 1936), he also emphasised many other types of ocular surgery.

After returning to Spain, he founded the Instituto Castroviejo and the Spanish Eye Bank in Madrid. The impact of Castroviejo's innovation was profound, applying his creativity and adaptation to new developments.

He once said: "What humans cannot do directly by themselves, they can do indirectly with the help of an instrument or a machine invented by them." Thus, he designed nearly 200 prototypes of instruments, including a new method of cataract extraction by suction, a cryoextractor.

* *Andrzej Grzybowski MD, PhD, MBA is Chairman at the Department of Ophthalmology, University of Warmia and Mazury, Olsztyn, Poland; Francisco J Ascaso MD, PhD is Chairman of the Medical & Surgical Retina Unit, Department of Ophthalmology, Hospital Clínico Universitario "Lozano Blesa", Zaragoza, Spain*

EUROTIMES | JULY/AUGUST 2015

Fig. 20.1 The Spanish influence in Ophtalmology. A. Grzbowski and J. Ascaso. Eurotimes. June 30, 2015. (Permission of Eurotimes)

A

Hermenegildo Arruga Liró was born on March 15, 1886, in Barcelona. In 1902, he began his medical studies, and just a year later, he commenced his training in ophthalmology by accompanying his father, Eduardo Arruga, who worked as an assistant at the clinic of Manuel Menacho [2, 3] (Fig. 20.2).

After completing his medical degree in 1908, Arruga was awarded a 2-year scholarship by the Barcelona City Council to pursue advanced training at leading European institutions with stays at the Hôtel-Dieu and the Pasteur Institute in Paris, the ophthalmology clinics of Hirschberg and von Graefe in Berlin, and, finally, with Jules Gonin in Lausanne, Switzerland—who would become both his mentor and close friend [2, 3].

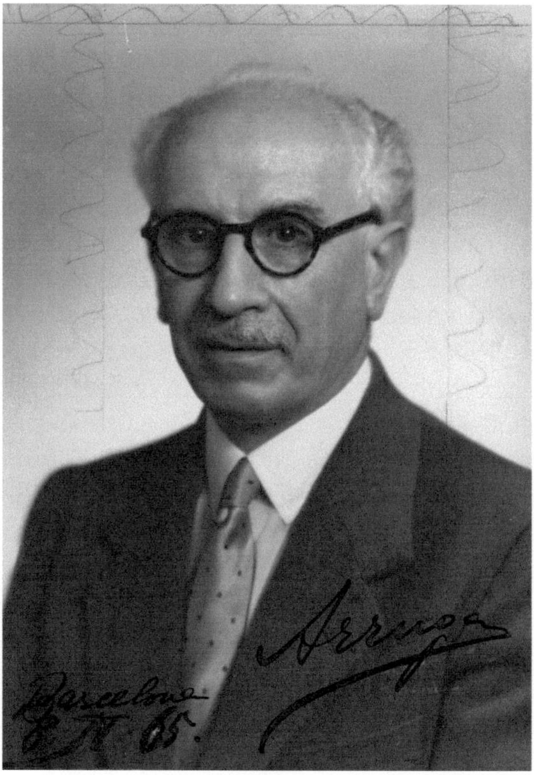

Fig. 20.2 Hermenegildo Arruga Liró (Portrait from a private collection)

Upon returning to Spain, Arruga joined his father's medical practice and became the first ophthalmologist outside Switzerland to apply Gonin's technique for the treatment of retinal detachment. He was also a pioneer in introducing the Wassermann reaction for the diagnosis of syphilis and the use of the tonometer for measuring intraocular pressure.

In 1914, he married Teresa Forgas, with whom he had four children. One of them, Alfredo Arruga, went on to continue the family's ophthalmological legacy.

In 1927, Arruga earned his doctoral degree with a thesis titled *"Una modificación sencilla y eficaz de la dacriocistorrinostomía"* ("*A Simple and Effective Modification of Dacryocystorhinostomy*"), a procedure that gained international recognition and became known as the "*Arruga's operation.*" This marked the beginning of his most productive professional period, during which he published extensively on lacrimal system disorders, cataract surgery, corneal transplantation, and—most notably—retinal detachment, the area in which he made his most significant contributions.

At the 1929 International Congress of Ophthalmology in Amsterdam, he presented his work "*The Treatment of Retinal Detachment*", in which he advocated for Gonin's technique—the first proven method to successfully treat the condition. He further disseminated these ideas at the meetings of the Spanish and French Ophthalmological Societies, through numerous scientific articles, and at the 1933 International Ophthalmology Congress held in Madrid. His findings were later compiled in his seminal book "*El desprendimiento de retina*", published in 1936. However, due to the outbreak of the Spanish Civil War, widespread recognition of his contributions was delayed for several years.

In 1946, he published "*Cirugía Ocular*" edited by Salvat, a comprehensive surgical treatise with nearly 900 pages and over 1000 illustrations

The work became a seminal reference in the field, with four editions in Spanish, three in French, and two in English. It was later recognized as one of the 100 most important ophthalmology books of the twentieth century [4, 5] (Fig. 20.3).

In 1957, he introduced the technique known as the "Lazo o hilo de Arruga" ("*Arruga's loop*" or "*Arruga suture*") for the treatment of retinal detachment, which involved encircling the eyeball with a non-extensible thread. Among his most notable contributions to surgical instrumentation was the development of the capsular forceps for intracapsular (total) cataract extraction—an instrument that would come to be known as "Arruga's forceps" [2] (Fig. 20.4).

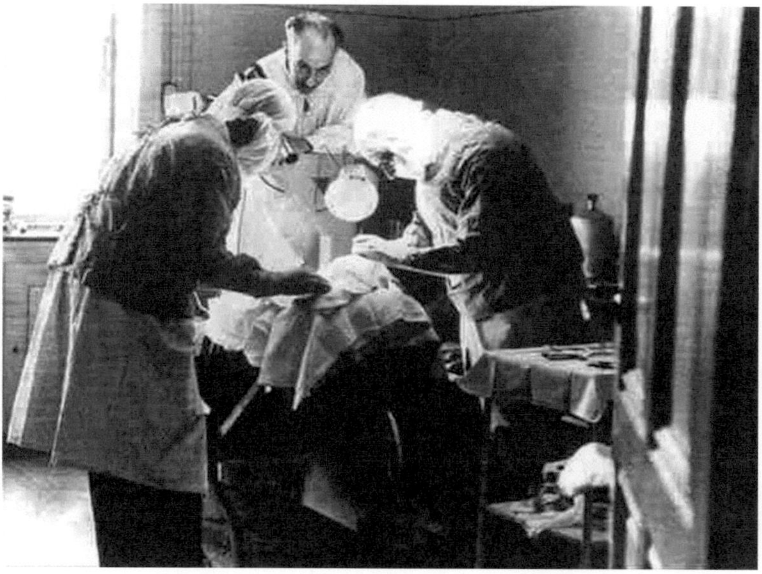

Fig. 20.3 Arruga participates with a camera in the first color films of the operations. Lausanne (Switzerland), 1936. From Museum of the History of Medicine of Catalonia

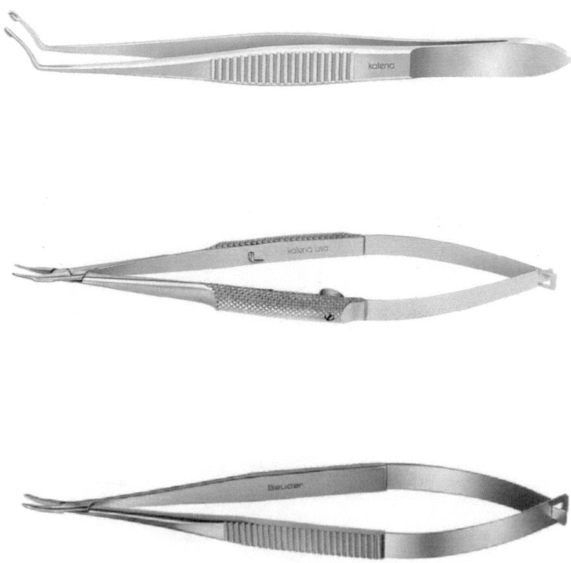

Fig. 20.4 Needleholders and forceps of Arruga, Barraquer and Castroviejo obtained from the catalogues of Katena and Geuder, both world's leading manufacturers of ophthalmic surgical instruments

Arruga died in his home-clinic in Barcelona on 17 May 1972 of a cerebrovascular accident; among the many distinctions he received were the Gonin Medal, the most important award in ophthalmology, the Cross of Alfonso X el Sabio and the title of Count of Arruga [2].

B

Ignasi Barraquer i Barraquer was born on March 25, 1884, in Barcelona, the son of José Antonio Barraquer Roviralta and his cousin Concepció Barraquer (Fig. 20.5).

His father was a prominent figure in Spanish ophthalmology and held the Chair of Ophthalmology at the University of Barcelona.

Ignasi earned his medical degree in 1907 and completed his doctoral thesis the following year. His dissertation, titled "*Dacryocystitis*", inflammation of the lacrimal sac, was based on his clinical experience, first as a general practitioner and later as an assistant physician at the Santa Creu and Clínic hospitals [2].

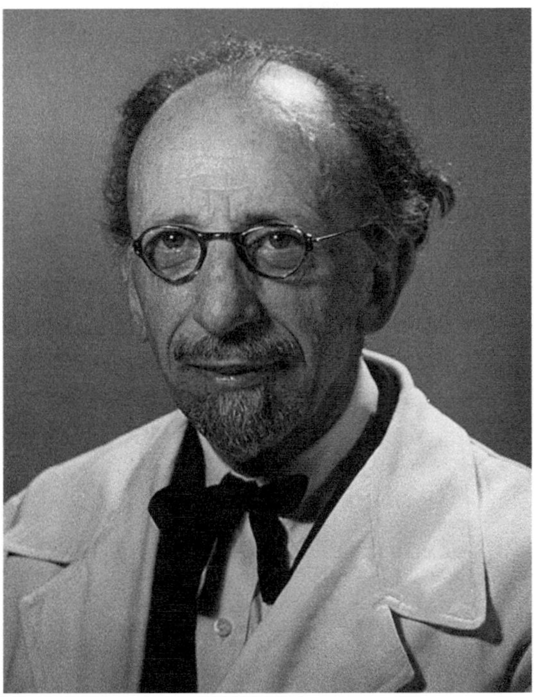

Fig. 20.5 Portrait of Ignasi Barraquer i Barraquer from Barraquer Ophthalmology Center photographic archive

In 1910 he married Josefina Moner, a marriage from which 7 children were born, with the two sons continuing his legacy: José in Colombia and Joaquín in Spain.

From 1909 to 1918, he served as assistant professor in his father's Chair of Ophthalmology at the University of Barcelona. After his father's retirement, he continued as interim professor but ultimately resigned the position, choosing not to compete for the permanent post through the formal examination process.

In 1917, at the Royal Academy of Medicine in Barcelona, Dr. Manuel Menacho, at the Royal Academy of Medicine of Barcelona, read a note of his titled "Ideal Extraction of the Cataract" that presented a new method to approach cataract surgery. This technique, which he called phacoerisis, also known as the "Barraquer operation," would be his great contribution to ophthalmology, since it allowed the complete extraction of the cataract using the erisíphaco, a pneumatic aspirator connected to a suction cup that was applied to the crystalline lens (Fig. 20.6).

As Barraquer said, the idea came to him during observation of his aquarium while watching how a leech apprehended a pebble from the bottom.

Barraquer had begun developing this technique as early as 1916, initially using a glass cannula, generating suction manually with his mouth. Over the following years, he refined and promoted phacoeresis through presentations at national and international congresses and in numerous scientific

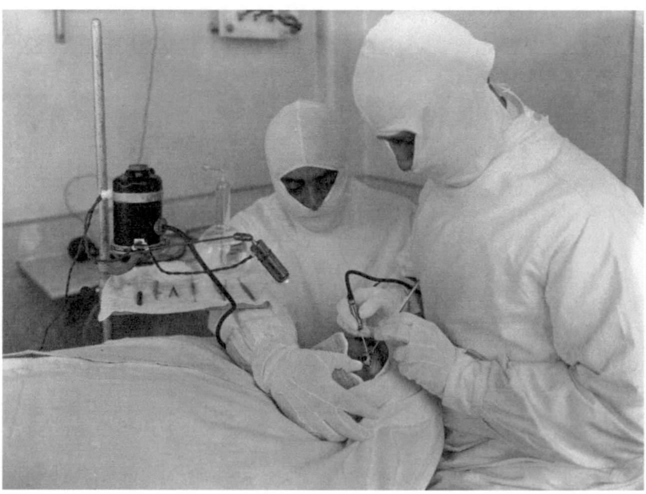

Fig. 20.6 Dr. I. Barraquer operating on cataracts with one of the first erysiphaque models, 1917 (from Barraquer Ophthalmology Center photographic archive)

publications. He documented exceptional visual outcomes and a remarkably low rate of complications across thousands of procedures.

Complete extraction of the crystalline lens—whether by phacoeresis or later techniques such as cryoextraction—became the preferred method for cataract surgery until the 1980s, due to its relative simplicity and minimal surgical risk [6].

Among his additional contributions to ophthalmic surgery was the design of the *Barraquer needle holder*, an instrument still widely used today (Fig. 20.4).

He also published influential work on glaucoma surgery, keratoplasty, and strabismus correction. For the latter, he developed a device called the *myocampter* for muscle shortening. Furthermore, he pioneered the use of labial mucosa grafts in the treatment of recurrent pterygium [2].

In 1928, Ignasi Barraquer was appointed a permanent physician at the Hospital de la Santa Creu i Sant Pau. In 1933, he returned as a professor at the Autonomous University of Barcelona and 2 years later he was appointed academic at the Barcelona Academy of Medicine.

Following his exile in Tangier during the Spanish Civil War, he was appointed as Head of the Ophthalmology Department at the Spanish Red Cross. During this period, he was also President of the *Societat Catalana d'Oftalmologia* (Catalan Ophthalmology Society) from 1929 to 1939.

In 1941, he founded the *Clínica Barraquer*, in Barcelona and in 1947, the *Instituto Barraquer*, dedicated to ophthalmic education and research. The *Clínica Barraquer* was the first monographic ophthalmology center in Spain and soon gained international recognition as a leading institution in the field. In 1973, the two entities were unified under the name *Centre d'Oftalmologia Barraquer*.

Ignasi Barraquer passed away in Barcelona on May 13, 1965, due to liver disease. In a final act of generosity, he donated his corneas for transplantation—an operation performed by his son, Joaquín Barraquer.

C

Ramón Castroviejo Briones, son of ophthalmologist Ramón Castroviejo, was born on August 24, 1904, in Logroño. He studied medicine at the Central University of Madrid and, in 1927, began his specialization in ophthalmology at San Carlos Hospital under Manuel Márquez and at the Red Cross Hospital under Francisco Poyales [7, 8] (Fig. 20.7).

In 1929–1930, he moved to the United States on a research grant at the *Eye, Ear, Nose, and Throat Hospital and College* in Chicago. He would go on to

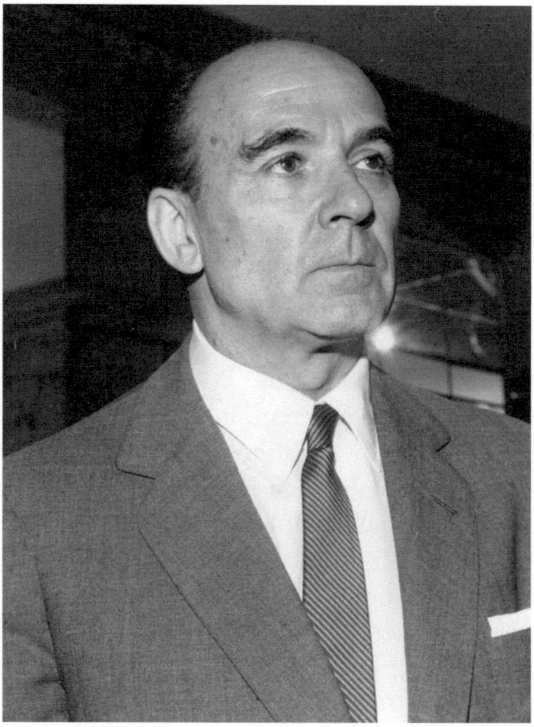

Fig. 20.7 Ramón Castroviejo Briones (Image Bank of Spanish Medicine. Royal National Academy of Medicine of Spain)

reside in the U.S. for nearly 50 years, obtaining American citizenship in 1936. After passing the *American Board Examination*, he visited major ophthalmological centers in Europe. It was during this tour that he saw the keratoplasty technique (corneal transplant) of Anton Elschnig in Prague—a pivotal experience that defined the trajectory of his career [8].

Upon returning to the United States, he worked at the *Mayo Clinic* in Rochester (1930–1932), where he began refining the keratoplasty technique using animal models. From 1932 to 1952, he was affiliated with the *Institute of Ophthalmology* at *Columbia-Presbyterian Medical Center* in New York, where he performed his first human keratoplasty. He later served as Director of the Department of Ophthalmology at *St. Vincent's Hospital and Medical Center* in New York, as well as Director of the Department of Special Corneal Surgery at the *New York Eye and Ear Infirmary*.

His growing experience with keratoplasties began to generate controversy and skepticism in the scientific community, which led him, in 1950, to rent a railway carriage to take more than 60 patients to the 52nd Meeting of the

American Academy of Ophthalmology and Otolaryngology, seating them at the back of the room and inviting the attendees to examine the results of his technique [2, 8].

In 1946, he married **Cintia Warren Smith**, the mother of his two children, Christopher and Alix. As his expertise in keratoplasty grew, so did skepticism from the medical community. In a bold move to counter this doubt, Castroviejo rented a railroad car in 1950 to transport more than 60 of his patients to the 52nd Meeting of the *American Academy of Ophthalmology and Otolaryngology*. Seated at the back of the lecture hall, patients were presented as living proof of the success of his surgical technique, which invited the audience to examine the outcomes firsthand [2, 8].

In 1946, he married Cintia Warren Smith, with whom he had two children, Christopher and Alix. In 1948, he opened his own private hospital in New York, which became a global reference center for keratoplasty. There, he trained over one hundred Spanish ophthalmologists and around thirty more from other countries through competitive fellowship programs [8, 9].

In 1976, due to health issues, Ramón Castroviejo relocated permanently to Madrid. A few years earlier, in 1972, he had founded the Instituto de Investigaciones Oftalmológicas Ramón Castroviejo (*Ramón Castroviejo Ophthalmological Research Institute)*, followed by the establishment of the Banco Español de Ojos (*Spanish Eye Bank)* in 1975. His passion for education and documentation led him to preserve an extensive archive of surgical recordings and explanatory notes at the Institute.

Among his prolific scientific output—comprising 247 publications—his most celebrated work is the "*Atlas de Queratectomías y Queroplastias" (Atlas of Keratectomies and keratoplasties)*, published by Salvat in 1964. This 446-page volume, richly illustrated and based entirely on his personal experience, is considered one of the most important texts in ophthalmology [4]. It was selected as the Official Presentation of the 40th Congress of the Spanish-American Ophthalmological Society and translated into English, French, and German [2, 10].

Over the course of his career, Castroviejo delivered more than 500 lectures, conducted 200,000 consultations, and performed over 40,000 surgeries—including 3000 keratoplasties [10].

Renowned for his inventiveness, he designed approximately 200 ophthalmic surgical instruments, particularly for keratoplasty—such as trephines, scissors, corneal clamps, and keratoprosthesis models. His most iconic design is the "*Castroviejo needle holder"* (Fig. 20.4), currently widely used in ophthalmic microsurgery and vascular surgery.

Among the many honors he received, two stand out: the creation of the "*Castroviejo Cornea Society*" in 1975 and the establishment of the *Castroviejo Award* by the Spanish Society of Ophthalmology in 1987, recognizing outstanding career achievements by ophthalmologists over the age of 40. In 2000, the *American Society of Cataract and Refractive Surgery* (ASCRS) named him one of the ten ophthalmologists who made the greatest contributions to the specialty in the twentieth century [9].

Ramón Castroviejo passed away in Madrid on January 1, 1987, at the age of 82, due to laryngeal cancer. In a final act of altruism, he donated his corneas; only one was viable and was successfully transplanted by his student and disciple, Dr. Juan Murube del Castillo [1, 9].

References

1. Enríquez Fuentes JE, Pascual Santiago MA, Montolío Marzo E, Santos Bueso E. The ABC of Spanish ophthalmology: Arruga, Barraquer and Castroviejo. Span J Hist Hum Ophthalmol. 2021;
2. Cotallo de Cáceres J, Hernández Benito E, Munoa Roiz J, Leoz de la Fuente G. History of ophthalmology. Madrid: Sociedad Española Oftalmología; 1993. (LXIX Presentation).
3. Royal Academy of History. Historia Hispánica. [cited 22 February 2025]. Hermenegildo Arruga Liró. Available at: https://historia-hispanica.rah.es/biografias/3961-hermenegildo-arruga-liro.
4. Thompson HS, Blanchard DL. One hundred important 20th-century ophthalmic books. Arch Ophthalmol. 2001;119(5):761–3.
5. Barbón JJ, Álvarez Suárez ML, Sampedro A. The three most important Spanish books in 20th century ophthalmology. Arch Soc Esp Oftalmol. 2007;82:385–7.
6. Barraquer J. History of intracapsular surgery. In: MR Lorente, Mendicute J. Surgery of the crystalline lens. Madrid: Spanish Society of Ophthalmology; 2008; 1: 30–42.
7. Virtual exhibition: Library of the Ramón Castroviejo Institute [Internet]. [cited 16 March 2025]. Available from: https://biblioteca.ucm.es/institutocastroviejo/exposicion-virtual.
8. Briones RC. 50 years since his admission to the Royal National Academy of Medicine - Anales RANM [Internet]. [cited 17 February 2025]. Available from: https://analesranm.es/revista/2023/140_02/14002_fdlm01.
9. Murube J, Muñoz Negrete F, Gutierrez Carmona F. Ramón Castroviejo. Centenary (part I). Studium Ophthalmologicum. 2004;XXII(3)
10. Murube J, Muñoz Negrete F, Gutierrez Carmona F. Ramón Castroviejo. His scientific legacy (part II). Studium Ophthalmologicum. 2004;XXII(4)

21

Francisco Grande Covián: Physiology of Nutrition

Miguel Pocoví Mieras

Francisco Grande Covián (Fig. 21.1), was born in Colunga (Asturias) on June 28, 1909, and passed away in Madrid on his 86th birthday, in 1995. His father, Emilio Grande de Riego, originally from Muros de Nalón (Asturias), moved to Colunga in 1905 to work as a doctor. In 1908, he married María Esperanza Covián, whom he had met through his friendship with her father, Ricardo Covián Junco.

Francisco Grande spent his early childhood in Colunga, in close contact with his grandmother who taught him to read and write before he began attending the local school run by nuns (Fig. 21.2). In 1918, his father moved to Oviedo to work at the Getino Sanatorium. In 1919, he enrolled in the secondary school in Oviedo, where he stood out as an excellent student, earning numerous honors.

From an early age, he was drawn to medicine, following in the footsteps of his grandfather Ricardo, his father, his maternal uncle Manuel Covián, and his paternal uncle Arcadio Grande. His biographer, Marino Gómez Santos, wrote of him: *"He was born a doctor by genetic inheritance."*

All pictures published with permission of the Foundation Francisco Grande Covian, Zaragoza.

M. P. Mieras (✉)
University of Zaragoza, Zaragoza, Spain

M. A. Cuesta, F. Mateo Vallejo (eds.), *Spain's Journey in Medicine*,
https://doi.org/10.1007/978-3-032-12221-6_21

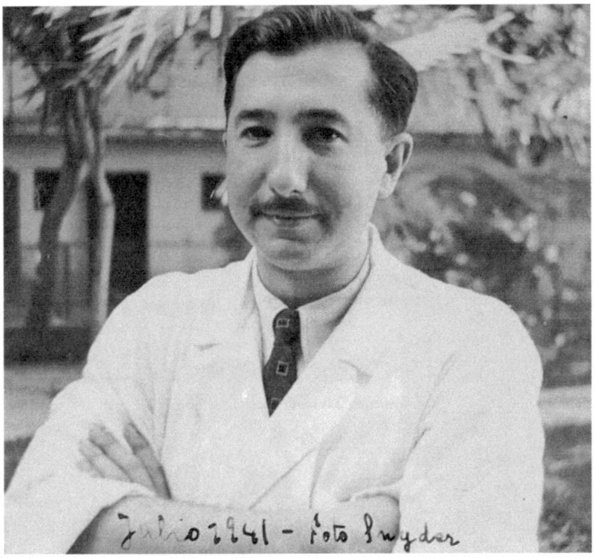

Fig. 21.1 Francisco Grande Covián July 1941 at the Institute of Medical Research

As a Medical Student

In 1926, he entered the Faculty of Medicine in Madrid Central University, residing at the *Residencia de Estudiantes*, which at the time was directed by Professor Alberto Jiménez Fraud. Founded in 1910 by the *Junta para Ampliación de Estudios*, the Residence was part of the *Institución Libre de Enseñanza* and served as an educational complement to the University.

Two of Francisco's great passions were awakened during his time there: on the one hand, his love for music, nurtured by fellow resident Jesús Bal y Gay—a musician and composer in charge of the music education of the students; and on the other, his passion for scientific research, sparked by his friend Severo Ochoa.

Grande Covián would later recognize the profound influence the Residence had on his life: *"My admission to the Residence marked my life, because it was there that I discovered my scientific vocation and decided to devote myself to research, giving up the practice of medicine."*

In 1928, his brother Ricardo—also a dedicated student—joined the Residence. Ricardo preferred to study in the early hours of the morning to review subjects from the School of Agricultural Engineering, while Francisco worked late into the night. Fellow residents would often remark that the light in the Grande brothers' room was never turned off.

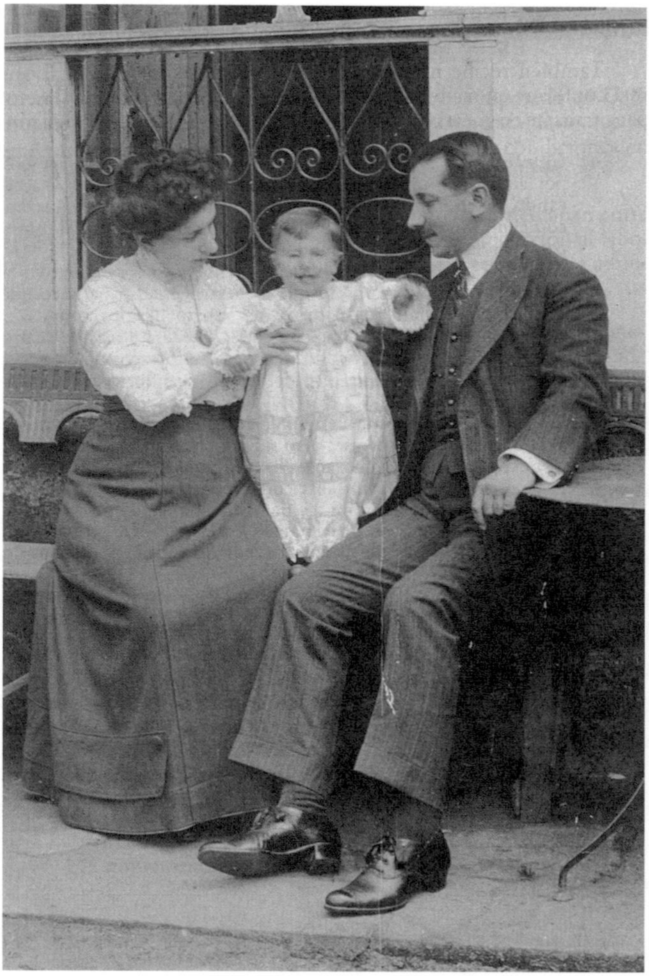

Fig. 21.2 Francisco Grande as a baby with his parents, María Esperanza Covián and Emilio Grande de Riego

In 1929, due to the political unrest and strikes, the dictatorship of General Primo de Rivera shut down temporarily the University of Madrid. Following the advice of his mentor, Juan Negrín, and with the support of his parents, Grande Covián moved to the University of Freiburg in Germany to continue his medical studies without interruption.

At Freiburg, he worked in the Laboratory of Neurophysiology under Paul Hoffmann, where he conducted research on spinal reflexes in freshwater turtles. This work would later form part of his doctoral thesis.

In 1931, he completed his medical degree and in 1932, he published his first scientific paper in collaboration with Severo Ochoa, on the concentration of phosphagen concentration after adrenal gland removal—almost simultaneously published in German as well [1].

In September 1932, at the age of 23, he defended his doctoral thesis titled "Sobre algunos fenómenos reflejos producidos en la médula por interferencia de excitaciones de distinta naturaleza" (*"On Some Reflex Phenomena Produced in the Spinal Cord by the Interference of Stimuli of Different Natures")* obtaining the maximal qualification.

Postdoctoral Stage

During this period, he worked in several laboratories, beginning at the Laboratory of Physiology of the Physical Exercise in Copenhagen, directed by Professor August Krogh, recipient of the 1920 Nobel Prize in Physiology or Medicine. Grande there spent 2 years (1932–1933), where he conducted studies on renal function during exercise, changes in plasma osmotic activity, and developed a micromethod for the determination of creatinine.

While in Copenhagen, he also conducted what was likely his first nutrition experiment: "Effect of Diet on Physical Exercise." In this study, he demonstrated that individuals fatigue more quickly during intense physical activity when consuming a diet high in fat. However, when glucose is administered, recovery is more rapid—even though the glucose is not oxidized. He concluded that fatigue was not due to a lack of metabolic fuel in the muscles, but rather to a deficiency of glucose in the nervous system.

Professor Krogh offered him the opportunity to continue his postdoctoral training in London, in the laboratory of Professor Sir Charles Lovatt Evans, one of the world's foremost authorities on carbohydrate metabolism.

Before joining Lovatt Evans' lab, Grande took advantage of this time to be admitted to Professor Torsten Thunberg's laboratory in Lund, Sweden. Dr. Thunberg was a renowned specialist in the study of dehydrogenases. There, Grande conducted intensive research and demonstrated that seeds contain specific dehydrogenases for palmitic and stearic acids—which is known today as delta desaturases. In fact, he discovered what are today referred to as delta-7 and delta-9 fatty acid desaturases [2].

In January 1934, he joined the laboratory of Sir Charles Lovatt Evans in London. There, he developed a heart perfusion system to measure oxygen and lactate consumption in both normal and diabetic dogs. This method became a classic and is still referenced in physiology textbooks. He also conducted important studies on the metabolic fuels of the heart and published several papers on the subject [3–5].

In early November 1934, Grande returned to Madrid, passed the competitive examination for assistant professor, and was appointed by Juan Negrín to teach lectures, seminars, and practical classes to second-year medical students at the Faculty of Medicine.

While continuing his laboratory research, he organized a physiology course on substances related to nutrition at the Faculty of Medicine of the Madrid.

In early 1936, due to the deteriorating state of university teaching and research in Spain, he applied for a grant from the Royal National Academy of Medicine to join Otto Meyerhof's laboratory in Heidelberg. Although the grant was awarded, he was unable to take advantage of it: on July 18 of that year, the Spanish Civil War broke out, and he was denied a passport.

Civil War Period

At Negrín's request, during the Spanish Civil War, Grande organized the Secretariat of the Faculty of Medicine, reorganizing the Laboratory of the Provincial Hospital. Suspended the classes, his work during this period was primarily administrative. When the fighting stopped in the University City, Grande took it upon himself to rescue the Faculty of Medicine's library—an invaluable bibliographic collection—to prevent its destruction. With the help of a security guard, he managed to move the entire library, book by book, through the trenches.

In 1937, he was offered a Rockefeller Fellowship by Professor August Krogh to return to Copenhagen. However, Negrín persuaded him to stay, for needing his expertise in Madrid. Grande was tasked with evaluating the nutritional needs of the population and was appointed Deputy Director of the National Institute of Food Hygiene.

At the Institute, he opened a consultation clinic for the diagnosis and treatment of nutritional disorders, attending to patients from different centers in Madrid. Together with doctors Francisco Jiménez, Manuel Peraita, and Márquez Cosín, he organized the distribution of vitamin supplements and cod liver oil. However, due to severe food shortages, nutritional deficiencies soon began to affect the entire population of Madrid.

At the beginning of 1938, the first patients began to present with skin lesions on the neck, the backs of the hands and feet, along with gastrointestinal, psychological, and neurological disorders. Grande immediately recognized the signs and symptoms of pellagra—or *mal de la rosa*—thanks to a book from his grandfather Ricardo's library in Colunga: *La Historia Natural y*

Médica del Principado de Asturias (The Natural and Medical History of Asturias) by Dr. Gaspar Casal, posthumously published in 1762.

Pellagra is a disease caused by a deficiency of nicotinic acid: the vitamin niacin (B3).

In 1937, Conrad Elvehjem of the University of Wisconsin had demonstrated that experimental pellagra that in dogs causes the blackening of the tongue (black tongue) could be cured with liver extract. Through fractionation of liver preparations, he identified nicotinic acid as the anti-pellagra vitamin [6].

His findings spread quickly, and by January 1938, Dr. Tom Spies of Cincinnati presented the first successful human clinical trial using nicotinic acid to treat pellagra at the *Central Society for Clinical Research*.

This discovery came to Grande through José Puche director of the Institute who received in la Universidad de Valencia foreign journals. With the help of a chemist at the Institute, Ángel del Campo, Grande managed to synthesize nicotinic acid from nicotine extracted from pesticide products—used to kill plant aphids—confiscated from agricultural and gardening suppliers. As the number of patients grew, so did the need to produce more nicotinic acid. Production was scaled up at the University of Valencia, in collaboration with Dr. Vicente Gómez Aranda.

The nicotinic acid was administered intravenously, allowing for near-immediate treatment. Over 3500 pellagra patients were treated at the Institute with nicotinic acid, with many more treated at the Psychiatric Clinic and the General Hospital

Despite all his efforts to improve the quality of life of the Spanish population during the Civil War, Grande was dismissed from the university at the end of the conflict and sanctioned with a 10-year ban from applying for professorships through competitive examinations. He was denounced as a "collaborationist" and came close to being arrested.

He took refuge for several months at Las Cañadas, an estate near Úbeda owned by his friend and collaborator Dr. Francisco Jiménez. There, in relative isolation, he wrote up his research on deficiency diseases during the war, which would later be published in the *Revista de Sanidad e Higiene Pública* and the *Revista Clínica Española* [7].

Post-War Period

After the war, Grande worked at the Ibys Institute, where he prepared vitamin supplements and published a treatise on vitamins. In 1940, Carlos Jiménez Díaz invited him to take over the position previously held by Dr. Severo Ochoa at the Institute of Medical Research. Jiménez Díaz knew Grande well—he had been a member of the panel that awarded him the Extraordinary Degree Prize and had closely followed his scientific career, as well as the humanitarian and scientific work he had carried out during the Civil War.

At the Institute, Grande conducted significant research on diabetes alongside José Carlos de Oya, José Luis Rodríguez Miñón, and Carlos Jiménez Díaz, publishing more than 30 papers on the subject. He was later appointed Director of the Institute's Department of Physiology.

It was during this period that he met Gloria Mingo, who would become his wife and his most valued collaborator in every sense—both scientific and personal. They were married on March 31, 1941 (Fig. 21.3).

In 1941, the Rockefeller Foundation awarded him the project *"Study of the Nutritional Situation in Europe,"* which enabled him to analyze nutritional deficiencies in children of the post-war period in the Puente de Vallecas district in Madrid comparing them to those of the Chamberi district. He published the results in several papers between 1943 and 1944 [8].

Walter Starkie, Director of the British Institute in Madrid, intervened by awarding him a grant of the British Council could travel to England. In 1949, he joined Dr. Derek Richter's laboratory in Cardiff, where he conducted a study on phosphorus transport in the spinal cord [9]. During his stay, he also completed the translation into Spanish of Starling's textbook on physiology [10].

In 1950, after to having served the unjust sanction that prevented him from applying for professorship, he obtained by competitive examination the Chair of Physiology and Biochemistry at the Faculty of Medicine of the University of Zaragoza. Upon his arrival, he found the department abandoned, which compelled him to rebuild it from the ground up. Despite significant economic and bureaucratic obstacles during his stay in Zaragoza, he managed to conduct some research work. Unfortunately, his time at the University of Zaragoza, though academically productive, was quite brief. He was compelled to resign from his professorship due to the political climate, institutional barriers, and financial hardships that hindered him from carrying out research aligned with his interests.

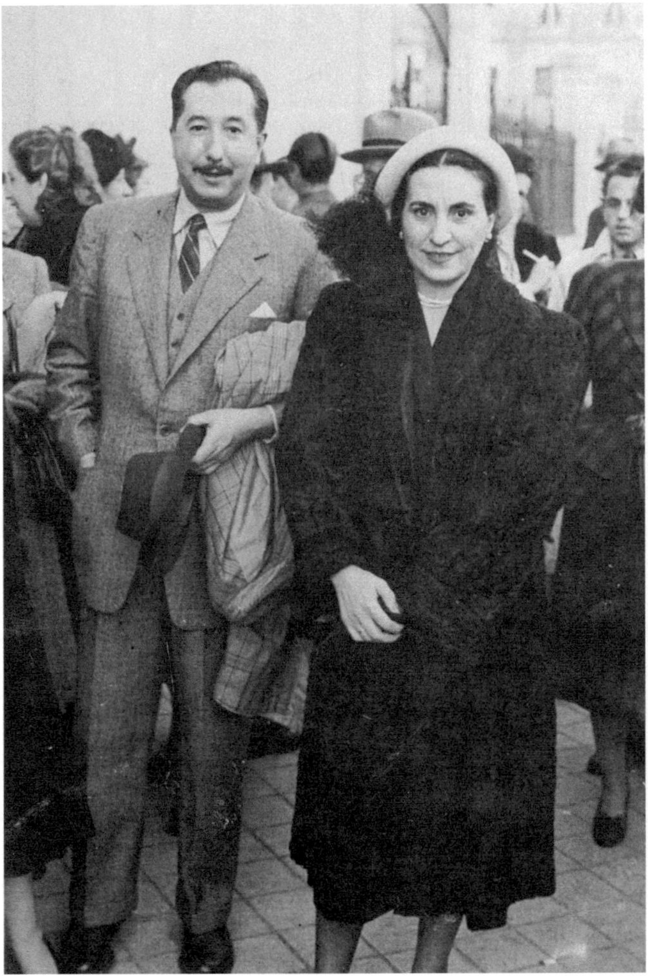

Fig. 21.3 Francisco Grande and his wife Gloria strolling through London, 1949

American Stage

In 1952, a meeting sponsored by the Food and Agriculture Organization of the United Nations (FAO) was held in Madrid to address issues of malnutrition. Among the attendees was Dr. Ancel Keys, a disciple of Krogh who had known Grande in Copenhagen during his time as a scholarship holder and was well acquainted with his work during the Civil War. Keys suggested that Grande consider moving to the United States. A few months later, Grande received a letter offering him a position as Associate Professor at the Laboratory of Physiological Hygiene at the University of Minnesota, where he would lead a program on dietary restriction commissioned by the U.S. Army—an extension of the renowned "Minnesota Experiment."

In December 1953, he embarked on his journey to Minneapolis, where he remained for over 20 years conducting research under the stands of the university's football stadium. His work focused on the following lines of research:

(a) Studies on calorie restriction and fasting, energy metabolism, body composition, and physical fitness;
(b) Comparative physiology, examining differences in lipolytic hormones between mammals and birds; and
(c) Development of the lipid hypothesis of atherosclerosis, investigating the effects of dietary fats and other components on plasma cholesterol levels.

The experiments that Grande conducted in Minneapolis on calorie restriction were carried out with young volunteers, most of them conscientious objectors. Don Paco demonstrated that the body can adapt to calorie restriction within certain limits and that our organism activates a series of mechanisms to cope with it, deciphering the various factors involved in caloric adaptation. He observed that part of the weight loss was due to the loss of body water. Furthermore, he showed that adequate water intake is essential and that adapting to water restriction is very difficult, as it causes severe disturbances in thermal regulation and in the elimination of nitrogen from proteins [11].

Thanks to these studies, it later became evident that many articles promoting "miracle" diets for weight loss contained significant miscalculations, often attributing fat loss where, in reality, the weight reduction was primarily due to water loss. Grande challenged these claims in a groundbreaking article published in 1968, which marked a milestone in the scientific investigation of dietary methods for weight reduction [12].

It had been shown that glucagon has a cholesterol-lowering effect in humans. Taking this into account, Grande initiated a series of studies comparing the effects of glucagon in birds and mammals. He demonstrated that, in birds, this hormone plays a crucial role in the mobilization of body fat, whereas its effect is less significant in mammals. Additionally, he observed that birds are not very sensitive to the effects of insulin and catecholamines [13].

During his stay at the Laboratory of Physiological Hygiene, Grande collaborated with doctors Ancel Keys and Joseph Anderson to study the effects of dietary fat on plasma cholesterol. Together, they developed an equation known as the "*Keys, Anderson, and Grande Equation*," which allows for the prediction of changes in plasma cholesterol based on alterations in the fatty acid composition and cholesterol content of the diet [14]. From this work, it

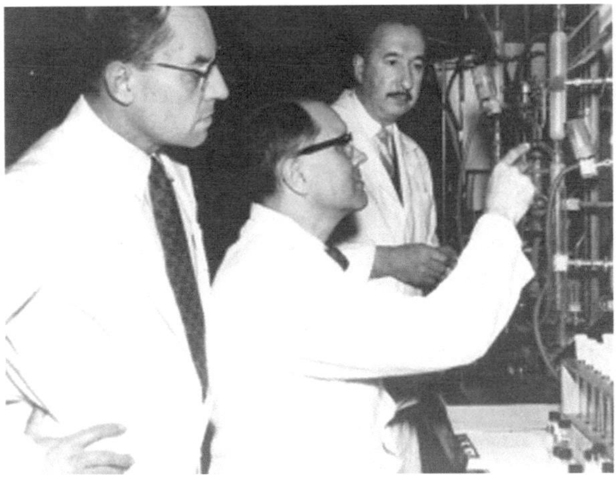

Fig. 21.4 Keys, Anderson, and Grande in the Physiological Hygiene Laboratory, 1960

is understood that saturated fats increase blood cholesterol levels, while monounsaturated and polyunsaturated fats tend to lower plasma cholesterol. The findings from his research on diet and the practical advice derived from his lipid theory have contributed to a significant reduction in cardiovascular mortality, saving millions of lives (Fig. 21.4).

Return to Spain

In 1974, he retired in the United States and returned to Zaragoza to take charge of the Juan Carlos I Institute of Nutrition. Shortly thereafter, he was appointed Extraordinary Professor at the University of Zaragoza. Many believed that his return from the United States marked a period of retirement in Spain, with his scientific activity limited to giving lectures and receiving tributes. However, nothing could be further from the truth. During this period, which he referred to as "my reincarnation," he produced a prolific and original body of scientific work, making it difficult to list all the research topics he addressed. One of his first projects upon returning was the study of the composition of human colostrum and mother milk. Throughout the 1970s, there was significant interest in analyzing the chemical composition of human milk, particularly its fatty acids, due to their potential influence on infant development and plasma lipid levels. Dr. Grande's studies provided original data on the composition of human milk in Spain and demonstrated that it differed in linoleic acid content compared to other nations—reflecting variations in dietary habits. An important aspect of this research was the identification of a high percentage of long-chain polyunsaturated fatty acids in the fat of human milk, which are undoubtedly crucial as a source of fatty acids for the developing child [15] (Figs. 21.5 and 21.6).

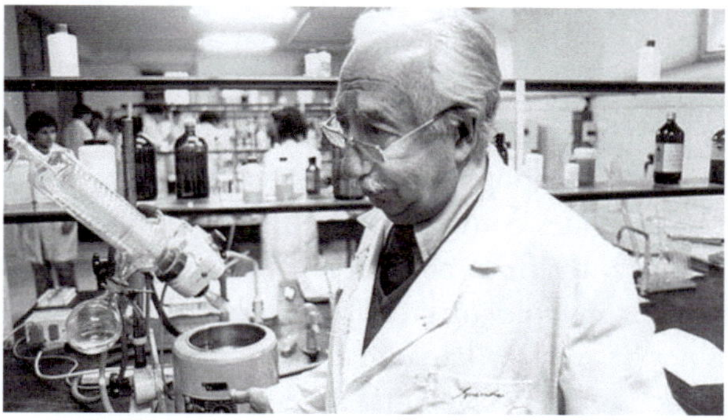

Fig. 21.5 Francisco Grande in his Biochemistry Laboratory, Faculty of Sciences, University of Zaragoza

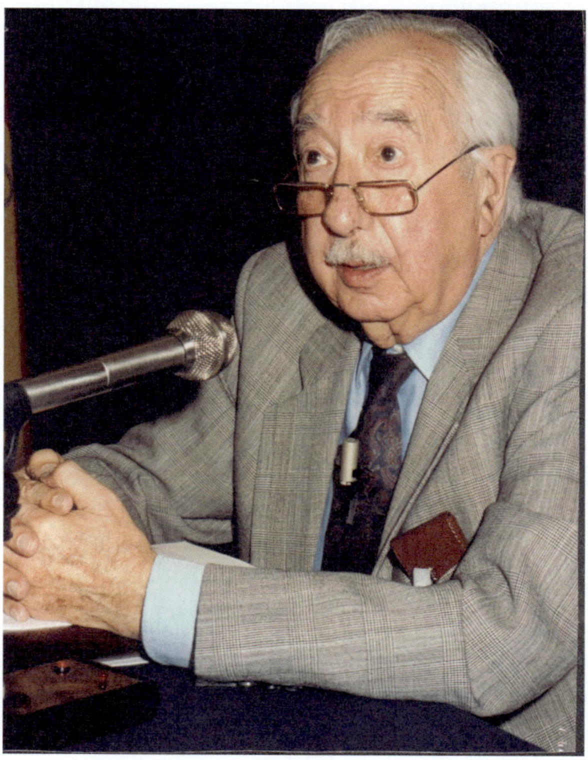

Fig. 21.6 Grande Covián giving a lecture at the first World Congress of Dairy Products in Human Health and Nutrition, Madrid, 1993

Other studies he conducted in collaboration with the Departments of Pediatrics, Obstetrics, and Gynecology at the Hospital Clínico Universitario de Zaragoza focused on lipid metabolism during gestation and in newborns. In his laboratory in Zaragoza, several doctoral theses were completed demonstrating that the plasma cholesterol levels of newborns were independent of race, place of birth, gender, and even maternal cholesterol and plasma lipid levels. An important finding was that high-density lipoprotein (HDL) cholesterol accounted for approximately 50 percent of total cholesterol in newborns, while plasma low-density lipoprotein (LDL) cholesterol levels ranged between 25 and 35 mg/dL—values considered optimal for uptake by LDL receptors, which differ significantly from adult levels [16]. Concurrently, he initiated research on changes in lipid metabolism during pregnancy. As he himself noted, this was not driven by a late interest in obstetrics but rather by the suitability of pregnancy as an experimental model. His studies demonstrated that gestational hyperlipidemia is more pronounced during the second half of pregnancy and is primarily due to hormonal factors that induce high lipolysis. This results in increased free fatty acids, allowing the mother to utilize fat as her main energy source while reserving glucose for the nutritional needs of the fetus [17].

The approach to studying lipid metabolism and its relationship with arteriosclerosis evolved significantly over the years. Initially, researchers in this field, including Grande Covián, focused primarily on the study of lipids themselves. However, it later became evident that the distribution of lipids among different lipoproteins and the enzymes involved in their metabolism played a crucial role. Concurrently, there was increasing interest in the protein component of lipoproteins—namely apolipoproteins—and the receptors responsible for removing these lipoproteins from blood plasma. The Grande Laboratory was a pioneer in adopting techniques for analyzing various lipoprotein fractions, characterizing apolipoproteins, and studying enzymes related to lipid metabolism.

Apoliproteins are proteins that binds lipids and fat soluble vitamins to form lipoproteins. They transport lipids in blood, and lymph.

In the 1980s and early 1990s, the genes encoding proteins involved in lipid metabolism had been mapped and sequenced. During this period, advances in molecular biology techniques made it possible to study these genes in greater detail. In 1987, under Grande's leadership and with the assistance of one of his most outstanding disciples, José M. Ordovás, they began investigating mutations in the genes of certain apolipoproteins. This research later expanded to include mutations in the LDL receptor gene, analyzing their relationship with various hereditary dyslipidemias and exploring gene-nutrient or gene-drug interactions.

Grande managed to establish an excellent laboratory in the basement of the Science Faculty at the University of Zaragoza. Despite his remarkable scientific stature, Grande Covián was content with modest resources; he successfully operated his laboratory at full capacity with very limited funding. Thanks to his enthusiasm and dedication, he quickly assembled a state-of-the-art facility equipped with advanced techniques for the time, including spectrophotometry, electrophoresis, immunochemistry, and chromatography. Professionals from other laboratories frequently visited it to learn these innovative methods.

We always learned from his teachings in a manner we called "by osmosis": simply listening to him speak was often enough. When he would say, "Como Vd. sabe" ("As you know"), it was essential to pay close attention, as it usually indicated a point you almost certainly did not know and that would be of great significance in the conversation. Grande Covián was one of those teachers who imparted not only knowledge but also a profound sense of humanity, always accompanied by his characteristic sense of humor. His Biochemistry class, which he taught to final-year Chemical Sciences students, was always well attended by his collaborators. I have yet to meet anyone who delivered classes as enjoyable and as clear as he did. He possessed an extraordinary memory, enabling him to recall anecdotes with remarkable detail—including dates—related to the subject he was explaining. His lectures were consistently popular, especially his doctoral course: "Nutrition and Food Chemistry," which attracted not only enrolled students but also other university professors who were passionate about the subject (Fig. 21.7).

At the University of Zaragoza, he is remembered as one of the most outstanding professors who have taught in their classrooms. No class or lecture was complete without a historical introduction providing context, often referencing Antoine Lavoisier as the father of biochemistry and the scientific understanding of nutrition; François Magendie for discovering the necessity of proteins in nutrition and identifying the essential amino acids; Claude Bernard, author of *Introduction to the Study of Experimental Medicine*; Eugene Chevreul for isolating cholesterol and demonstrating that fats are esters of glycerol and fatty acids; and, of course, his friend and colleague Severo Ochoa

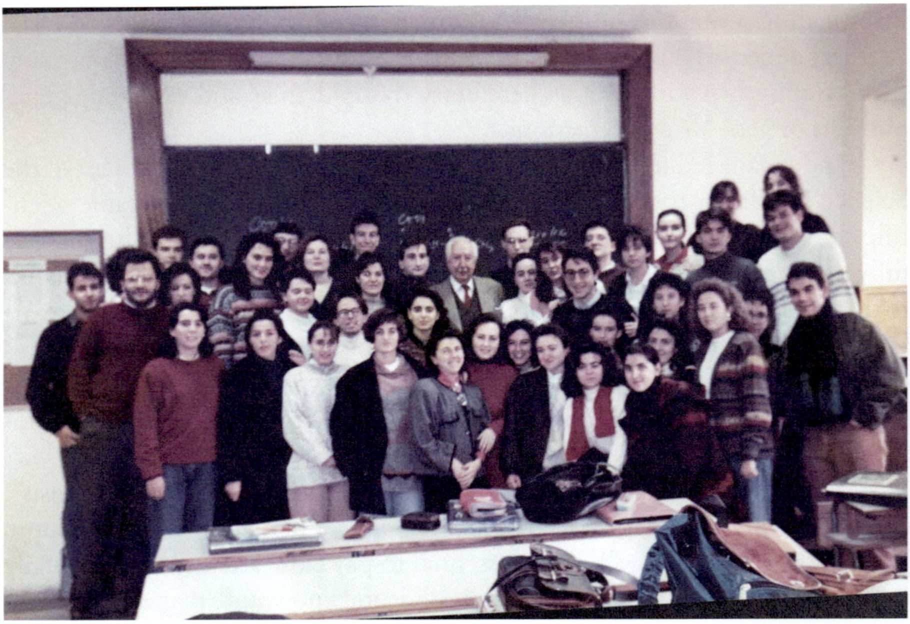

Fig. 21.7 Grande Covián with his Biochemistry students, University of Zaragoza, academic year 1991–1992

for deciphering the genetic code and conducting pioneering studies on phosphorylation (Fig. 21.8).

After returning from the United States, he succeeded in establishing a scientific school known today as "*La Escuela de la Reencarnación de Grande*," (Grande's school of reincarnation) which has spread throughout Spain and abroad. He supervised a total of 18 doctoral theses. Thanks to Grande Covián's efforts, biochemistry studies at the University of Zaragoza received a significant boost. The nucleus he created in the basement of the Faculty evolved into what is now the Department of Biochemistry, Molecular and Cellular Biology at the University of Zaragoza. Currently, the foundation bearing his name aims to preserve his legacy and continue the scientific activity he championed. Dr. Grande Covián was also a passionate popularizer of nutrition science, delivering hundreds of lectures and receiving numerous tributes from both Spanish and international societies. Undoubtedly, he was one of the great scientists of the twentieth century. His friend and collaborator, Professor Gregorio Varela, remarked: "*Dr. Grande Covián was the best and cleverest man I have ever known.*"

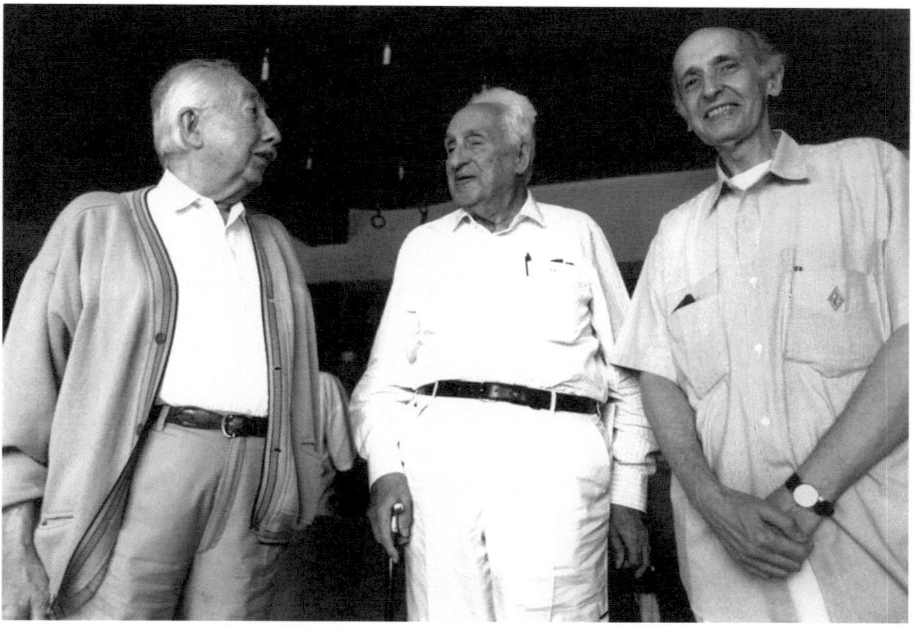

Fig. 21.8 Severo Ochoa, Francisco Grande Covián, and Santiago Grisolía at the summer school in La Granda (Asturias) in 1987

References

1. Ochoa S, Grande F. Nota sobre el contenido en fosfágeno de los músculos del cobaya después de la extirpación de las suprarrenales. Rev Esp Biol. 1932;1:75–6.
2. Grande F. Uber das Vorkonmen von Palmitico-und Srearicodehi-drogenasen in einigen Pflanzensemen. Skandinavischen Archiv fur Physiologie. 1934;69:189.
3. Evans CL, Grande F, Hsu FY. The glucose and lactate consumption of the dog's heart. Q J Exp Physiol. 1935;24:347.
4. Bogue J, Elvehjem CR, Madden RJ, Strong FM, Woolley DW. Relation of nicotinic acid and nicotinic acid amide to canine black tongue. J Am Chem Soc. 1937;59:1767.
5. Evans CL, Grande F, Hsu FY. The effect of adrenaline and of increased work on the carbohydrate metabolism of the mammalian heart. Q J Exp Physiol. 1935;25:213.
6. Grande F, Hsu FY. The distribution of blood sugar. J Physiol. 1935;84:29.
7. Grande Covián F, Jiménez García F. El tratamiento de la pelagra por el ácido nicotínico. Rev Clin Esp. 1940;2:144–52.

8. Grande Covián F, Rof Carballo J, Jiménez García F, Morata Cernuda A. Alimentación y desarrollo infantil. I. El estado nutritivo de los niños en edad escolar de un suburbio madrileño. Rev Clin Esp. 1944;12:87–94.
9. Grande F, Richter D. The effect of electrical stimulation on the transport of radioactive phosphorus in the frog sciatic nerve. J Physiol. 1950;111:57.
10. Starling EH. Principios de fisiología humana. Traducción de Grande F y Vivanco F. Editorial Aguilar; 1952.
11. Grande F, Anderson JT, Taylor HL. Effect of restricted water intake on urine nitrogen output in man on a low calorie diet devoid of protein. J Appl Physiol. 1957;10:430–5.
12. Grande F. Energy balance and body composition changes. A critical study of three recent publications. Ann Intern Med. 1968;68:467–80.
13. De Oya M, Prigge WF, Swenson DE, Grande F. Role of glucagon on fatty liver production in birds. Am J Phys. 1971;221:25–30.
14. Grande F, Anderson JT, Keys A. Diets of different fatty acid composition producing identical serum cholesterol levels in man. Am J Clin Nutr. 1972;25:53–60.
15. Villacampa MJ, Casaus Pemán C, Grande Covián F. Fatty acid composition of human milk. An Esp Pediatr. 1982;16:324–35.
16. Diaz M, Leal C, Ramon y Cajal J, Jimenez MD, Martinez H, Pocovi M, Grande F. Cord blood lipoprotein-cholesterol: relationship birth weight and gestational age of newborns. Metabolism. 1989;38:435–8.
17. Ordovas JM, Pocovi M, Grande F. Plasma lipids and cholesterol esterification rate during pregnancy. Obstet Gynecol. 1984;63:20–5.

22

The Gil Vernet Saga in Urology

José María Gil-Vernet Sedó

The Gil Vernet family is an outstanding medical dynasty from Barcelona that has left a profound mark on the history of urology.

The story begins with Salvador and continues with his son José María.

Salvador Gil Vernet

Surgical Technique and Urological Anatomy (Fig. 22.1)

Salvador was born on 10 August 1892 in Vandellós (Tarragona), in his own words: "A very small farming village, a mountain village of much work and little profit". He attended the village school and in 1903 he began the baccalaureate at the Institut General i Tècnica de Tarragona (Tarragona General and Technical Institute). In his adolescence he showed a great interest in botany and took advantage of the summer holidays to collect and study a large number of plant species. In the summer of 1909 he moved to Barcelona, where he would witness the events of the Tragic Week shortly before

All pictures with permission of José María Gil-Vernet Sedó.

J. M. G.-V. Sedó (✉)
Gil-Vernet Urology Centre, Barcelona, Spain

M. A. Cuesta, F. Mateo Vallejo (eds.), *Spain's Journey in Medicine*,
https://doi.org/10.1007/978-3-032-12221-6_22

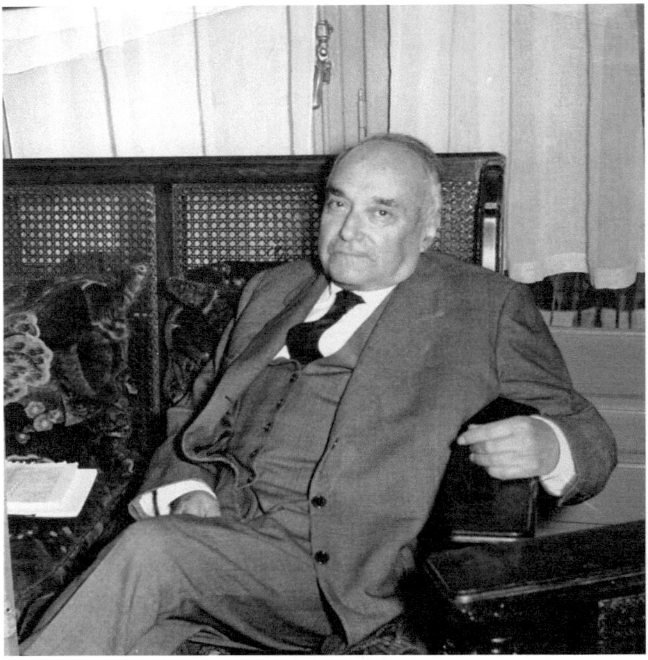

Fig. 22.1 Salvador Gil Vernet

beginning his studies at the Faculty of Medicine. During his time as a student at the Hospital de la Santa Cruz, he met Dr. Pedro Esquerdo Esquerdo (1851–1922), professor of Pathology and Clinical Medicine, who entrusted him with performing autopsies; he also worked there as an anatomical preparator with Dr. Alejandro Planellas and as intern student of Surgical Pathology with Dr. Ramón Torres Casanovas at the Hospital Clínic (Fig. 22.2).

In this way he became an intern student at both hospitals, earning a salary that he supplemented with what he earned administering anaesthesia. Interested in urology, he worked as an intern student in the Urology Department of Dr. Joaquín Mestre at the Hospital de la Santa Cruz. On 30 June 1915 he graduated with distinction and continued his training as a urologist in the private clinic of Dr. Gabriel Estapé, who was also a surgeon at the Hospital de la Santa Cruz.

In 1918 he read his doctoral thesis "Contribución al estudio de la anestesia local" "*Contribution to the study of local anaesthesia*" and in 1919 he obtained by examination the post of assistant professor of Anatomy and Anatomical Technique at the chair of Dr. Emilio Sacanella who was the introducer of transvesical prostatic adenomectomy in Spain. I In 1920, he married Mercedes Vila Sanromá (1891–1953). From this union were born two sons — Salvador

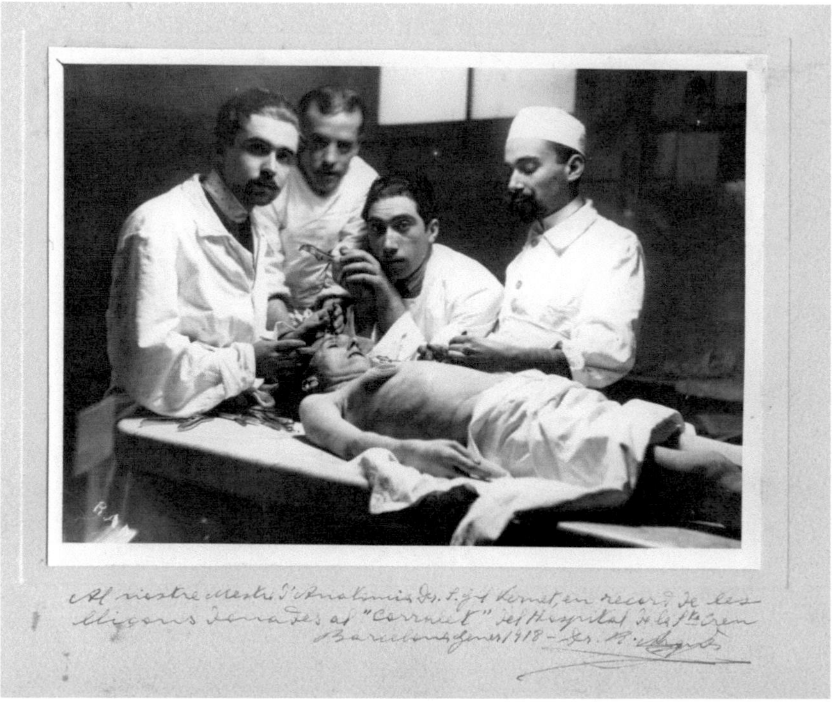

Fig. 22.2 Anatomy class. Hospital de la Santa Cruz. Barcelona 1918. Salvador Gil Vernet is on the right without taking his eyes off the dissection table. The dissection room was known as the "Corralet"

(1921–1964) and José María (1922–2020) — both of whom would later distinguish themselves as urologists (Fig. 22.3).

That same year, he began preparing for the national competitive examinations at his family country house in Hospitalet del Infante. The absence of electric lighting there compelled him to study by candlelight. Although he was unsuccessful in obtaining the chair of Anatomy at the Faculty of Medicine of Madrid, the experience allowed him to establish a cordial and intellectually fruitful relationship with Santiago Ramón y Cajal (1852–1934), then serving as president of the examining board.

In 1926, he was awarded the chair of Anatomy at the University of Salamanca, a position he ultimately chose not to occupy, having requested a leave of absence to continue his professional work in Barcelona. Two years later, following the death of Dr. Manuel Serés (1888–1928), he successfully competed for a transfer and assumed the chair of Anatomy at the University of Barcelona. There he was entrusted with the specialized teaching of *Diseases of the Urinary Tract and their Clinical Practice* within the Urology Clinic of the

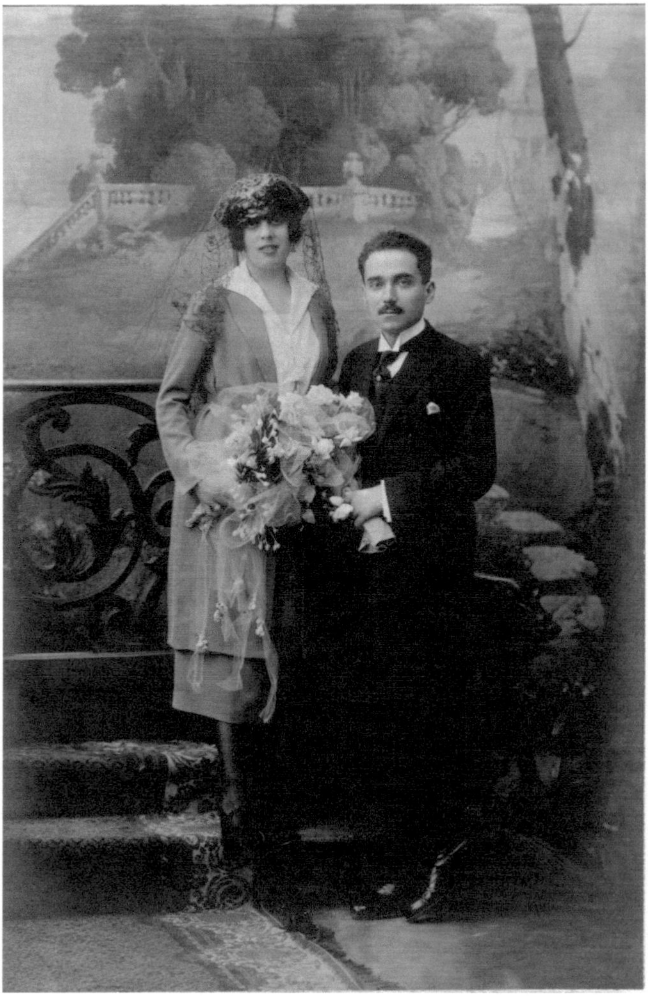

Fig. 22.3 Salvador Gil Vernet and Mercedes Vila on their wedding day. Barcelona. 1920

Hospital Clínico y Provincial, which commenced operations that same year. In 1929, a formal specialization program in Urology was inaugurated under his supervision, structured as a two-year course with a maximum enrollment of six students.

In 1931, he became one of the founding members of the Catalan Society of Urology, serving on its first governing board under the presidency of Narciso Serrallach Mauri (1875–1951). Committed to advancing his field and recognizing the unique value of international collaboration, he attended as many medical congresses abroad as circumstances permitted. Thus, in 1933, accompanied by urologist Leonardo de la Peña Díaz (1875–1957), he took part in the fifth Congress of the International Society of Urology held in London, where he performed a pararectal prostatectomy at Saint Paul's Hospital. That same year, he was appointed Professor of Urology at the University of Barcelona—an institution known between 1933 and 1939 as the Autonomous University of Barcelona—a role which required him to resign the chair of Anatomy to dedicate himself fully to the new discipline.

On 12 August 1936, the Civil War began in July 1936, he was dismissed and removed from his posts by a decree law signed by Manuel Azaña, minister president of the II Spanish Republic, and 2 days later, persecuted for his conservative ideas—his son Salvador was arrested and taken to the prison in Calle de San Elías for questioning about his father's whereabouts—he took the road to exile, something he would recall years later: "*When, at dusk on 14 August 1936, from the French ship Corté II, I thought I was saying goodbye to my country forever, I experienced emotions I had never known before. Suddenly I had lost everything a man can lose except his honor and his life, and his life had been saved thanks to the representatives of Nicaragua and France*".

At the beginning of his exile he lived in Toulouse, Narbonne, Nice, Montpellier and Marseille, and it was in the latter city, attending the meetings of the Urological Society of South-East France, where he made friends with Italian urologists from Turin, Genoa and Milan. As a result of this relationship with colleagues from France and Italy, they will establish the Society of Urology of the Latin Mediterranean. He then moved to Italy, where he spent the last 2 years of his exile. In 1939 he returned to Barcelona where he could resume his teaching and professional activity.

In 1948 he was appointed full member of the Royal Academy of Medicine and Surgery of Barcelona, occupying the chair of Dr. Ángel Ferrer Cajigal with the inaugural speech "*Divertículos vesicales*" (Bladder diverticula) responded by Dr. Pedro Nubiola Espinós. In 1955 he inaugurated the Professional School of Urology in the chair of Urology with the lecture "*Conceptos fisiopatológicos del adenoma de próstata y tratamiento abortivo*". (*Physiopathological concepts of prostate adenoma and abortive treatment*). In 1953 he received the Medal of Mérito Sanitario (Health Merit) and the Medal of Alfonso X el Sabio. In 1963 he was appointed honorary professor at the University of Madrid and together with Dr. Agustín Pedro Pons he received the title of "doctor honoris causa" from the University of Toulouse.

In 1966 he was awarded with the "Pedro Virgili" National Prize for Surgery, the "Antoine Portal" Prize from the French National Academy of

Medicine and was named Knight of the French Légion d'Honneur and Stella de la Soliedaritat Italiana di Primera Classe. In 1967 he was elected President of the Societé International d'Urologie, a position he held until 1973. In 1967 he was appointed Honorary President of the Asociación Española de Urología (Spanish Society of Urology). In 1973 he chaired the International Congress of Urology in Amsterdam, being his inaugural speech on the "Origen y desarrollo del cáncer de próstata". (*Origin and development of prostate cancer*). In 1977 he was appointed Honorary member of the Real Academia Nacional de Medicina, where he entered with the speech "Divertículos bulbouretrales y reflujo vesicoureteral" (*Bulbourethral diverticula and vesicoureteral reflux*). He was also recognized as an honorary member of the Societies of Urology of France, Italy, Greece, Mexico and Colombia and as visiting professor at the universities of Chicago, Columbia, Autónoma de México, Buenos Aires, Bogotá, Tolouse, Tokyo, Amsterdam, Athens, Johannesburg and Munich.

On 4 February 1987, together with his son José María, he received the *Narcis Monturiol Prize* awarded by the Generalitat de Catalunya. At the age of 75 he retired from his professional activity and devoted his last years to growing roses and lemon trees at his home in Castelledefels. He died in Barcelona on 24 October 1987.

The Scientific Work

In 1917, the clinical application of his anatomical studies of the pelvis allowed him to describe a new technique of sacral epidural anaesthesia, which became known as "*Gil Vernet's extradural anaesthesia*" and which was very useful in prostate surgery. In 1919, in collaboration with Francisco Gallart Monés, he studied the abdominal neurovegetative plexus and described, for the first time in humans, the inferior mesenteric ganglion.

From 1920 onwards, his research focused on the topographic and microscopic anatomy of the pelvis and the male perineum, with special attention to the bladder, prostate and pelvic neurovegetative plexus, as well as on the pathological anatomy of the prostate. Interested in functional anatomy, he considered that it was not enough to know the "*what*" and the "*how*" of an anatomical structure, he needs to find out the "*what for*". Thus, by developing a

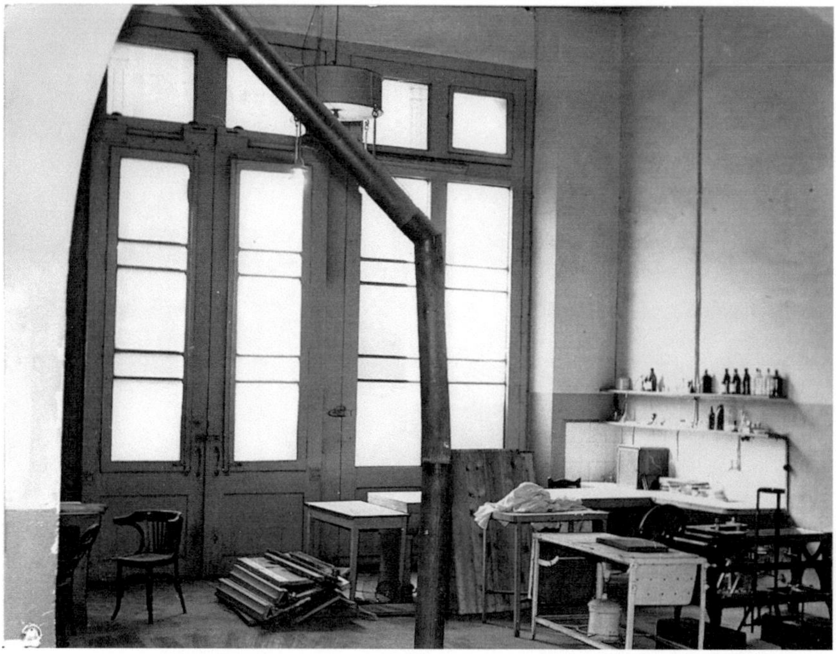

Fig. 22.4 Uroanatomy Laboratory at the Barcelona Medical School, ca. 1957. The giant Sartorius-Werke microtome can be seen at the bottom right

functional urogenital anatomy he wanted to understand the physiology of urination, erection and ejaculation and, at the same time, to go deeper into a topographical anatomy that will allow him to develop more precise and less invasive surgical techniques [1–4].

A tireless worker with exceptional talent, he applied the method of serial anatomical sections described by the German anatomist Otto Kalischer. In the Laboratorio de Uroanatomía in the Hospital Clínico and with the help of the giant Sartorius-Werke microtome, he obtained freezing sections of the pelvic visceral block, both normal and pathological (Fig. 22.4).

From each specimen, about 200 preparations measuring 12 × 9 cm and with a thickness of 20–50 microns were obtained, which were then examined with a magnifying glass or microscope. In this way it was possible to carry out a thorough dissection of the muscular and nervous elements that

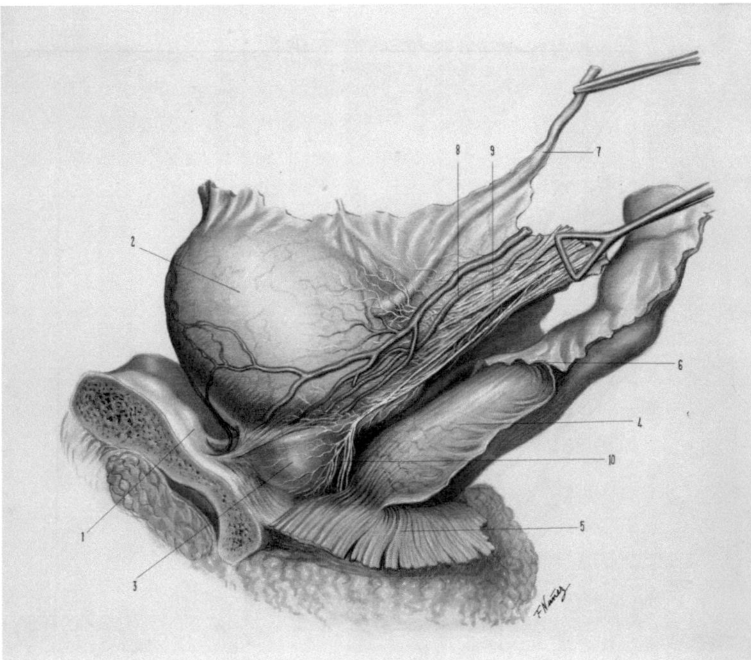

Fig. 22.5 Pelvic plexus and neurovascular bundles. Mixed media on paper 28 × 31 cm. by Francisco Núñez. 1944

were invisible during the macroscopic dissection. The most relevant findings were noted down in his field notebooks and subsequently drawn in pencil and Indian ink by the second-year students of the Faculty of Medicine. All this graphic work, together with the drawings of two exceptional medical illustrators, Francisco Núñez and Rafael Alemany, now constitute the Salvador Gil Vernet Collection of Urological Drawings [4] (Fig. 22.5).

Between the 1950s and 1960s, prestigious international urologists interested in learning about Salvador Gil Vernet's morphological research visited his Urology Department. These included W. Gregoir, René Küss, Ian Thompson, Ermanno Mingazzini and Charles B. Huggins. Ch. Huggins, winner of the Nobel Prize for Medicine in 1966, for his discoveries concerning hormonal treatment of prostatic cancer", maintained a close friendship with him beyond the professional sphere (Fig. 22.6).

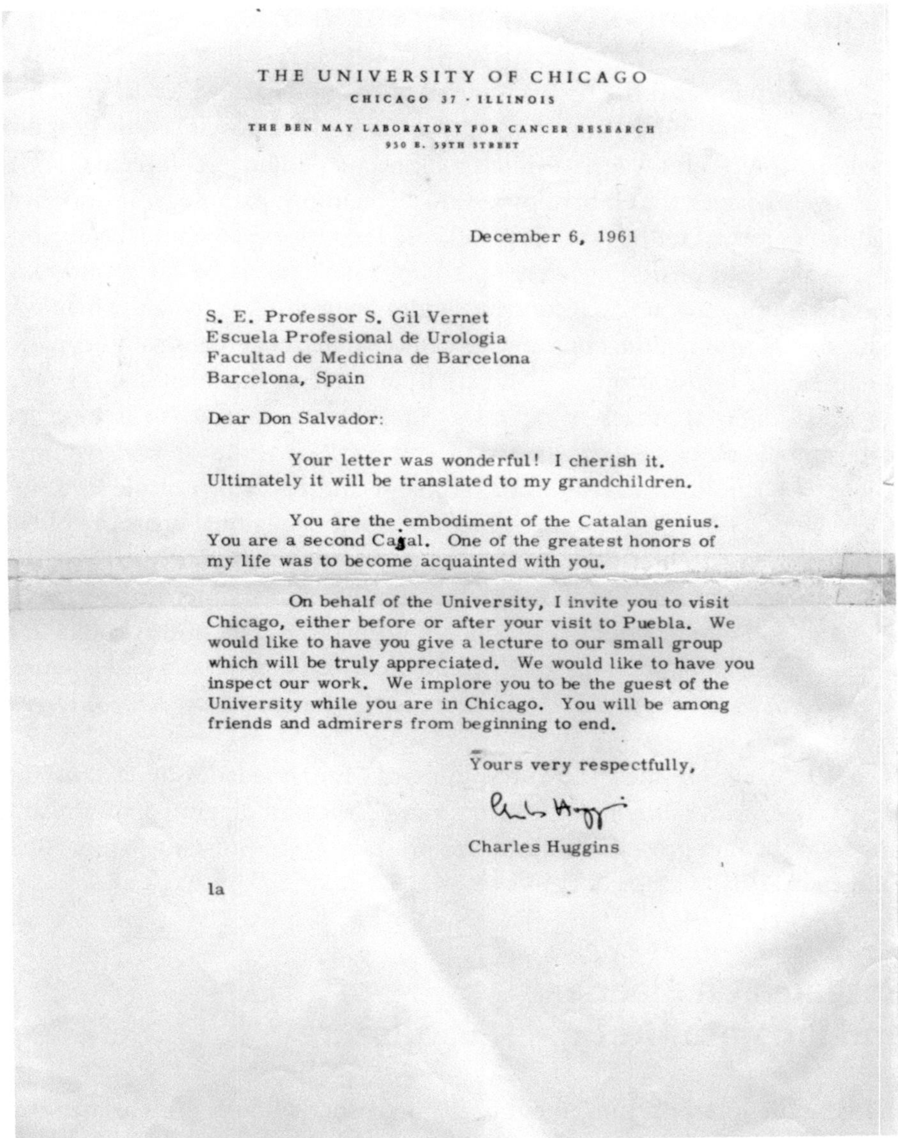

THE UNIVERSITY OF CHICAGO
CHICAGO 37 · ILLINOIS

THE BEN MAY LABORATORY FOR CANCER RESEARCH
950 E. 59TH STREET

December 6, 1961

S. E. Professor S. Gil Vernet
Escuela Profesional de Urologia
Facultad de Medicina de Barcelona
Barcelona, Spain

Dear Don Salvador:

Your letter was wonderful! I cherish it. Ultimately it will be translated to my grandchildren.

You are the embodiment of the Catalan genius. You are a second Cajal. One of the greatest honors of my life was to become acquainted with you.

On behalf of the University, I invite you to visit Chicago, either before or after your visit to Puebla. We would like to have you give a lecture to our small group which will be truly appreciated. We would like to have you inspect our work. We implore you to be the guest of the University while you are in Chicago. You will be among friends and admirers from beginning to end.

Yours very respectfully,

Charles Huggins

la

Fig. 22.6 Letter from Dr. Charles B. Huggins with an invitation to Salvador Gil Vernet to come as a visiting professor to the University of Chicago. 1961

Urogenital Pathology: His Great Work

In 1944 he published the first volume of his comprehensive work, Patología Urogenital (Urogenital Pathology), titled Cáncer de Próstata. This groundbreaking, three-volume series, which took over a decade to complete (1955), extensively covered the embryology, regional anatomy, pathology, and surgical techniques related to the prostate gland, and is considered a seminal contribution to the field of urology. Patología Urogenital was to be his great work, considered the most notable contribution of Spanish Urology and which was to have great international impact. He demonstrated that malignant neoplasia has its origin in the prostate gland itself and not in the adenoma. He also described a new approach to radical perineal prostatectomy, the ischiorectal juxta-sphincteric approach. In 1953 he published the second volume: "Biología y Patología de la Próstata" (Biology and Pathology of the Prostate) where he described, for the first time, the zonal or regional anatomy of the prostate based on a urethrocentric model, dividing the prostate into two main regions, the "*cranial gland*" and the "*caudal gland*" and an intermediate gland. Dr. Hugh H. Young, a pioneer of modern urology, has said of this book: "*It is a monumental work, with the most striking illustrations that have ever appeared in a medical text. Its contribution to the study of prostate pathology and surgery is truly great.*

In 1955 he published the last volume of "Enfermedades de la Próstata" (*Diseases of the Prostate)* in which he reviewed the pathological anatomy and surgery of benign prostatic hyperplasia, prostatic cysts, prostatitis and genital tuberculosis [5].

Research on Bladder and Prostato-Urethral Musculature

In his studies on the arrangement of the detrusor, (smooth muscle layer that forms the main muscular wall of the urinary bladder), he described the trigonal muscular loop, the precervical transverse arch and the posterior longitudinal fascicle. In the prostatic urethra, he demonstrated the existence of the posterior prostatourethral muscular fascicle that forms the urethral crest. As a result of his interest in preserving urinary continence after radical prostatectomy, he carried out an exhaustive study on the neuroanatomy of the pelvic plexus, describing the prostatic neurovascular bundles and the dual somatic and neurovegetative innervation of the external urethral sphincter, his great contribution. In 1968 appeared *Morphology and Function of the Vesico-prostato-urethral musculature*, which would be his major work originally in English and which would be cited in the scientific literature 50 years after its publication. In this work he introduced important new concepts like a three-part external urethral sphincter and specific arrangements of smooth and striated muscle in the pelvic floor that are determining for urinary continence and ejaculation [6].

José Maria Gil-Vernet Vila

Excellence in Urology (Fig. 22.7)

Born on 9 December 1922 in Barcelona, he was the son of Salvador Gil Vernet (see above) and nephew of Emilio Gil Vernet (1905–1970), professor of Obstetrics and Gynecology and founder of a dynasty of gynecologists. The outbreak of the Civil War interrupted his baccalaureate studies at the Jesuit school San Ignacio de Sarriá, and, later at the Institute. He witnesses the persecution suffered by his father at the hands of the Popular Front and that led

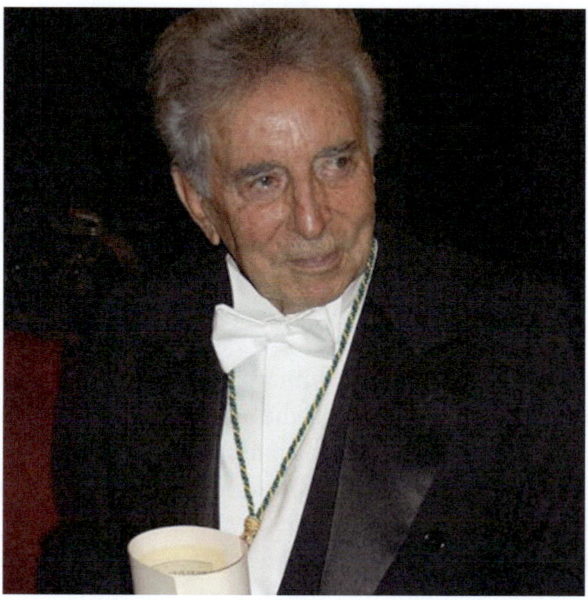

Fig. 22.7 José María Gil-Vernet

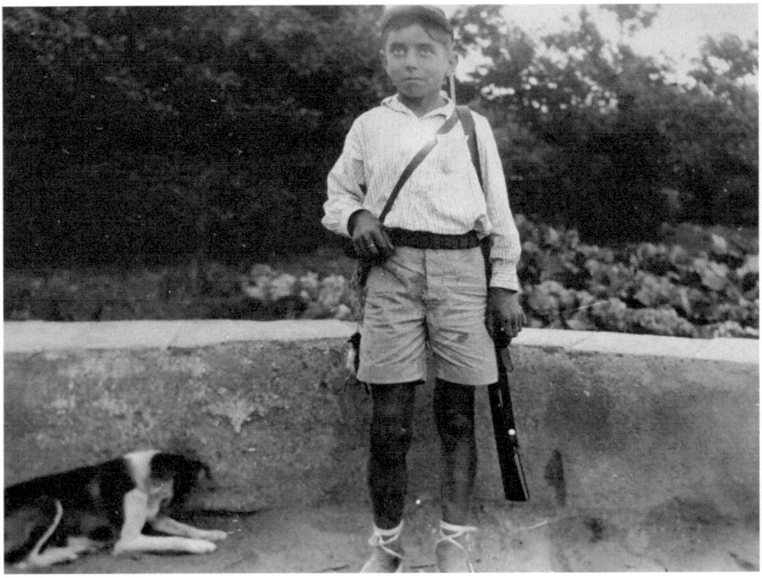

Fig. 22.8 José María Gil-Vernet. With his dog and shotgun on his shoulder. Vandellós (Tarragona). 1936

to his exile. Thus, with his mother Mercedes Vila Sanromá (1891–1953) and his brother Salvador (1921–1964), he left Barcelona for the village of Vandellós (Tarragona), where they lived in the house of his paternal grandparents until the end of the war. During these forced holidays, José María became a passionate hunter and always accompanied by his dog, he roamed the mountains in search of rabbits, partridges and quails (Fig. 22.8).

The shortage of ammunition forced him to sharpen his wits, and he invented a system for recovering the piston of the cartridges. When the war ended and his father returned from exile in Italy, he returned to Barcelona, where in 1947 he graduated in Medicine and Surgery. During his time as a high school student, he accompanied his father to the dissection room—it was not unusual to meet him on Sunday afternoons when the young José María was thinking only of going to the Barça football stadium—where he learnt the secrets of the topographical anatomy of the pelvis and perineum.

In 1951 he obtained his doctorate from the University of Madrid with the thesis *Estudio de la reimplantación de uréteres en el intestino (Study of reimplantation of ureters in the intestine)*, a work in which he showed his interest in the use of intestinal segments in urology for the reconstruction of the ureter and bladder in urinary tuberculosis and in bladder replacement in the treatment of bladder cancer. This innovative work was the result of the application of his knowledge of digestive surgery which he learnt in the Department of

Surgical Pathology of Dr. Ramón Arandes Adán, with whom he performed the first colocystoplasty in urology. (use of a colon segment for bladder replacement). He wrote of Dr. Arandes: "I always received a positive, sincere and learned impulse from him". In 1956 he qualified as a specialist in Urology at the University of Barcelona and that same year he married Olga Sedó (1935–2014), the best man at the wedding being the urologist Dr. Alfonso de la Peña Pineda (1904–1971). Three children were born of the marriage and two of them, José María (1957-) and Alfredo (1959-) are currently urologists.

Gil-Vernet was in charge of teaching the Urology in the Surgical Pathology III until Dr. Arandes retired. That same year he attended the European Congress of Surgery held in Nantes as a speaker, accompanied by Dr. Rafael Gosálbez and Dr. Arturo Soler Roselló. It was his first scientific trip abroad and he wrote: "The journey was a real odyssey, half in a utility vehicle, part by train and part on foot, we went through hardships of all kinds, but we returned from there with great satisfaction as scientists".

In 1958 he won the gold medal at the first "Scientific film" congress in Brussels. In 1961 he was elected member of the French Academy of Medicine and from 1961 to 1967 he was a visiting professor at Columbia University (New York), Johannesburg, Rochester, Missouri, California, Sao Paulo, Bucharest, Berlin, Cook County Hospital (Chicago), Moscow, London School of Medicine, Nigata (Japan), Salysbury (Rhodesia). In 1964 he was appointed director of the Transplant Unit of the Hospital Clinic of Barcelona. In 1967 he received the National Surgery Award and was invited by Dr. Willard E. Goodwin (1915–1998), director of the Department of Urology at the University of California, Los Angeles as a visiting professor where he performed several operations, being the only Spanish urologist, without the ECFMG certificate, who has been able to operate in the USA. There he became friends with Dr. Joseph J. Kaufman and Jean B. DeKernion, whom he invited to collaborate in the International Urology Courses held at the Hospital Clínico de Barcelona from 1958 to 1981 (Fig. 22.9).

In 1972, at the proposal of Dr. Fabián Estapé, rector of the University of Barcelona, he was appointed full professor of Urology and from 1973 as director of the Professional School of Urology. From 1973 to 1980 he was vice-rector of the University of Barcelona. In 1972 he was president of the National Commission of the Specialty of Urology.

In 1974 he was awarded the title of Commendattore dell'Ordine al Mérito by the President of the Italian Republic. In 1980 he was awarded the "Golden Eagle" prize by the Council on International Non-Theatrical Events in New York. In 1981 he was appointed member of the Royal Academy of Medicine of Catalonia, occupying the chair of Dr. Joan Puig-Sureda Sais. His

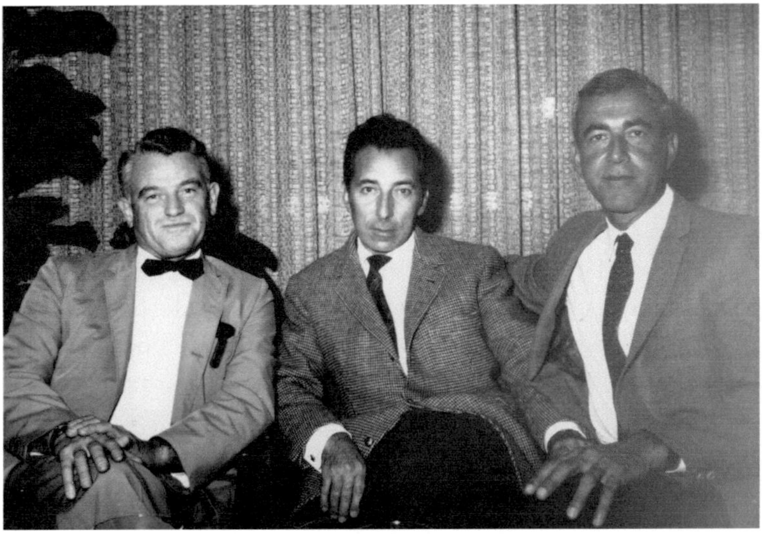

Fig. 22.9 José María Gil-Vernet (centre) at UCLA during his stay as a visiting professor. On the left Dr. W. Goodwin and on the right Dr. J. Kaufman. Los Angeles 1967

acceptance speech, *Renal transplantation*, was answered by Dr. Moisés Broggi Vallés. In 1986 he received, together with his father, the Narcis Monturiol Prize. In 1997 he received the Josep Trueta medal for health merit. In 2001 he received the Gold Medal at the 29th International Exhibition of Inventions in Geneva for the development of a device for the treatment of female urinary incontinence.

In 2002 he was awarded the Francisco Diaz Medal of the Spanish Urology Association. In 2008 he was appointed as an elected member of the Real Academia de Medicina (Royal Academy of Medicine of Spain) with a speech on" *Trasplante de órganos. Su repercusión en cirugía urológica*" (*Organ transplantation. His impact on urological surgery)* being answered by Dr. Hipólito Durán Sacristán. In 2009 he received the *Distinguished Career Award* from the Société International d'Urologie and in 2016 the Innovators in Urology Award from the EAU (European Association of Urology).

At the age of 65 he retired from public office and in 1988 he was appointed professor emeritus by the University of Barcelona. A tireless worker, he continued to work as a urologist until he was well into his 90 s and continued to collaborate with the Royal Academy of Medicine of Barcelona and the Royal Academy of Medicine of Spain until the end of his life. He died in Barcelona on 5 March 2020 [7, 8].

The Scientific Work

In 1957, for the first time in the history of urology, he used the large intestine—the sigmoid colon—to create a neobladder in a patient with infiltrating bladder carcinoma. Also, the use of small bowel allowed him to perform bladder enlargements in tuberculous cystitis. The technique was published in the Journal of Urology in 1960 and 4 years later he used the ileocolic segment to replace the ureter and bladder at the same time. In 1964, with the collaboration of the Barcelona Zoo veterinarian, Miguel Luera Carbó, he started the experimental programme of renal transplantation in dogs. On 23 July 1965, with the collaboration of the nephrologist Antonio Caralps Riera and the immunologist Jordi Vives Puiggrós, he performed the first successful kidney transplant in Spain.

Other pioneering operations in Urology [9, 10]:

1965: New approach to the renal pelvis, the intrasinusal approach, to extract coralliform stones through a transverse pyelolithotomy. The technique will be called "extended pyelolithotomy or Gil-Vernet operation".
1966: A new two-stage technique for the treatment of complex urethral strictures.
1975: He introduced renal hypothermia techniques that allowed extracorporeal surgery and renal autotransplantation in cases of complex vascular, tumour or congenital anomalies that did not allow conventional surgery.
1976: A new retroperitoneal approach to the splenic vessels, which allowed splenorenal anastomoses to be performed without the need for a median laparotomy.
1978: he performed the first cadaveric testicular transplant on a 21-year-old male, the graft remained viable for 2 months and had to be removed due to a rejection crisis.

In the same year he described orthotopic renal transplantation, used in those patients in whom it is not possible to use the aorto-iliac axis and also described the descent of the right renal vein for the treatment of stenosis of the proximal ureter.

1979: he introduced the operating microscope in urological surgery for the treatment of infertility and in vascular anastomoses in renal transplantation.

1981 he used three-dimensional intraoperative radiology for surgery of renal lithiasis, an exploration that allowed him to know the exact location of renal stones.
1983 he performed the first pancreas transplant in Spain with the surgeon Laureano Fernández-Cruz, the graft worked correctly, and the patient died after 10 years.
1984 he described a new, minimally invasive operation for the treatment of vesicoureteral reflux in children, the so-called trigonoplasty or Gil-Vernet anti-reflux technique.
1990 he described a technique of bladder autoplasty with a posterosuperior bladder flap used in the treatment of complex vesico-vaginal fistulas and named after its author.
1994 he published a new urethroplasty technique using a vascularised scrotal flap, and in
1998 he invented an adjustable hydraulic prosthesis for the treatment of female urinary incontinence.

José María Gil-Vernet was also an innovator in teaching, since 1954 he has been the co-director, in collaboration with Dr. W. Gregoir (1920–2000) of ten international urology courses at the Hospital Clínic, a congress attended by hundreds of urologists from all over the world (Fig. 22.10).

The interventions were broadcast live to the Montjuic Conference Centre. In its last edition, in 1981, it brought together more than 2000 urologists (Fig. 22.11).

In order to make his different surgical techniques known, he filmed his operations with a 16 mm camera and thus, through his films, he continued to present his work at national and international congresses. An extraordinary surgeon, with more than forty procedures and several surgical instruments bearing his name, he is possibly the best urological surgeon of the twentieth century and today his work is an indissoluble part of the universal history of urology.

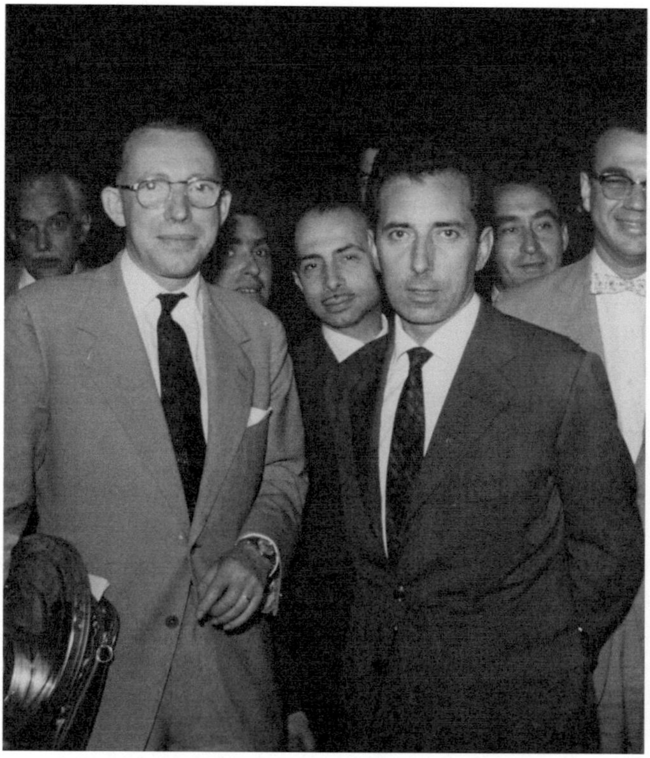

Fig. 22.10 José María Gil-Vernet (right) with Dr. W. Gregoire. At the V International Urology Course. Hospital Clínico. Barcelona 1968

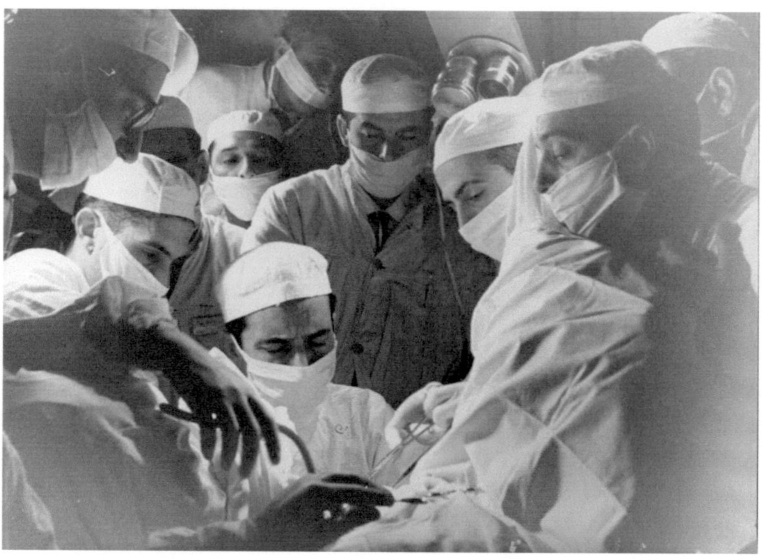

Fig. 22.11 José María Gil-Vernet performing a colocystoplasty at the III International Urology Course. Hospital Clínic. Barcelona 1962

Bibliography

1. Gil-Vernet Sedó JM, Gil-Vernet Vila JM. History of urological anatomy. In: Huri E, Veneziano D, editors. Anatomy for urologic surgeons in the digital era. Cham: Springer; 2021.
2. Gil-Vernet Sedó JM. Salvador Gil Vernet a pioneer in urological anatomy. De Historia Urologiae Europaeae. 2017;24:48–77.
3. Gil-Vernet JM, Arango O, Álvarez-Vijande R. Topographic anatomy and its development in urology in the 20th century. The work of Salvador Gil Vernet. Eur J Anat. 2016;20:231–47.
4. Gil-Vernet JM. The art of transforming science. Salvador Gil Vernet's modern understanding of urologic anatomy. Pamplona: Next Door Publishers; 2015.
5. Gil Vernet S. Patología urogenital. Three volume: 1- Prostate Cancer, 1944, Miguel Servet, editor, Barcelona; 2-Biology and Pathology of the Prostate, 1953, Paz Montalvo editor, Barcelona; 3-Diseases of the Prostate, 1955, Paz Montalvo, editor, Barcelona.
6. Gil Vernet S. Morphology and function of the Vesico-prostato-urethral musculature. Treviso: Edizione Canova; 1968.
7. Letter to Josep María Gil-Vernet. Hasta siempre, padre. (Farewell, father). José María Gil-Vernet Sedó. El Periódico, Barcelona, Tuesday 10/3/2020.
8. Fernández-Cruz Pérez A. Obituary session in memory of Prof. José María Gil-Vernet. An RANM. 2021;138(suppl 01):25–7.
9. Guardiola E, Baños JE. Josep María Gil-Vernet Vila. Gil-Vernet operations. Catalan physicians' contributions to medicine: a historical view through eponyms. Barcelona: Dr. Antoni Esteve Foundation; 2021. p. 257–67.
10. Angulo J, Otero I, Pérez M. Las bases de la cirugía moderna. José María Gil-Vernet Vila and urological surgery; Ed. Asociación Española de Urología; 2025. p. 241–256.

23

Sara Borrell Ruiz: Steroid Hormones

José Borrell Andrés

Sara Borrell Ruiz was born in September 1917, in Madrid, within a well-to-do middle-class family with a liberal character. On her father's side there was a long family tradition of pharmacists, since the beginning of the eighteenth century in Amer, Girona. But it was Sara's great-grandfather, Félix Borrell i Font born in Malgrat de Mar, Barcelona in 1822, who moved to Madrid in 1854 and opened a pharmacy, which remained open at number 5, Puerta del Sol until the 1960s, run by Sara Borrell's grandfather (Félix Borrell Vidal) and uncle (Félix Borrell García Lastra). Sara's grandfather, Félix Borrell Vidal (Madrid, 1858–1926), in addition to his dedication to pharmacy, developed an intense cultural activity in the world of music, painting and bullfighting. The Borrell Pharmacy was known during all those years for its intense social, cultural and political activity, intervening in a decisive and responsible way in the scientific and political sphere of those decisive years of the late nineteenth and early twentieth century in Spain. Sara's father, José Borrell García (Madrid, 1889–1986), did not follow the footsteps of his predecessors in the field of pharmacy. After high school, he took the exams to become a surveyor at the Instituto Geográfico y Catastral de España and later became an inspector at the Banco Hipotecario de España (Mortgage Bank of Spain)(Fig. 23.1).

All pictures published with permission of Family Borrell.

J. B. Andrés (✉)
Emeritus Professor, Researcher CSIC, Madrid, Spain

M. A. Cuesta, F. Mateo Vallejo (eds.), *Spain's Journey in Medicine*,
https://doi.org/10.1007/978-3-032-12221-6_23

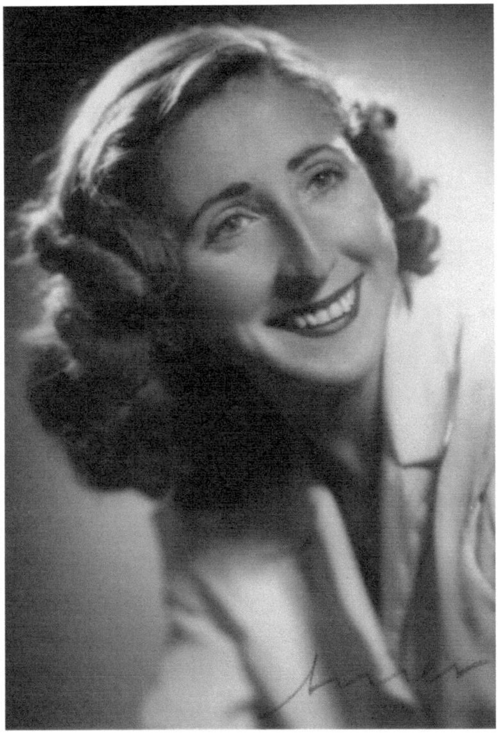

Fig. 23.1 Sara at the age of thirty

Sara's maternal family distinguished itself by supporting the higher education of women. Her grandmother, Clementina Albéniz Pascual, born in 1853 in Madrid, sister of the Spanish composer Isaac Albéniz, had studied teaching. She was a teacher at the Asociación para la Enseñanza de la Mujer, (Association for the Education of woman) founded in 1870 by Fernando de Castro Pajares, (pedagogue and priest).

After finishing her studies, she moved to Puerto Rico to direct one of the schools of the Sociedad de Instrucción de Mayagüez. Before her move to Puerto Rico, she had married physician Víctor Ruiz Rojo, with whom she had two children, Sara and Víctor, but unfortunately, he passed away when the children were young, so she decided to return to Spain. Here, she went back to work for the Asociación until her death in 1946. As educator, she was awarded with the Medalla del Trabajo.

Sara Ruiz Albéniz, daughter of Clementina and mother of Sara Borrell, also studied at the Association for the Education of Women, where she studied teaching, as well as piano and harp. She combined these studies with her great love of painting, being an assistant to the master Cecilio Pla. It was precisely in Pla's studio where she met the man who would become her husband and Sara's father, José Borrell García.

Sara began her university studies at the School of Pharmacy in 1933, but, due to the Spanish Civil War, she had to interrupt them in 1936. She resumed her studies in 1939 and finished her degree in 1940. To do so, she took all the pending subjects through regular exams, without resorting to the so-called "patriotic exams", which required an express declaration of loyalty to the new Franco's regime.

The years after the Civil War were especially difficult for Sara, as her father, a militant of the Republican Left party, was arrested and imprisoned on two occasions, although he was finally acquitted [1].

In September 1940, after finishing her degree, she was appointed assistant professor of practical classes in chemical analysis, a position she held for several years. Her doctoral thesis, directed by Professor Román Casares, consisted of an analytical study of the waters of the Tagus River. For more than a year, she collected about 150 samples from the river and its tributaries, performing 2500 analyses that allowed him to study the composition of the water depending on the terrain and the time of year. His thesis obtained the Extraordinary Doctorate Award [2].

In 1941, the School of Pharmacy incorporated a new discipline: Bromatology and Toxicology (B and T), being Sara appointed as assistant teacher for practical classes and the following year as assistant professor in B and T, a position she held until January 1949. In 1949, she resigned from this position after obtaining the position as scientific collaborator at the CSIC.

First Stays Abroad: Scotland and England

To further her studies, she applied for a scholarship from the Cultural Relations Board of the Ministry of Foreign Affairs and in October 1946, almost at the end of World War II. She moved to Great Britain, where he spent 10 months researching dairy products. Eight of those months were at the Hannah Dairy Research Institute in the town of Ayr in Scotland (Fig. 23.2). He also worked at the Chemical & City Analysts Department of the Glasgow Corporation and at the Dairy Research Institute in Reading. Her objective was to study the problems of dairy from a scientific and practical approach, covering production, sanitary control, British legislation and the manufacture of dairy products. In 1947, he returned to Spain to his

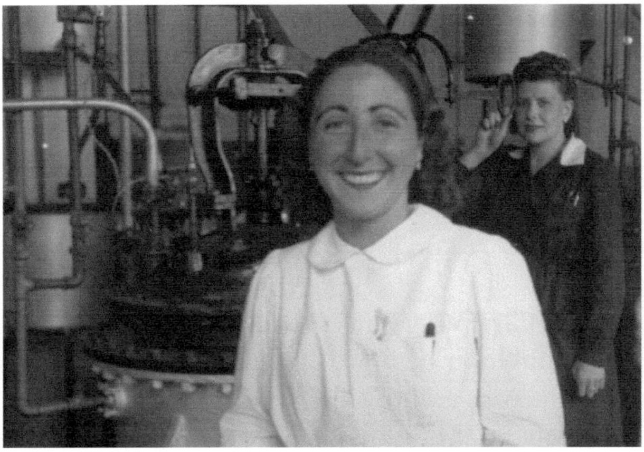

Fig. 23.2 Sara during her stage at the Hannah Dairy Research Institute in Air, Scotland, 1946

laboratory at the Faculty of Pharmacy in Madrid with a comprehensive view of the industrial sector and a solid basis for starting research in this field.

With the purpose of applying the knowledge acquired in the UK, she accepted a position as assistant inspector in the municipal laboratory of Madrid, in the milk section. However, she was unable to implement the techniques she had learned in Scotland, since her work was limited to routine tasks, such as the determination of milk density. And in the absence of opportunities to advance in her field of research, she decided to leave the post.

Her experience in the study of food chemistry awakened in her a growing interest in endocrinology. In 1950, she began working in the Experimental Endocrinology Laboratory of the CSIC, (directed by Gregorio Marañón) and located in the former Cajal Institute in the Cerro de San Blas, in the Retiro in Madrid, combining this work with her position as a scientist in the CSIC.

Eager to learn new methods emerging in the scientific literature—not only for the determination of amino acids, but also of sugars, steroids and other compounds—in 1951 she applied for a CSIC grant to study in Cambridge, at the Low Temperature Research Station, under the direction of Dr. Lea, whom she had met in the spring of 1947. There she learned, among other modern techniques, the chromatography for the determination of organic acids. Her work led to several publications in scientific journals, including a previous note in the journal *Nature* in 1952 [3].

With the intention of returning with as much preparation as possible, she applied for an extension of his fellowship, working at the Dunn Nutritional Laboratory of the University of Cambridge with Leslie J. Harris over the

ACTH, (adrenocorticotropic hormone) where she was initiated in the investigation of glucocorticoid hormone metabolism and the use of small rodents as experimental models. Subsequently, she spent several months at the Courtauld Institute of Biochemistry of the Middlesex Hospital in London with Edwards C. Dodds, Nobel Prize 1948, for his work on the synthesis of estrogens, where she specialized in the determination of adrenal corticosteroids and in the chromatographic separation of 17-ketosteroids. Finally, in July 1952, she returned to Madrid.

Her training in the prestigious research centers of the United Kingdom consolidated her interest in Endocrinology and her link to the Institute of Experimental Endocrinology of the CSIC directed by Gregorio Marañón.

At the Worcester Foundation for Experimental Biology

Prior to her return from Great Britain, Sara had applied for a fellowship at the Institute of International Education of New York to work at the Worcester Foundation for Experimental Biology (WF).

The Worcester Foundation for Experimental Biology was founded in 1944 in Shrewsbury, Massachusetts, by Gregory Pincus and Hudson Hoagland as an independent research center, devoted primarily to basic biomedical studies on the relationship between hormones and diseases such as cancer, heart disease and schizophrenia. However, WF is primarily recognized for the development of the first birth control pill, approved in May 1960 by the U.S. Food and Drug Administration (FDA). This revolutionary method changed women's lives and transformed society not only at the time, but even today.

Based on a natural product found in the barbasco plant, used ancestrally by indigenous women in Mexico as a contraceptive, the Mexican scientist Luis E. Miramontes Cárdenas, synthesized in 1951 the norethindrone, a synthetic progesterone at the UNAM university in Mexico, and after many changes of companies and scientists, Pincus, with Min Chueh Chang, WF senior scientist, demonstrated that progesterone acted as an ovulation inhibitor in humans. Their pioneering studies revolutionized the understanding of contraceptive medicine and led to the development of the combined oral contraceptive pill. In 1953, fertility specialist John Rock joined the team, and together they initiated clinical trials in Massachusetts that by the end of the decade expanded to Puerto Rico, Haiti, Mexico and Los Angeles.

Upon her arrival at WF, and in agreement with G. Pincus, she started working at Dorfman's laboratory with Betty Rubin. In that laboratory, the determination of 17-ketosteroids was investigated by means of a paper chromatography technique, innovative in its quantitative application, developed by Rubin herself. The stay at the WF was also an opportunity for Sara to deepen the methodology for the determination of estrogens by comparing the sensitivity of different methods and reagents. But beyond her work in the laboratory and the direct contact with the research being carried out in the different sections of the WF, her training was enriched by attending the conferences that were held regularly at the institute given by specialists in different fields of Endocrinology, with the participation of prestigious researchers from various centers in the United States and Europe. She also made several visits to research centers in New York and other cities, all of them dedicated to the study of steroid hormones, which allowed her to return to Spain with a current and broad vision of Endocrinology and in particular of steroid hormone research, making her a pioneer Spanish researcher in this area.

During her stay at the WF, Sara maintained a fluid correspondence with Gregorio Marañón, which reflected his interest as director in guaranteeing her the best possible conditions for her incorporation into the Institute that was being planned to be incorporated into what years later would become the Centro de Investigaciones Biológicas (CIB) of the CSIC in Madrid. In these letters, both Marañón and his direct collaborator, the physiologist José Luis Arteta, expressed their willingness to equip a laboratory in the best conditions. In a letter dated August 21, 1953, Marañón wrote to her:

> Make a list of the material required for the work.... We will find a way to pay for it and transport it.

Before her return to Spain, Pincus offered Sara a job at WF to join Dorfman and Rubin's group and participate more directly in the research on the production of oral contraceptives. However, Sara declined the offer and decided to return to Spain with the intention of starting and developing her own line of research at the new Institute of Experimental Endocrinology, with the purpose of contributing, as far as possible, to the incipient scientific development of the country in those 1950s.

It is possible that her decision to return to Spain was also influenced by the distance that would separate her from her parents if she accepted the position, as her mother was recovering from a recent accident. Likewise, it cannot be ruled out that Sara considered the possible repercussions that her participation in the research and development of the contraceptive pill might have had with the CSIC authorities—especially its Secretary General, Albareda, a member of Opus Dei—in the event of a later return to Spain.

Sara maintained always optimal contact with Pincus, Dorfman and Rubin. In fact, Dorfman visited Madrid in 1954 during a trip to Europe and even gave a lecture in March of that year at the CIB. At that time Sara was facing serious difficulties in setting up her laboratory in the new Institute. It was then that Pincus and Dorfman, aware of Sara's difficulties in setting up her laboratory, reiterated their offer for her to rejoin the Worcester Foundation in a more formal contract position. Since Sara had repeatedly expressed to Pincus her desire to remain close to her parents, he sent her a letter dated March 8, 1956, formally offering her:

> ...a position with the rank of assistant professor. This carries with it a salary of $5,750 per annum.... for exclusively biochemical research

in the Department of Pharmacology at the University of Puerto Rico School of Medicine. In a later letter, dated March 20 of the same year, Pincus wrote to her:

> I think that your family would specially appreciate the freedom and an atmosphere in which progress is being made. So many things are going on that they should be able to find much of interest for them.

It was clear that Pincus was very interested in having Sara join the research development at WF. However, he was not the only one: Dorfman also contacted her to offer her a position in his research group. However, in letters to Dorfman and Pincus in July 1956, Sara regretfully told them of her decision to continue working in Spain and to accompany her parents. Nevertheless, she maintained personal contact for years with both scientists and especially with Betty Rubin, whose friendship remained until her death.

Return to Spain

Upon her return to Madrid at the end of 1953 to the Laboratory of Experimental Endocrinology, she began to implement the methods learned for the determination of corticoids and 17-ketosteroids. After the bad experiences after her first return to Spain, when she could not put into practice what she had learned during her stays in the United Kingdom, Sara showed a clear concern and worry about the possibility of applying in the best conditions the

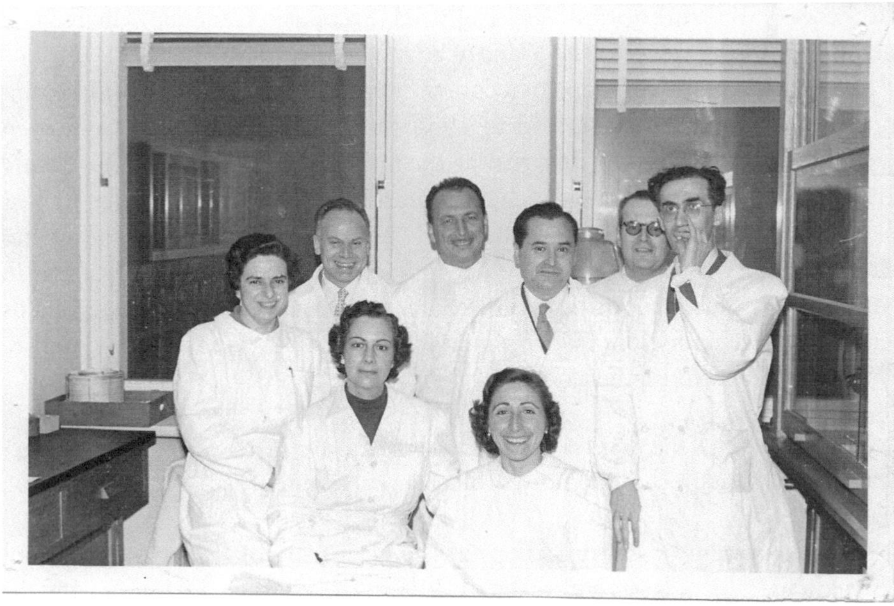

Fig. 23.3 The Marañón Group at the Instituto de Endocrinología Experimental in the new Centro de Investigaciones Biológicas. *Sara sitting in the middle, from the left to the right: Aurora Carvallido, Puchol, Carmen López (worker with Arteta), Zamorano, Arteta, Rodrigo, Albarracín*

knowledge acquired in the WF. Already in 1954, at the Institute of Experimental Endocrinology, she continued to work with the methods learned in the United States, adapting them to the conditions and materials available at that time. This process was slow due to the technical and reagents limitations of the time, but thanks to the support of both Marañón and Arteta, she was able to develop her own lines of work. Between 1954 and 1957, she devoted much of her time to the implementation of paper and column chromatography methods for the separation and analysis of different steroid metabolites (Fig. 23.3).

However, on October 15, 1955, a laboratory accident nearly cut short her scientific career. While distilling to purify ethyl alcohol with potassium hydroxide (necessary for steroid determination), the flask exploded and injured her eyes. During the first days after the accident, it was feared that she might lose her sight, and it took him months to recover, which she expressed in a letter addressed to the Secretary General of CSIC on March 27, 1956. In this letter, in addition to thanking her colleagues and especially Arteta for the help received both at the time of the accident and in the months that followed, she expressed to Albareda the need to:

The CSIC should study the creation of an insurance against accidents at work to protect us financially, since the salaries that most of us receive do not allow us to cover extraordinary expenses.

There is no record of any response or action by CSIC management to this request.

In 1957, shortly after the transfer of the Institute from Cerro de San Blas to the new CIB in calle Velázquez, Arteta passed away at the age of 55. His loss was a hard blow for Sara, as he had been a fundamental pillar both in the creation of the new institute and in its integration. Sadly, it was not long before Marañón passed away on March 27, 1960. The death of her teacher, together with that of Arteta, represented an extremely difficult moment for Sara, because from then on, she perceived a change in the spirit that Don Gregorio (as she called Marañón) had planned to promote at the Institute of Experimental Endocrinology.

In 1957, she obtained the position of senior scientific researcher of the CSIC presenting a research project focused on the "study of hormonal metabolites in different physiological and pathological states."

The new institute integrated into the CIB had incorporated new and outstanding research groups, such as those led by Gabriela Morreale and Francisco Escobar, Alberto Sols and José Luis Rodríguez Candela. After Marañón's death, the institute adopted his name, becoming known as the "Instituto Gregorio Marañón", with Rodríguez Candela as its director. In the same year of its creation (1960), Sara was appointed Secretary of the Institute, a position she resigned in 1962 due to disagreements with the Institute's management.

In 1963 the Steroid Section of the Marañón Institute was created, which under Sara's direction consolidated several lines of research related to steroid metabolism in special physiological situations, such as pregnancy, lactation and menopause, as well as in endocrine and metabolic pathologies. In her laboratory the training of young doctors was implemented through the completion of doctoral theses, consolidating the reputation of the laboratory as a reference center in the study of steroid hormones in Spain. But Sara always maintained a special interest in transposing the laboratory techniques as much as possible to the human clinic. This led her to establish contacts with Spanish hospitals and clinical endocrinologists to perform specific hormone determinations, in many cases exclusive to the technology that the laboratory possessed, in clinical cases of special relevance. Obviously, the elaboration of such determinations entailed an expense that could not be covered by the laboratory itself. For this reason, and in the spirit of honesty and respect for the public service that always characterized Sara, she requested authorization from the General Secretary of the CSIC to carry out such work; on March 20, 1963, the Deputy General Secretary of the CSIC sent an official letter authorizing Sara Borrell at the Gregorio Marañón Institute carry out the following work

> *collaboration work that has been repeatedly requested by prestigious clinicians, and to receive for such collaboration work such amounts as may be stipulated, amounts to be received through the Administration of the Biological Research Center, and intended to defray some of the expenses of the research work to be carried out.*

During those years Sara maintained close collaboration with research groups in other countries, especially in the United Kingdom, France and the United States, which allowed her to keep abreast of scientific and technological advances in the field of endocrinology. In 1963, the *International Study Group for Steroid Hormones* was created in Rome, and Sara was nominated as a member of the International Committee of this group. That same year, in the United States, Elsevier began publication of the scientific journal *Steroids*, in whose foundation Sara participated as a member of the Editorial Committee and Chief Executive Officer in Spain. In 1964, she was appointed *Affiliate Member* of *the Royal Society of Medicine* in London. During those years, the laboratory of the Steroids Section was visited by national and foreign researchers from different countries, with the aim of updating in the modern techniques for the determination of steroid hormones developed there (Fig. 23.4).

Sara always attached great importance to the training of both new researchers and technical staff, which led her to maintain a relatively small working group, allowing her to develop appropriate training processes of the highest scientific quality. She used to make the completion of a doctoral thesis coincide with the start of a new one, always in relation to the research lines of the Steroids Section. As a result of this selective approach, throughout his scientific career he supervised only six doctoral theses.

The research work in the Steroid Section, under Sara's direction, evolved over time. An important leap in the development of the work was the acquisition in the mid 60's of an Aminco-Bowman spectrophotofluorimeter, which allowed the determination of both steroid hormones and bioamines in a much more efficient and selective way than with the techniques that had been developed in the laboratory until then. The acquisition of this equipment, given its very high cost, the need for a special location and the difficulties of importing equipment from abroad in those years was a hard and arduous task for Sara, who, knowing the importance it had for

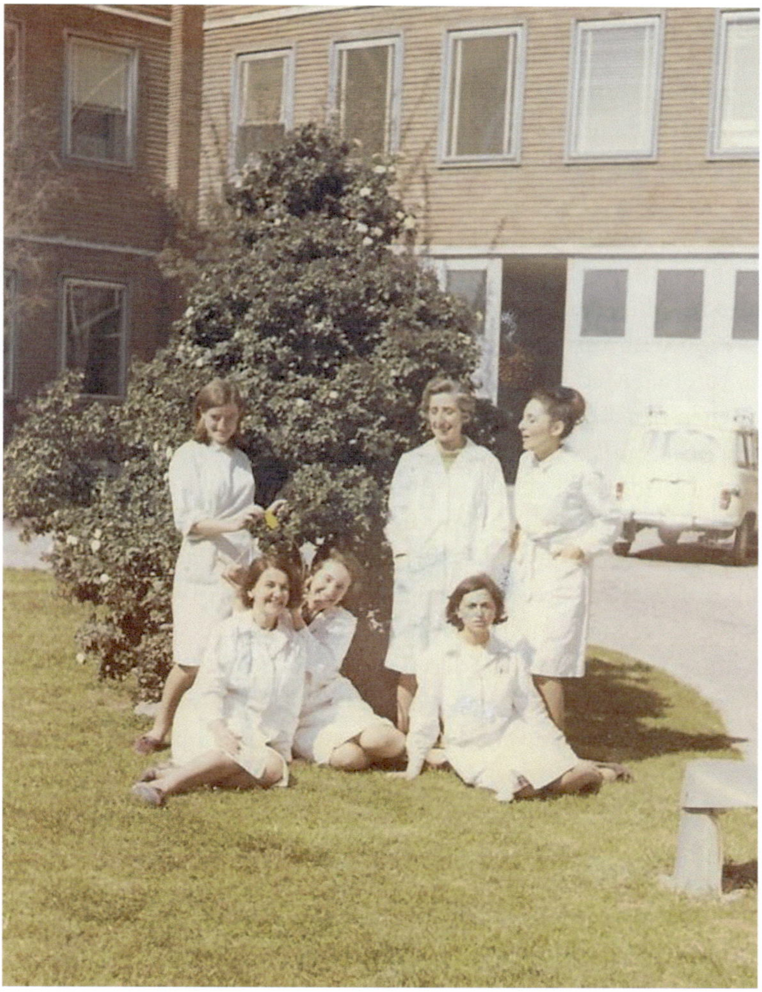

Fig. 23.4 1967, The Unit of Steroids in the Centro Investigaciones Biológicas, Madrid

the development of the work in the Steroid Section, did not stop until she got it. In the beginning, the work focused on the study of steroid metabolism, both in humans [4] and in the cat [5] (used as an experimental model due to its similarity to humans in the metabolism of glucocorticoids). Subsequently, research was directed towards the study of the interactions between steroid hormones in the adrenal cortex and catecholamines in the adrenal medulla [6]. This line of work derived, in the 1970s, with the emergence of Neuroendocrinology, in the investigation of the mechanisms of control of these hormones by the cerebral monoaminergic systems.

Cerebral monoaminergic system refers to a group of neurotransmitter systems in the brain that use monoamine neurotransmitters, such as dopamine, norepinephrine, serotonin and histamine (see Chap. 29).

These studies focused on stress [7] and on the processes of dependence and tolerance to drugs such as morphine [8] and ethanol [9], using the cat and the rat as experimental models.

The development of new determination techniques also allowed an important advance in the development of methods for the determination of these hormones in samples from human patients, which meant a period of fruitful collaboration with various clinicians and health institutions and in particular with the Internal Medicine Department of the Hospital Clínico San Carlos in Madrid, then directed by the internist José Casas Sánchez and the Pediatrics Department of La Paz Hospital in Madrid.

Sara combined the direction of the research group with her participation in national and international congresses, as well as with further stays in foreign laboratories. An example of this was her stay in 1962 at the *Istituto Superiore di Sanità* in Rome, where she carried out studies on "Two-dimensional chromatographic techniques with isotopes applied to the study of intermediary carbohydrate metabolism", under the direction of the Nobel Prize winner Ernst Boris Chain. In 1967, she made a research stay at the Pasteur Institute in Paris, where she worked for 6 months on the development of radioimmunoassay techniques applied to steroid hormones. On his return to Madrid, she tried to implement this methodology in the Steroid Section, but it was impossible because she could not get the basic equipment necessary to work with radioisotopes in safe conditions. In addition to his activity in the laboratory, she was a consultative member of different organizations: Commission for the Evaluation of Active Ingredients of major consumption in the Seguridad Social or National Member of the General Council of the Spanish College of Pharmacists.

In 1975 the Centro de Biología Molecular (CBM) was inaugurated at the Universidad Autónoma de Madrid as a center coordinated with the CSIC. This meant the transfer of different research groups from the CIB to this center and in particular the group of Eladio Viñuelas and Margarita Salas, who belonged to the Instituto Gregorio Marañón since their return from the United States. This brought with it an important remodeling of the Marañón Institute and Sara became Vice-Director of the Institute.

With the arrival of democracy in this country, at the end of the 70's the CSIC began a period of remodeling and restructuring of its Centers and

Institutes. Based on the new CSIC organic regulations (Royal Decree 34501, 1977), the Steroids Section disappeared in November 1979 and its staff was integrated into Research Teams, one of them the Neuroendocrine Team headed by Sara. The new CSIC organic regulations also brought with them a new mechanism for appointing institute directors in the institution, by vote of all the doctors linked to each center. On this basis, Sara was elected and appointed Director of the Gregorio Marañón Institute of Endocrinology on February 1, 1980, possibly being the first woman to reach this position in the CSIC through a democratic system of election.

In 1983 Sara retired and left all research activity at CSIC. From that moment on she dedicated herself with special attention to the care of her father, who died 3 years later in 1986 at the age of 97. Sara died in May 1999 and her remains lie next to those of her parents in the municipal cemetery of her beloved town of El Escorial in Madrid.

Sara Borrell's professional career for almost 50 years was marked by a deep passion for knowledge, scientific rigor and commitment to the training of new generations and represents the vocation of a lifetime dedicated to study and research in the field of Endocrinology, with the constant desire to contribute to scientific progress and social welfare. Her contributions have been pioneering on the analysis and metabolism of steroids hormones, with emphasis on sex steroids and their influence on reproductive health. In recognition of her work, over the years the Instituto de Salud Carlos III of the Ministry of Health gave her name to a postdoctoral contract program that is still in force.

References

1. Santesmases MJ. Género, afición y mérito: una biografía de Sara Borrell Ruiz. Arenal. 2017;24:287–318.
2. Borrell S. Estudio analítico de las aguas del rio Tajo. Anal Real Acad Farm. 1944.
3. Lea CH, Rhodes DN, Borrell S. A reaction of D-glucosamine in the presence of "dry" protein. Nature. 1952;169:1097–8.
4. Borrell S. The excretion of Pettenkofer chromogens by healthy subjects and patients with various endocrine disorders. J Clin Endocrinol Metab. 1961;21:1321–7.
5. Borrell S. Urinary steroids of cats: corticosteroid-like substances. J Biochem. 1963;89:54–7.

6. Borrell J, Borrell S. Alterations of adrenal corticosteroids and catecholamines during amino-glutethimide feeding. Hor Metabol Res. 1974;6:414–7.
7. Borrell J, Torrellas A, Guaza C, Borrell S. Sound stimulation and its effects on the pituitary-adrenocortical function and brain catecholamines in rats. Neuroendocrinol. 1980;31:53–9.
8. Guaza C, Torrellas A, Borrell J, Borrell S. Effects of morphine upon the pituitary-adrenal system and adrenal catecholamines: a comparative study in cats and rats. Pharmacol Biochem Behav. 1979;11:57–63.
9. Guaza C, Borrell S. Effect of naloxone administration upon responses of adrenal hormones to withdrawal from ethanol. Psychopharmacol. 1984;82:181–4.

24

Joan Oró: The Origin of Life

Joan Oró Trilla

Joan Oró I Florensa was born on October 26, 1923, in Lleida, Spain, within a family of bakers. From his childhood he showed an insatiable curiosity for the great questions of existence. He reflected on the origin of life, the purpose of humanity and the possibility of life outside the Earth. His formation in the Marist Brothers provided him with a religious basis that nourished his intellectual restlessness, although it did not provide him with the answers he was looking for. This dissatisfaction led him to explore philosophy, but he did not find convincing explanations either. It was then that, definitively, he turned to science, immersing himself in books that deeply enlivened his fascination. Among them, two works were key in his life: The Origin of Species by Charles Darwin and The Plurality of Inhabited Worlds by Camille Flammarion. At the age of 16, while walking near his home, he had a revelation. He decided that his life would be dedicated to the study of the origin of life. That day, Oró exclaimed with firmness and conviction: "I know what I will do, I will study the origin of life". In 1942, he entered the University of Barcelona to study Chemistry for this purpose. During his training, he excelled especially in

All pictures published with permission of the Fundació Joan Oró.

J. O. Trilla (✉)
President of the Foundation Joan Oró, Lleida, Spain

M. A. Cuesta, F. Mateo Vallejo (eds.), *Spain's Journey in Medicine*,
https://doi.org/10.1007/978-3-032-12221-6_24

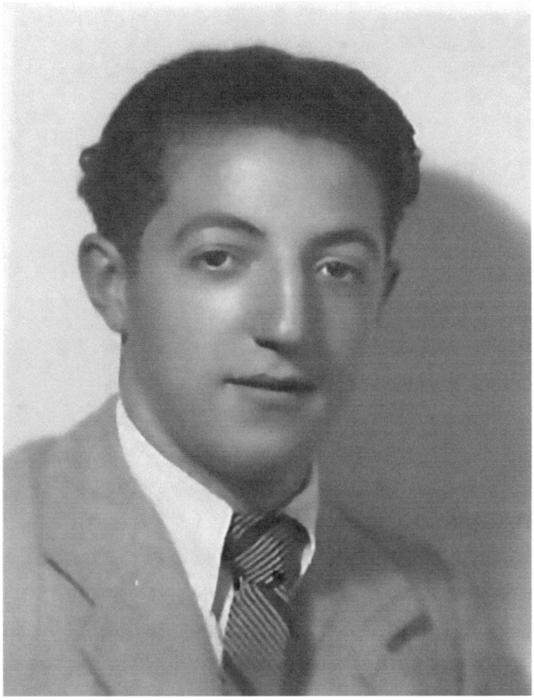

Fig. 24.1 Joan Oró before starting University Studies in Chemistry in University of Barcelona, 1942

organic chemistry and became interested in biochemistry, a discipline still in its infancy in Spain [1–5] (Fig. 24.1).

His eagerness to learn led him to set up his own laboratory at home, another sign of his determination and passion. In 1947, after graduating, he married Francesca Forteza and returned to Lleida. There, the scientific opportunities were limited, so he tried several businesses that failed. In the end, he went back to work in the family bakery to support his slowly growing family. Despite the economic hardships, his interest in the origin of life never waned, especially fueled by long nights watching the starry sky. He knew that, to fulfill his dream, he needed opportunities beyond Spain, so, in 1949, he wrote to more than fifty universities in the United States seeking support to continue his studies in Biochemistry. In 1951, he received a positive response from the Rice Institute in Houston to pursue graduate studies in Chemical Engineering. Despite his limited economic resources and his poor command of English, he emigrated alone to the United States, leaving his wife and three children in Lleida. In Houston, he obtained his Ph.D. in biochemistry in 1956 from Baylor College of Medicine [6]. During that period, he also began teaching Chemistry at the University of Houston, where he founded his own laboratory. There, he gathered a group of young scientists and began to develop his pioneering studies on the origin of life. In 1959, he achieved one of the greatest achievements of his career: the abiotic synthesis of adenine, an essential component for life.

Abiotic relates to things in the environment that are not living.

Abiotic synthesis of adenine refers to the formation of adenine, a key component of nucleic acids (DNA and RNA), from non-living matter.

His work was published in Nature in 1961 [7]. This discovery, together with Stanley Miller's 1952 experiment, was a major milestone in the search for the origin of life.

The Stanley Miller experiment was a pivotal study in the field of abiogenesis, exploring how organic molecules could have formed from inorganic precursors under prebiotic Earth conditions [8].

Oró was a pioneer in connecting the study of the origin of life on Earth with the exploration of the universe. In 1961, he published a second article in the journal *Nature*, in which he presented a revolutionary hypothesis that prebiotic material, essential for the emergence of life on Earth, could have arrived from space via comets, challenging established ideas and opening new frontiers in science [9].

He continued the research to clarify the synthesis of these organic compounds through special circumstances such as electrical discharges, under high energy conditions and other studies on the Murray meteorite [10–12].

Throughout his career, he worked closely with NASA, participating since 1963 in the Apollo program, where he was in charge of analyzing the lunar samples brought back by his missions, contributing to confirm the absence of signs of life on the Moon. He also participated in the Viking program during the 1970s, an ambitious scientific challenge with the aim of detecting signs of life on Mars. Thanks to their collaboration, the results that initially suggested the possibility of life in the Martian samples were correctly interpreted. Although he lived in the United States, he played a key role in promoting scientific research in our country since the 1970s. After his retirement in 1994, he returned definitively to Spain where he continued to promote research, innovation and scientific projects. He passed away in Barcelona in 2004, leaving a legacy of remarkable scientific contributions and deeply human values [13].

The Path to the Origin of Life on Earth

The origin of life is one of the most intriguing scientific questions, and several theories have been developed to explain how life arose from inert matter. Among the most significant are the ideas of Aleksander Oparin and J.B.S. Haldane, which gave rise to the primordial soup hypothesis [14, 15].

Oparin, a Soviet biochemist, was one of the first to propose in 1924, a model for the chemical origin of life. He suggested that the Earth's primitive atmosphere, devoid of oxygen and rich in methane, ammonia and hydrogen, favored the formation of organic molecules from simple compounds, driven by energy sources such as ultraviolet light and lightning. These molecules would accumulate in the oceans, forming the primordial soup from which, through gradual chemical evolution, life emerged. Almost simultaneously, the British biologist John B. S. Haldane proposed in 1929 a similar idea, centered on a reducing atmosphere (with very low amounts of free oxygen) that favored the formation of organic compounds. He introduced the term prebiotic soup to describe the oceans where these chemicals were concentrated. According to him, life could have originated in warm, shallow pools, where chemical reactions accelerated the formation of complex molecules, eventually giving rise to life. These ideas induced later experimental work, such as Stanley Miller's experiment of the 1950s. Simulating primitive chemical earth conditions, they recreated an atmosphere with electrical sparks that mimicked lightning. The result was the formation of organic molecules, supporting the primordial soup hypothesis and demonstrating that the building blocks of life could form under primitive Earth-like conditions. The primordial soup hypothesis, formulated by Oparin and Haldane, together with Miller's experiment, represented a fundamental milestone in understanding how life could have arisen from simple chemical compounds. These studies inspired the young scientist Joan Oró, who, motivated by these advances, began to investigate how the building blocks of life could have formed in primitive conditions on Earth. As Oró expressed, "I understood that if Darwin said that the most complex beings come from the simplest ones, it was a matter of descending until reaching the simplest being that could exist. Then, I would surely arrive at the last question: well, where does such a simple being come from?"

The Discovery of the Abiotic Synthesis of Adenine; an Essential Molecular for Life

Thus, with his characteristic determination, in 1959, at the University of Houston, Joan Oró began to develop a series of experiments inspired by Miller's work, but focused mainly on hydrogen cyanide, which he thought could play an important role in the prebiotic chemistry of the Earth.

Prebiotic chemistry is the study of the chemical reactions that led to the origin of life on Earth, focusing on the formation of organic molecules from non-living matter.

This extremely reactive molecule had appeared in Miller's experiment as an intermediate by-product, which aroused Oró's interest. Fascinated by its ability to polymerize, he was initially able to successfully synthesize several amino acids (including glycine, serine and alanine) from a mixture that included hydrogen cyanide, ammonia and water. When he subsequently analyzed the mixture obtained in his experiments, he noticed a small dark spot on the paper chromatography, in the expected place for adenine. Although at the time he considered the signal too weak to be significant, he decided not to discard it. That clue led him to question whether hydrogen cyanide might have acted as a precursor to the essential purines on early Earth. To test his hypothesis, the Lleida-born scientist conducted an experiment that would lead to one of the most important discoveries of his career. On Christmas night 1959, he could synthesize genetic molecules from hydrogen cyanide, water and ammonia, common components in stars and interstellar space. He let the product dry overnight and the next day, analyzed the chromatogram under a UV lamp at 250 nm. To his surprise, a large dark spot appeared. Analysis of the components made it clear that he had succeeded in synthesizing adenine, one of nitrogenous bases of nucleic acids (DNA and RNA). That moment, as the Catalan biochemist later recalled, was one of the most exciting of his life: "I got goose bumps. I was alone, in the dark, seeing what was in front of me, and I couldn't believe it". The chemical reaction consisted of the spontaneous polymerization of five hydrogen cyanide molecules to form adenine. The discovery was published in the Biochemical and Biophysical Research Communications in June 1960 under the title "Synthesis of adenine from hydrogen cyanide", and in Nature in September 1961, under the title "Mechanism of adenine synthesis from hydrogen cyanide under possible primitive Earth conditions" [7]. In August 1961, he presented his findings at the fifth International Congress of Biochemistry in Moscow. He had just achieved what, deep down, he most desired and inspired his life: on the one hand, he had managed to advance in the study the mechanisms leading to the origin of life, and, on the other hand, he had given a decisive step to begin to establish himself as a scientist with a name of his own in world science [16]. Together with Miller's experiment, the abiotic synthesis of adenine is one of major breakthroughs in the study of the origin of life, paving the way for future generations of scientists in prebiotic chemistry (Fig. 24.2).

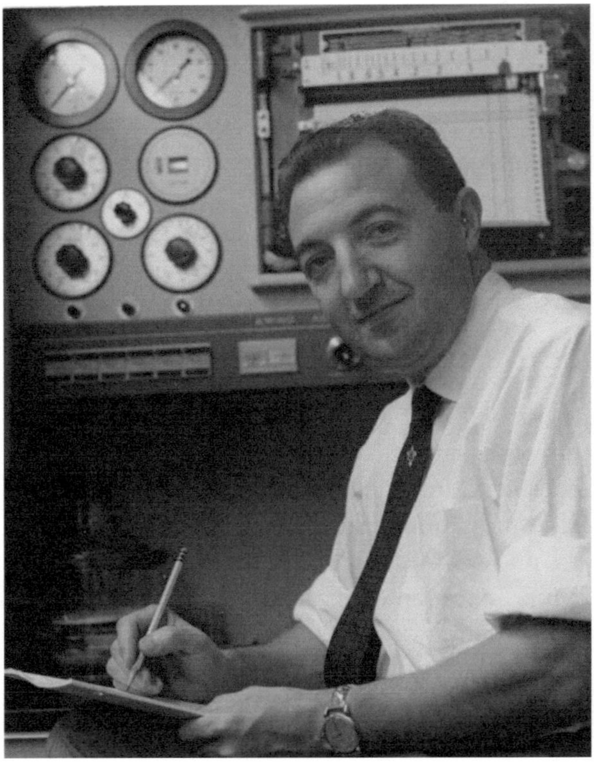

Fig. 24.2 1959. Joan Oró in his Lab in Houston, performing the experiments leading to the abiotic synthesis of Adenine

Comets and Basic Compounds for Life

The finding of the adenine synthesis formed the basis on which Oró took a riskier and more speculative step than those he had taken until then in his research on the origin of life. In this sense, he was a pioneer in integrating research on the origin of life on Earth with the exploration of the universe, suggesting that comets could have played a crucial role in this process. In 1961, in his article in Nature, "Comets and the Formation of Biochemical Compounds on the Primitive Earth," he postulated that comets could have brought to Earth prebiotic compounds fundamental to origin of life. This theory was based on the idea that comets, laden with carbon-rich materials such as hydrogen cyanide, amino acids and other organic molecules, could have impacted with the early Earth in large quantities, increasing the number of organic compounds available for prebiotic chemistry. According to Oró, comets not only contributed these basic compounds, may also have helped create a suitable environment for the chemical reactions that gave rise to life to take place. In fact, hydrogen cyanide, which he had previously identified as a key component in the abiotic synthesis of complex molecules, was present in comets and was considered a crucial ingredient for the creation of essential organic molecules [9]. This hypothesis was groundbreaking because it extended the frontiers of prebiotic chemistry beyond Earth's primitive oceans, suggesting that life might not only have originated on Earth, but also have been favored by cosmic processes. Oró made the following reasoning: "If comets carry hydrogen cyanide, if it seems proven that they fell on the primitive Earth with much more profusion and frequency than they do now, it is very logical to think that those comets brought the organic material from which biochemical molecules fundamental for life can be generated". The idea that comets might be carriers of prebiotic molecules became a major focus of astrobiological research. In later years, studies of the composition of comets confirmed that these celestial bodies contain large amounts of carbon, hydrogen and other elements essential life, providing strong support for his biochemist's theory. Oró's vision opened a field of research that today is crucial in astrobiology.

Astrobiology is a scientific field within the life and environmental sciences that studies the origins, early evolution, distribution, and future of life in the universe by investigating its deterministic conditions and contingent events.

His proposal not only challenged the traditional view that prebiotic compounds originated exclusively on Earth, but also laid the groundwork for the exploration of how organic matter could have spread throughout the solar system, influencing the chemistry of other planets and, potentially, life on other worlds. Over the decades, Oró's hypothesis on comets and prebiotic molecules has established itself as one of the most interesting proposals for understanding the origin of life on Earth and its possible existence in other corners of the universe. The link between organic chemistry and astrobiology, which he advanced in the 1960s, continues to be one of the main lines of research for scientists studying the origin of life and the possibility of extraterrestrial life. Just after the publication of this article, Joan Oró began to collaborate with NASA and, in 1963, he began to propose scientific research proposals to the Agency itself (Fig. 24.3).

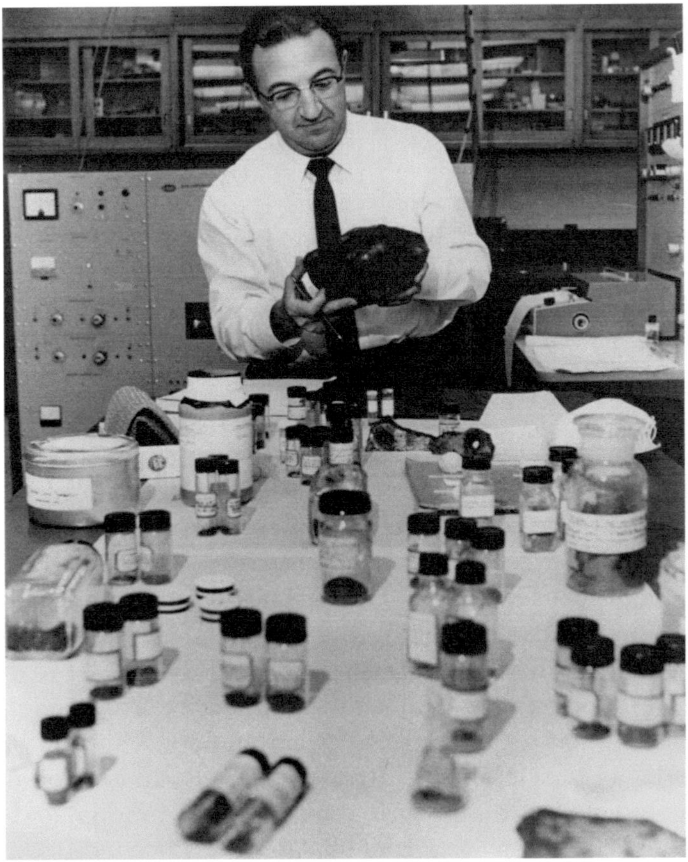

Fig. 24.3 Joan Oró analyzing meteorites in Depth because he believed they could carry prebiotic molecules to Earth

Apollo and Viking Program

In 1963, Oró's association with NASA, the organism created by the U.S. government in 1958 as an independent agency to coordinate and conduct aerospace research, began. NASA, an acronym for the National Aeronautics and Space Administration, was established to counter the advantage gained by the USSR in the space race in late 1950s. To this end, NASA called upon the most outstanding scientists to collaborate in its space programs. Thus, Joan Oró joined the agency's research with a group of scientists from seven U.S. universities working on the Apollo program, specifically in the area of organic chemistry. He assumed the role of Principal Investigator, a position that placed him at

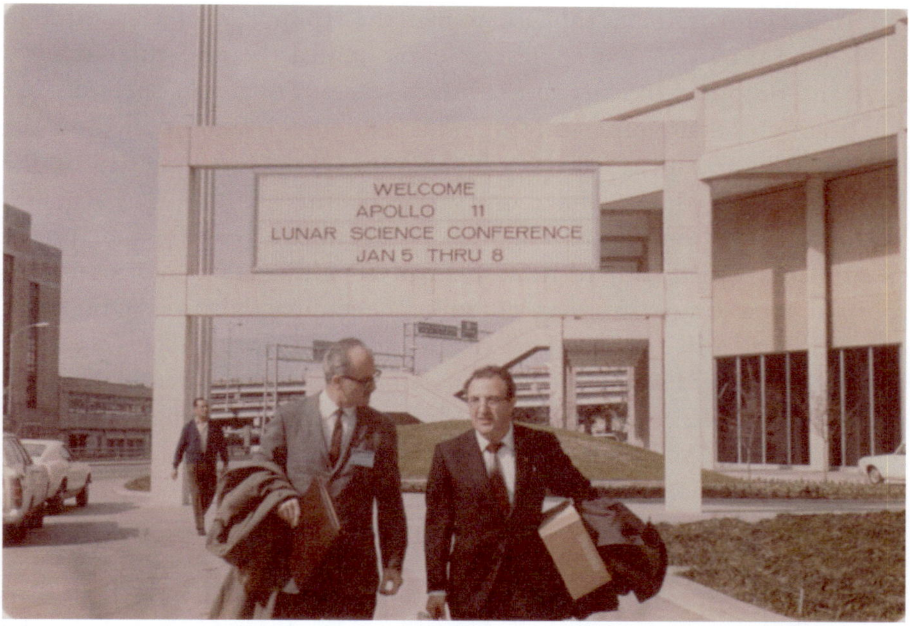

Fig. 24.4 Joan Oró was a key figure in the First analysis of the lunar simples from the Apollo program. On the picture going to the "Apollo 11 Lunar Science Conference Jan 5 1970"

the head of the University of Houston team, collaborating directly with NASA. The intervention of the Spanish biochemist in the Apollo program, the historic space mission that led Neil Armstrong and Buzz Aldrin to set foot on the Moon on July 20, 1969, was crucial, since he had the privilege of accessing the lunar samples brought back by the Apollo 11 mission and also from subsequent missions. His laboratory, equipped with advanced technology such as a gas chromatograph and a mass spectrometer, allowed thorough analysis of these samples. However, no evidence of life on the Moon was detected, as no significant presence of organic material was found in the samples obtained. In Oró's own words: "There is hardly any organic matter on the Moon", and he acknowledged that these results of the analysis of the lunar samples were not a disappointment for the researchers; they were already expected. "The Moon is a satellite with very little gravitational mass, the gravity is very low and, since its formation, it cannot retain water or any volatile matter. In addition, it has hardly any atmosphere," said the Catalan biochemist (Fig. 24.4).

In 1964, during the development of the Apollo program, a meeting was held in Stanford University in California, with the participation of a hundred scientists, including Oró, to plan the exploration of Mars through the Viking program. The Spanish scientist joined the molecular analysis team and proposed to carry miniaturized versions of a mass spectrometer and a gas chromatograph to Mars. This equipment was installed on the landers, which also carried three biological experiments designed by the Biology team. Viking 1 landed on Chryse Planitia on July 20, 1976, and Viking 2 landed on Utopia Planitia on September 3, 1976. One of the experiments, called Labeled Release, involved adding an aqueous nutrient solution to a sample of Martian soil. The radioactivity detectors were designed to identify emissions of gaseous substances with 14 C (radiocarbon), which would be interpreted as possible evidence of microbial metabolism. The results were positive on both landers, detecting CO2. This finding was received with enthusiasm at NASA and the U.S. Congress immediately authorized its announcement. Just before the event, a meeting was organized to finalize the details of the presentation. However, during the meeting, Oró quickly identified a plausible cause for the positive result. He recalled that sodium formate, a molecule he had studied years earlier, was present in the nutrient mixture. From his knowledge, he deduced that any oxidizing substance in the Martian soil could have oxidized the formate, leading to the detected CO2 emissions. His explanation surprised his colleagues and helped to cool initial excitement. Finally, it was decided that, at the press conference, it would be announced that there was some evidence suggesting the presence of life on Mars, but that Oró had proposed an abiotic alternative for the result. "I asked permission to speak, requesting the consent of the biologists, and offered to explain what I thought. There were tense faces in the room, a stony silence, because, of course, I was breaking that excitement about having discovered life on Mars, which was a prospect that excited everyone. But no, it was the formic acid, when it oxidized, chemically and not biologically, that produced that confusion, that feeling of the existence of life that was actually false," explained Oró. Seen from today's perspective, it is impressive how Joan Oró managed to maintain a dissonant stance in the face of the general excitement. His attitude reflected the scientific rigor that must prevail when dealing with extraordinary claims. Since the time of the Viking program, the general consensus has been that the positive response of the Labeled Release experiment was caused by a non-biological process (Fig. 24.5).

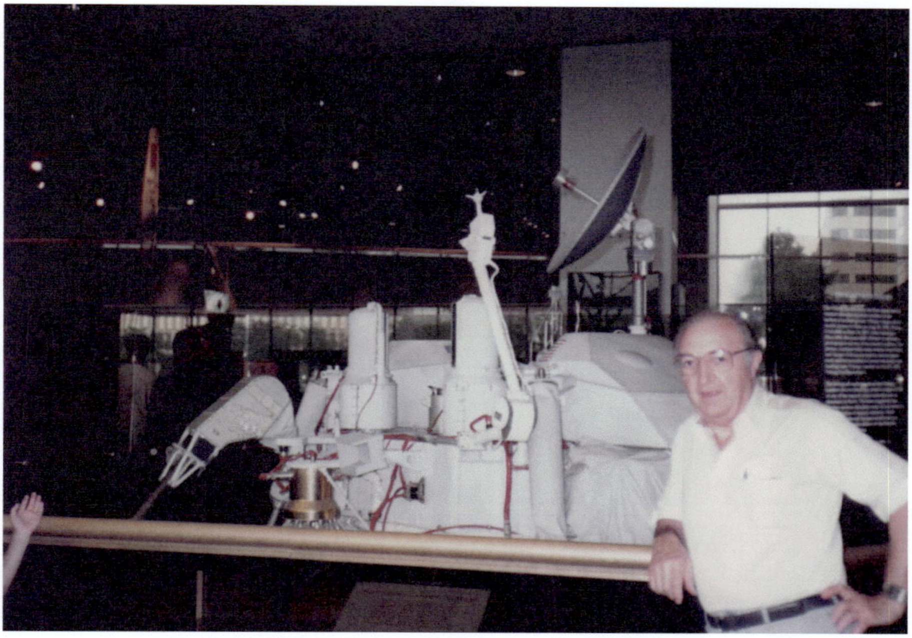

Fig. 24.5 Joan Oró participated in the design of the Scientific experiments of the Viking (I and II) program

Boosting Research in Spain

Oró had a long and distinguished career in the United States, but throughout his life he maintained a strong link with Spain, despite living and developing his career mainly in Houston. Recognized for his research on the origin of life, he was the object of multiple attempts by Spanish institutions to facilitate his return to the country and to integrate him in outstanding scientific projects. His contribution to the promotion of Spanish science began in the 1960s, when his participation in meetings of the Spanish Society of Biochemistry made him known as a scientist who emigrated to the United States. Thanks to his international success, he was invited by the University of Granada and the Universitat Autònoma de Barcelona to lead academic projects. In 1971 he accepted a Chair of Biophysics at the Universitat Autònoma de Barcelona, and founded the Institute of Fundamental Biology, but unfulfilled promises made him return to Houston after a few months. In 1975, Joan Oró was involved in the creation of the Severo Ochoa Institute of Molecular Biology in Madrid and the Institute of Biophysics and Neurobiology in Barcelona, projects promoted by Federico Mayor Zaragoza. Although the Institute of Biophysics and Neurobiology was linked to the CSIC and served as an embryo for future research centers, Joan Oró withdrew from the project due to

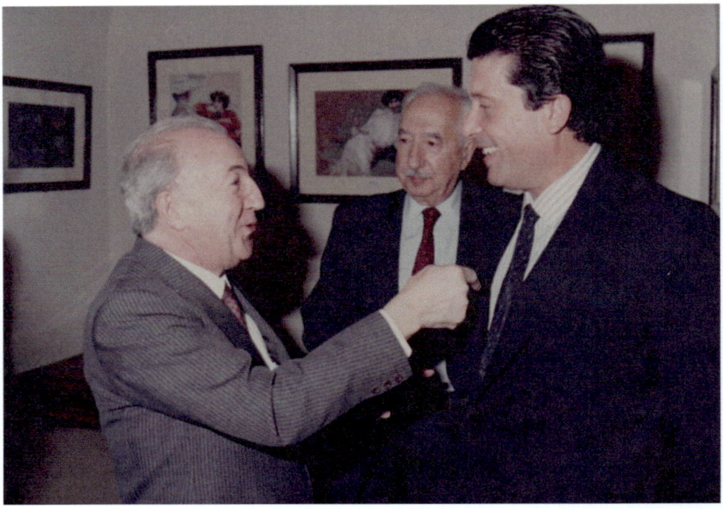

Fig. 24.6 Joan Oró with Federico Mayor Zaragoza and Francisco Grande Covián boosting the Scientific Research in Spain from the 1970s onwards

lack of adequate support and resources. This reinforced his decision to continue his career in the States, where academic freedom and means were more favorable. He also promoted the creation of the Mediterranean Center for Research and Development (currently the Centre d'Estudis Avançats de Blanes), inaugurated in 1984, to promote oceanography and other related scientific fields. In the political sphere, in 1980, he ran for election to the Parliament of Catalonia with Convergència i Unió, where he was elected deputy for the demarcation of Lleida to try to strengthen the scientific competences of the Generalitat de Catalunya, but the slowness of the transfer of competences slowed down his initiatives and he abandoned his seat in 1981. Despite the difficulties, he maintained an active link with Spain and Catalonia. He founded the Associació Amics de Gaspar de Portolà, in 1981, to foster scientific relations between Catalonia and California, and in 1986 he participated in the creation of the Fundació Catalana per a la Recerca (currently Fundació Catalana per a la Recerca i la Innovació) to promote research and innovation in Catalonia. In Lleida, he created the Fundació Joan Oró in 1993, dedicated to promoting his scientific legacy and fostering research. Since 1994, it has focused on promoting the construction of the Parc Astronòmic del Montsec and the Observatori del Montsec, both located in the territorial demarcation of Lleida, which finally became a reality in 2008. With these words Oró summed up perfectly the importance he attached to research and innovation in Spain: "The economic, social and cultural development of a country depends on its capacity for scientific creation and innovation" (Fig. 24.6).

The Legacy of an Universal Scientist

Joan Oró i Florensa was a visionary pioneer in biochemistry, whose influence transformed the study of the origin of life on Earth and the search for life on other planets. His work laid the foundations for new lines of research that continue to define the direction of science. Although he spent much of his career outside Spain, his initiatives left an indelible mark on Catalan and Spanish science and research. He stood out for his ability to unite international and national efforts in search of answers. In addition, he was a strong advocate of scientific dissemination, understanding the importance of communicating science to the public, and actively participating in congresses and symposia, both in Spain and abroad, where he shared his valuable findings. His legacy, both scientific and human, lives on. Today, he inspires new generations to explore the enigmas of life on our planet and in the universe, and to use science as a powerful tool to build a better world.

To conclude, and as a summary of his profound vision of humanity, Oró left us these words that today remain more revealing than ever: "We must be humble, because life comes from very simple molecules; we must be supportive, because we all share same common origin; and we must be cooperative, because, from the Moon, the Earth is seen as a small grain of sand lost in the immensity of the universe" (Fig. 24.7).

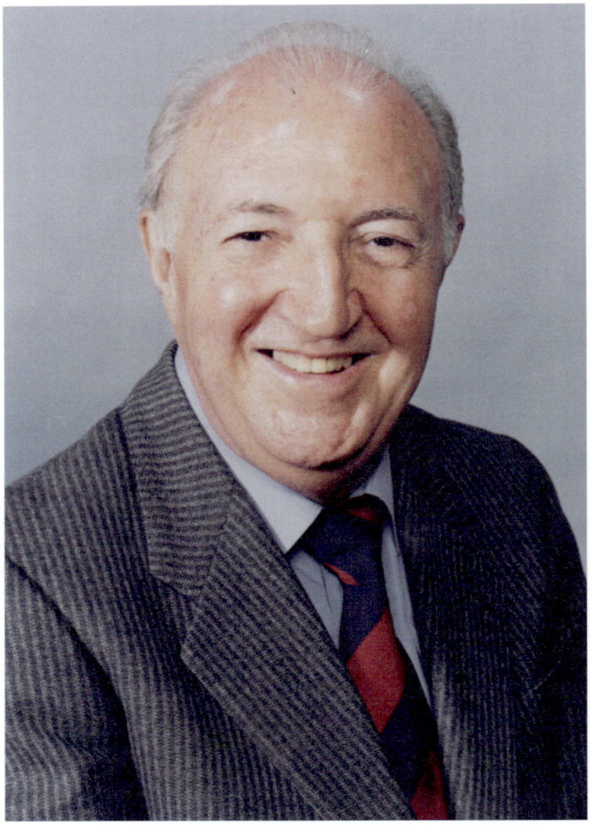

Fig. 24.7 Joan Oró, Scientist and strong advocate of Science as a tool to create a better World

References

1. Pairolí M. Joan Oró. Fundació Catalana per a la Recerca i la Innovació; 2022.
2. Valldeoriola M. Joan Oró. El científic de la vida. Angle Editorial; 2001.
3. Guerrero R. Joan Oró (1923–2004): Una vida dedicada a la ciència i a la cultura catalana. València: XVII Congrés de Metges i Biòlegs de Llengua Catalana; 2004.
4. López I. Joan Oró Florensa: centenario de un científico universal. Arbor. 2024;200:2625–30.
5. Pérez-Poch A, Català JA, Joan OT. A memoir of professor Joan Oró on the centennial of his birth. 58th IAA History of Astronautics Symposium, Milan 2024.
6. Oró J. 14C-Formate metabolism in animal tissues with special reference to the mechanism of formic acid oxidation [Doctoral Thesis]. Baylor University College of Medicine, Houston.

7. Oró J. Mechanism of synthesis of adenine from hydrogen cyanide under possible primitive earth conditions. Nature. 1961;191:1193–4.
8. Miller S. A production of amino acids under possible primitive earth conditions. Science. 1953;117:528–9.
9. Oró J. Comets and the formation of biochemical compounds on the primitive earth. Nature. 1961;190:389–90.
10. Oró J. Synthesis of organic compounds by electric discharges. Nature. 1963;197:862–7.
11. Oró J. Synthesis of organic compounds by high energy electrons. Nature. 1963;197:971–4.
12. Oró J. Ultra-violet-absorbing compounds(s) reported present in the Murray meteorite. Nature. 1963;197:756–8.
13. Guerrero R. Obituary of Joan Oró I Florensa. Int Microbiol. 2005;8:63–8.
14. Oparin A. The origin of life. Dover Publications; 2003.
15. Haldane JBS. The origin of life. Dover Publications; 2010.
16. Oró J, Kamat SS. Aminoacids synthesis from hydrogen cyanide under possible primitive earth conditions. Nature. 1961;190:442–3.

25

Carmen Gil Fernández: Virology in Spain

Rolando Pérez Álvarez and Víctor García Gil

Carmen Gil Fernández was born in La Granja de San Ildefonso (Segovia), where her family spent the summer, on August 31, 1929. She received from her parents an education based on solid moral principles and, at the same time, very tolerant and modern. His father, Juan Gil Collado, was an entomologist of international prestige before the Civil War. She went from living a happy and well-to-do childhood to seeing it torn apart by war and transforming her life into the exodus of a refugee and, later, into the existence of someone without resources, which led her to develop a sense of solidarity with the most disadvantaged; an attitude she

R. P. Álvarez
Science Research Centre, Universidad Autónoma del Estado de Morelos, Cuernavaca, Mexico

V. G. Gil (✉)
Architect. AUG-Architects, SLP, Castellón de la Plana, Spain

M. A. Cuesta, F. Mateo Vallejo (eds.), *Spain's Journey in Medicine*,
https://doi.org/10.1007/978-3-032-12221-6_25

maintained throughout her life. At school, and later in high school, she received a rather disjointed education, as a consequence of the events of the Civil War and the post-war period, but, in spite of this, she entered the Faculty of Sciences of the Central University of Madrid, brilliantly completing her degree studies in 1952. He received his doctorate from the Faculty of Sciences with a thesis entitled "Cultivo de los simbiotas del Argas persicus", (Culture of the simbiotas of the Argas Persicus) on the spread of Q fever in Spain, which won him the Torres Quevedo Prize of the CSIC in 1957. This work was only published internally by the Consejo Superior de Investigaciones Científicas (CSIC) in Spanish. The success achieved with her doctoral thesis allowed her to obtain a scholarship from the Fundación March in 1957 to continue her postgraduate studies in Cambridge (UK), something that very few young people of her time were able to achieve. In Cambridge she met another Spanish research fellow, who was doing his doctorate in Physics and who would be her future husband: Federico García Moliner, whom she married on April 6, 1959, and had three children, in 1960, 1961 and 1965 (Figs. 25.1, 25.2, and 25.3).

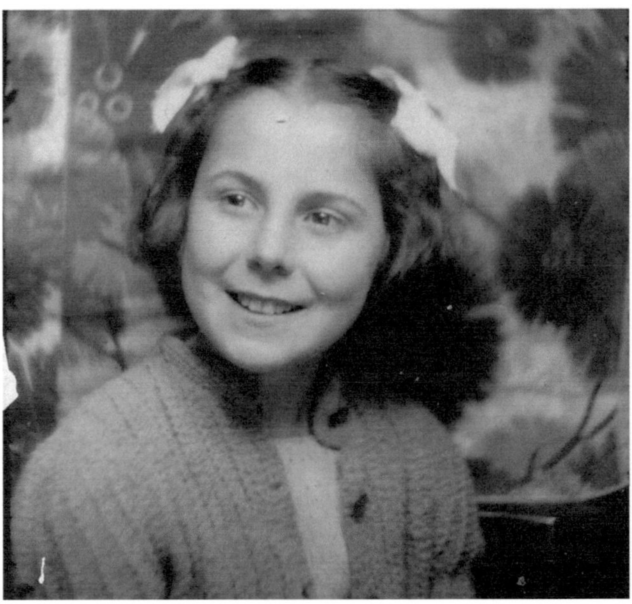

Fig. 25.1 Carmen Gil at 6 years old. (V. García Gil file)

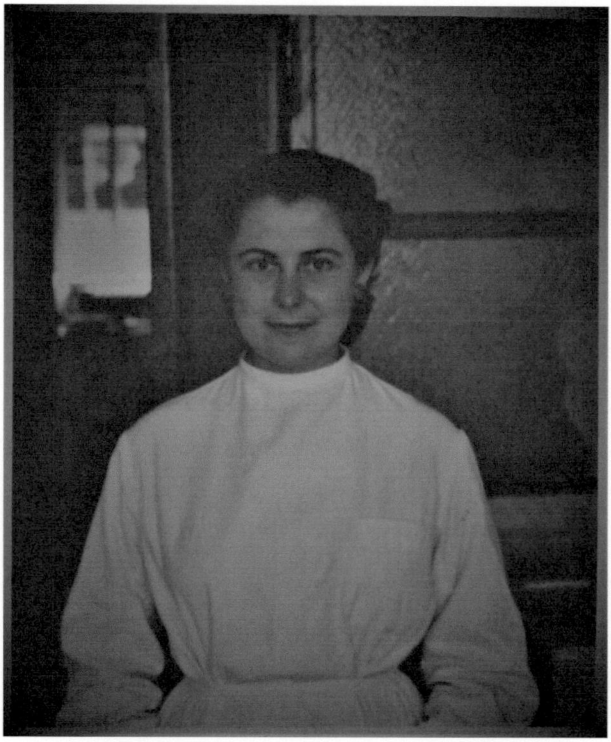

Fig. 25.2 Carmen Gil in the Jaime Ferrán Institute of the CSIC. Madrid, 1954. (V. García Gil file)

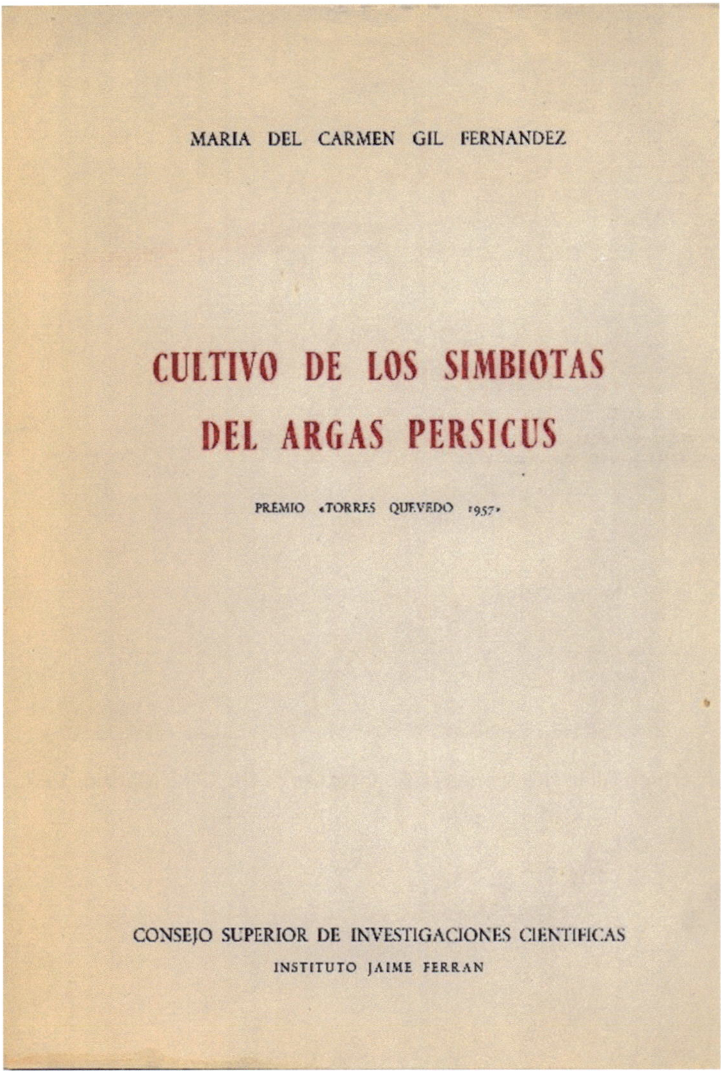
MARIA DEL CARMEN GIL FERNANDEZ

CULTIVO DE LOS SIMBIOTAS
DEL ARGAS PERSICUS

PREMIO «TORRES QUEVEDO 1957»

CONSEJO SUPERIOR DE INVESTIGACIONES CIENTIFICAS
INSTITUTO JAIME FERRAN

Fig. 25.3 Cover page of the doctoral thesis, "Cultivo de los Simbiotas del Argas Persicus", directed by Arnaldo Socías. Madrid, CSIC, Instituto Jaime Ferrán, 1957. (V. García Gil file)

Her Professional Work

Carmen Gil Fernández worked in different fields, in which she made important contributions. She began her career in the second half of the 1950s, when the World Health Organization (WHO) was concerned about a disease called Q fever, which, being common in cattle and poultry farms, although it caused symptoms similar to those of tuberculosis, had a different cause. This disease had first been described in 1935 in Australia by Edward Holbrook Derrick, who documented an outbreak of the disease in a group of workers in a cattle slaughterhouse. The causative factor was determined by Macfarlane Burnet [1] to be a Rickettsia, later identified as Coxiella Burnetti. Knowledge of Q fever in Spain dates back to the seminal studies of Florencio Pérez Gallardo in 1949, with the isolation of Coxiella Burnetii in ticks and the subsequent description in wild (dormice and rabbits) and domestic (bovids) reservoirs. However, this knowledge was scarce, and it was not known for sure how this disease could be acquired from ticks. Carmen Gil, working in the Laboratory of animal viruses at the Jaime Ferrán Institute of Microbiology of the CSIC in Madrid, identified the cause of the disease produced by Rickettsia; she described how it infected a tick, which transmitted it to domestic animals such as chickens, which, in turn, infected their caretakers, thus spreading the disease to humans. In the United Kingdom, at the Virus Laboratory of the Department of Pathology of Cambridge, directed by Professor M.G.P. Stoker, Carmen Gil worked on the latency of the Herpes Simplex virus. There she discovered the phenomenon of latency of a human virus. The latency of human viruses was already known in vivo, but there were no studies in vitro with virus-infected humans. Her discovery opened the possibility of investigating it with the help of the microscope in the laboratory. Therefore, her work, published in Nature [2] aroused worldwide interest, receiving more than 350 requests for reprints from all over the world. In her abstract she points out:

> Persistence of herpes virus in cells cultured in vitro might provide a suitable model for investigating the phenomenon of latent herpes infection in humans. During a study on the interaction between herpes virus and HeLa cells [3], it was observed that an extensive cytopathic effect eventually resulted from inoculation of a monolayer culture with the HFEM strain of herpes virus. A few isolated cells sometimes survived, however, and if growth medium containing antiviral serum was added, colonies grew from these surviving cells, leading eventually to a large population. These recovered cells were apparently healthy and grew as well as the original HeLa cells: there were no gross morphological differences such as those described by Marguerite Vogt and Renato Dulbecco [4], who studied cells recovered after poliomyelitis infection.

In her study on viral latency, she defined the phenomenon of herpes virus latency in HeLa cells cultured in vitro, thus corroborating the possibility of working with other human viruses under experimental conditions in the laboratory. Due to her great experience, acquired in Cambridge, she introduced the in vitro cell culture technique on his return to Spain [5]. Postgraduate training allowed her to become familiar with cell culture techniques and various immunological techniques with figures such as Eduardo Gallardo, Robin Coombs, Michael Stoker and Lindsay Black. In 1961, the couple moved to the University of Illinois at Chicago (1961–1964) where Carmen Gil's husband had been appointed Professor of Physics. At that university, Carmen Gil obtained a Postdoctoral Training Fellowship in Microbiology from the Public Health Service of the USA in 1962 to continue her research as a Research Associate in 1963 and 1964. During this period at that university she focused her research on animal and plant viruses, working with distinguished botanist Professor Lindsay Black. The established belief among botanists was that there are some viruses that reproduce in animals and others in plants. Black launched the idea, then heterodox, that there are viruses that can reproduce in both animals and plants. When Carmen Gil arrived at Black's laboratory, she found that they did not use cell cultures, since they were working with a greenhouse, an expensive and very inefficient technique. Carmen Gil proposed to Black to use another, much more efficient method. This involved obtaining cell tissue cultures of Agallia constricta, a tiny 3 mm insect that carries the tobacco mosaic virus.

Using specific immunofluorescence techniques, she identified the various tissues of the insect in which the virus reproduced and then infected the plant. With this, a young Spanish researcher opened a new research view for Lindsay Black and his collaborators [6] (Fig. 25.4).

When she returned to Madrid in 1964, Carmen Gil joined again the Jaime Ferrán Institute of Microbiology of the CSIC. The cell culture technique that she had introduced in Spain allowed her to carry out interesting studies with very few resources [7]. Her most productive periods were between 1970–73 and 1983–93. Publishing most of her work in international journals [8–11] (Fig. 25.5).

In May 1981, a massive food poisoning occurred in Spain by adulterated rapeseed oil that provoked a serious health crisis, and the Spanish government dedicated the most advanced laboratories and equipment to the study of its cause and effects. It was what later became popularly known as toxic oil syndrome (TOS) or rapeseed disease. TOS is a chronic multisystemic disease caused by a massive intoxication associated with the consumption of rapeseed oil denatured with 2% aniline, imported for industrial use and subsequently diverted for human consumption. The disease affected more than 20,000 people and caused the death of some 330 people. When the problem arose, many Spanish researchers, including Carmen Gil, generously stopped what

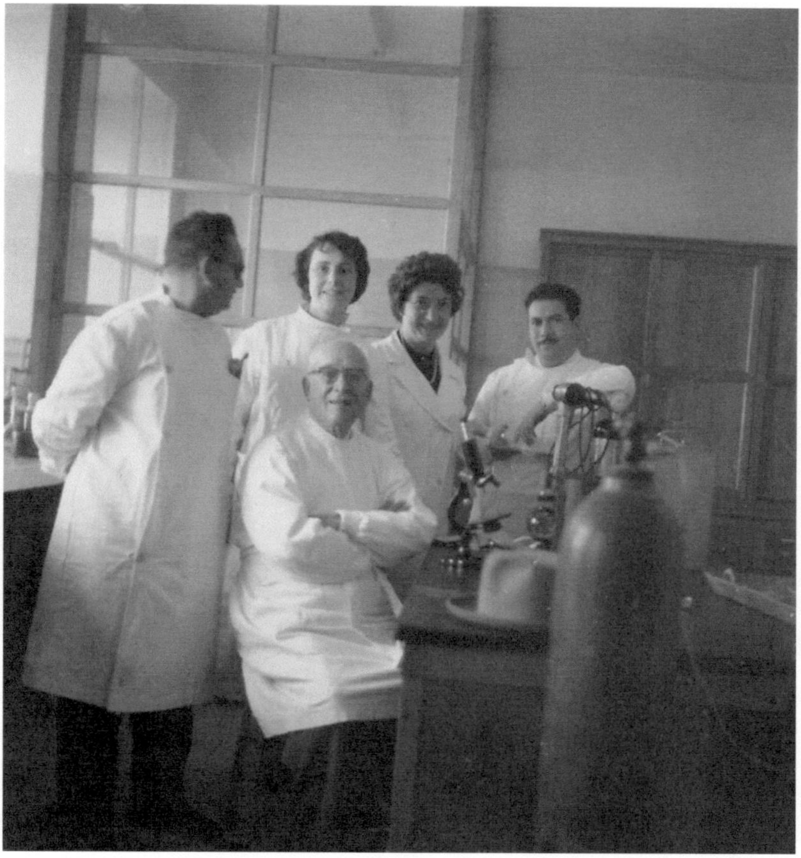

Fig. 25.4 Staff of the Department of Virus of the Jaime Ferrán Institute of the CSIC. (Eduardo Gallardo Martínez, stand Emilio Ronda Laín, Carmen Gil Fernández, María Luisa Alonso Puertas y Ángel García Gancedo). Madrid, 1961. (V. García Gil file)

they were doing and set to work on it. In a very short time the origin of the poisoning was established.

In the case of the Carmen Gil's research, by inoculating rapeseed oil in chicken embryos, managed to reproduce exactly and completely the whole syndrome. Equivalent results were obtained by other CSIC researchers. To supervise in some way this excellent work, Dr. Alan Woolf from the USA came to Spain, invited by the government of the time (Felipe Gonzalez, president of the government). Once he had seen all that he was shown, in an interview on Spanish TV he said that he really did not know why he had been called, since the Spanish researchers had worked in an exemplary way, they had irrefutably demonstrated that rapeseed oil was the culprit of the toxic syndrome, and they had done a much better job and in much less time than

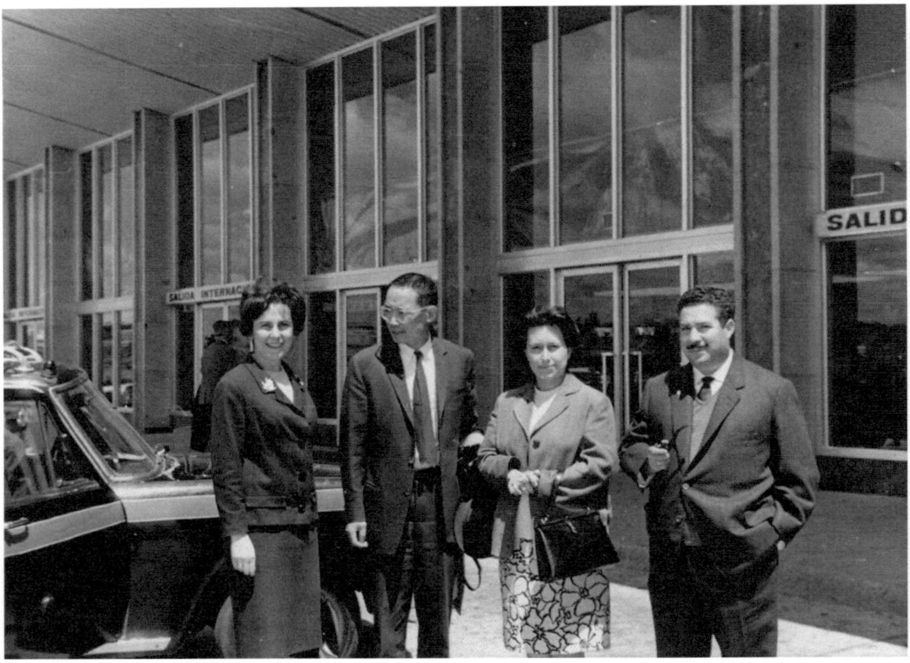

Fig. 25.5 Carmen Gil Fernández, Monto Ho, Pilar Vilas and Ángel García Gancedo in the airport of Barajas, (Madrid, 1971). (V. García Gil file)

the Americans when they had the Legionella problem. The CSIC, who had done their work so generously and brilliantly, did not get any recognition from the State.

Carmen Gil also made important contributions to research on African swine fever (ASF) [9–11]. The ASF virus is not harmful to humans, but it causes a great economic impact, forcing the slaughter and burning of pigs in large numbers. For several years, as a consequence of the spread of the disease in Spain, many countries closed their borders to the import of pork products from our country. As in the case of rapeseed oil, several researchers stopped what they were doing and dedicated themselves to researching ASF. Carmen also participated in this work, researching the ASF virus for 3 years. The first difficulty was to obtain samples of the ASF virus from the laboratories of the Dirección General de Veterinaria (Directorate of Veterinary Medicine). Faced with the refusal to provide them, they had to go to Portugal, where some colleagues provided them, passing them hidden to Spain. The Belgian researcher Erik De Clercq, who had the financial means to carry out antivirus research, visited Carmen Gil's laboratory on several occasions to discuss with her the progress of their research. Thanks to this relationship, Carmen was able to obtain funding for further research [9–11]. The ASF episode ended with an improper gesture in the scientific world, as the researchers who had worked on the ASF virus were ordered by the then president of the CSIC to give to him a scientific report of their work. The president, with all this material, published a paper under his name for an international journal, without the slightest reference to the real authors. These researchers, including Carmen Gil, were unable to publish anything they had been working on for so long.

In short, a professional life dedicated to establishing new experimental protocols of wide use with which she helped to consolidate virology not only with her personal and group activity, but also through the organization of periodic courses within the CSIC itself and in connection with the faculties of Biological Sciences and Pharmacy. And all within a framework of scarcity, lack of recognition or, directly, relegation of women [12].

She passed away on April 11, 2018, in Castellón de la Plana, the city to which she had moved with her husband in 1996.

Her obituary (Mediterráneo, April 13, 2018) noted that:

Carmen was distinguished by her simple and sincere manner, her proverbial modesty, her predisposition to humanitarian aid from the field of research and, especially, her generosity.

Their Attitude Towards Research

Carmen Gil lived relatively inhibited by the scientific stature of her life partner, Federico García Moliner, who, among other important recognitions, received the Prince of Asturias Award for Technical and Scientific Research in 1992. However, for him, Carmen Gil's scientific contributions had been superior to his own (Fig. 25.6).

As a wife and mother of three children, she covered for her husband's frequent absences for professional reasons, damaging her own projection, but without expressing any discomfort about it. Her attitude towards research was very disinterested in terms of the visibility of her results, while at the same time highlighting her dedication and collaboration in team tasks. Carmen Gil, as a researcher, was characterized by her absolute dedication, sparing no effort to research. She did not mind passing by her laboratory at night, even on holidays, to monitor the progress of the HeLa cells and to check the status of her cultures. He belongs to the generation of microbiologists who made virology grow, to which he contributed decisively with his technical

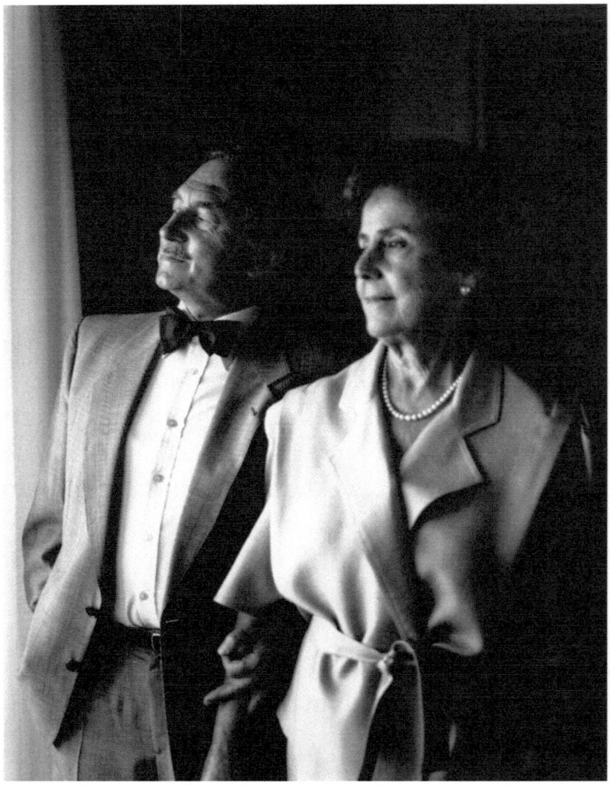

Fig. 25.6 Carmen Gil and her husband Federico García Moliner. 1997. (Permission: C. Solís Santos)

contributions. In her career she suffered from the rigidity of the administrative and scientific culture of the sixties to eighties, embodied in the formation of very closed working groups that competed for resources, chronically scarce, through their capacity for institutional or political influence and with promotion criteria equally mediated by the will of the bosses in office and a notable gender bias. She gave no importance to publications and yet she was highly esteemed by those who knew her and those who worked with her. She was very clear that science can and should help the world, but to help it one must first understand it. It took a long time for her to begin to understand that if a researcher does not publish his work, the world does not know she exists, so she is less likely to continue to do useful work. She began to understand this in Illinois, but nevertheless, she did not hesitate to neglect her personal projection when years later problems arose that she thought she could help with

the research was carried out in the field of Toxic Oil Syndrome, African swine fever, etc. and forced the group to abandon its ongoing research and move on to other fields.

When Carmen Gil retired, she donated part of her articles and books to the Faculty of Biology of the University of Havana, including not only her personal scientific production, but also the books and articles she had bought and photocopied over the years. The rest of her scientific material, together with that of her husband, was donated to the Universitat Jaume I and the Diputación Provincial de Castellón.

Throughout her life, she generously welcomed many scientists and researchers from different fields and nationalities to his home, attending young people who were just starting out as well as internationally recognized and consecrated personalities. The scientists who visited the couple found joy, altruism and love in their home. It was therefore not surprising that, in her last days, a good number of them bid her farewell with deep affection.

Her Facet As a Painter and Sculptor

In addition to her professional work as a virology researcher, Carmen Gil was a very good painter and sculptor. As a painter, she had an amazing ability to capture the light of each moment. She would quickly set up her easel as if it were the tripod of a camera, and then paint with the right mix of oils to capture the tones and intensity of the light in the image her eyes captured. His favorite subject was nature (Fig. 25.7).

He also produced excellent sculptures on an astonishing variety of subjects, themes, characters, ideas and experiences. Her work contains maternities, couples, groups of people embraced and united in a shared pain or abstractions about the landscape and social inequalities. All this shows us a woman committed to her time, in constant evolution and eager to continue learning. Carmen Gil was a great woman who always worked with efficiency, abnegation and modesty, a researcher who, with her efforts, helped to begin to raise Spanish science in years of isolation and scarcity. She was always highly appreciated by her work and for her human qualities, including her elegance and discretion. Her legacy remains in the memory of all those who had the good fortune to know her.

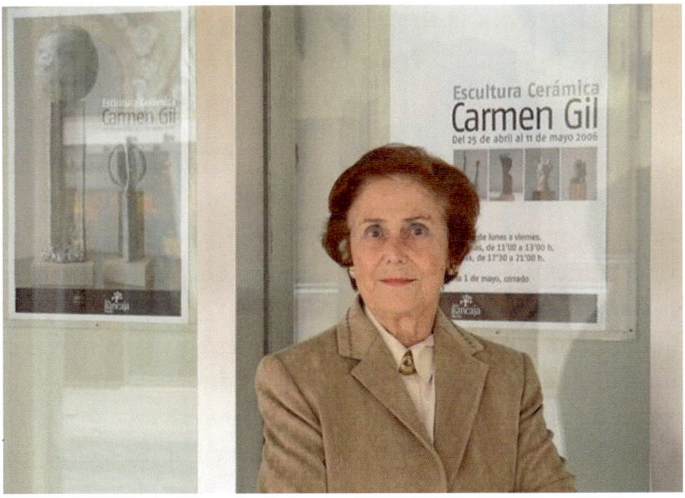

Fig. 25.7 Carmen Gil, exposing her work in Bancaja, Castellón 2006. (V. García Gil file)

References

1. Macfarlane Burnet received the Nobel Prize in 1960, together with P. Brian Medawar, for the discovery of tolerance to transplanted tissues.
2. Persistence of herpes simplex virus in HeLa cells. Nature 1960; 185: 4708.
3. HeLa cells (also known as "Hela cells" or simply "Hela") are a particular type of cell culture cell used in scientific research. They are the oldest and most used human cell lineage. The lineage to which these cells derive from a sample of cervical cancer obtained on February 81951 from a patient named Henrietta Lacks (hence the acronym He{nrietta} La{cks}), who died on October 4 of the same year due to cancer. Unlike noncancerous cells, HeLa cells can be cultured in the laboratory constantly, which is why they are referred to as "immortal cells".
4. Vogt M, Dulbecco R. Properties of a HeLa cell culture with increase resistance to Poliomyelitis virus. Virology. 1958;5:425–34.
5. During a trip back to Spain, Carmen Gil bought in Cambridge, with money from her own pocket, a collection of Pyrex bottles to continue her scientific work in Spain. These bottles presented the ideal conditions for cell culture work and did not exist at that time in Spain.
6. 6 Years later, while enjoying a vacation in Costa Rica, Federico and Carmen went to visit the National Biodiversity Center, which had been awarded the Prince of Asturias Prize, in whose jury Federico had participated. The researchers of this center received them very kindly and shared a pleasant lunch with them. There they learned that the director of the center had worked in Illinois with Professor Black. When Carmen told him that she had worked there, the director exclaimed with great vehemence: "So you are "the Carmen" that Black talked about every day!

7. Proof of the precarious means with which Carmen Gil carried out her work is reflected in the fact that, as she had no money to buy serum with which to feed the cells, both she and her colleagues had to bleed themselves to feed them. When they were visited by American researchers who wanted to meet her, seeing the scarcity of means with which she worked, they sent them money to buy a special ultracentrifuge and a special stove, very expensive and essential to be able to work effectively on these subjects.

8. Gil Fernández C, Black LM. Some aspects of the internal anatomy of the Leafhoper Agallia constricta (Homoptera: Cicadellidae). Ann Entomol Soc Am. 1965;58:275–84.
9. Gil Fernández C. Plaque formation by African swine fever virus in chick embryo fibroblasts in the absence of CO2 atmosphere. Arch Virol. 1976;52:207–15.
10. Sola A, Rodríguez Saint-Jean S, Gil Fernández C, Carrasco L. New agents active against African swine fever virus. AAC. 1986;29:284–8.
11. García-Villalón D, Gil Fernández C, De Clercq E. Activity of several S-adenosylhomocysteine hydrolase inhibitors against African swine fever virus replication in Vero cells. Antivir Res. 1993;20:131–44.
12. Rodríguez O. Esteban: "Mujeres y ciencia del CSIC: Carmen Gil Fernández (1929- 2018)". Dpto. History of Science. Faculty of Medicine Universidad de Granada.

26

The Spanish National Transplant Organization: A Model for the World

Rafael Matesanz

The Spanish "Organización Nacional de Trasplantes" (ONT) National Transplant Organization is a technical body dependent on the Ministry of Health, created in 1989 by the nephrologist Rafael Matesanz to coordinate the donation and transplantation of organs, tissues and cells (Fig. 26.1). Its implementation radically changed the fate of thousands and thousands of patients waiting for an organ or tissue to continue living or to improve their quality of life, and at the same time it changed forever the world of transplants in Spain and, by extension, in many other countries that have followed our organization model. Their functions can be summed up by saying that, as with any other part of our healthcare system since it was transferred to the 17 autonomous communities in Spain, these communities are responsible for managing care for citizens—including transplants—while the Central Ministry, through its technical body, the ONT, mainly acts as a coordinator and facilitator. The ONT takes care of everything that individual hospitals or regions cannot handle on their own. It supports them in their daily work, connects them with other centers across Spain, and, in short, provides the backing needed to carry out and improve organ donation and transplant activities. As part of the Spanish Ministry of Health, it represents the State in any international forum.

What we have achieved together in the field of transplants can be summarized in a very clear way: any Spanish citizen, from any community that has

R. Matesanz (✉)
National Organization of Transplants, Madrid, Spain

M. A. Cuesta, F. Mateo Vallejo (eds.), *Spain's Journey in Medicine*,
https://doi.org/10.1007/978-3-032-12221-6_26

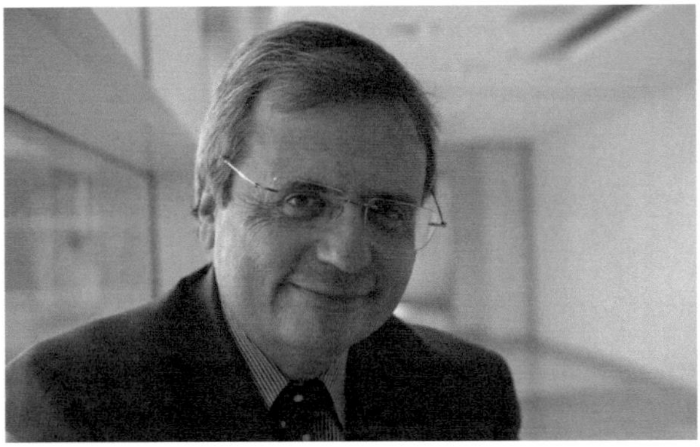

Fig. 26.1 Rafael Matesanz Acedos

needed a heart, liver, kidney or any other organ transplant in order to continue living, has been during the last 32 years, since 1992, the citizen of the world with the best chances of getting it, and moreover, within a public, universal system, without positive or negative discrimination for reasons of economic, social, geographical or any other kind of position. Nothing more than that, nothing less than that. This is by far the most splendid reality of Spanish healthcare, looked upon with envy by half the world. If we want to illustrate it, there are data that are simply overwhelming: since these therapies began in Spain more 140,000 Spaniards or residents in our country have received an organ transplant, and almost a million if we add tissues and cells [1, 2]. We are the only medium to large state in the world in which there are more patients with chronic renal failure with a transplanted kidney than on dialysis, and in some age groups, such as those under 45 years of age, more than three quarters of the patients are transplanted. Or, for example, when comparing comparable populations Spanish and American our 10-year survival results in renal transplantation were more than 20 points higher than in the United States, both in terms of the patient and the transplanted organ, mainly as a result of the improved post-transplant care provided by our health system [3].

Few Spanish institutions enjoy such national and international prestige. The ONT has received awards such as the Prince of Asturias Prize and is part of the "Marca España" initiative. It has chaired major global transplant forums—including the Council of Europe for 12 years and the Ibero-American Council on Donation and Transplantation since 2005—and led key EU regulations, such as the 2010 Transplant Directive and the 2023 Regulation on Substances of Human Origin.

As a WHO partner and adviser to many countries, the ONT helps improve organ donation and transplantation systems worldwide. The "Spanish Model" has likely saved more lives abroad than in Spain itself, earning the Prince of Asturias Award for International Cooperation in 2010. Recently, The Lancet highlighted the ONT as a global reference in transplant organization [4].

The Beginnings

The first renal transplants in Spain were performed in the 1960s in Barcelona, Madrid and Pamplona. They then went through a long desert crossing in which only the Hospital Clinic in Barcelona and the Fundación Jiménez Díaz in Madrid maintained an appreciable activity that until the mid-70's was between 20 and 40 interventions per year. From 1975 onwards, other centers were added all over Spain, as new Social Security hospitals were opened, with the result that activity increased progressively, especially after the approval in 1979 of the transplant law with its corresponding royal decree of 1980 that developed it [5].For the first time, the conditions for diagnosing brain death or for proceeding with live donation were established, procedures which until then had been based on protocols taken from the practice of other countries, but which lacked a legal basis (Fig. 26.2).

Activity increased at a good rate until 1986, but a prolonged hospital conflict in 1987 led to a 20% drop in transplant activity, which in Madrid reached 50% and not recover in the following 2 years. All this, together with the appearance in the 80's of heart and liver transplants lacking any organizational infrastructure, led to great unease among patients and professionals, with complaints to the ombudsman and great repercussions in the media. These were the reasons why the Ministry of Health decided that something had to be done and brought to light an old project that had remained buried throughout the 80's: the NATIONAL ORGANIZATION OF TRANSPLANTS (Fig. 26.3).

What this organization has become today has fortunately nothing to do with what was originally planned in the Official State Gazette—a merely auxiliary, highly centralized body designed for a time before healthcare was transferred to the Autonomous Communities, and clearly unsuitable for today's Spain.

The early years were very challenging, but within just 3 years we became world leaders, and in the first half of the 1990s transplant activity grew by

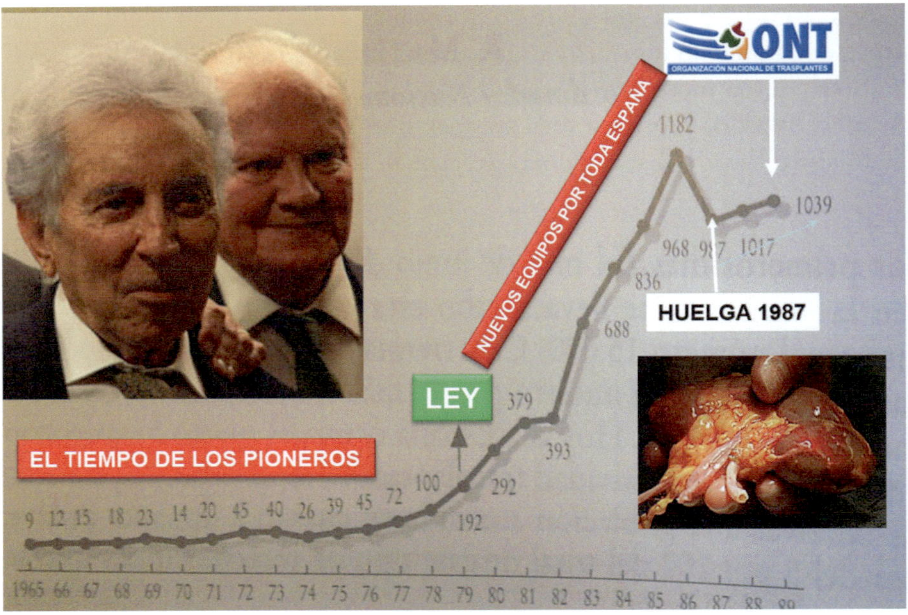

Fig. 26.2 Beginning of the organ's transplant in Spain. First renal transplant in 1965 by José María Gil-Vernet y Antoni Caralps in the Clinic Hospital of Barcelona. Increase of the activity with the Law 30/79, increase with the new equipment in the 80's, the impact of strike in 1987 and subsequent stagnation, what is the origin of creation of the ONT in 1989

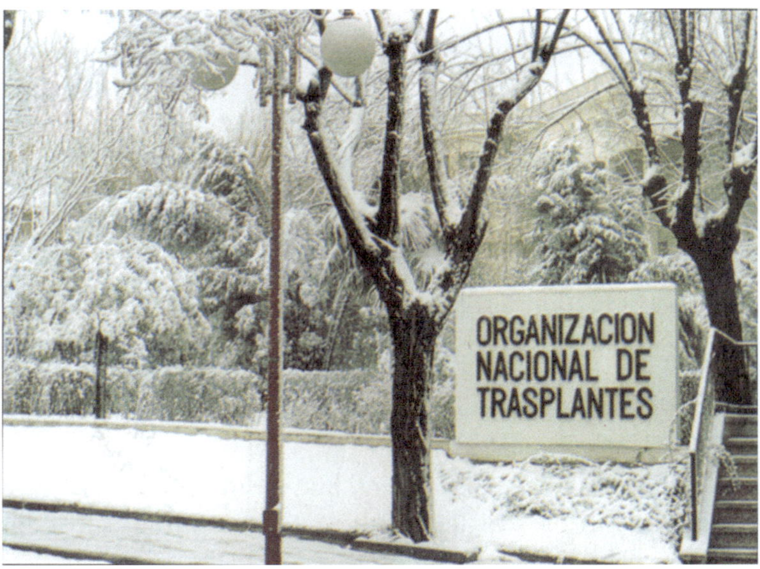

Fig. 26.3 First headquarter of the ONT on the grounds of the Health Institute Carlos III in Madrid

more than 50%. From then on, the project gained full momentum and evolved into the successful reality it is today.

The Basis of the System

Fortunately, our system has very solid foundations. The first and foremost is our National Health System, of remarkable quality, although it is not going through its best moments, from which the entire donation and transplantation system emanates and in which our mission has been to extract the best. The second is the deep connection with the society that ultimately makes transplants possible with their donations on the one hand and the support of the system with their taxes on the other. Our transplantation system is based on solidarity and altruism: everyone must donate in an altruistic way because everyone may need it in the future and then they will get it without admitting any positive or negative discrimination [5].

In Spain, presumed consent applies: we are all considered organ donors unless we have explicitly stated otherwise in writing during our lifetime. The law aims to ensure that donation is a voluntary and altruistic act, and the deceased person's family is always consulted to confirm their wishes regarding donation.

Therefore, the mission of the ONT is to get the best out of Spanish healthcare in this field. To achieve this, it has a great staff, not a large staff, at the central office of the ONT: 8 doctors,16 nurses and the entire management structure, IT, etc., a total of some 50 people trained over the years and who are currently at the peak of their professional careers, in a job that cannot be improvised or learned from outside: we have been creating and reinventing it every day and it is one of our main assets (Fig. 26.4). Moreover, I dare say that one of the keys to the success of this organization is its smallness in what amounts to agility. But this staff by itself would be nothing if it were not perfectly complemented by a peripheral structure formed not only by the 17 autonomous coordinators and the approximately 500 hospital coordinators including doctors and nurses throughout Spain, but also by the more than 20,000 professionals of all categories that we have been training throughout this quarter of a century, and the hundreds organ, tissue and cell transplantation teams, which together constitute the best guarantee for the future. The ONT is a coordinating body of horizontal management that reaches its greatest significance in a decentralized state such as the one we live in, in which each autonomous

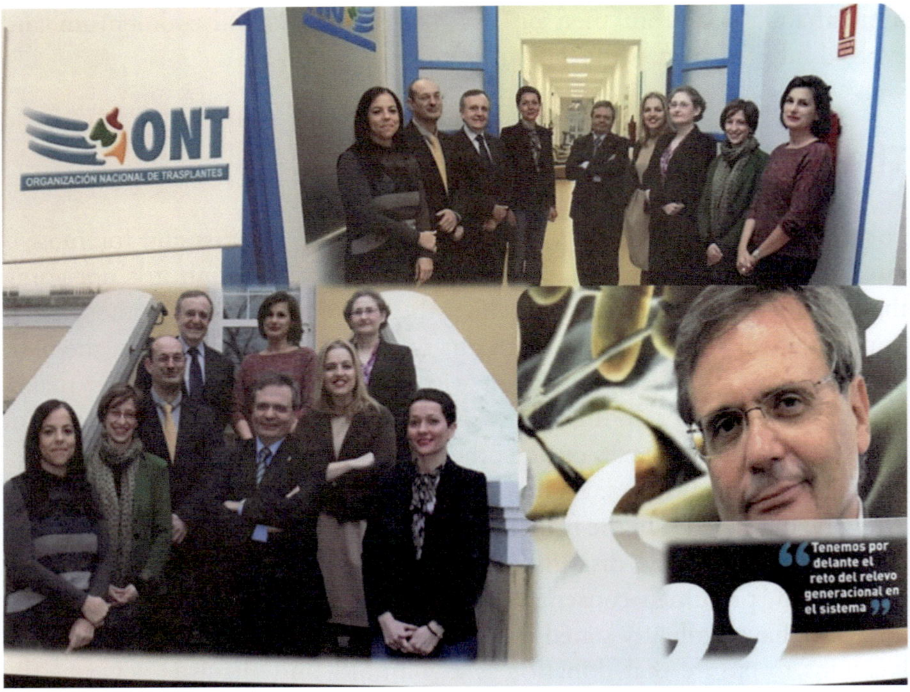
ONT
ORGANIZACIÓN NACIONAL DE TRASPLANTES
Tenemos por delante el reto del relevo generacional en el sistema

Fig. 26.4 Medical team of the ONT, 2015

community has its full competencies, but needs the collaboration of the others to achieve its maximum performance. Any relevant decision on donation and transplantation is taken by agreement of the 17 Autonomous Communities, without distinction of political color and often after extensive discussions, but one can count on the fingers of one hand the number of times in a quarter of a century that a vote has had to be taken due to lack of agreement. This is how, we manage people, resources, information, professional training, public awareness, etc., everything that is necessary to keep the system running perfectly 24 h a day. In short, what has been achieved has been possible thanks to the loyal and continuous collaboration of everyone, in which no one alone could have achieved anywhere near the quantitative or qualitative results that we have achieved together. Each community has at some point been a reference point in some aspect of donation and transplantation and has made its own contribution to this field, and it has made its experience at the disposal of others while learning from them in other fields so that in the end the only beneficiaries have been the patients throughout Spain. I dare say that if this way of acting had been applied to many other aspects of our public life, everything would be much better [6].

The Need to Innovate

The creation of the ONT in 1989 meant that we went from being in the lower middle range of donation in Europe to being world leaders in just 3 years, in 1992. Naturally, this was not the result of chance but of the application of a different method to what we had been doing until then and to what the rest of the countries around us were doing. The usual practice was that all the attention was focused on transplantation, while donation was placed in a secondary position, dependent only on the generosity of the population, theoretically fed by awareness campaigns. We turned the scheme around, we focused our efforts on donation, we realized that campaigns only serve to convince those who are already convinced, and in short, we dedicated our resources to professionalizing the process of organ donation through transplant coordinators, intensivist physicians who are perfectly trained to successfully carry out even the most difficult donations. It was a matter of putting the right person in the right place at the right time and extending this approach community by community and hospital by hospital throughout the country. With this model, continuously improved over time, we have been a world leader for 32 years. In all these years, the need for innovation has continued to be evident at various times. If we analyze the evolution of Spanish donation rates over the years, we can see how during the first decade of this century, although the absolute number of donors continued to grow moderately, so did the population, more or less at the same rate, so that organ donation rates had stagnated at 32–34 donors pmp (per million population) and the model showed signs of wear and tear. From our in-depth analysis of the situation, it was found that the number of brain deaths showed a clear downward trend throughout Spain, not only due to the continuous reduction of traffic accidents, which had already been established since the 1990s, but also due to a better management of hypertension and other processes. And above all, due to an evolution in the limitation of life support treatment (LST) in intensive care units, which in turn is the result of changes in society and in the clinical practice of intensivists themselves. It became clear that, in order to keep growing, it was necessary to innovate and make a major change in what we were doing. More than ever, the phrase attributed to Einstein and repeated in multiple versions became more valid: "If you want different results, do different things". As a result of these reflections, the "PLAN DONACIÓN 40" (DONATION PLAN 40) was conceived in 2008, as 40 donors pmp (per million inhabitants) was the target to be achieved at that time, which has now been amply surpassed (in 1989 we had only 14). Although there were many recommendations, two of them were fundamental for the future of donation and transplantation in Spain: on the one hand, training and collaboration with emergency physicians to detect potential donors outside the ICU, and on the other, the establishment of controlled asystole donation, a practice then limited to very few countries, almost all Anglo-Saxon and none of them predominantly Catholic. In fact, the two lines of action were necessarily convergent, since a good number of potential donors detected outside the ICU could only become donors through asystole extraction. These two lines of action represent today more than half of the organ donors in Spain and if they had not been tackled at the time, we would have lost the world leadership and the privileged position we have held since 1992 many years ago. It was not easy to make the decision to address controlled asystole, which even required a very sensitive legal change since it had to touch the concept of death. The SEMICYUC (Spanish Society of Intensive Care Medicine and Coronary Units) data were fundamental, showing that more than half of the patients who died in the ICU at that time were dying after LSTL and that this percentage had only increased in previous years. These data and the majority opinion of intensivists (nearly 90% of coordinators in Spain) led us to take the step. A joint decision was made with all the regions in 2008, followed by a pilot study carried out in Vitoria in 2009–2010 under the supervision of the Basque Health Service and the ONT. A consensus process with all the professionals involved took place in 2010–2011, and in 2012 a legal amendment was introduced—without the slightest public or political controversy, probably thanks to the great prestige of our transplant system. Finally, the initiative was rolled out across Spain with intensive team training from then on, which still continues today [7] (Fig. 26.5).

All this has meant that we have long since surpassed the hundred or so hospitals where this type of donation has been incorporated into the daily routine and now represents 45% of all organ donors, with a tendency to continue growing. Citizens have accepted it quite naturally, even with a percentage of family refusals of less than half that of brain death donation. Controlled asystole has definitely become part of the landscape even in situations as sensitive as donation in cases of euthanasia, and this is probably the maximum to which we could aspire when we started the process.

Controlled asystole donation, or donation after circulatory death (DCD), involves organ retrieval after a patient's heart has stopped beating, but under

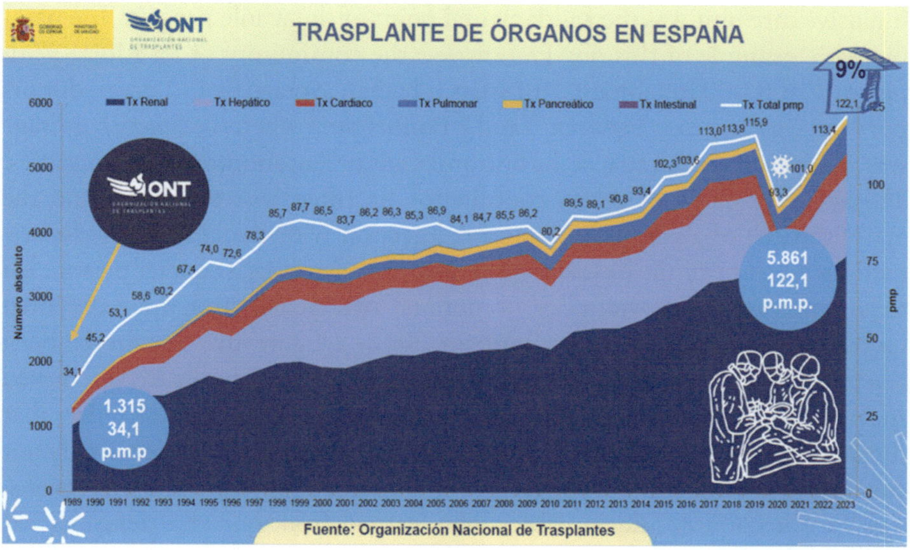

Fig. 26.5 Organ transplantation in Spain since the creation of the ONT to 2023 in absolute numbers and pmp. The chart shows different types of transplants, including renal, hepatic, cardiac, pulmonary, pancreatic and intestinal. In this period the donors have multiplied by a factor of 4 and the transplants per million inhabitants by a factor of 4,5. The source is the ONT

controlled circumstances. After death is declared, the organs are preserved, using an extracorporeal device to maintain their viability for transplantation. This contrast with donation after brain death (DBD), where the donor is still on life support but meets neurological criteria for death [8].

Similarly, collaboration with emergency physicians in organ donation has been, together with asystole, the fundamental factor that has boosted transplantation in Spain in the last 15 years. The reasons are very simple: the vast majority of potential donors enter the hospital through the emergency department, but whereas 20 years ago only those who were transferred to the ICU and died in a situation of encephalic death crystallized as real donors, today they are approached as donors by the emergency physician, who assesses them together with the intensivist and activates the protocol of what is known as "donation-oriented intensive care" either after brain death or in cardiac arrest [9]. The perfect understanding between the ONT and the group of emergency physicians developed many years ago when we investigated the factors that could allow us to continue to grow in the number of organ donors through an analysis with a strict benchmarking methodology in all hospitals authorized for donation, we found that the role of the emergency physician, or rather, the coordination between the emergency physician and the intensive care unit was the fundamental point of the whole process. The paradigmatic example of this observation was the community of La Rioja. With just over 300,000 inhabitants, for years it had an average of 1–2 organ donors per year, which meant between 3 and 6 donors pmp when the Spanish average was 33–35, which placed it at the bottom of all the Autonomous Communities. The arrival in 2004 of a new coordinator, an intensivist physician, and the establishment of a perfect system of connection with the emergency department, where one of the physicians was also nominated as a contact person, led to an increase in the number of donors, spectacular and unprecedented increase to reach 74.2 donors pmp in 2007, a figure that has never been reached anywhere in the world and which has taken many years to be achieved sporadically in some communities (never outside Spain). The realization that the detection in the emergency department of potential donors previously not considered as such was the key factor for continued growth was a true revolution in our country and in others who learned from our experience. It has involved the training by the ONT of thousands of emergency physicians from all over Spain in organ donation over the years and, together with the other fundamental and complementary measure, the donation to a stopped heart, has made it possible to go from 30–35 to the 50 pmp donors we have today in the last 15 years [10]. Without emergency physicians, Spain would not have been able to maintain its undisputed world leadership for more than 30 years and it is only fair to acknowledge this [11]. In these more than three decades of life of the ONT, many things have changed radically in the world of transplantation, starting with the profile of organ donors. The idea of the typical donor in the 1980s was that of a young motorcyclist without a helmet, something that today is little more than an urban legend, but which still persists in the beliefs of many people. Although the first year we were able to obtain the complete characteristics of donors was 1992, and very probably in the 80's traffic accidents accounted for more than two thirds of donors, we started that year with 43% of traffic accidents as the cause of death of donors, which in 2000 had dropped to 21.3% and today is 4.7%, mostly due to road traffic accidents and not exactly young people (Fig. 26.6).

Similarly, donors over 60 years of age were only 10% in 1992, had risen to 31.3% in 2000 and today are 56.8%, that is, more half, and of these, 29.7% are over 70, and 4.6% are over 80 years of age. The oldest donors are mainly liver donors and, to a lesser extent, kidney donors, although all organs, including heart and lung, participate in this aging trend of donors, as do the recipients. Livers of 93 and 94 years of age have been transplanted and in Italy, a 97 year old has been transplanted. Age barriers have definitely ceased to exist

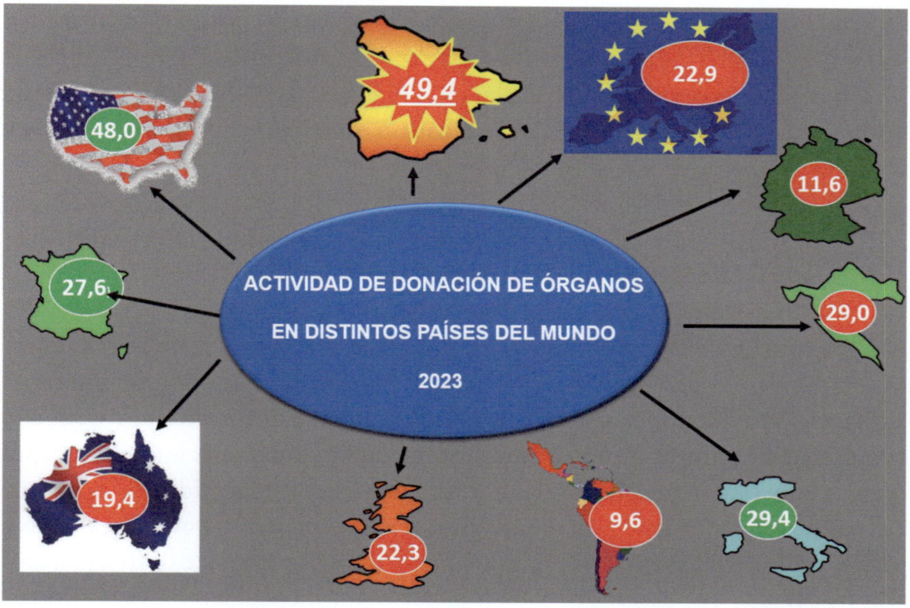

Fig. 26.6 Organ donation activity per million population in selected countries and areas worldwide during 2023. Data from the European Commissions' Organ Donation Council (ODA)

in transplantation, both for the donor and the recipient, and this is one of the fundamental ways of expanding the procedure that allows more and more lives to be saved or improved every year.

An Integrated Model of Donation and Transplantation

It is important, as a general consideration, to emphasize that our donation and transplantation model constitutes an Integrated Management System for the Donation and Transplantation of Organs, Tissues, and Cells. This integrated structure defines and distinguishes us; it is the original feature that has made our system unique worldwide. Any attempt to deregulate or privatize any of its components could jeopardize its integrity and effectiveness.

This is not to say that the public and private sectors cannot coexist—indeed, they have done so without significant difficulties in certain areas of tissue and cell transplantation. Nevertheless, a process as sensitive and ethically complex as organ and tissue donation and transplantation must remain under the regulation and oversight of health authorities. Numerous international experiences have clearly demonstrated the risks associated with inadequately controlled privatization practices, risks that must be avoided at all costs.

Final Conclusions: Solidarity and Cooperation

And to conclude these reflections, I would like to say that transplants reflect many things. As has been said, our donors are aging because our society is aging and as a developed country, it avoids avoidable deaths in the young. We have received a flood of immigrants in the last two decades and as a consequence between 10% and 12% of our donors were born outside Spain, practically the weight of this population in our country as a whole. They reflect society and help it to look in the mirror and learn to recognize both its virtues and its defects. The actions of the ONT are a not inconsiderable factor in the cohesion of the national health system. Every year the balance of both organs and patients transplanted between communities is analyzed and systematically around a quarter of the transplants performed each year in Spain are performed with organs donated in other communities, exactly 23% in 2023. There are communities such as Madrid, Catalonia or Cantabria that receive more organs than they send because they have more centers of reference, where patients from other parts of Spain go, or their teams have more advanced criteria and transplant organs that are not used in their places of origin. Others, such as Euskadi, Rioja, the two Castillas, etc., have high rates of donation and send them to other places where their patients go to receive treatment. A quarter of the transplants performed in Catalonia, almost half of the transplants in Madrid, or more than half of those in Cantabria are performed with organs donated in other communities.

The conclusion is very clear: No community on its own would achieve anywhere near the quantitative and qualitative results achieved by working with the other 16 in the same direction, and all this for the benefit of our sole objective: the best care for the patient. We all win when we are united and transplants contribute day by day to prove it, saving thousands of lives.

References

1. Organización Nacional de Trasplantes: Dossier de actividad de donación y trasplante; 2023. https://www.ont.es/wp-content/uploads/2024/03/ACTIVIDAD-DE-DONACION-Y-TRASPLANTE-ESPANA-2023.pdf.
2. Registro Español de Enfermos Renales. (Spanish Register of renal patients) Informe; 2022. https://www.ont.es/wpcontent/uploads/2023/11/Memoria_REER_2022.pdf.
3. Ojo AO, Morales JM, González Molina M, et al. Comparison of the long-term outcomes of kidney transplantation: USA versus Spain. Nephrol Dial Transplant. 2013;28:213–20.
4. Organ donation: lessons from the Spanish model. Editorial. Lancet. 2024;404:1171.
5. Ley 30/1979, de 27 de octubre, sobre extracción y trasplante de órganos. (Spanish Law about extraction and transplantation of organs). https://www.boe.es/eli/es/l/1979/10/27/30.
6. Matesanz R. El Milagro de los Trasplantes. De la donación de órganos a las células madre (The miracle of transplants. From organ donation to stem cells). Ed. La Esfera de los Libros; 2005.
7. Matesanz R. Gestión con alma. Las claves del éxito de la organización nacional de trasplantes y su aplicación a la empresa (Management with soul. The keys to the success of the ONT and their application to business). Ed. La Esfera de los Libros; 2019.
8. Matesanz R. Otra forma de donar: a corazón parado (Another way to donate: from the heart stopped). 03-23/formas-de-donacion-a-corazon-parado_3395971/.
9. Martínez Soba F, Masnou N, de la Rosa G, Povar J. El profesional de urgencias y el proceso de donación. Recomendaciones del grupo colaborativo ONT-SEMES. (Emergency personnel and the donation process). Emergencias. 2016;28:193–20.
10. Matesanz R, Domínguez-Gil B, Coll E, et al. How Spain reached 40 deceased organ donors *per* million population. Am J Transplant. 2017;17:1447–54.
11. Matesanz R, Domínguez Gil B, Coll E, et al. Spanish experience as a leading country. What kind of measures were taken? Transpl Int. 2011;24:333–42.

27

Conversations with Mariano Barbacid: A Life of Fighting Cancer

Nacho Meneses

Mariano Barbacid Montalbán was born in Madrid on 4 October 1949 (Fig. 27.1). He studied Chemical Sciences at the Complutense University in Madrid. In 1974, he obtained his PhD in Biochemistry, under the supervision of Prof. David Vázquez at the Institute of Cell Biology of the CSIC, with the thesis: "Interacción de antibióticos con el centro activo peptidil transferasa del ribosoma eucariótico" [1], (Interaction of antibiotics with the active peptidyl transferase centre of the eukaryotic ribosome). He then went to the USA, first as a fellow at the National Cancer Institute (NCI) in Maryland, where he became director of the Department of Oncology. He returned to Spain in 1998 to head the Spanish National Cancer Research Centre (CNIO) until he left in 2009, remaining as a researcher at the same centre.

When, 1 day in 1974, Mariano Barbacid left Dulles airport in Washington D.C., he did so aboard a small plane flying behind a massive Boeing 747. He was on his way, at the invitation of a colleague, to a cancer conference in Hershey, Pennsylvania, but little did he know that the first talk he would hear would forever change the course of his scientific career. "I didn't have money for a hotel, so we had to get there and back in a day; it was a beating. But [my colleague] said to me, 'Let's go by plane. As I'm from an aeroclub, we can rent it just like renting a car," he recalls, with a half-smile, from his small,

N. Meneses (✉)
Journalist newspaper "El País", Madrid, Spain

M. A. Cuesta, F. Mateo Vallejo (eds.), *Spain's Journey in Medicine*,
https://doi.org/10.1007/978-3-032-12221-6_27

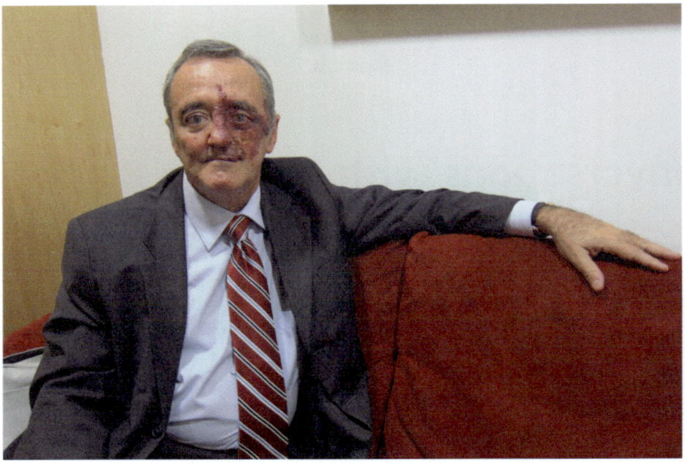

Fig. 27.1 Mariano Barbacid

elongated office at the headquarters of the Spanish National Cancer Research Centre (CNIO) in Madrid.

Barbacid, then a young biochemist who had recently arrived in the United States as a postdoctoral researcher, accepted the proposal without thinking twice: "I love flying, so I told him let's go to the congress, or we'll go for a beer, but I'm going". He was already showing the same initiative and determination that, at the age of 13 and under the guidance of two good teachers (Carmen Michelena, one, and Rosario, whose surname he does not remember) awakened his curiosity and interest in science.

The opening lecture, delivered by Mike Bishop and Harold Varmus (recipients of the 1989 Nobel Prize in Physiology or Medicine), presented a discovery that challenged long-standing ideas: retroviral oncogenes — cancer-causing genes first identified in viruses — were in fact mutated versions of normal genes already present in the human genome.

"This opened up the possibility that human cancer might also be caused by similar oncogenes, without the involvement of viruses, instead triggered by spontaneous mutations or external carcinogenic agents," he explains.

At that moment, I asked myself: *Could human cancer be caused by those same oncogenes, not requiring the participation of a virus, but rather arising from spontaneous mutation?*

The hypothesis was powerful, but it was not enough to formulate it: it had to be shown that these genes, when activated by mutation, could cause cancer in humans. "In physics, you can predict the Higgs boson and wait 60 years for it to be found. In biology that doesn't work. If you don't prove it, it's useless".

In *El camino inverso (The reverse path)*, the documentary about his career by Mediapro and the Quintero Brothers Foundation (Spain), Mariano Barbacid recalls that the first documented case of cancer caused by an external element was that of the chimney sweeps in London: they developed cancer of the scrotum because soot accumulated there, they also did their business without washing their hands, and the soot had carcinogenic agents [2].

The opportunity to empirically demonstrate his hypothesis came 8 years later, in 1982. Barbacid — by then at the National Cancer Institute in Maryland, which he would later direct — applied a technique developed by Ángel Pellicer at Columbia University (New York) to identify transforming genes in cell lines. After several experiments with human cells, he obtained positive results.

"We saw that human cells contained these genes, which needed to be cloned and then isolated," he explains. "I worked with 20 or 30 cell lines, and once I got a positive result… I isolated it, cloned it, and characterized it." He had just identified and isolated the first human oncogene. From this work emerged the RAS genes, the first human oncogenes, which subsequently became the focus of extensive research to understand their mechanisms of action.

An oncogene is an altered or mutated gene (proto-oncogene) that can promote uncontrolled cell growth ultimately resulting in the formation of cancer [3].

In molecular biology, transformation is the genetic alteration of a cell by the direct action and expression of DNA from its surroundings.

The finding, published that same year, was a paradigm shift: "When I went to the United States, absolutely nothing was known about how cancer was produced. It was a black box," he says. The discovery (then received with incredulity) served to demonstrate, for the first time, that a specific mutation in a human gene, HRAS, could be the origin of a cancer process: "It was not a complete answer, but it was an open door" [4, 5].

RAS, from "Rat Sarcoma virus" is a protein encoded by genes. The instructions for making the RAS protein are found in the DNA of genes. The protein is involved in cell signaling pathways that regulate cell growth and division and differentiation (from ScienceDirect). Mutation in the RAS genes produce abnormal RAS proteins that can contribute to the uncontrolled growth of cells (from National Cancer Institute). Mutation in RAS genes can lead to cancer.

There are multiple RAS genes, like H-RAS, K-RAS and N-RAS, that code for similar but distinct RAS proteins [6].

K-RAS Oncogene and the Scientific Frontier

After the discovery of H-RAS, Barbacid continued to explore the role of other oncogenes in different types of cancer. In the 1990s, his career took a new turn with the identification of the TRK gene (Tyrosine Receptor Kinase) and, in parallel, he began a line of work that would end up focusing his attention on one of the most frequent and difficult-to-treat mutations in oncology today: the K-RAS oncogene (the K stands for Kirsten rat sarcoma virus), responsible for 25% of lung cancers, 50% of colon cancers and 95% of pancreatic cancers. "In a nutshell: if we could one day manage to control or cure the action of this oncogene and have an impact on the tumor, it would be wonderful. Especially with pancreatic tumors… And that is what we are working on". Barbacid is not selling smoke or false hopes but speaks with the sobriety and knowledge of someone who has spent more than 50 years dedicated to research (and those that remain).

For decades, KRAS was considered unapproachable from a pharmacological point of view. "KRAS is like a tiny heart, very round, and for many years it was thought that no inhibitor could be placed there," he explains. Despite being one of the most frequent mutations in tumors such as lung, colon and pancreatic cancer, no one was able to design a molecule capable of fitting into its structure: "It took 30 years to identify a small hole where you could put a molecule, an inhibitor. The drug was approved in 2021. We discovered KRAS in humans in '82, so 40 years had passed". That first inhibitor, Sotorasib, approved by the FDA, has been a clinical milestone, although his results, he says, have been limited. "The median survival is seven months. It has no advantage over chemotherapy, except that it is less toxic".

The identification of TRK was made in Stuart Aaronson's laboratory at the US National Cancer Institute. A discovery that, as is often the case in science, was a bit of chance and a bit of intuition.

One Friday afternoon, a sample of colorectal tumor tissue arrived at the laboratory as part of the routine workflow maintained with Memorial Sloan Kettering. Barbacid recalls the moment vividly: "I saw that it was on ice and thought this is no longer suitable for establishing cell lines; it needs to be frozen." Instead of discarding the sample, he decided to cut a fragment and isolate its DNA.

"I had a hypothesis: perhaps oncogenes were consistently detected because cell lines remained in culture for extended periods of time. So I thought: if I analyze a freshly obtained tumor, I might find something different."

And he found it — despite the fact that the probability of such an event was estimated at one in a thousand. The tumor harbored a fusion involving the NTRK1 gene and the gene encoding the receptor for nerve growth factor (NGF) [7, 8]. This discovery not only led to the description of a new oncogene but also enabled the first identification of the receptor for NGF, whose existence had already been recognized when Stanley Cohen and Rita Levi-Montalcini were awarded the Nobel Prize in 1986.

"The receptor was unknown — and, unexpectedly, this was it," he recalls, still with a sense of wonder.

Decades later, this specific mutation gave rise to an entirely new class of targeted antitumor therapies — the TRK inhibitors — notable for their ability to act regardless of the tissue of origin of the tumor. This represents one of the earliest examples of genetically driven targeted therapy: among these agents, larotrectinib has demonstrated clinical efficacy even in pediatric patients [9, 10].

Barbacid learned of this impact first-hand at a dinner organized by the CRIS Cancer Foundation in Spain. Sitting next to Antonio Pérez, head of Pediatric Oncology at La Paz Hospital in Madrid, he heard a story that touched him very closely. "He told me that he had a baby with fibrosarcoma, and in the biopsy they found a mutation for which they had just come out with a syrup. He didn't even call it a drug. A syrup. And he says to me: it's a new oncogene, I don't know if you've heard of it, TRK. I say: well, yes. We discovered it ourselves!

The crossover between basic science and clinical experience then became tangible. "Seeing a basic discovery become an effective treatment is one of the greatest satisfactions of my career," he says. Since then, he has maintained a friendship with the oncologist, and a deep admiration for what they have achieved in that pediatric unit. "This guy's work is top-notch. And in an environment like the public health system, and what La Paz is, it's wonderful".

TRK, unlike KRAS, was a discovery that found its way to the patient relatively early; perhaps because the mutation was easier to target and perhaps because someone like Barbacid did not pass up that sample that arrived on a Friday afternoon, when many others would have discarded it.

In his CNIO laboratory in Madrid, Barbacid works with genetically modified animal models to faithfully reproduce the behaviour of human tumors. They have identified two other therapeutic targets that when acting together with KRAS, cause complete tumor regression in mice. "They disappear, it's spectacular," he says. But again, there is a gap between this finding and the clinical application: "An inhibitor is not a drug. An inhibitor is a molecule that works, whereas a drug is a molecule that does not kill the patient. And that requires a whole other stage of development.

The challenge is technical, economic and regulatory. And it also has a political dimension that often does not understand the timing of science, whose basic research needs long periods of time and constant funding. But in a country like Spain, where - according to him - "researchers no longer even protest", this type of science is difficult to sustain: "The government has given me 150,000 euros a year. And the maintenance of our mice alone costs around 300,000. If I had to live with this, I would have retired!.

That discovery, he recalls, was not theirs alone, since two other laboratories had demonstrated it in parallel. And he recalls a conference in Squaw Valley, California, to which these two labs were invited: "I wasn't invited because, of course, nobody knew me. But I went and presented my poster with my findings; that's something that is still being done now: people who are not invited present their data like that".

So there was Dr. Barbacid, standing next to his poster, when a man came up who turned out to be Peter Rigby, a scientist and editor of *Nature,* and continue Barbacid*:* "I had on there on the poster, that we had cloned the gene, the structure of the restriction map.... We knew that the mutation that activated it wasn't very big, but we wouldn't discover that until October of that year (this was March). Rigby congratulated him on his work and, as he was leaving, asked him which of the two labs (Robert A. Weinberg's or Michael Wigler's) he had done his work with. Barbacid replied that he had done neither: just him nor a couple of *postdocs.* "And, with his characteristic English phlegm, he said, "You're telling me you've done all this, and I've never heard of you?"

A Race Against Time and the System

The limitations of the Spanish research system have been a constant theme in his statements for years, and Barbacid has never disguised his disenchantment with the way science is organized and funded. One of the elements that irritates him most is the lack of structural and continuous funding. "You have to ask for projects every three years. I have a 50-year career, and I have to justify every three years what I'm going to do," he laments.

The anecdote that illustrates this disagreement may seem minor, but it sums up the heart of the problem: a collaborator of his, already with a place at the university, continues some experiments in his laboratory, "and she has been given 50,000 euros a year. What do you do with that? Nothing. You can't hire anyone. Nothing. You can't hire anyone. Well, yes, you hire one and you don't have a single euro left. It's just that we spend 300,000 on mice alone. Only in maintaining and genotyping them".

Barbacid frequently refers to animal models as an essential tool for validating the efficacy and toxicity of possible treatments. "Now there are those who argue that organoids are enough; that we don't have to use mice, but if it is toxic for the brain, how do you see it? The first ones to die? Because an organoid has no brain, no heart and no kidneys".

Organoids are three-dimensional mini-organs grown in the laboratory that mimic the structure and function of human organs. They are used to investigate diseases, treatments and biological development, offering an alternative to animal models.

To what extent are the results obtained with laboratory mice extrapolated? Barbacid points out two major differences: first, that the tumor in mice is much smaller; and second, time: in lung cancer, for example, it takes about 30 years from the moment you start smoking until the tumor appears. "If we cure lung or pancreatic cancer in a mouse, we are not naïve enough to think that we can cure human cancer with the same thing. But because the mechanism of tumor formation is the same, we do expect it to have an impact.

His experience in the pharmaceutical industry - he worked for 10 years at Bristol-Myers in Princeton - allows him to speak with first-hand knowledge of the approval process for new drugs. "A company won't bring out a compound if it hasn't been tested on animals. Because if there is toxicity, the company is going to be responsible. And in the United States they get smashed. They get a lawsuit that sinks them".

Since returning to Spain in the late 1990s, after two decades in the United States, Barbacid has tried to build more stable structures. In 1998 he founded the Spanish National Cancer Research Centre (CNIO), with the support of the Ministry of Health. And he did it, he says, from scratch. "I asked for two things: that the budget should come directly to us, without going through the CSIC or the university, and that we could manage it independently. Ana Pastor, the minister, told me: 'OK'. I asked her for 20 million and she gave it to me. Without doing any study; without memory. She trusted me".

But there is no room for triumphalism in his account. He admits that he made a mistake by not legally shielding the CNIO's Board of Trustees, the centre's governing body. "When the government changed and Celia Villalobos came in, it became clear to me that some politicians don't care about the CNIO. And if they have to be president of the Board of Trustees, they are, but they don't really care" [11, 12].

That raw, unfiltered tone is as much a part of his public persona as his scientific curriculum vitae. Far from moderating it, he embraces it. He speaks as he thinks, even when doing so distances him from certain prevailing currents. "Nowadays, there are things that feel out of place," he says, referring — with a touch of provocation — to broader social debates that sometimes surface in his discourse.

Yet when the conversation turns back to cancer and science, his demeanor changes. He speaks with precision — at times with fatigue — but never with indifference.

No Time to Retire

Throughout his five-decade career, Barbacid has defended basic research as the only solid path to real advances in the fight against cancer. The road, he says, is long and full of obstacles, but it is the only one that allows us to understand the mechanisms of the disease in order to eventually offer clinical answers. A conviction that has kept him active even when, at his age, others would have opted for a comfortable and well-deserved retirement: "That's what I'm going to devote the rest of my life to, as long as I have funding and have a bit of brain left," he promises.

Other Contributions

In 2003, Barbacid showed that the CDK2 enzyme, which until then was thought to be essential for cell division, was not needed for the initiation of replication, and that even without it, cells could replicate their DNA and divide. His group is currently working on new therapeutic combinations against KRAS, a front that is still open. "We are now finishing revising the manuscript for *Nature.* One of the reviewers is one of the people who developed the KRAS inhibitors, and he doesn't like it when we say they don't work well. But they don't work well. That's what the data show.

Over the years, Barbacid has adopted an increasingly direct way of speaking. He does not hide it, nor does it bother him. "I am 75 years old. I'm not going to shut up anymore," he defends. This way of expressing himself has grown with his career. He does not soften the nuances when he refers to political decisions, to scientific practices that he considers erroneous or to the lack of institutional ambition. “There are some things that are grating,” he says quietly, without elaborating on them, but making it clear that he doesn't care about everything.

What has not changed is his loyalty to those he considers fundamental to his career. When he talks about David Vázquez, his thesis director, the tone changes: “He taught me to do research, to follow the scientific method, to be rigorous and honest”. Sadly, Vázquez died of colon cancer at the age of 56, shortly after receiving the Prince of Asturias Award in 1985.

In parallel to this career, his personal life was often relegated to the background, but Barbacid accepts this without drama: “I have given priority to my career, that's true. I'm not going to hide it. When he left for the United States, he broke off a relationship with a person he loved, convinced that such a change would make it impossible for them to live together in a healthy relationship. “In Spain we would have been compatible, but in the United States, without speaking the language, without friends, without a network, it would have been a disaster. There he lived for 14 years with an American woman, whom he could not marry because divorce did not exist in Spain at that time. “I was married in inverted commas,” he says. “Now everyone says, ‘my partner’, but in my time they didn't use that word”.

The demands of a lifetime devoted to science are clear to see when he is asked what he does to switch off, because he simply doesn't do it: “This is what I like”, he admits, although of course he also has other passions. He played football until he was 40, in university and neighborhood leagues, even in the United States. “I was very bad, but I was very keen,” he admits with a smile. Later, he took up skiing - “I ski down the black ones, even if it's through the hole” - and maintains a strong devotion to classical music and opera. He sometimes regrets modern stagings, which in his opinion betray the spirit of the works: “I went to Verona to see Aida, and in the Triumphal March they came out with bicycles disguised as camels. An aberration”.

Humor and irony, which appear without warning, are also part of the character. But they never cloud the underlying seriousness. When talking about his work, the gaze is focused, and the message is direct; Barbacid does not seek unnecessary ornaments. He wants the science to speak for itself. “We are not here to do experiments with little cells that are worthless. We are here to understand cancer. And for that we have to keep searching”.

References

1. Mariano Barbacid Montalbán. Interaction of antibiotics with the active peptidyl transferase centre of the eukaryotic ribosome. Complutense University of Madrid; 1974.
2. El camino inverso (The reverse path). Fundación QUAES Youtube 6/11/2023.
3. Reddy EP, Reynolds RK, Santos E, Barbacid M. A point mutation is responsible for the acquisition of transforming properties by the T24 human bladder carcinoma oncogene. Nature. 1982;300:149–52.
4. Sukumar S, Notario V, Martin-Zanca D, Barbacid M. Induction of mammary carcinomas in rats by nitroso-methylurea-involves malignanat activation of H-ras-1 locus by single point mutations. Nature. 1983;306:658–61.
5. Zarbl H, Sukumar S, Arthur AV, Martin-Zanca D, Barbacid M. Direct mutagenesis of HA-RAS-1 oncogenes by N-Nitroso-N-Methylurea during initiation of mammary carcinogenesis in rat. Nature. 1985;315:382–5.
6. Barbacid M. Ras genes. Ann Rev Biochemist. 1987;56:779–827.
7. Klein R, Jing SQ, Nanduri V, O'Rourke E, Barbacid M. The TRK proto-oncogenes encodes a receptor for nerve growth factor. Cell. 1991;65:189–97.
8. Lamballe F, Klein R, Barbacid M. trkC, a new member of the trk family of tyrosine protein kinases, is a receptor for neurotrophin-3. Cell. 1991;66:967–79.
9. Malumbres M, Ortega S, Barbacid M. Genetic analysis of mammalian cyclin-dependent kinases and their inhibitors. Biol Chem. 2000;381:827–38.
10. Hennessy EJ, Sheedy FJ, Santamaria D, Barbacid M, O'Neill LA. Toll-like Receptor-4 (TLR4) Down-regulates MicroRNA-107, Increasing Macrophage Adhesion via Cyclin-dependent Kinase 6. Biol Chem. 2011;286:25531–9.
11. Sampedro J. El Pais (29 September 2009). Barbacid leaves CNIO directorship to focus on research. Retrieved 29 September 2009. "The scientist has already expressed his intention to leave his post after the start-up of the cancer centre".
12. Meneses N. El Pais (23/6/2023). Mariano Barbacid, biochemist: In Spain people don't talk about science; it's something that doesn't matter. And if it doesn't matter, why are you going to invest in it?

28

In Search of the Secret of Sudden Death: The Brugada Syndrome

Pedro Brugada, Josep Brugada, and Ramón Brugada

In 1992 we published an article entitled "Right bundle branch block, persistent ST segment elevation and sudden cardiac death: A distinct clinical and electrocardiographic syndrome. A multicenter report." [1] (Figs. 28.1 and 28.2).

In this publication we describe eight patients who survived documented sudden death due to ventricular fibrillation. All had a macroscopically normal heart, with no heart valve lesions, perfectly functioning heart muscle, normal biopsies, and completely patent coronary arteries, and no other abnormalities. Three patients were children, two of them siblings. Six were men and two were women. In five of them ventricular fibrillation was the first manifestation of the disease. In two others there had been previous episodes of syncope

P. Brugada (✉)
Free University of Brussels, Brussels, Belgium

Medical Centre Brugada, Aalst, Belgium

Hospital Medical Helicopters, Puerto Banús, Málaga, Spain

J. Brugada
Universidad de Barcelona, Barcelona, Spain

R. Brugada
Universidad de Girona, Girona, Spain

M. A. Cuesta, F. Mateo Vallejo (eds.), *Spain's Journey in Medicine*,
https://doi.org/10.1007/978-3-032-12221-6_28

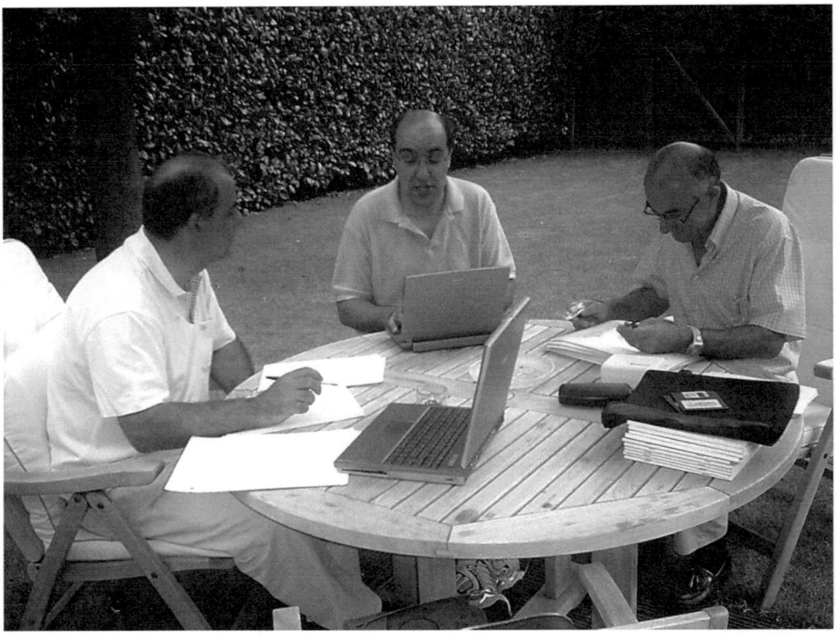

Fig. 28.1 The Brugada's brothers (Josep left, Ramón center and Pedro, right) correcting the book: "Nuestros electrocardiogramas más queridos" (Our most loved ECG), 2003

before the sudden death averted, and in the third (eight-year-old girl) atrial fibrillation had been discovered since birth.

Sudden cardiac arrest averted, or sudden death averted suggest a scenario where someone has narrowly escaped death, often due to a medical event or intervention.

Their cardiac arrest was not preceded by previous syncope. Four patients had a family history of sudden death of unknown cause at a young age (less than 42 years). In the first patient, a boy, episodes of ventricular fibrillation were triggered during fever. What did these patients have in common to suggest a distinct, new cardiac syndrome? All of them had a curious pattern resembling right bundle branch block, but with marked ST segment elevation in the right precordial leads. Additional findings were atrial fibrillation, sinus dysfunction, conduction disturbances with prolongation of the PR intervals in the ECG and HV (His-ventricular interval) in the electrophysiological study, and induction of ventricular fibrillation or sustained polymorphic tachycardia with programmed stimulation in the seven patients in whom the study could be performed. With the data collected, we postulated that it was a purely electrical disease of the

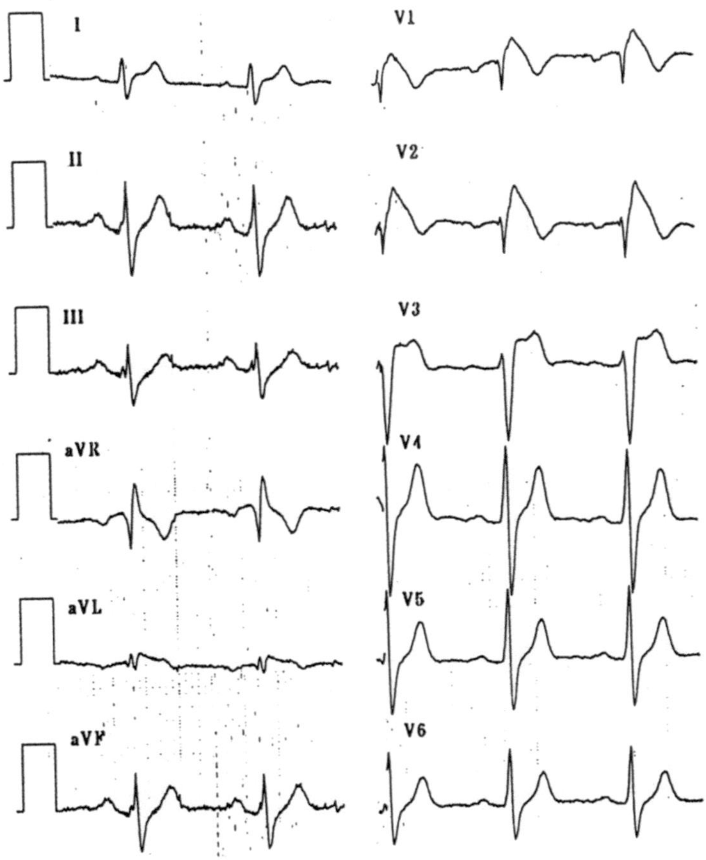

Fig. 28.2 Typical ECG of the Brugada Syndrome. Right bundle branch block, persistent ST segment elevation in the right precordial leads

heart, with a clear hereditary factor, with arrhythmias caused by functional reentry with or without a component of anisotropy in the conduction of the cardiac electrical impulse. At that time we thought that our publication was nothing more than a mere scientific curiosity that would be quickly forgotten. The passage of time showed us that we were very wrong. With currently almost 5000 citations received by the original article and more than 50,000 citations of the related articles, we have to conclude that the publication was not a curiosity, but a true revolution in the world of sudden death. In fact, we had just discovered one of the secrets of death. To understand this phrase in all its fullness, we have to go into the past, ...

Prehistory

"Those who are going to study medicine, and young physicians, should light their torches with the fire of the ancients." (Rokitansky in the introduction to the translation of the Papyrus Ebers by Cyril P. Bryan). In the Ebers papyrus (named after its discoverer, the German Egyptologist Georg Ebers), the oldest book in the world (4000 B.C.E.), the picture of sudden death is clearly described: "If a patient has pain in his arm and left side of the chest, there is an immediate risk of death". Progress on this medical picture was very slow. For a new description of sudden death it took 3500 years until Chio (China) explains that: "an irregular pulse is a predictor of immediate death" and Hippocrates writes in his aphorisms: "an intense pain in the chest and clavicle and dorsum is a sign of poor prognosis," to continue with: "obese individuals die more frequently suddenly than the thin," and: "those with episodes of syncope die suddenly." The first known graphic illustration of sudden death came to us with a tombstone carved with the body of Pheidippides (or Philippides), the hemerodromos or "day runner" or "news-bearing runner" who died after running from Marathon to Athens. The second illustration was the engraving showing Count Gaston de Foix in the fourteenth century, who, sensing the bad time coming, said to those close to him, "I am a dead man, may God have mercy on me." (Fig. 28.3)

It was not until the eighteenth century that sudden death began to be understood. Giovanni M. Lancisi established the relationship between sudden death, chest pain and heart disease, but without specifying anything concrete. A few steps forward were made with William Heberden's description of angina pectoris, and in the nineteenth century with Albert von Bezold's observation that occlusion of a coronary artery could produce cardiac arrest. Already in the twentieth century, James B. Herrick fully developed the concept of myocardial infarction, but it is only at the end of the twentieth century that non-ischemic causes of sudden death began to be recognized, starting with long QT syndrome (1957 and 1963), polymorphic adrenergic tachycardia (1982), and the arrhythmogenic right ventricular dysplasia (1982) [2]. Despite these advances, in a large group of patients with sudden death the exact cause of the problem remained unknown, and these were classified as patients with idiopathic ventricular fibrillation, i.e., of unknown cause [3]. In these patients all tests were normal. However, as we shall see, falsely normal in many, if not all, patients.

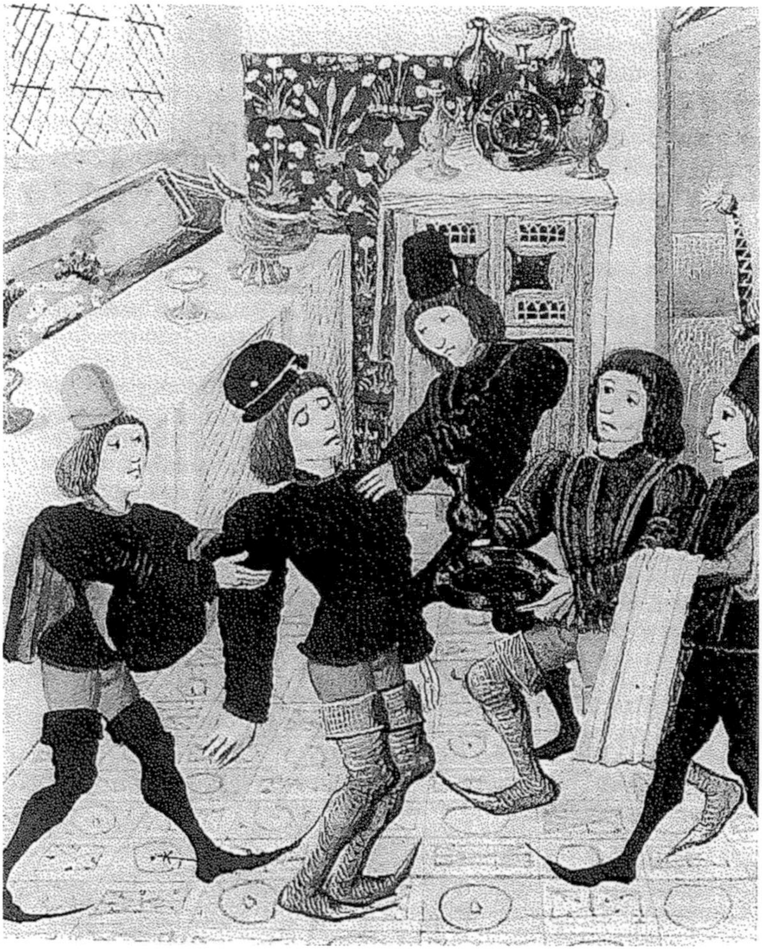

Fig. 28.3 Count Gaston de Foix in the fourteenth century, who, sensing the bad time coming, said to those close to him, "I am a dead man, may God have mercy on me

Progress in Technology and Physiology

Not surprisingly, progress in unmasking the secrets of sudden death advanced in parallel with technological progress. The most important "Millennial Stones" in cardiology were:

- The discovery of electricity by William Gilbert (1600).
- Discovery of conduction between nerves and muscles by Jan Swammerdam (1668).

- In 1774 William Hawes and Thomas Cogan recover a three-year-old girl from sudden death with the application of electricity to her body and prophetically declare, "No person should be given up for dead until all possible means of recovery have been used."
- 1775. Peter Ch. Abildgaard resuscitates chickens with electric shocks.
- In 1791, the invention of the galvanometer by Luigi Galvani made it possible to measure the intensity of electric current, an essential step for the later development of electrocardiographs.
- 1972. In his experiments with executed criminals, Giovanni Aldini revives them with electric shocks.
- In the middle of the nineteenth century, Emil du Bois-Reymond discovered the muscle action potential, A. von Hoffa described fibrillation in animals, and Rudolph A. von Kolliker and Heinrich Muller confirmed for the first time the relationship between electric current and heartbeat.
- William Thompson develops the galvanometer with mirror that allows to write down the results of the measurements, which will lead A. Waller to record the first human ECG in 1887. It will be Willem Einthoven with his string galvanometer who will make possible the reliable and easy recording of the ECG a few years later (1895).
- In 1926, anonymous authors published for the first time the use of a "pacemaker" to resuscitate a newborn. The authors kept the publication anonymous fear of being criticized, even punished, by their colleagues, as the patient was a newborn.
- In 1980 M. Mirowski and M.M. Mower implanted the first internal defibrillator in a human being. B. Lown criticized them in such esteemed journals as Circulation as promoters of demonic ideas. Fortunately, it did not take long to recognize that M. Mirowski and M.M. Mower had started a true revolution in the treatment and prevention of sudden death.

These developments in the clinical field were driven by the great advances in physiology during the nineteenth and twentieth centuries:

- The sinus node and the normal conduction system of the heart and the abnormal (pathways accessory) are described by A. Keith and M.W. Flack, L. Aschoff and S. Tawara, Bachmann, W. His, J.E. Purkinje, Kent, I. Mahaim and James.
- A theory about the cell membrane is presented (Hermann and J. Bernstein) while A. Hodgkin and A. Huxley show the existence of local currents in cells and demonstrate the presence of cellular channels that open and close creating the electrical activity of the heart and nerves.

From ECG to Clinical Electrophysiology and Genetics of Arrhythmias

It was in 1952 that this knowledge of the electrical activity of the heart led to the development of clinical electrophysiology in the following years. Dirk Durrer in Amsterdam and Philippe Coumel in Paris independently demonstrated in 1967 the possibility of initiating and terminating tachycardias in the human heart by programmed electrical stimulation. Twenty years later (1987) a meeting is held in Maastricht (Fig. 28.4) in which almost 800 of the world's top experts in cardiac arrhythmias participate.

The purpose of the meeting was not to celebrate what had been achieved, but to outline the lines of research to be followed in order to accelerate

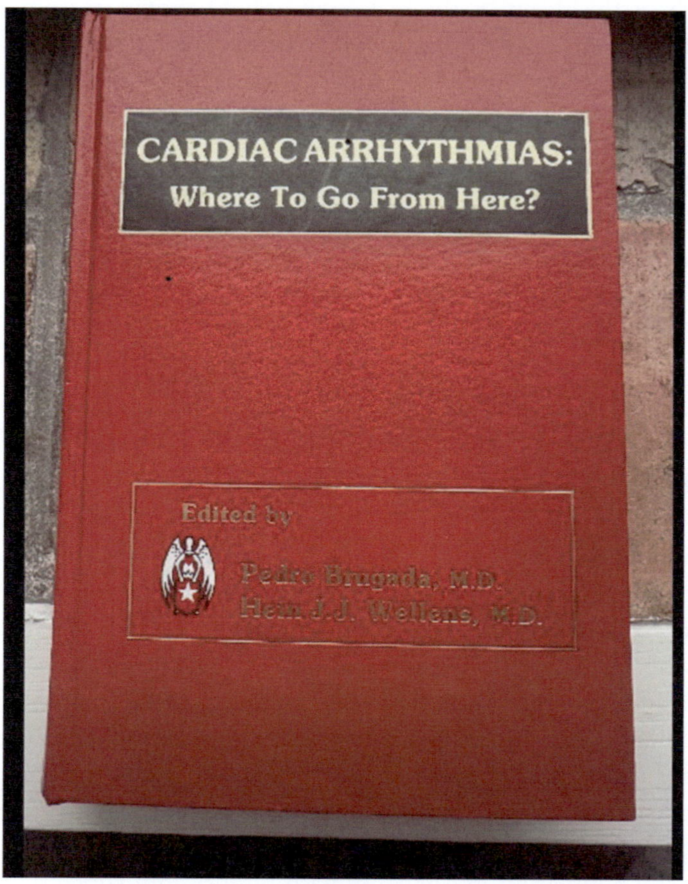

Fig. 28.4 Cover of the book, published on the occasion of the congress about arrythmias in Maastricht, "Cardiac Arrhythmias: Where to Go from Here" Edited by Pedro Brugada and Hein J.J. Wellens, 1987

exponentially our knowledge and thus achieve optimal treatment of patients with arrhythmias. The results of the meeting were quickly felt in practice: close collaboration arises between basic and clinical researchers, engineers, pathologists, and surgeons. They even discussed topics as diverse as the control of scientific research and such sensitive issues as the relationship between universities and industry. It was in the early 1990s that genetics made its full entry into the world of arrhythmias, starting with the discovery of the first gene responsible for the heritable long QT syndrome [4]. As the mechanisms of arrhythmias became better understood, catheter ablation became universal, accompanied by the development of better surgical ablation techniques for more complex arrhythmias such as ventricular tachycardia after myocardial infarction. The use of implantable defibrillators is now widespread. Curiously, despite so much progress with new technologies used in cardiology, one of them, perhaps the cheapest, the ECG, continues to show its immense value. It is the ECG that leads to the discovery of two new diseases: in 1992 the Brugada syndrome (so named by Japanese authors) [1], and in 2000 the short QT syndrome [5].

Discoveries that almost completely erase the concept of idiopathic ventricular fibrillation. But how is it possible that it took so long for these entities to be recognized? Particularly Brugada syndrome, the most frequent cause of sudden death in patients with normal heart, much more frequent than long QT syndrome, catecholamine-dependent polymorphic tachycardia, and short QT syndrome? [6].

A Retrospective History of Brugada Syndrome: What Folklore and Traditions Tell Us

In Northern Thailand there is a tradition that is believed to date back more than a century. During the night after his wedding, the groom dresses up as a woman to go to sleep. The idea of the disguise is to fool the witch (called Batibat) who, according to the popular saying, becomes jealous of the bride and comes at night to suffocate the groom by sitting on his mouth (Fig. 28.5).

These beliefs (there are other popular versions, of course) have their origins in the high prevalence of sudden death nocturnal arrest in young men in Southeast Asia, the Philippines and Japan. Subsequent studies have shown a high prevalence of Brugada syndrome in these areas, as high as 5 per thousand of the general population in Thailand, with publications suggesting even 1% [7]. Brugada syndrome has also been clearly shown to be the cause of sudden

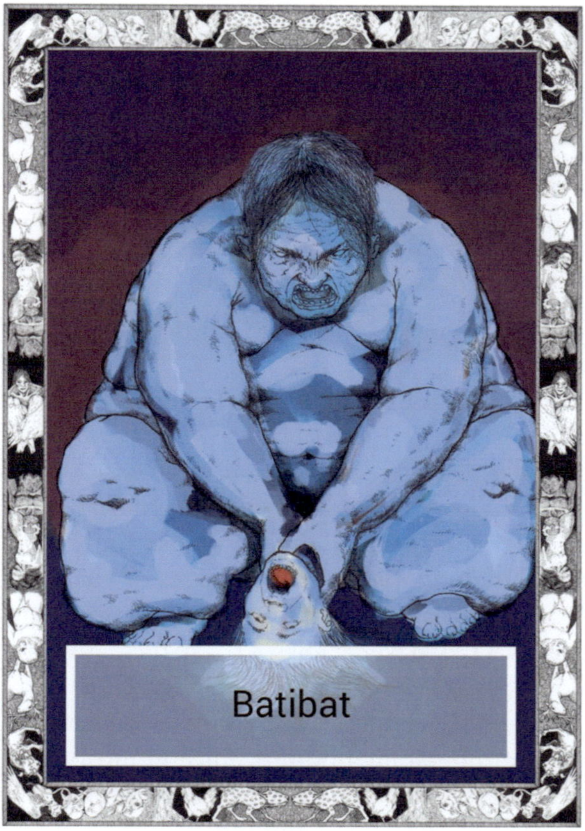

Fig. 28.5 One of the different forms that take Batibat according to the traditional beliefs

death in what used to be called sudden unexpected death syndrome (SUDS or SUNDS) known as "Bangungut" in the Philippines. Bangungut is called Pokkuri in Japan, Tsob Tsuang in Vietnam, Laos and Cambodia and Lai Tai in Thailand. These are areas of high prevalence of Brugada syndrome. The different names describe the same thing: snoring during sleep and dying. This is the typical situation where a patient with Brugada syndrome dies. It was Maria Paz Mendoza-Guazon who first described Bangungut in 1917 in the Philippine Journal of Medicine and Pharmacy (Fig. 28.6).

She referred to it writing, "In this country, the victims are young men (average age 33 years) in apparent good health, who after a hearty meal at night, wake up with symptoms of snoring, with agonal respiration and difficulty in breathing." Dr. Mendoza did not have an electrocardiograph and could not find any clear cause for the Bangungut [8]. In the following

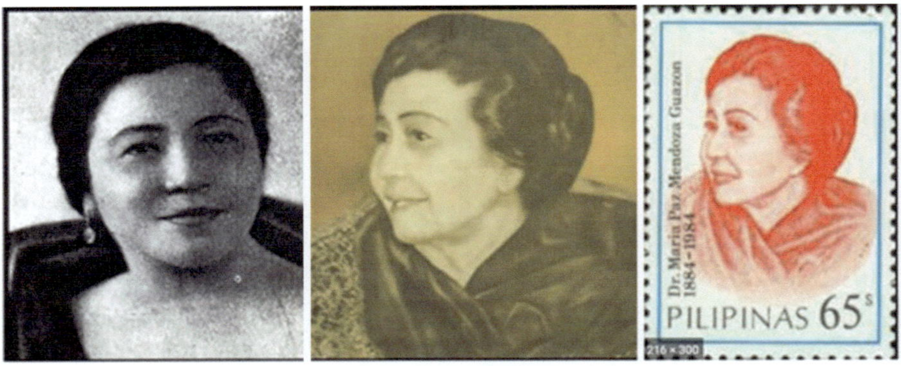

Fig. 28.6 Dra. Maria Paz Mendoza-Guazón who first described Bangungut in 1917

decades, many studies related to sudden unexpected death in young patients in apparent good health were published: A.R. Moritz and N. Zamcheck studied 140 military men with SUDS in whom findings during autopsy were normal. A.V. Majoska published 120 cases of young Filipino men in the Hawaii Medical Journal, without finding the cause. There were publications on Mexicans (J. Chavez Nolasco), Japanese (M. Sugai), Hmong (A. Adler), followed by studies on emigrants in the United States of America (Baron), and Singapore (Goh). In none of the studies was a correlation made with electrocardiographic findings, since in most of them there were no records because they were apparently healthy people with no previous symptoms. The lack of substantial findings led to incredible speculation about the cause of death, from the Batibat story to suspicions of suicide, allergies, or murder by intoxication or suffocation [8]. The Bangungut inspired Wes Craven to make one of the best horror movies ever made "A nightmare on Elm street" where Johnny Depp made his acting debut. Parallel to these studies that did not clarify the cause of sudden death, publications appeared on ECGs that, retrospectively, corresponded to patterns that today we would recognize as diagnostic of Brugada syndrome. Curiously, no connection was made between the electrocardiographic findings and sudden death. Thus, an intense search by Andrés Riera [8] suggests that the first ECG published compatible with Brugada syndrome would be one by H.L. Osher and L. Wolff in 1953. These authors published only one case and considered the pattern as a variant of normal. The same was concluded by L. Calo in another case he published. Numerous articles on SUDS followed without finding a cause for the syndrome. In 1989 B. Martini published six cases of idiopathic ventricular fibrillation where, retrospectively, one patient could be identified with an ECG that we would now consider typical of Brugada syndrome. He concluded that his patients had structural heart disease, similar to right ventricular dysplasia. No specific mention was made of the electrocardiographic pattern.

The Encounter, New Patients and Difficulties in Publishing

It was in 1986 when the first patient in our series appeared with his father in our office. The child was at that time 3 years old. He had already suffered several episodes of syncope and had been resuscitated several times. His sister had died of ventricular fibrillation at the of 3 years. The child had suffered several episodes of syncope and cardiac arrest despite wearing a pacemaker and being treated with amiodarone. The child's syncope episodes were triggered during fever. Admitted to the hospital all his examinations were normal, except for the ECG in Fig. 28.2. During his stay in the coronary unit he presented an episode of spontaneous ventricular fibrillation that we treated with external electric shock. Thanks to the father's help, we were able to obtain the ECGs of the deceased sister. The father smuggled the documents himself across the Berlin Wall to the university hospital in Warsaw and returned with the girl's documents. The ECGs were identical to those of her brother. This could no longer be a coincidence, and the ECGs could not be a variant of normal. Over the course of the next 4 years we were able to recognize two additional unrelated patients (one Belgian and one Dutch). Both had suffered ventricular fibrillation. Their ECGs were identical to those of the two children. The findings during cardiological examinations were otherwise completely normal. It was in 1991 that we presented a poster with the four patients at the NASPE (North American Society of Pacing and Electrophysiology) meeting in Washington, D.C. During the meeting, a multitude of our former students reviewed the poster. Many of them thought they had seen something similar and promised to send us the data and ECGs of their cases. Thus was born one of the most heterodox multicenter studies that ever existed: no research protocol, no ethics committee (at that time there were none in most research centers either), no financial support of any kind from public or private institutions. It was simply a study based on the scientific interest of the participants. Among the various cases that were sent to us, we found four patients with the same characteristics as ours. Thus the first manuscript was born. Manuscript yes, but publishing it was another story. The study was rejected by almost all existing cardiology journals. The reviewers' comments were always the same: that it was a variant of normal, that it was a variant of long QT syndrome, that it was Printzmetal's angina. From the repetitive comments, the similar English grammar, the misspellings, even from the typeface of the typewriters of the time, it was clear that we were continually running into the same reviewers in the different journals. We had to change our strategy, or we would never see our study published. "A bald opportunity is a bald one", says the saying, a saying that originates from the Goddess of the Occasion, with beautiful long hair in front, but bald behind, indicating that when she passes in front of us, we must take the hair, because when she finishes passing there is nowhere to hold it. And so we did. Armed with all the material in the article, including the reviewers' comments, we went as guests to the opening of the arrhythmia center of an ex-fellow, Dr. Karl-Heinz Kuck in Hamburg. We knew that Melvin Scheinman, associate editor of the Journal of the American College of Cardiology (JACC) was going to be present. During the rapporteur dinner we sat next to him in the Italian restaurant and after a few grappa's, we attacked him with our problem. We presented the data to him as a simple scientific curiosity, urging him to publish it as such. Mel promised to personally review the article, which he did. After rejecting the repetitive arguments of the previous reviewers, and with some accurate corrections suggested by him, the article saw the light of day in November 1992. What followed, and continues to follow, is one of the most fascinating adventures of the scientific history.

After 1992

After publication in 1992 [1], knowledge about Brugada syndrome grew exponentially. An important milestone was the discovery of the genetic defect causing the disease in the SCN5A gene [9]. Although up to 20 different genes have subsequently been identified, the SCN5A gene, which encodes the cardiac sodium channel, is where mutations responsible for Brugada syndrome are most frequently found. These investigations resulted in the full entry of genetics into cardiology, which made it possible to understand the great variety of pathologies that a single gene can produce, depending on whether there is an increase or a decrease in the function of the corresponding channel (Fig. 28.7).

The consequences of the publication were not long in coming. Immediately the new knowledge made us understand other clinical pictures, such as the cause of sudden death of the newborn, the possible relationship with sudden nocturnal death, sudden death after exercise (perhaps Pheidippides?) and

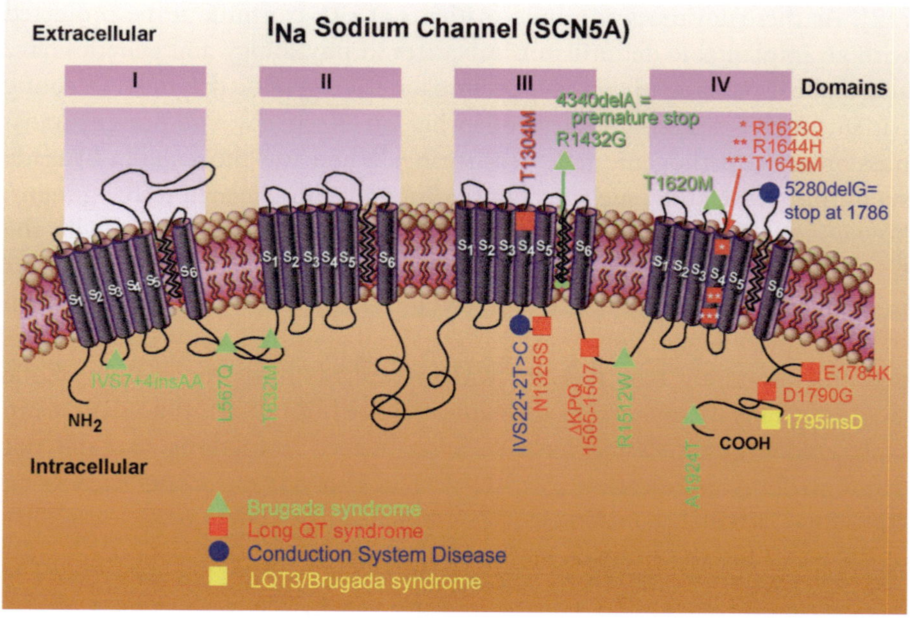

Fig. 28.7 Diagram of the sodium channel, 2000, showing different diseases caused by mutations known in this year. Today, more than three-hundred different mutations are known in the Brugada Syndrome

naturally the cause of many syncopes of unknown cause. The etiology of Bangungut and so-called "sudden Voodoo death" was also understood. The implications of the syndrome were reflected in all areas of medicine, from pediatrics, gynecology, to forensic medicine, to occupational medicine, sports medicine, epidemiology, veterinary medicine [10] and even medical history. How many unexpected deaths in history were caused by Brugada? The sudden deaths of many well-known athletes? For example, the case of Tommy Morris Jr. famous Scottish golfer, who dies at the age of 24 in his sleep? Many deaths are suspected of this. After understanding the detrimental effects of drugs and medications on Brugada syndrome (see www.brugadadrugs.org) one may wonder if the death of singer Michael Jackson was not caused by Brugada syndrome unmasked by the Propofol he was receiving. Brugada syndrome had important implications for physiology. Numerous publications studied the mechanisms of arrhythmias, with sometimes opposing theories. The findings led to the development of ablation techniques aimed at curing Brugada syndrome [11]. Over time and with very long follow-up of our patients, an algorithm could be developed to stratify the risk of sudden death based on truly scientific data rather than subjective feelings

[12]. As these advances continue, patients at risk continue to be protected with an implantable defibrillator. Advances in physiology and genetics have also made it possible to consider preimplantation genetic diagnosis in young patients with a desire for healthy offspring, an effective way to prevent transmission of the pathogenic gene to offspring. Where was the secret in Brugada syndrome? If we know such ancient traditions as those related to Bangungut, how is it possible that it took so long to define this syndrome? Naturally, the first problem for diagnosis is related to the fact that the heart of these patients is macroscopically normal. Despite seeing so many cases and studying them in detail, pathologists could never make the diagnosis. Firstly, an ECG was needed, something that was not widely available until the middle of the twentieth century, once seen the typical ECG (Fig. 28.2), the relationship with sudden death should have been established, something that did not occur until our publication in 1992. But in Brugada syndrome there is an additional factor that makes diagnosis difficult: the spontaneous variability of the ECG and the Brugada pattern (Fig. 28.8).

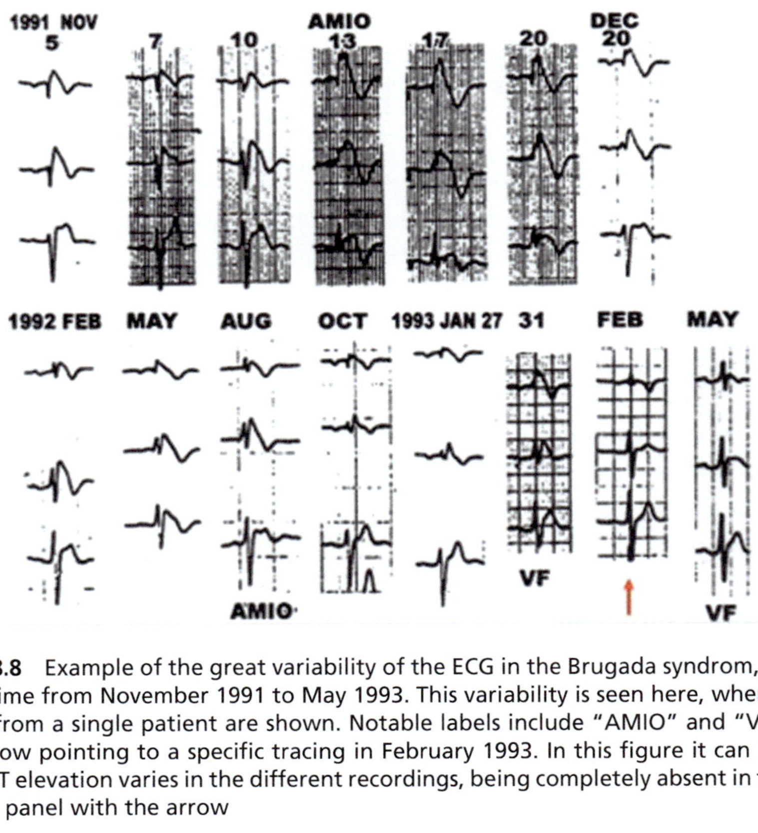

Fig. 28.8 Example of the great variability of the ECG in the Brugada syndrom, tracing over time from November 1991 to May 1993. This variability is seen here, where serial ECGs from a single patient are shown. Notable labels include "AMIO" and "VF" with an arrow pointing to a specific tracing in February 1993. In this figure it can be seen how ST elevation varies in the different recordings, being completely absent in the ECG of the panel with the arrow

This variability is seen in Fig. 28.8, where serial ECGs from a single patient are shown. In this figure it can be seen how ST elevation varies in the different recordings, being completely absent in the ECG of the panel with the arrow. An analysis of our patients with Brugada syndrome showed that the ECG normalizes at a given time in virtually all of the recordings, implying that if the patient is seen at the time when the ECG is normal, the diagnosis is neither suspected nor made. Mutations in the sodium channel in Brugada syndrome cause a decrease sodium current. This is the basis for conduction disturbances and ST elevation. Cardiac currents are influenced by many factors. In the case of Brugada syndrome, vagal stimulation increases ST elevation and adrenergic stimulation decreases it. Increased body temperature (fever and exercise) can increase ST in patients with temperature-dependent mutations [13]. Drugs that influence the electrical currents of the heart also have an effect on the appearance of ST. Thus, administration of sodium current blocking drugs increases ST elevation and may cause ventricular fibrillation. These effects, if well controlled, can be used to unmask the syndrome in patients in whom it is suspected but the ECG is normal. The suspicion may come because the patient is a relative of another with Brugada syndrome or because there is history of sudden death in the family of unknown cause, someone with syncope of unknown cause or with idiopathic atrial fibrillation (especially at a young age). Sodium channel blockers, such as ajmaline, procainamide, flecainide or pilsicainide, are used to unmask the ECG pattern. Because of its greater diagnostic sensitivity and short half-life, ajmaline is the drug of choice for this pharmacological test. As it is not available in all countries, one of the alternative drugs can be used, considering a lower sensitivity for procainamide and the danger of late arrhythmias with flecainide due to its long half-life.

Figure 28.9, shows an example of a positive test in a patient with syncope and a family history of sudden death at a young age, in whom the ajmaline test shows that he is a carrier of Brugada syndrome. It has been suggested by some authors [14], that these tests could be false positives, without clarifying why they would be false positives, i.e., what is the alternative explanation. This reminds us of the ease with which in the past it was accepted that the electrocardiographic pattern of Brugada syndrome was simply a variant of the normal ECG, without any scientific basis, nor any response from other scientists, without further explanation. A positive ajmaline test in the absence of alternative explanations (of which we are unaware) is diagnostic of Brugada syndrome. It is evident that ECG variability in Brugada syndrome greatly complicates the diagnosis. With a normal ECG, the diagnosis may go unnoticed, unless the physician suspects it and procures a pharmacological test to

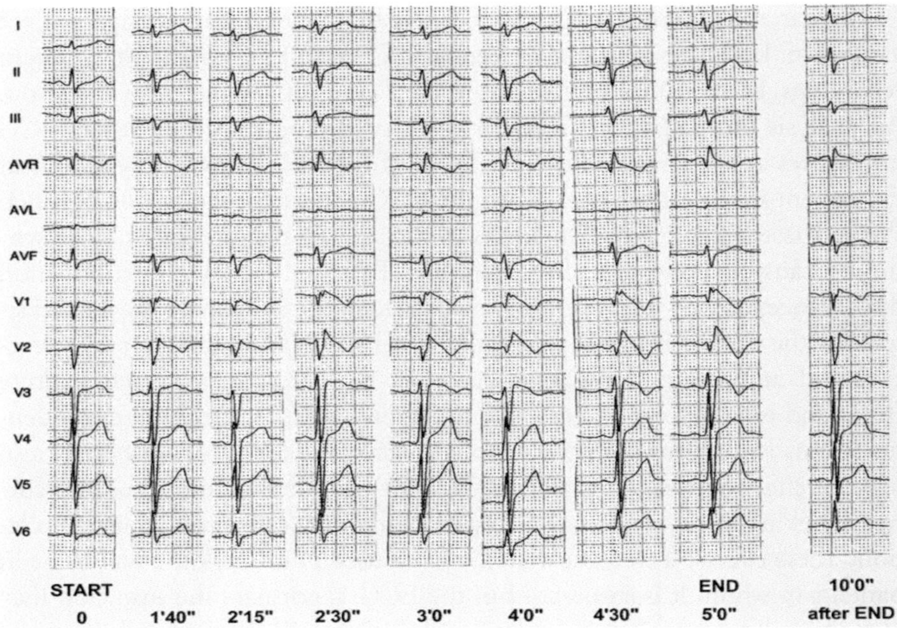

Fig. 28.9 Example of a positive test in a patient with syncope and a family history of sudden death at a young age, in whom the ajmaline test shows that he is a carrier of Brugada syndrome (Elevation of the ST during administration of the ajmaline)

confirm or rule it out. Thinking about and making a diagnosis of Brugada syndrome depends, like everything else in medicine, on the physician's determination. This explains the apparent variability in the diagnosis of cases in different countries. The statistics we know about regional prevalence are influenced by the physician's willingness to seek the diagnosis. If no ajmaline test is performed in patients with a normal ECG, with syncope of unknown cause, or with idiopathic atrial fibrillation, the cause will never be found to be Brugada syndrome

Brugada Syndrome, Philosophy, and Well-Being of Our Patients

Brugada syndrome has also led us to the field of philosophy, particularly ethics and logic. The most important philosophical and practical problem is illustrated in Fig. 28.10, with the paradox of "the physician as a risk factor" [15]. When considering the possible risk of sudden death we can use Sieira's algorithm to get an objective idea of the risk to the patient, but in doing so we may fall into the

The physician as a risk factor

1 **Risk assessment**	2 **Physician's appreciation of risk**	3 **Action by physician**	4 **Result in case of event**
Low	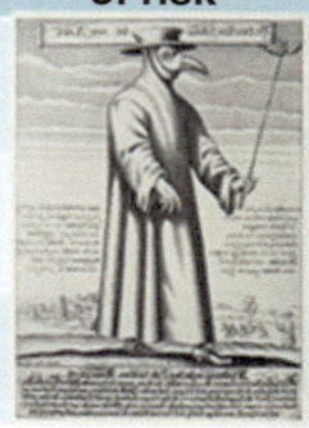	Do nothing, passive attitude	Death
Intermediate		Protect?	Death if not protected
High		Protect!	Alive

Fig. 28.10 Stratification of the risk, when considering the possible risk of sudden death we can use Sieira's algorithm to get an objective idea of the risk to the patient, but in doing so we may fall into the paradox of the physician as risk factor

paradox of the physician as risk factor. Why? What is this paradox? By considering the different risk categories we will classify our patients into low and high risk groups. In doing so, we try to decide who is and who is not a candidate for treatment of the syndrome, through implantation of a defibrillator with or without accompanying ablation, either preventively because of high risk (primary prevention), or because the patient has already suffered a previous cardiac arrest (secondary prevention). It will not be difficult for the physician to convince himself and the patient of the need for treatment when the patient is considered high risk. Thus, high-risk patients are treated and protected. In case of an episode of ventricular fibrillation, the defibrillator will terminate the arrhythmia and the patient will survive. The situation is very different if the patient is classified as low risk. The physician's approach to the patient will be very different. When considering the patient as low risk, the tendency will be not to treat and wait, apart from the usual recommendations such as avoiding potentially proarrhythmic drugs and treating fever. But what will happen to the patient if he/she go into ventricular fibrillation? Not being protected by the implantation of a defibrillator, the probability of surviving a cardiac arrest is less 10% in Europe. In other words, the high-risk patient is protected and survives the arrhythmia, whereas the low-risk patient inevitably dies due to lack of protection in the event of developing a malignant arrhythmia. This is the paradox of the physician as a risk factor. Actually, this paradox is even more relevant if we consider what "high and low risk" really means. High risk, no problem, but low risk? Low risk compared to what? Yes, low compared to the high-risk group with Brugada syndrome, but if we compare the effective risk of the low-risk patient with Brugada syndrome with the risk of sudden death in a healthy population without the syndrome and the same age, the risk of patients with Brugada syndrome and "low risk" is 300 times higher than in the population without the syndrome. This does not indicate that all patients should be treated, including those at low risk, but it does indicate that in the decision to treat or not, the patient should be involved and his or her wishes should always be respected. A problem linked to ethics and psychology that we should discuss is related to the consequences of the diagnosis of the syndrome, especially in patients in whom it is discovered by causality or during family examination and who are asymptomatic. The impact of the diagnosis should not be underestimated. The psychological impact and insecurity of the diagnosis (what will happen to me and my children?) are enormous. Feelings of guilt about having passed on the disease to offspring often develop. These negative feelings about hereditary diseases lead to divorce and even suicide [16]. The diagnosis can lead to loss of employment (train or bus drivers, airline pilots, professional athletes), loss of life and health insurance protection, or unacceptable increase in fees. During the process of diagnosis and development of the treatment strategy, the wishes of the patients should always be at central point. The medical team should act only as an informant and supporter of the patient's wishes. This is a very complex task that requires dedication and time and medical team that is willing to help, not to confuse the patient with doubts about the diagnosis or the plan to follow. The physician's doubts do not help the patient. Therefore, the approach to the patient and family members with Brugada syndrome is a process that should be left in the hands of highly specialized centers equipped to face the problems of diagnosis, prognosis, treatment and psychological and social support. Centers where the medical team is willing to make clear decisions, knowing that any decision always carries the risk of error.

The Future and Final Notes

The technological revolution continues to make giant strides. The development of the CRISPRcas17 or "genetic scissors" technique has opened the door to the possible manipulation and cure of hereditary diseases (see Chap. 35) [17]. The theoretical part is very simple: cut out the genetic defect with the scissors and "sew" in its place a piece of healthy genetic material. Although in practice we encounter major problems (such as the side effects of the vector used to transport the genetic material), there is no doubt that this is the real future for the cure of Brugada syndrome. If in the future this cure can be offered in an effective and uncomplicated manner, all the present discussions will seem ridiculous. There will be no need for risk stratification after diagnosis. There will be no need for electrophysiological studies, ablation techniques or defibrillator implantations. We will simply cure our patients by correcting the problem, not the consequences of the problem as we do now. We can only hope that this future is not far away. Although the future may not exist (Dean Buonomano), it is clear that we are the ones who create it.

Acknowledgments It would be laughable to think that the discovery of Brugada syndrome was made as if by magic. Nothing is less true. Many circumstances, and certainly some coincidences, allowed us to look with different eyes at a type of ECG that until then had been considered normal. Our eyes had been trained by our teachers. With the same eagerness we trained the eyes of our students, learning again in the process. With the support of both teachers and fellow students, our eyes were lucky enough (and trained) to look differently. But this would not have been possible without the support of our environment; including our families. The people who participated directly or indirectly in this story are so many, it is impossible to name them one by one, but they all know to what degree we have and continue to appreciate their support. In the now more than 30 years after the original publication, the concept of a new disease was not accepted overnight. On the contrary, discussions at scientific congresses, in the medical literature and even in the were tough, even exasperating. Like any discovery, Brugada syndrome went from a phase of surprise to an immediate phase of denial on the part of many colleagues, followed by another of enthusiasm, to lead us back to a period of doubts and even reproaches, until we reached calm waters. Frankly, these hard times were precisely the greatest encouragement for us to move forward. For this, we are enormously grateful to all those who criticized us so harshly in the past. This is the great advantage of science; with time it corrects itself and in the end the truth prevails. We would like to apologize for the limited number of references presented due to space limitations. The references do not reflect the extensive bibliography and the immense work of many colleagues who have contributed to the current reality of Brugada syndrome. Therefore, we encourage the reader to search for more information on the Internet.

References

1. Brugada P, Brugada J. Right bundle branch block, persistent ST segment elevation and sudden cardiac death: a distinct clinical and electrocardiographic syndrome. A multicenter report. J Am Coll Cardiol. 1992;20:1391–6.
2. Bezzina CR, Wilde AAM, Roden DM. The molecular genetics of arrhythmias. Cardiovasc Res. 2005;67:343–6.
3. Lemery R, Brugada P, Bella PD, Dugernier T, Wellens HJJ. Ventricular fibrillation in six adults without overt heart disease. J Am Coll Cardiol. 1990;13:911–6.
4. Hedley PL, Jørgensen P, Schlamowitz S, Wangari R, Moolman-Smook J, Brink PA, Kanters JK, Corfield VA, Christiansen M. The genetic basis of long QT and short QT syndromes: a mutation update. Hum Mutat. 2009;30:1486–511.

5. Gussak I, Brugada P, Brugada J, Wright RS, Kopecky SL, Chaitman BR, Bjerregaard P. Idiopathic short QT interval: a new clinical syndrome? Cardiology. 2000;94:99–102.
6. Papadakis M, Papatheodorou E, Mellor G, et al. The diagnostic yield of Brugada syndrome after sudden death with normal autopsy. J Am Coll Cardiol. 2018;71:1204–14.
7. Veerakul G, Khongphatthanayothin A, Nademanee K. Brugada syndrome in Thailand: three decades of progress. Heart Rhythm. 2022;16:743–51.
8. Riera AR, Schapachnik E, Ferreira C. Brugada disease: chronology of discovery and paternity. Preliminary observations and historical aspects. IPEJ. 2003;3:253–60.
9. Chen Q, Kirsch GE, Zhang D, Brugada R, Brugada J, Brugada P, Potenza D, Moya A, Borggrefe M, Breithardt G, et al. Genetic basis and molecular mechanism for idiopathic ventricular fibrillation. Nature. 1998;392:293–6.
10. Brugada-Terradellas C, Hellemans A, Brugada P, Smets P. Sudden cardiac death: a comparative review of humans, dogs and cats. Vet J. 2021;274:105696.
11. Nademanee K, Veerakul G, Chandanamattha P, Chaothawee L, Ariyachaipanich A, Jirasirirojanakorn K, Likittanasombat K, Bhuripanyo K, Ngarmukos T. Prevention of ventricular fibrillation episodes in Brugada syndrome by catheter ablation over the anterior right ventricular outflow tract epicardium. Circulation. 2011;123:1270–9.
12. Sieira J, Conte G, Ciconte G, Chierchia GB, Casado-Arroyo R, Baltogiannis G, Di Giovanni G, Saitoh Y, Juliá J, Mugnai G, La Meir M, Wellens F, Czapla J, Pappaert G, de Asmundis C, Brugada P. A score model to predict risk of events in patients with Brugada Syndrome. Eur Heart J. 2017;38:1756–63.
13. Dumaine R, Towbin JA, Brugada P, Vatta M, Nesterenko DV, Nesterenko VV, Brugada J, Brugada R, Antzelevitch C. Ionic mechanisms responsible for the electrocardiographic phenotype of the Brugada syndrome are temperature dependent. Circ Res. 1999;85:803–9.
14. Tadros R, Nannenberg EA, Lieve KV, Škorić-Milosavljević D, Lahrouchi N, Lekanne Deprez RH, et al. Yield and pitfalls of ajmaline testing in the evaluation of unexplained cardiac arrest and sudden unexplained death: single-center experience with 482 families. JACC Clin Electrophysiol. 2017;3:1400–8.
15. Brugada P. On risk stratification and its paradoxes. Eur Heart J. 2021;42:715–6.
16. Niaz T, Saunders M, Bos J, et al. Prevalence of suicide among patients with sudden death–predisposing genetic heart diseases. JACC Clin Electrophysiol. 2021;7:253–5.
17. Bhatia S, Pooja, Yadav SK. CRISPR-Cas for genome editing: classification, mechanism, designing and applications. Int J Biol Macromol. 2023;238:124054.

29

Neuroendocrinology: The Race to Discover Hypothalamic Hormones

Antonio Gómez-Pan

I was born on July 4, 1946, in Laxe, La Coruña, into a family of three children. My father, Antonio, was the owner of the Capitol Cinema, while my mother, María del Carmen, worked as a dressmaker. From the early age of three, I already longed to "be a doctor". In 1957, when I started high school, my parents, in search of a better life that would allow them to pay for my higher education, emigrated to Caracas, Venezuela. Thus, the stone house with a garden facing the sea and my childhood were left behind. I finished high school at the Colegio Fray Luis de León in Caracas, becoming the youngest high school graduate in the republic. In 1964, I returned alone to Spain to begin my Medical Degree at the University of Santiago de Compostela. I secured a position as an Anatomy intern with Prof. A. J. Echeverry, obtaining honors, in Histology, where Dr. Diego Ribas Mujal congratulated me for having memorized the book "Cell Biology" by De Robertis/Nowinski/Sáez. I finished my medical degree in 1970, with outstanding rating. Endocrinology fascinated me because of its pathophysiological approach and its potential for great advances in the future. With the desire to delve deeper into this area, in 1971, I was admitted as Honorary Clinical Assistant in the Endocrinology group of Prof.

A. Gómez-Pan (✉)
Professor in Endocrinology, Madrid, Spain

M. A. Cuesta, F. Mateo Vallejo (eds.), *Spain's Journey in Medicine*,
https://doi.org/10.1007/978-3-032-12221-6_29

T. Russel Fraser at the Hammersmith Hospital in London. There I performed advanced techniques in treatments, such as Yttrium pituitary implants. In 1972, after passing the official British end-of career examination and with the aim of obtaining a more complete training in Endocrinology, I was admitted as Resident Physician in the Endocrinology Unit in Newcastle upon Tyne, after the return to England of Prof. Reginald Hall from the Massachusetts General Hospital in Boston. In that unit, attached to the University of Newcastle, I carried out my clinical and research training. In 1975, I was appointed Research Director of the Neuroendocrinology Group. My training period coincided with the discovery of hypothalamic hormones, to which I will devote this chapter. I returned to Spain in 1977, with the position of Head of Neuroendocrinology at the Iberoamerican School of Endocrinology and Nutrition of the Complutense University of Madrid. In addition, I was appointed as Associate Professor of Experimental Endocrinology under the direction of Prof. Alberto Oriol Bosch at the Faculty of Medicine in Madrid and In 1990, as head of the Endocrinology and Nutrition Department at the Hospital Universitario La Paz in Madrid, a position I held until 1998. Subsequently, until my retirement, I worked as Head of the Endocrinology Department at the Hospital de La Princesa in Madrid.

Neuroendocrinology

In 1948, Geoffrey Harris, considered the father of modern neuroendocrinology, studied the control of the anterior pituitary and proposed that its regulation was due to factors produced in the neurons of the hypothalamus, which reach the adenohypophysis through the hypophyseal portal system. This theory predicted the later discovery of hypothalamic hormones that regulate adenohypophysis hormones [1]. The search for hypothalamic factors with hypophysiotropic activity, as well as their subsequent characterization and synthesis, represented a monumental task in which researchers Andrew Victor Schally and Roger Guillemin in the United States soon took the lead. Both researchers, although initially sharing a common goal, separated professionally due to personal disagreements, which started a competition between them to be the first to identify, isolate and synthesize hypothalamic hormones [2]. For almost two decades, they obtained, from several thousand ovine and porcine hypothalamus, only a few milligrams of

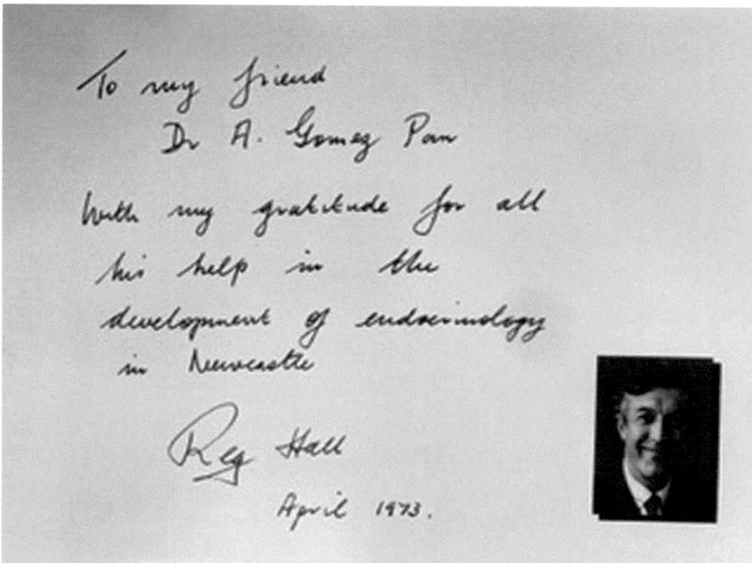
To my friend
Dr A. Gomez Pan
With my gratitude for all
his help in the
development of endocrinology
in Newcastle
Reg Hall
April 1973.

Fig. 29.1 Reginald Hall. Dedication to Antonio Gómez-Pan for his help in the development of Endocrinology in Newcastle, April 1973

active principles, which were later purified, characterized and synthesized. The hypothalamic hormones turned out to be small peptides, as they had postulated. In 1970, Reginald Hall (who years later would become my great friend Reg), Head of the Endocrinology Unit at Newcastle University, was already a recognized authority on thyroid pathology. He had worked with John B. Stanbury at the Massachusetts General Hospital and had a laboratory that analyzed, by very sensitive techniques, thyrotrophin (TSH) values. These reasons contributed to his receiving the first samples of hypothalamic thyrotrophin-releasing hormone TRH, which Andrew V. Schally had recently succeeded in synthesizing in his laboratory in New Orleans. Thus was born a long and fruitful collaboration between Newcastle, where I worked, and New Orleans, in which the actions and clinical applications of all the hypothalamic hormones that were identified over time were tested, as Schally acknowledges in his book "The Pursuit of Hypothalamic Hormones" [3] (Figs. 29.1 and 29.2).

There was also a strong collaboration between the Neuroendocrinology groups at Newcastle (Prof. Reginald Hall) and St. Bartholomew's Hospital in London (Prof. Michael Besser). From 1970 to 1977, we performed hundreds of experiments on volunteers, patients and experimental animals. These were

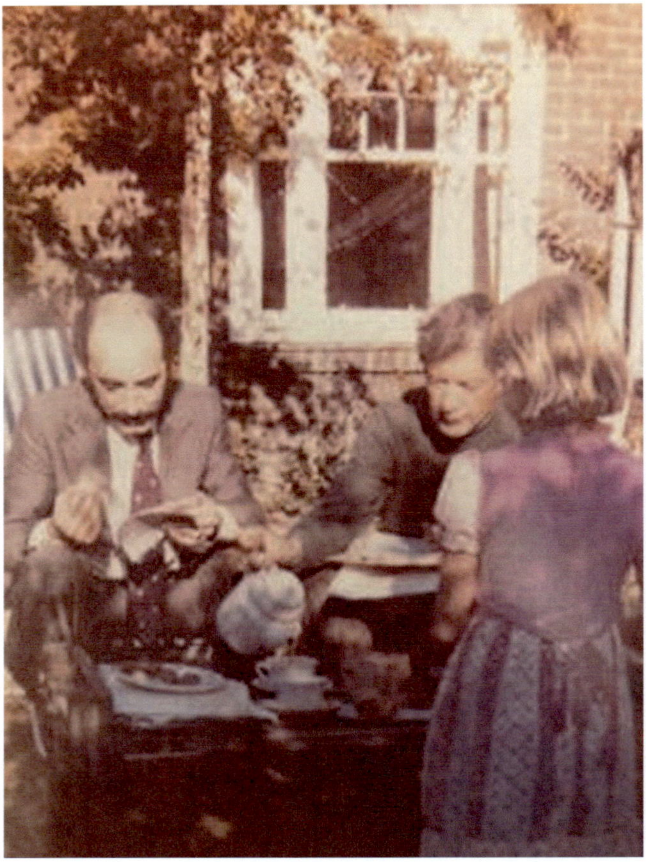

Fig. 29.2 Discussing Research projects with Reginald Hall in the garden of his house in Newcastle

years of very intense work, during which we also cared for the department's patients, conducted clinical sessions, taught and published numerous scientific articles. Thanks to the collaboration of all the members of the different teams involved, we achieved significant advances in the field of Neuroendocrinology. These joint efforts culminated in the award of the Nobel Prize in Physiology or Medicine in 1977 to Andrew V. Schally and Roger Guillemin (Fig. 29.3).

I would like to discuss the actions and clinical applications of the various hypothalamic hormones that were progressively identified and which we investigated at Newcastle, in collaboration with Schally's group in the United States.

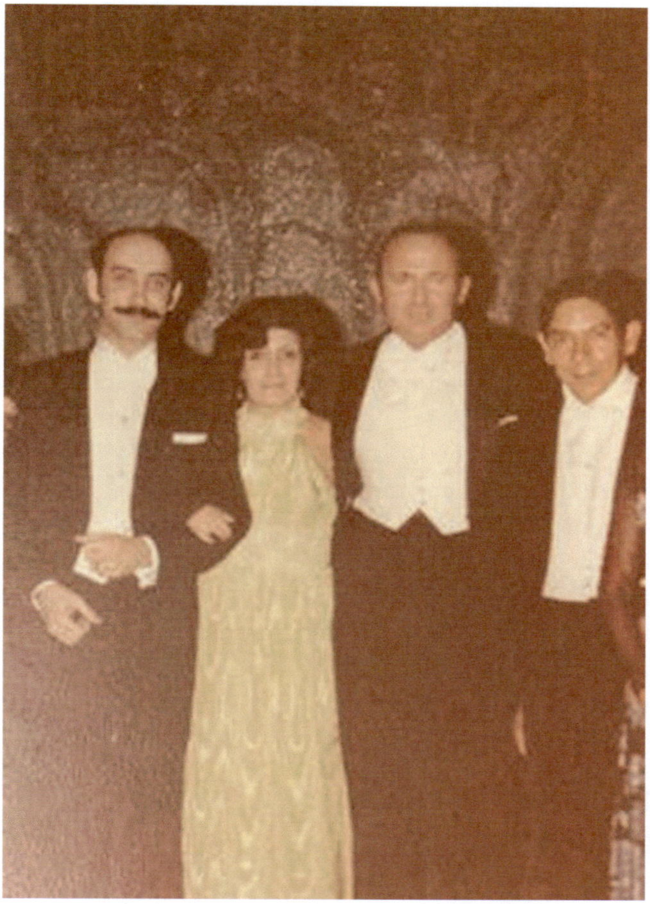

Fig. 29.3 Gala dinner after the Award ceremony of the Nobel Prize 1977. With Ana María Comaru-Schally, Andrew V. Schally and González Bárcena

Thyrotrophin-Releasing Hormone (TRH)

TRH was the first hypothalamic hormone whose structure was elucidated in 1969 from porcine hypothalamus by Schally's group. As expected, it is a small molecule, a tripeptide: PyroGlu-HisPro-NH2 [4]. Roger Guillemin, loser of the first phase of the race, although he synthesized it from ovine hypothalamus with little time difference, elegantly recognized that the characterization of TRH is the event with which Neuroendocrinology becomes an established science [5]. Administration of synthetic TRH in humans causes a dose-response release of pituitary TSH, in addition to activating prolactin secretion.

The standard TRH test was published in 1971. The tripeptide was administered parenterally at a dose of 200 mcg, with TSH determinations at baseline and at 20 and 60 minutes. This test proved to be of great clinical diagnostic utility in thyroid pathology, since it contributed to identify different degrees of hypothyroidism and to diagnose hyperthyroidism in situations where there were no ultrasensitive plasma determinations of TSH, triiodothyronine or thyroxine. The TRH-induced TSH response is modulated by circulating thyroid hormone levels. In hyperthyroidism, the TSH response to TRH is absent, and a normal response excludes this diagnosis. This absence of response to TRH is also observed in euthyroid patients with ophthalmic Graves' disease, being a relevant diagnostic finding. In primary hypothyroidism, it is not necessary to perform the TRH test, it is sufficient to determine baseline TSH levels, which will be elevated. Patients with hypothyroidism secondary to pituitary disease generally do not respond to the TRH test, whereas those with hypothalamic involvement have a positive but delayed TSH response, with values greater at 60 minutes instead of the normal response at 20 minutes. In patients with renal insufficiency, the TRH test can provoke a decreased, absent or delayed TSH response, without alterations in the hypothalamic-pituitary axis or thyroid function. As for the therapeutic role of TRH in thyroid dysfunction, it offers no advantages over other treatment methods [4].

Gonadotrophin Releasing Hormone (GnRH or LHRH)

Gonadotrophin-releasing hormone (GnRH or LHRH) was identified and synthesized by Matsuo of Schally's group in 1971 [6].

It is a decapeptide, with formula PiroGlu-His-Trp-Ser-Tyr-Gly-Leu-Arg-ProGly-NH2.

It stimulates both pituitary folliculotropin (FSH) and luteinizing hormone (LH). The LHRH test, using 100 mcg administered intravenously, produces greater increase in LH than FSH in adults. The studies, both with native LHRH and with its analogues, were carried out on volunteers, the first to receive the molecules being the members of the Unit. In patients with central hypogonadism of hypothalamic-pituitary origin, the LH/FSH response to LHRH administration does not allow differentiation of etiology. In contrast, in patients with primary hypogonadism, it is sufficient to determine basal gonadotrophins, which will be elevated. The LHRH test also allows differentiation between prepubertal and pubertal or adult subjects: administration of LHRH in prepubertal subjects elevates both gonadotropins, with a predominance of FSH over LH. In addition, LHRH is used in the Triple Stimulus

Test, where the simultaneous administration of TRH, LHRH and insulin is very useful to evaluate the patient's pituitary reserve, determining in blood the response of TSH, GH, cortisol, prolactin, LH and FSH [7]. The administration of LHRH induces a potent release of gonadotrophins, albeit temporarily; subsequently, it inhibits their synthesis and release. For this reason, the use of long-acting analogues as blockers of gonadotrophin synthesis and release has become established, which are suitable for "reversible medical castration".

Andrew Schally's group led the study of the clinical utility of these long-acting analogs.

The most widely used is possibly D-Trp6-LHRH (Decapeptyl), although more than 200 analogues have been developed by hypothalamic hormone research groups. These analogues are the treatment of choice in patients with precocious puberty, both of idiopathic central origin and due to hypothalamic hamartomas, as well as in cases of testosterone-dependent hormone (prostate cancer) or estrogen-dependent cancer (breast cancer, endometriosis) [7, 8].

Somatostatin

Somatostatin (S-S or GHRIH, initially identified as a growth hormone release inhibitory hormone, GH) is a tetradecapeptide: H-Ala-Gly-Cys-Lys-Asn-Trp-Lys-Thr-Thr-Ser-Cys-OH Its linear structure was reported by Brazeau and collaborators in 1973, from Guillemin's group, based on studies in ovine hypothalamus. In the same year, Coy and collaborators of Schally's group described the cyclic (native) structure in porcine hypothalamus [9]. Somatostatin is the most widely distributed hypothalamic peptide in the body.

Its presence has been detected in numerous organs, especially in the central nervous system.

Somatostatin-containing neuronal bodies are located mainly in the anterior periventricular nuclei. The axons of these neurons project to the median eminence, where their fibers are located in the outer layer, with terminals adjacent to the capillaries of the pituitary portal system.

In addition, somatostatin is widely distributed in the gastroenteropancreatic system.

Somatostatin: Actions on Adenohypophyseal Hormones

The physiological and pathological significance of somatostatin, as well as its therapeutic applications, have been extensively studied by our group [8–11]. Somatostatin acts as a potent inhibitor of growth hormone (GH) secretion and suppresses the GH response to various stimuli, such as exercise, insulin hypoglycemia, arginine, levodopa, and nocturnal GH spikes [8, 9].

Elevated growth hormone (GH) levels in patients with acromegaly can be suppressed by somatostatin administration. In addition, the GH response after TRH stimulation in these patients is also blocked by somatostatin [10]. In the case of paradoxical GH secretion in patients with carcinoid syndrome, somatostatin can inhibit this production [11]. Likewise, somatostatin exerts an inhibitory effect on TSH: it inhibits elevated levels of this hormone in patients with primary hypothyroidism and inhibits the TSH response to TRH. TSH has a circadian rhythm, reaching peak values at 23:00 h, which are also inhibited by somatostatin infusion [9].

Prolactin (PRL) and corticotropin (ACTH) are not affected by somatostatin, either at basal levels or after stimuli such as insulin hypoglycemia, arginine or stress. However, somatostatin can suppress elevated ACTH levels in Nelson's syndrome. On the other hand, gonadotropins (LH and FSH), both at their basal levels and after stimulation with LHRH, are also unaffected by somatostatin [9].

Somatostatin: From the Hypothalamus to the Gastrointestinal Tract

Somatostatin is present in the D cells of the pancreatic islets, dispersed in humans in all areas of the islets of the pancreas. This distribution allows somatostatin to exert local and paracrine control over pancreatic hormones, mainly insulin and glucagon, in addition to maintaining its endocrine action on them through the arterial pathway. In humans, somatostatin secreting cells present a gradient from the stomach to the colon, with the gastric antrum being the area of highest concentration. In the intestinal wall, somatostatin interacts with other secretory cells, such as gastrin, glucagon, secretin and cholecystokinin, as well as with pepsin and gastric acid, exerting an inhibitory action on them. Somatostatin released into the interstitial space also exerts an autocrine action [9].

Gastrointestinal Actions of Somatostatin

Exocrine secretions: Somatostatin inhibits gastric secretion of pepsin, hydrochloric acid and intrinsic factor, as well pancreatic secretion of bicarbonate and enzymes, and intestinal and biliary secretions [12].

Endocrine secretions: It also acts by inhibiting the secretion of various hormones, including gastrin, secretin, CCK-PZ, GIP, VIP, enteroglucagon, pancreatic polypeptide, motilin, neurotensin and substance P.

Motility: Somatostatin inhibits gastric emptying, intestinal motility and gallbladder motility.

Blood flow: Decreases mesenteric blood flow and increases mesenteric vascular resistance.

In addition, somatostatin reduces the absorption of calcium, glucose, galactose, fructose, lactose, xylose, amino acids, triglycerides and water.

Actions of Somatostatin in the Endocrine Pancreas

Somatostatin inhibits basal insulin secretion, as well as that induced by stimuli such as glucose, arginine, glucagon and tolbutamide.

In addition, it also acts by inhibiting basal glucagon secretion and its response to stimuli. Both actions are carried out through the action of somatostatin on the membrane receptors of the alpha and beta cells of the pancreatic islets, using a negative feedback mechanism, mainly in the alpha cells [9].

Actions of Somatostatin on Gastric Secretion

Gastrin secretion: Somatostatin administration causes a delay in the rise in blood glucose after an oral glucose overload, although this effect is not observed when the overload is administered intravenously. This dissociation of effects suggests that somatostatin acts directly on the gastrointestinal tract, not only on insulin and glucagon.

Somatostatin decreases gastrin levels (basal and after stimulation). It inhibits, by direct action on gastric parietal cells and gastric principal cells, the secretion of hydrochloric acid and pepsin, respectively. In addition, it reduces acid and pepsin secretion in response to pentagastrin stimulation, as well as acid secretion in response to food intake, as demonstrated in studies in experimental animals (cats) with chronic gastric fistula [12]. These studies [12] established for the first time that this hormone exerts exocrine effects in addition to endocrine effects, as commented by Andrew Schally [6].

Clinical Applications of Somatostatin

Intravenous administration of somatostatin has a short duration. On the other hand, long-acting analogues are very useful in the treatment of patients with acromegaly, as is the case of octreotide (SMS 201–995). These analogs are also used in the treatment of insulinomas, neonatal nesidioblastosis, glucagonomas, gastrinomas and carcinoid tumors [13–15]. Upper gastrointestinal bleeding caused by duodenal or gastrointestinal ulcers can be treated with somatostatin, which has been shown to be even more effective than cimetidine. This is due to its ability to decrease mesenteric blood flow, increase gastric mucus production and exert a cytoprotective effect, as well as inhibit gastrin and gastric hydrochloric acid secretion. Somatostatin has also been used preoperatively in patients with Zollinger-Ellison syndrome and in the treatment of gastrointestinal bleeding due to esophageal varices. Good results have been obtained using somatostatin in the treatment of pancreatic fistulas. In addition, somatostatin has a prophylactic usefulness in preventing pancreatitis after endoscopic retrograde cholangiography (ERCP). It is considered the treatment of choice in cases of acute pancreatitis and in the management of pancreatic pseudocysts [16].

The Nobel Prize in Medicine or Physiology 1977

Neuroendocrinology reached its peak when both researchers Andrew V. Schally and Roger Guillemin were awarded the Nobel Prize in Physiology or Medicine in 1977. This recognition was due to their "enormous contribution to the understanding of the structure of hypothalamic hormones and the interrelationship between the brain and the endocrine system" (Presentation Speech, Prof. Rolf Luft, December 10, 1977). They shared the award with Prof. Rosalyn Yalow, who was recognized for the development of the radioimmunoassay technique for peptide hormones. In their Nobel Prize acceptance lectures, Roger Guillemin and Andrew V. Schally highlighted how hypothalamic hormones have given rise to the new Endocrinology: Neuroendocrinology [5, 6].

Roger Guillemin, born January 11, 1924, in Dijon, France, and died in San Diego on February 21, 2024, was a member of the French Resistance during his youth. He studied medicine at the University of Burgundy and later moved to Canada, where he worked at the University of Montreal alongside Hans Selye. In the United States, he began his career at the Baylor Institute in Houston (1953–1970) and, in 1970, he founded the Laboratory of Neuroendocrinology at the Salk Institute in La Jolla, San Diego, California.

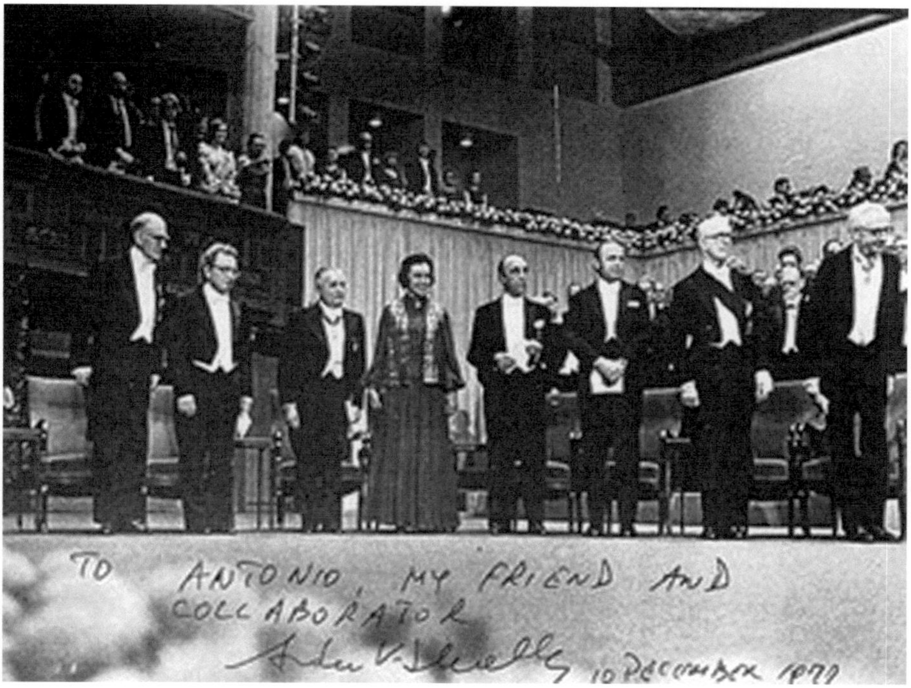

Fig. 29.4 Ceremony of the Nobel Prize, dedication of Andrew V. Schally : "To Antonio, my friend and collaborator, 10 December 1979"

Andrew V. Schally was born on November 30, 1926, in Vilnius, Poland (now Lithuania). His father was a general and head of the Cabinet of the President of Poland. In 1939, the family was exiled to Romania, while his father went into exile in Great Britain. In 1945, Schally continued his studies in England and later received his doctorate in Endocrinology from McGill University in Montreal. From 1957 to 1962, he worked at the Baylor Institute in Houston with Roger Guillemin, before moving to the Veterans Hospital of Tulane University in New Orleans. Vicente Aleixandre was awarded the Nobel Prize in Literature in the same year, unable to collect it, it was done by the poet Justo Jorge Padrón.

As mentioned above, I participated very actively in the design, realization and publication in journals of some of the papers that merited this Nobel Prize. The honor of having collaborated was immense. The Swedish Academy appointed me as a personal guest of Andrew V. Schally, receiving the invitation through the Spanish Royal House, attending all the events of the celebration and the award ceremony in Stockholm (Figs. 29.4 and 29.5).

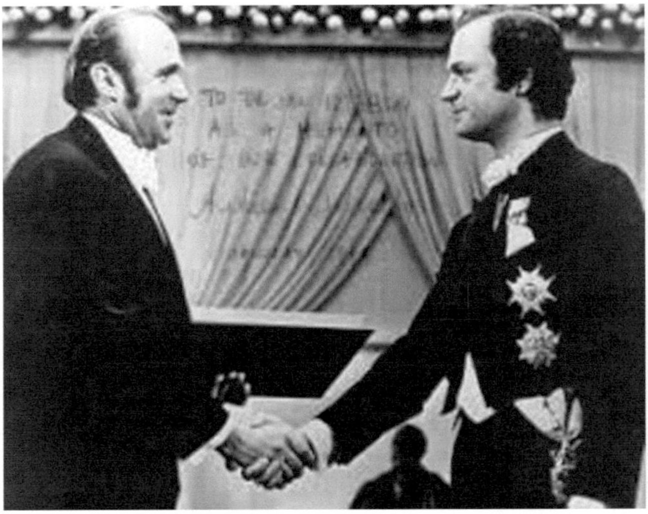

Fig. 29.5 Andrew V. Schally receives the Nobel Prize from the King Carl XVI Gustaf of Sweden

Neuroendocrinology Anecdotes

1. I made several trips to New Orleans to discuss with A.V. Schally and his team the achievements of their experiments. The atmosphere at Tulane University was very cordial, with Andrew Schally, Akira Arimura and Aba Kastin. In 1975, after I had given several lectures, Andrew proposed me to stay a few more days in New Orleans for sightseeing. Obtaining Reg Hall permission, I changed the airline ticket to extend my stay and enjoyed the wonderful city. Unfortunately, the plane that was initially supposed to take me to New York was involved in a terrible accident, with only 11 survivors out of 124 people on board. Thanks to my officially granted leave, my parents and relatives did not receive any adverse notification. At that moment, I felt like I was born again (Fig. 29.6).
2. In 1974, I presented initial data on the gastrointestinal actions of somatostatin in humans during the General Clinical session at my hospital in Newcastle. At the end of the lecture, David Reed, Professor of Physiology in the Newcastle University Medical School, came up to congratulate me on the results and commented, “We have a colony of cats, the animal whose digestive tract is most similar to humans, with chronic gastric fistula. They are at your disposal.” The cats, excellently cared for, were named Pixie and Dixie, and allowed us to demonstrate that somatostatin inhib-

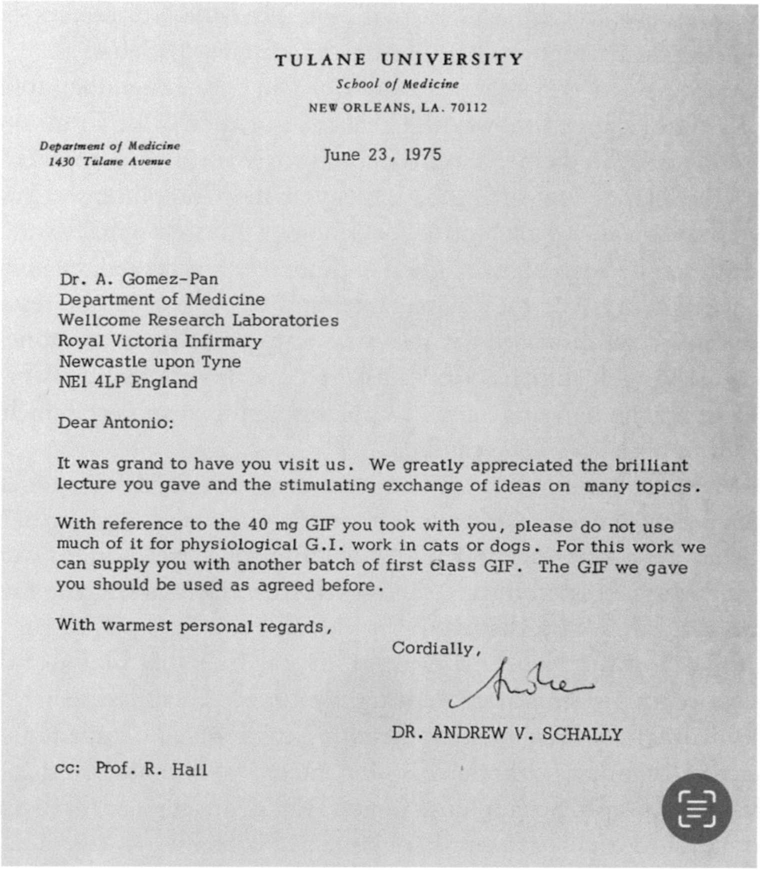

TULANE UNIVERSITY
School of Medicine
NEW ORLEANS, LA. 70112

Department of Medicine
1430 Tulane Avenue

June 23, 1975

Dr. A. Gomez-Pan
Department of Medicine
Wellcome Research Laboratories
Royal Victoria Infirmary
Newcastle upon Tyne
NE1 4LP England

Dear Antonio:

It was grand to have you visit us. We greatly appreciated the brilliant lecture you gave and the stimulating exchange of ideas on many topics.

With reference to the 40 mg GIF you took with you, please do not use much of it for physiological G.I. work in cats or dogs. For this work we can supply you with another batch of first class GIF. The GIF we gave you should be used as agreed before.

With warmest personal regards,

Cordially,

DR. ANDREW V. SCHALLY

cc: Prof. R. Hall

Fig. 29.6 Letter from Andrew V. Schally on my return from the lectures given in New Orleans

ited both gastric acid and gastrin (exocrine action). The collaborations between the two departments were crucial in facilitating the acquisition of these relevant data.

3. I traveled frequently, once a month, to London as a doctor at the Spanish Embassy. I took advantage of these trips to exchange results with members of Michael Besser's team and to work on our joint publications. On one occasion, after discussing the findings with Michael Thorner, who would later discover growth hormone releasing hormone (GHRH), we tried to stay overnight at Mortimer's house, who had invited us, but the house was occupied. It was very late; Mike's house was quite far away, and we had a

team meeting early the next day. In the end, we ended up sleeping in ENT cubicles at St. Bartholomew's Hospital, admitted as patients.

4. In the spring of 1977, Professor Rolf Luft, an eminent endocrinologist at the Karolinska Institute, was the chairman of the Nobel Committee for Physiology or Medicine. He had come to Madrid as a speaker at the Iberoamerican School of Endocrinology at the Complutense University, where I was in charge of Neuroendocrinology. Andrew Schally was also in Madrid, so I decided to invite them to dinner. Luft accepted the invitation; we picked him up at the Palace Hotel and went to a nearby restaurant. Over dinner, we discussed the relevance of hypothalamic hormones (Luft had worked with somatostatin) and the possible serious illness of Roger Guillemin, who had undergone complex abdominal surgery, which could jeopardize his Nobel Prize candidacy.
5. Ana Maria Comaru-Schally, wife of Andrew, was a Brazilian endocrinologist at Tulane University, of great kindness, an immense support for Victor, as she always called him, and an outstanding collaborator in his work. We spoke Portuguese, and during the Nobel Prize celebrations, she took care of me as if I were a brother.
6. On the day of the Nobel Prize ceremony, the cabs that took us from the hotel to City Hall followed very tightly timed schedules, which almost coincided. The young men from both Schally's and Guillemin's teams greeted each other with the "V" for victory and other hand gestures. However, Andrew Schally and Roger Guillemin avoided even crossing their gazes; the duel between them remained palpable.
7. Queen Silvia of Sweden was a beauty, very intelligent and a great polyglot. We spoke in Spanish, and she told me that they used to come incognito on vacation to Spain. She was surprised when I explained where I was born. However, she did not grant me the honor of dancing with her, the first dance was to be inaugurated with King Gustav.

Andrew Schally is, above all, a tireless worker. Even at his advanced age, he continues to make excellent scientific contributions, especially in the field of oncology. Educated in a very disciplined manner and a great sportsman, he maintained a daily swimming routine in his pool and had a great fondness for soccer. His favorite team is Real Madrid, and he enjoyed enormously when we visited the Trophy Museum at the Santiago Bernabeu Stadium in Madrid (Fig. 29.7).

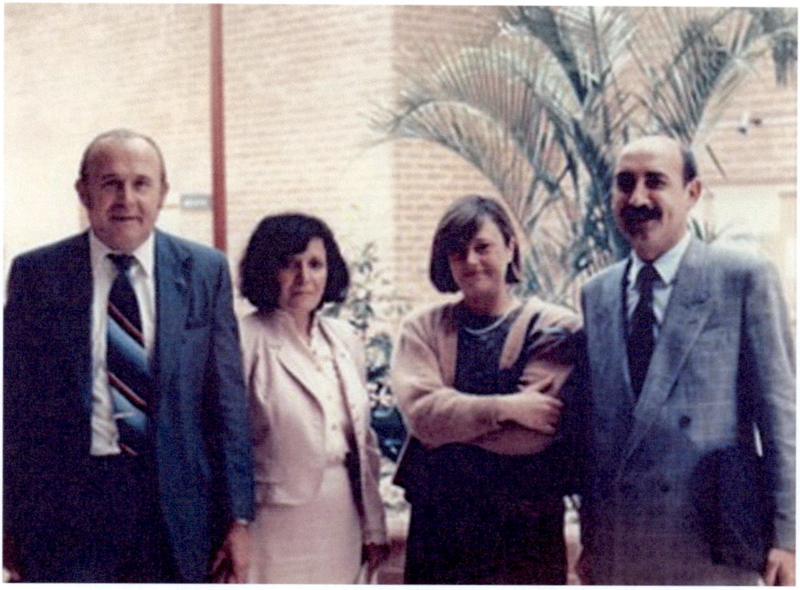

Fig. 29.7 Andrew V. Schally, Ana María Comaru-Schally, María Dolores Rodríguez-Arnao and Antonio Gómez-Pan, in Madrid

Roger Guillemin was a very competitive professional in his work, elegant and with a French touch. He traveled to Paris on the Concorde during his trips to Europe. He was also a passionate winemaker, with large vineyards in California. As a guest speaker at the 25th anniversary of the Hospital La Paz in Madrid, he asked to visit La Rioja. I was fortunate to meet the doctor of the Marqués de Creixell, owner of the winery, he so admired, "Marqués de Murrieta". We were invited to a delicious meal which culminated with Guillemin's signature in the book of honor and the presentation of a special gift: a bottle from the year of his birth in 1924. Great art scholar and very interested in the Monastery of San Lorenzo of El Escorial, we had the opportunity to make a memorable private visit with him, thanks to the Regional Minister of Environment of Madrid, Luis Maestre (Figs. 29.8 and 29.9).

In 1982, together with Emilio del Pozo and Maurice F. Scanlon, we founded the European Neuroendocrine Association (E.N.E.A.), and I was appointed First Secretary General. I also assumed responsibility for Scientific Policy and European Integration of the European Society of Clinical Investigation (E.S.C.I.), of which I was appointed Vice-President in 1991.

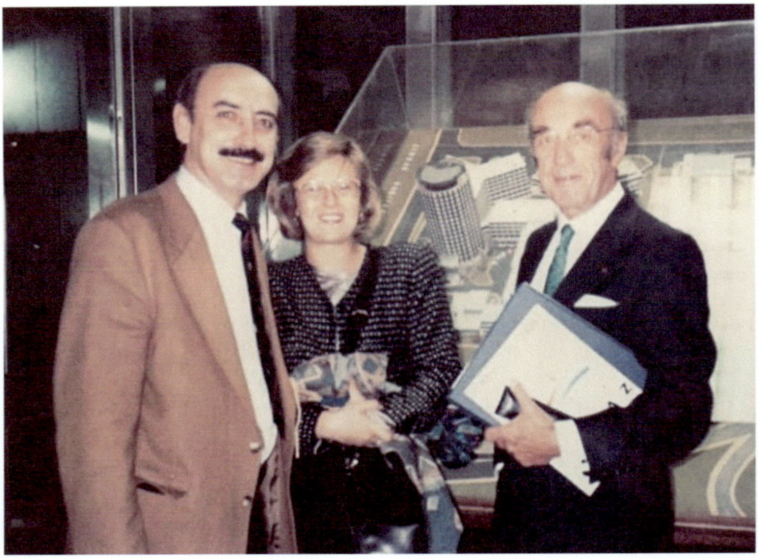

Fig. 29.8 Roger Guillemin, Antonio Gómez-Pan and María Dolores Rodríguez-Arnao, in the University Hospital La Paz in Madrid 1990

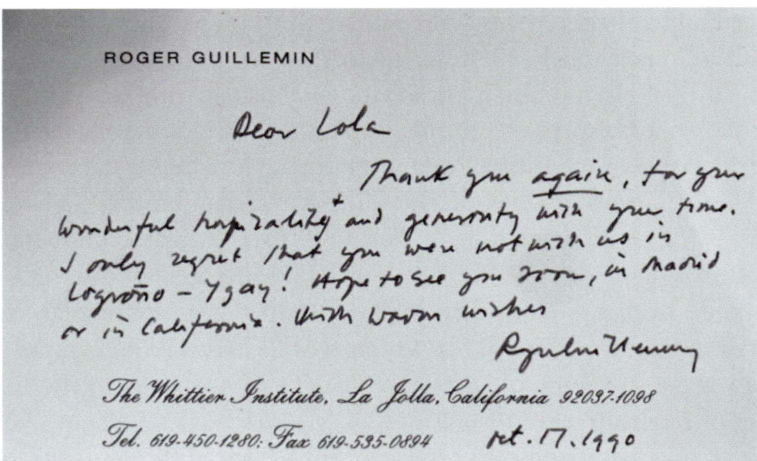

ROGER GUILLEMIN

Dear Lola

Thank you again, for your wonderful hospitality and generosity with your time. I only regret that you were not with us in Logroño - Ygay! Hope to see you soon, in Madrid or in California. With warm wishes

Roger Guillemin

The Whittier Institute, La Jolla, California 92037-1098

Tel. 619-450-1280; Fax 619-535-0894 Oct. 17, 1990

Fig. 29.9 Thank you handwritten card from Roger Guillemin October 17, 1990, for Lola Rodriguez Arnao, for hospitality and generosity during his stay in Madrid and for the trip to Ygai in La Rioja

Addendum. Research Projects Carried out in Neuroendocrinology

- Clinical Applications of Hypothalamic Thyrotrophin Stimulating Hormone (T.R.H.) and Hypothalamic Gonadotrophin Stimulating Hormone (L.H.R.H.).
- Physiological, Adenohypophyseal and Gastrointestinal Actions of the Hypothalamic Hormone Somatostatin (G.H.R.I.H.).
- Actions of Somatostatin (G.H.R.I.H.) on Gastric Acid and Gastrin Secretion under Basal Conditions and Stimulation in Experimental Model.
- Clinical and Therapeutic Applications of Somatostatin (G.H.R.I.H.).
- Clinical and Therapeutic Applications of Somatostatin Analogues.
- Study of Somatostatin Receptors in Intestinal Mucosa and Brain.
- Neuropharmacology of Hypothalamic Hormones.
- Neuroregulation of Adenohypophyseal Hormone Secretion.
- Adenohypophyseal actions of the hypothalamic hormone prosomatostatin (Somatostatin-28).
- Dopaminergic Treatment in Patients with Acromegaly.
- Dopaminergic modulation of Thyrotrophin (T.S.H.) and Prolactin.
- Dopaminergic modulation in functional and tumor hyperprolactinemia.
- Physiological Actions of Hypothalamic Gonadotropin Stimulating Hormone Analogues (L.H.R.H.).
- Therapeutic Actions - Reversible Medical Castration - of Hypothalamic Gonadotropin Stimulating Hormone Analogues (L.H.R.H.) in Precocious Puberty, Endometriosis and Prostate Carcinoma.
- Physiological Actions of Hypothalamic Growth Hormone Stimulating Hormone (G.H.R.H.).
- Pharmacological Actions of Hypothalamic Growth Hormone Stimulating Hormone (G.H.R.H. 1–44) in G.H. Deficiency.
- Pharmacological Actions of Hypothalamic Growth Hormone Stimulating Hormone (G.H.R.H. 1–29) in G.H. Deficiency.
- Pharmacological Modulations of Hypothalamic Growth Hormone Stimulating Hormone (G.H.R.H. 1–29 and G.H.R.H. 1–44).
- Actions of hypothalamic growth hormone stimulating hormone (G.H.R.H.) on behavior.
- Neuroendocrinological Actions of Opioid Peptides.
- Therapeutic Actions of Somatostatin Analogues (Octreotide) in Carcinoid Syndrome.
- Therapeutic Actions of Somatostatin Analogues (Octreotide) in Nesidioblastosis.

Epilogue

After my return to Spain, I continued research and publications with all the groups cited in Neuroendocrinology. Hypothalamic hormones have continued to mark significant milestones in scientific progress. In 1981, corticotrophinreleasing hormone (CRH) was identified, isolated and synthesized, and in 1982, growth hormone-releasing hormone (GHRH). The actions of somatostatin and prosomatostatin gave rise to further research work focused on both pituitary and gastrointestinal areas. The diagnostic and therapeutic applications of hypothalamic hormones, the basis of Neuroendocrinology, are multiple. and their usefulness has been demonstrated in the treatment of hormone-dependent medical oncology. Andrew V. Schally continues to work on its applications in the field of medical oncology.

Acknowledgments To Dr. María Dolores Rodríguez-Arnao, my teammate and wife. To Professor Miguel Ángel Cuesta, for the great distinction, which makes me proud and grateful.

References

1. Harris GW. Neural control of the pituitary gland. Physiol Rev. 1948;28:139–79.
2. Wade N. The Nobel Duel. Two scientists' 21-year race to win the worlds's most coveted research prize. Garden City, New York: Anchor Press/Doubleday; 1981. ISBN 0-385- 14981-6
3. Schally AV. In the pursuit of hypothalamic hormones. In: Meites J, Donovan BT, McCann SM, editors. Pioneers in neuroendocrinology II. New York: Plenum Press; 1978.
4. Gómez-Pan A, Hall R, Besser GM, Mortimer CH, Schally AV, Kastin AJ, Coy DH. Thyrotropin-releasing hormone: clinical studies. In: Charro AL, Fernández-Durango R, del Campo JGL, editors. Basic and clinical aspects of hypothalamic hormones, vol. 374. Amsterdam: Excerpta Medica, I.C.S; 1976. ISBN 90-219-0305-9.
5. Guillemin R. Peptides in the brain. The new Endocrinology of neuron. Nobel Lecture, December 8, 1977. The Nobel Prize in Physiology or Medicine. https://www.nobelprize.org/prizes/medicine/1977/summa ry
6. Schally AV. Aspects of hypothalamic regulation of the pituitary gland with major emphasis on its implications for the control of reproductive processes. Nobel Lecture, December 8, 1977. The Nobel Prize in Physiology or Medicine. https://www.nobelprize.org/prizes/medicine/1977/summary.

7. Hall R, Gómez-Pan A. The hypothalamic regulatory hormones and their clinical applications. In: Bodansky O, Latner AL, editors. Advances in clinical medicine. Nueva York: Academic Press, Inc.; 1976. ISBN 0-12-010318-4.
8. Schally AV, Coy DH, Arimura A, Redding TW, Meyers CA, Vilchez-Martínez J, Pedroza E, Gordin A, Molnar J, Kastin AJ, Labrie F, Hall R, Gómez-Pan A, Besser GM. Structure-activity relationship of hypophysiotropic hormones. In: James VHT, editor. Endocrinology. Amsterdam: Excerpta Medica; 1977. ISBN 978-9021903316.
9. Gómez-Pan A, Hall R. Somatostatin (growth hormone-release inhibiting hormone). J Clin Endocrinol Metab. 1977;6:181–200.
10. Gómez-Pan A, Tunbridge WMG, Duns A, Hall R, Besser GM, Coy DH, Schally AV, Kastin AJ. Hypothalamic hormone interactions in acromegaly. Clin Endocrinol. 1975;4:455–60.
11. Gómez-Pan A, Scanlon MF, Thorner MO, Hall R, Rees LH, Besser M, Schally AV. Effects of somatostatin on abnormal growth hormone and prolactin secretion in patients with the carcinoid syndrome. Clin Endocrinol. 1979;10:575–81.
12. Gómez-Pan A, Reed JD, Albinus M, Shaw B, Hall R, Besser GM, Coy DH, Kastin AJ, Schally AV. Direct inhibition of gastric acid and pepsin secretion by growth hormone-release inhibiting hormone (somatostatin) in cats. Lancet. 1975;305:888–90.
13. Gómez-Pan A, Rodríguez-Arnao MD. Somatostatin and growth hormone releasing factor: synthesis, location, metabolism and function. Clin Endocrinol Metab. 1983;12:469–507.
14. Schally AV, Coy DH, Murphy WA, Redding TW, Comaru-Schally AM, Hall R, Rodríguez-Arnao MD, Gómez- Pan A, González-Bárcena D, Millar RP, Konturek S. Physiological and clinical studies with somatostatin analogs and prosomatostatin. Distinguished Nobel Prize lectures. In: Raptis S, Rosenthal J, Gerich JE, editors. Somatostatin. Germany: Verlage Tubingen GMBH; 1984.
15. Gómez-Pan A, Rodríguez-Arnao MD, del Pozo E. Advances in somatostatin research. In: del Pozo E, Fluckiger E, editors. Dopamine and neuroendocrine active substances. London: Academic Press; 1985. ISBN 0-12-209045- 4.
16. Gómez-Pan A, Sastre J, Díez JJ. Somatostatina: Desde el Hipotálamo hasta el Eje Gastro-entero-pancreático. In: Blázquez E, Tamarit J, editors. Péptidos reguladores gastrointestinales y recepción y transducción de señales generadas por hormonas polipeptídicas tiroideas y esteroideas. Madrid: Editorial Centro de Estudios Ramón Areces; 1992. ISBN 84-8004-028-9.

30

Margarita Salas: The Polymerase and DNA Amplification

Iole Ferrara Romeo

> Science is the knowledge of everything that surrounds us, there are people who think that science is dogma, but it is not (...) in science there are no dogmas. One does experiments, obtains results, interprets those results in the most precise way possible, but in a year, two years, ten years, someone may come along who contradicts the results you have interpreted (...). (M. Salas Falgueras)

The Germ of Her Scientific Vocation

In the gardens of the Hospital Universitario "12 de Octubre" in Madrid blooms a unique white rose with simple petals, the Margarita Salas rose (Fig. 30.1). Created by Matilde Ferrer —recognized expert in these flowers— this variety was planted in the hospital gardens as a tribute to one of Spain's most brilliant scientists, whose career has left its mark on the world [1].

Margarita Salas was born in 1938, in the middle of the Civil War, in the small town of Canero in Asturias. When she was 1 year old, once the war was

I. F. Romeo (✉)
Institute of Medicinal Chemistry (IQM-CSIC), Spanish National Research Council (CSIC), Madrid, España

M. A. Cuesta, F. Mateo Vallejo (eds.), *Spain's Journey in Medicine*,
https://doi.org/10.1007/978-3-032-12221-6_30

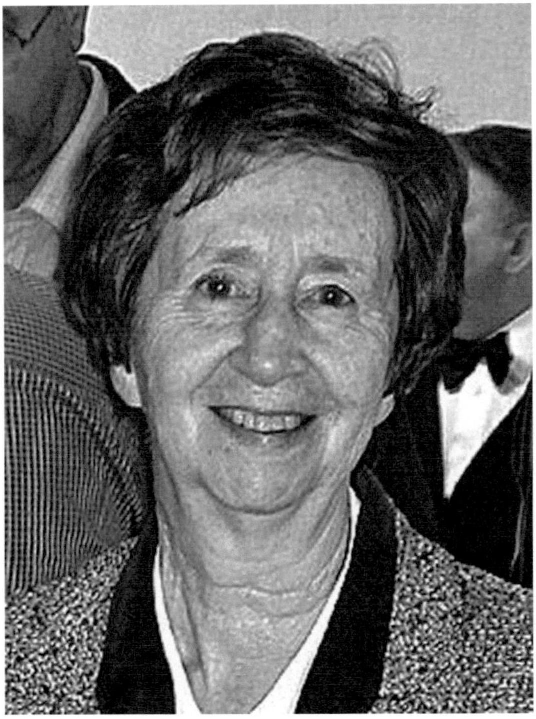

Fig. 30.1 Margarita Salas in 2009. (Permission Fundación Margarita Salas)

over, her family moved to Gijón, where Margarita spent her childhood and early youth. Her parents had three children, two girls and a boy, and they were very clear that all three were going to pursue a university career, something very uncommon at the time, women were destined to the family and home. With the frankness that characterized her, Margarita always emphasized this circumstance and the privilege it entailed [2]. Interviewed by researcher Jesús Ávila, who had been her disciple [3], she said: "My father always told us: the best inheritance I will leave you is a university degree, and indeed, that was our best inheritance". Once she had high school and pre-university studies, young Margarita was faced with the decision of what career to follow. She hesitated between medicine and chemistry and as the former was not available at the University of Oviedo —the closest to Gijón—, she decided to move to the capital and enroll in what is now the Complutense University of Madrid, to follow a one-year course that was common to both careers. She finally decided on chemistry and quickly became passionate about it. In the third year she tackled organic chemistry and deeply fascinated by the long hours spent in the laboratory. The summer of 1958 was the summer that changed her life. She went to Gijón for vacation and was lucky enough to meet Severo Ochoa, who would have a decisive influence on her future. Margarita's father and the future Nobel laureate related (an uncle of Ochoa's was married to an aunt of Margarita's father) and, in addition, they had been medical school classmates. Ochoa worked at the New York University (NYU) School of Medicine, and although he had not been to Spain for a long time, he went to the peninsula to spend the vacations. The biochemist and molecular biologist and his wife Carmen went to have lunch with the Salas family. During the meal, Ochoa invited Margarita and her father to attend a lecture he was going to give in Oviedo the next day. After listening to the talk, Margarita was deeply fascinated; "He was a magnificent lecturer. So, I had the chance to talk with him. I was a little 'plugged in', because of Ochoa's friendship with my father," she told Jesús Ávila, adding that the scientist promised to send her a book on biochemistry as soon as he returned to New York. "I was very excited when I received the book 'General Biochemistry' by J.S. Fruton and S. Simmonds, with a dedication from Severo Ochoa," she wrote in an article about her scientific career. When she finished her studies in chemistry, Margarita was already determined to devote herself to biochemistry [4]. Ochoa advised her to do her doctoral thesis in Madrid with Alberto Sols, a brilliant scientist who had returned to Spain after several years in the United States (U.S.), and then to go to his laboratory at NYU for a postdoctoral stay. Ochoa wrote her a letter of recommendation and Sols accepted the request. Margarita always recognized the good fortune of having known Severo Ochoa closely, whom she described on several occasions as a teacher and friend. In her conversation with Ávila, she said: "I went from chemistry to biochemistry and molecular biology thanks to Severo Ochoa". Thus, in 1961 Margarita Salas began her doctoral thesis. At the end of her chemistry studies, she became engaged to Eladio Viñuela, a brilliant scientist who also worked in Sols' laboratory and who would become her life partner. Two years later, Margarita Salas defended her doctoral thesis directed by Alberto Sols about the metabolism of the carbohydrates at the University of Madrid (today's Complutense University) with the qualification *cum laude*. The same year, after obtaining a grant from the Juan March Foundation, she and Eladio married. Both had a strong vocation for molecular biology and biochemistry, and the following year they moved to New York to join Ochoa's laboratory. In her autobiographical article, Margarita writes: "I have very good memories of my stay in Severo Ochoa's laboratory. The three years I spent there were the best of my scientific life. Ochoa taught us (Eladio and me) not only molecular biology, which we would later develop and teach in Spain, but also his experimental rigor and enthusiasm for research". After three exciting and fruitful years, Margarita and Eladio decided to return home to develop the molecular biology they had learned in the U.S. "We knew that Spain was going to be a scientific desert and that it was going to be difficult to start molecular biology research," she said, but still, armed with determination and passion, they decided to give it a try. At that time in Spain, there was hardly any funding for research, so the Viñuela-Salas couple had to look for American money. "We obtained the funds with the help of Severo Ochoa. It was only thanks to this grant that we were able to start our work in Spain," wrote Margarita. The couple decided to work together to join forces in the face of difficulties that awaited them. The previous summer, during a course in the U.S., they had learned to work with bacteriophages (viruses that infect only bacteria, also called 'phages') and chose one of these viruses as a subject of study; specifically, phage Φ29 (phi29). "It had the characteristics we were looking for: it was small in size, had a complex morphology, and very little was known about it," explained the scientist. They returned to Madrid in 1967 to begin their scientific adventure in Spain and started working at the Centro de Investigaciones Biológicas (CIB) of the Consejo Superior de Investigaciones Científicas (CSIC; CIB-CSIC), where they were appointed research scientists. A few months after their arrival, the first predoctoral fellowships were awarded and Margarita and Eladio were able to offer a contract to their first students. The director of the Biochemistry Department of the Faculty of Chemistry at the Complutense University of Madrid invited them to teach a course on molecular genetics. Thus, for the first time, this discipline was taught at a university in Spain (Fig. 30.2).

This is how the story begins of the woman who would become undisputed icon of Spanish science [2–4].

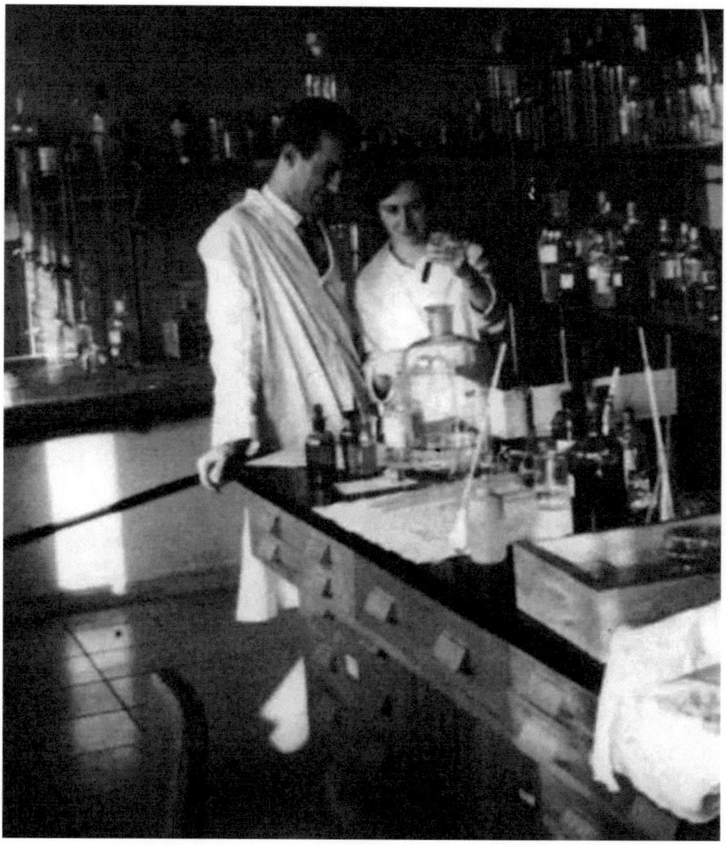

Fig. 30.2 Margarita Salas and Eladio Viñuela in the CIB in 1962. (Permission of the Asociación Torre Isunza)

First Scientific Discoveries

A deep passion for research, coupled with firm rigor and tireless perseverance characterized Margarita Salas' scientific life from the very beginning. During her postdoctoral stay in Ochoa's laboratory, 1964–67, Margarita made decisive discoveries that marked fundamental milestones in molecular biology, a discipline that, at that time, was still in its infancy. Just a few years earlier, the so-called 'central dogma of molecular biology' had been established, which states that genetic information flows from DNA to RNA and from RNA to proteins. However, during the stay of Margarita Salas in NYU, very little was still known about the mechanisms that transfer the genetic message, an area in which Ochoa's group was working. RNA molecules have two distinct ends, which are defined as 3′ and 5′. Margarita's first research project after her arrival in Ochoa's laboratory was to determine in which direction the translation of an RNA into a protein occurs, i.e., whether the RNA molecule is read in the $3' \rightarrow 5'$ direction, in the opposite direction, or in both directions [5]. Margarita demonstrated that the reading direction of RNA is unique and proceeds from the 5′ to the 3′ end. Let's not forget that details of the different types of RNA (tRNA and mRNA) and their reading by ribosomes were not known at that time.

On the other hand, RNA has signals in its structure that indicate exactly to what point each molecule has to be translated into a protein. Today it is known that there are three different signals that stop translation, and Margarita contributed to identify one of them: the so-called UAA triplet. Both the directionality in reading the genetic message and the identification of the UAA triplet as a translation termination signal—both discoveries made by Margarita when she was not yet even 30 years old—are part of the basic notions of molecular biology, and appear in all biology textbooks [5].

How Margarita Salas Changed Genetics Research Forever

In the late 1970s, after 10 years working at the CIB-CSIC, Margarita moved to the newly founded Center for Molecular Biology Severo Ochoa (CBM-CSIC). It was at this Institute where—in the mid-1980s—she obtained the most important scientific discovery of her career: the identification and characterization of the DNA polymerase of phage Φ29, the protein responsible for duplicating the genetic material of this bacterial virus. Φ29 infects the bacterium *Bacillus subtilis*. Infection occurs in such a way that the virus binds to the bacterial cell surface and injects its DNA into the cell. Once inside, the viral genetic material takes control of the cell and triggers a series of processes leading to the production of numerous clones of the phage. Subsequently, these exact copies of the virus kill the bacterium from within so that the bacterium breaks down and releases the new viruses into the surrounding environment thus spreading the infection.

One of the first steps in the generation of viral clones consists of creating copies of phage DNA, a task carried out by the enzyme discovered by Margarita Salas and her disciple Luis Blanco (Fig. 30.3).

There are countless types of DNA polymerase, and these enzymes are in fact found in all living organisms. These enzymes are used in laboratories

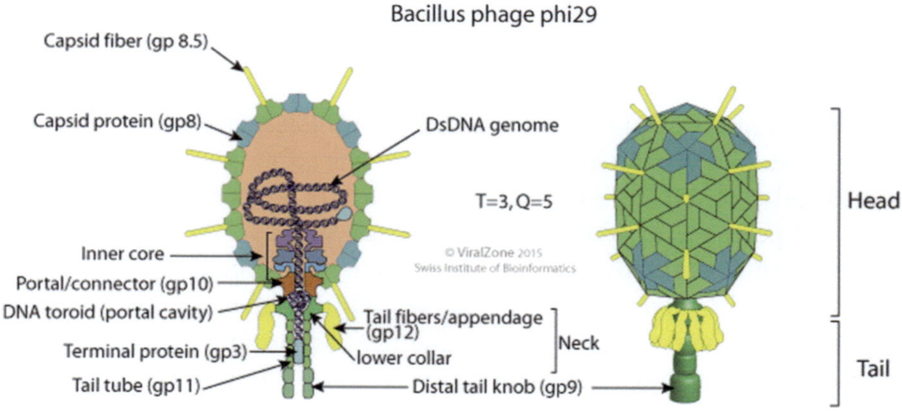

Fig. 30.3 Schematic drawing of a Bacillus phage Φ29 (cross section and side view)

around the world to amplify DNA, i.e. to create millions of copies from a few starting molecules, so that it can be studied.

Just 1 year before the Spanish scientists isolated the enzyme from Φ29, in 1984, the American biochemist Kary Mullis (Nobel Prize, 1993) had developed in 1983 the so-called polymerase chain reaction (PCR), a technique that takes advantage of the natural capacity of these enzymes to amplify DNA *in vitro*, in the laboratory. This tool was a true revolution for genetic analysis and studies, and is still used extensively on a global scale, however, it has some limitations.

Margarita Salas and Luis Blanco found that the Φ29 enzyme polymerase possesses exceptional features in comparison to the previously known DNA polymerases, giving it an extraordinary capability to amplify DNA. They soon realized that, thanks to these excellent properties, the enzyme had great potential for use in biotechnology [6].

A phage is short for a bacteriophage virus, so called because it infects bacteria, very simple and easy to work with in the laboratory. And for that matter, Φ, is the Greek letter Phi ("fi"). The DNA polymerase of Φ29, discovered by Margarita Salas and her collaborators, turned out to have some very interesting properties. It eventually came to be used to develop an alternative technique to PCR called Multiple Displacement Amplification (MDA). In recent years, MDA has become a true alternative to PCR, being widely used to amplify and read entire genomes, even from a single cell. DNA polymerase of Phage Φ29 is much faster and more accurate than other DNA polymerases.

Many years after this discovery, during an interview, Margarita compared PCR to an old photocopying machine, which can only copy pages one at a time, makes a limited number of copies and, in addition, produces typographical errors. Similarly, the PCR technique has a limited amplification capacity, so it can only amplify small molecules, and requires a certain threshold amount of starting DNA. In addition, it introduces errors in the copies it generates and for the amplification reaction to take place, the sample has to be heated and cooled many times, which complicates the experimental process. The Φ29 polymerase, on the other hand, can amplify DNA samples from extremely small amounts, is much more precise when copying, so it reproduces the DNA more accurately and, in addition, allows amplification of large molecules and at a constant temperature. This enzyme is therefore a very useful tool for studying DNA samples as it allows them to be amplified more quickly, reliably and easily than PCR. This finding radically transformed genetic analysis and today the enzyme of this small phage is used worldwide for medical, forensic and archaeological applications, among others. "When you have small amounts of DNA, such as a hair found in a crime or archaeological remains, this DNA polymerase amplifies the DNA millions of times so that it can be analyzed, sequenced and studied," explained Margarita. In the clinical context it is used, for example, for the diagnosis of infectious diseases; in fact, its high sensitivity makes it possible to detect infections in early stages, sometimes even before symptoms appear. It is also a key tool in oncology, since, on the one hand, its high fidelity makes it possible to detect tumor mutations very reliably, and, on the other hand, its high sensitivity makes it possible to analyze tumor DNA without the need for invasive biopsies, which facilitates both diagnosis and monitoring of the disease.

In 1989, Margarita Salas, Luis Blanco, Antonio Bernad and José María Lázaro patented the Enzyme [7]. The CSIC, as owner of the patent, granted an American company the license to exploit it, and the company developed and marketed kits for DNA amplification. This patent was the most profitable in the history of the CSIC, in fact, between 2003 and 2009 — years in which it was active— it accounted for more than half of the income obtained by the organization. In the following years, Margarita's team continued working on this enzyme and succeeded in developing improved variants of the original enzyme, which in turn were patented for application in biotechnology.

Margarita believed deeply in the value of basic research, that is, in the pursuit of knowledge as an end in itself. She always stood out as the patent of Φ29 was an example of a practical application derived, unexpectedly, from the desire to know. In her interview with Jesús Ávila she commented: "From a purely basic research, such as the research with phage Φ29, we have reached biotechnological applications. I think this is important to emphasize, because nobody gave a dime for Φ29 from a practical point of view". Quoting her mentor Severo Ochoa, the scientist repeatedly stated: "We must carry out quality basic research and leave the researcher free to do it, because practical results will come out of it that are not predictable *a priori*, but that will be of benefit to society".

The Legacy of Margarita Salas in Spain

Margarita Salas' legacy goes beyond her important scientific discoveries. Together with her life and professional partner, Eladio Viñuela, the Asturian scientist has the great merit of having started the School of Molecular Biology in Spain (Fig. 30.4).

Many researchers have been trained in her laboratory; over time, several of them have founded their own research groups and are now widely recognized in their respective areas of work, both nationally and internationally. Margarita, who from 1968 to 1992 was Professor of Molecular Genetics at the Complutense University of Madrid, believed deeply in teaching and in the value of training new generations of researchers. When Jesús Ávila asked her if you have to have a lot of patience, or hobby, to create a school, she replied, "You have to have a lot of dedication and a lot of enthusiasm to transmit the teachings to your disciples," and added, "I feel very proud of all the students I have had, because they have been excellent students and so it is not difficult to make a school." In 2017, the scientific journal *Nature* awarded her the Nature Award for Mentoring in Science in recognition of her exceptional work as a mentor, which boosted the training and development of numerous scientists and researchers [8].

Every 4 years, from 1980 to 1996, she organized the International Workshop on Bacteriophages in Salamanca, in which the best phage

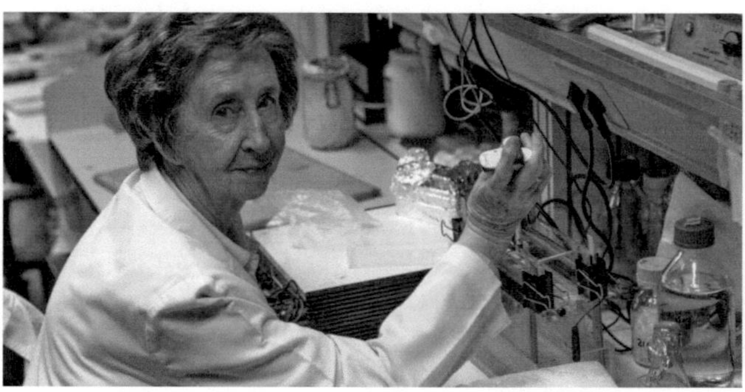

Fig. 30.4 Margarita Salas in the Laboratory. (Permission Fundación Margarita Salas)

researchers from Europe and the USA participated. In her autobiographical article she wrote: “In the first workshop, I demonstrated to my foreign colleagues that in Spain we could do good science. I think this was the beginning of my international recognition”.

A Pioneer Woman

“Salas was a model of courage,” wrote Jesús Ávila, Federico Mayor and Lourdes Ruiz Desviat in the journal *Nature* a few weeks after the scientist’s death [9]. Margarita was educated during the regime of the dictator Francisco Franco, a social and historical context in which women did not enjoy equal conditions. Despite this, the young woman pursued her professional interests, and although she would eventually become an internationally recognized scientist, at that time difficulties were not long in coming to arrive. In her autobiography she wrote: “During the phase of the doctoral thesis I had a hard time. It so happened that Eladio and I were meeting with Sols, our thesis director, and while we were talking about my work, he addressed Eladio, he never addressed me, I was like invisible, which was terrible for me”. Years later, when he was awarded the Severo Ochoa Research Prize from the Ferrer Foundation, Sols commented: “When Margarita came to the laboratory to ask me to do a doctoral thesis I thought, bah, a girl, I’ll give her something that is not important because if she doesn’t get it done it doesn’t matter”. Undoubtedly, Sols’ way of thinking was not exceptional. It was the 1960s and in the mentality of the time the place for women was not the university or the laboratory, but the home and the family. In the U.S. the situation was different; “With Severo Ochoa I felt like a person for the first time from a scientific point of view, regardless of my status as a woman,” Margarita told Jesús Ávila (Fig. 30.5).

However, when she returned to Spain at the end of the 1960s, she again felt discriminated against. She and her husband worked together, both had PhD students under their care and were professors at the Complutense University of Madrid, but in the eyes of the world she was only Eladio’s wife. Thus, in 1970 her husband decided to change his field of study: “Eladio was very generous, and there came a time when he decided to stop working with phage Φ29 and start a new research topic”, the scientist said, adding: “So, little by little, he left the study of phage Φ29 to me, so that I could be independent and demonstrate whether or not I was worthy of doing research. And then, little by little, I became Margarita Salas”.

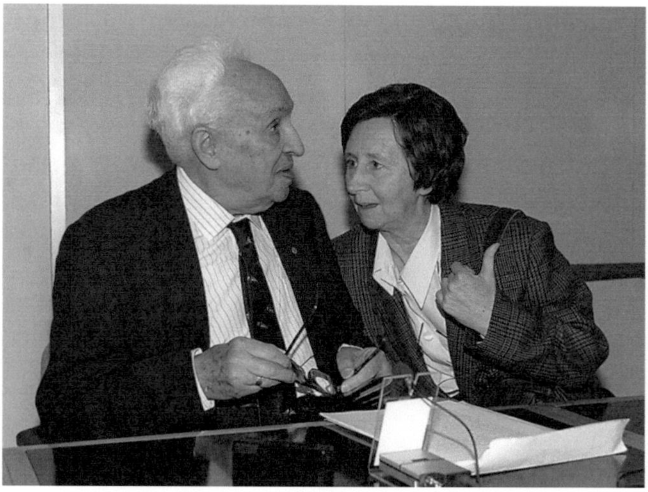

Fig. 30.5 Margarita Salas and Severo Ochoa. (Permission Fundación Margarita Salas)

The Asturian scientist received an extraordinary number of awards and recognitions, not only nationally but also outside Spain. In many of them, as well as in several of the positions she held, she was a pioneer as a woman. "It is not my merit to be a pioneer; there were so few women when I started that it was easy to be one," she told Jesús Ávila. In 2007 she became the first Spanish woman member of the National Academy of Sciences of the States, "I think it is the most important thing that has happened to me," she said in an interview. Between 1992 and 1994 she was director of the CBM-CSIC, being the first woman in Spain to direct a large biomedical research center. She was also the first woman president of the Institute of Spain, the first scientist to join the Royal Spanish Academy and the first to be elected by several scientific academies. In 2019, just a few months before her death, she received the Inventor of the Year award, given by the European Patent Office, in two categories: 'Lifetime Achievement' and 'Popular Vote'; it was the first time in the history of the award that the double recognition was given to the same person [10].

Conclusions

Throughout her career, Margarita Salas registered eight patents and published more than 350 papers in national and international journals and books. After retiring at the age of 70, she was able to continue working thanks to her appointment by the CSIC as an *ad honorem* professor at the Centro de Biología Molecular Severo Ochoa. An advocate that in science there should be no retirement, during a conference she stated that she wanted to be like Rita Levi-Montalcini who went to the laboratory until she was 100 years old. Margarita passed away on November 7, 2019, at the of 80, and until a few weeks before she was still going to the lab every day.

Acknowledgements I would like to thank Alicia del Prado for her time, dedication, and the enthusiasm she has shared with me. I would also like to thank Miguel A. Cuesta for involving me in the book and giving me the opportunity to write this chapter.

References

1. El Hospital 12 de Octubre planta una variedad de rosal dedicado a Margarita Salas. Comunidad de Madrid; 2021. enlace.
2. Salas M. My life with bacteriophage phi29. J Biol Chem. 2012;287:44568–79.
3. Margarita Salas entrevistada por Jesús Ávila, no 13 de la revista CIC Network; 2013.
4. Salas M. My scientific life. Bacteriophage. 2016;6:1271250.
5. Last JA, Stanley WM, Salas M, Hille MB, Wahba AJ, Ochoa S. Translation of the genetic message, IV. UAA as a chain termination codon. Proc Natl Acad Sci USA. 1967;57:1062–7.
6. Salas M, Blanco L, Lázaro JM, de Vega M. My favorite Enzyme. The bacteriophage Φ29 DNA polymerasa. IUBMB Life. 2008;60:82–5.
7. Margarita Salas Falgueras - DNA amplification for genomics. European Patent Office; 2019. enlace.
8. ICFO receives 2017 Nature Mentoring Award. Nature Research; 2017.
9. Ávila J, Mayor F, Ruiz-Desviat L, Salas M. (1938–2019) - Biochemist whose discoveries led to faster, more-accurate DNA testing. Nature. 2019;576:208.
10. Margarita Salas gana el Premio al Inventor Europeo de 2019. SINC; 2019. enlace.

31

Valentín Fuster: A Life with Purpose

Antonio San José

Every morning, at four o'clock sharp, Dr. Valentín Fuster jumps out of bed ready to face the new day (Fig. 31.1). It is an inveterate habit that leads him to sleep only 4 h a day, but he explains that this time is enough for him because his sleep induction is as instantaneous as it is profound. Getting up and running so far ahead of the rest of the humans leads him to know perfectly well the night cleaning staff at Mount Sinai Hospital in New York and also the maintenance staff at the CNIC, the Centro Nacional de Investigaciones Cardiovasculares (National Center for Cardiovascular Research) in Madrid. No one is surprised to see, long before dawn, a vocational physician who, as soon as he occupies his office on either side of the Atlantic, dedicates the first 15 min of his long day to meditate, to think about the new day and what he is doing at any given moment. This time of reflection constitutes his way of being in the world, the defensive barrier against the incessant bustle of daily issues, the mental air he needs to breathe to continue feeding his vital purpose, which he defines as "move on". There are few human beings capable of enduring jet lag as well as Dr. Fuster. Every week, he flies from New York to Madrid to spend a day at the CNIC, which he has presided over since its foundation in 1999 [1]. We are talking about a center of research and scientific excellence that depends on the Ministry of Science and Innovation of Spain and the Carlos III Institute of Health, with the support of the private

A. S. José (✉)
Journalist. Political Analyst, Madrid, Spain

M. A. Cuesta, F. Mateo Vallejo (eds.), *Spain's Journey in Medicine*,
https://doi.org/10.1007/978-3-032-12221-6_31

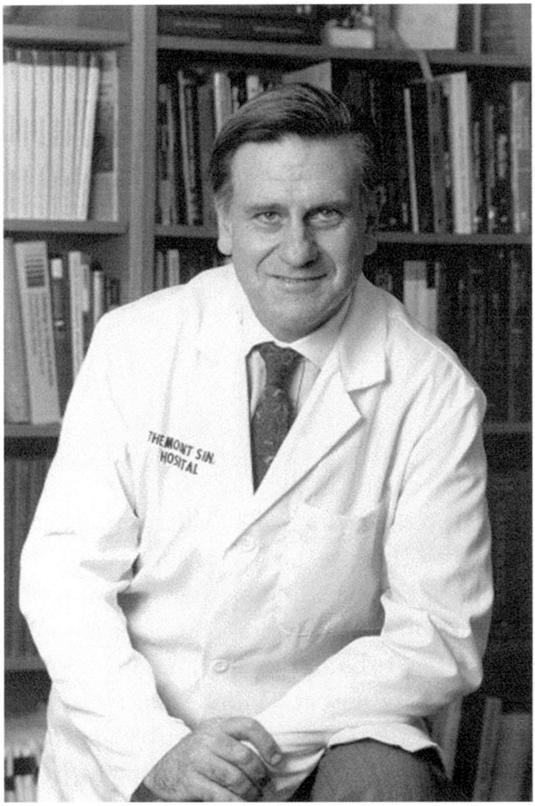

Fig. 31.1 Valentín Fuster, Mount Sinai Hospital

sector through the PROCNIC Foundation. There he attends meetings, directs those responsible for the different projects and, above all, he leaves the imprint of his experience and the teaching of many years at the forefront of the knowledge of all the secrets of the heart.

An Intense Life

Valentín Fuster Carulla, born in Barcelona on January 20, 1943, holds the title of Marquis of Fuster, although this is a circumstance that does not affect him at all because his field is Medicine and also Philosophy, a discipline in which he later obtained his doctorate as a complement to the scientific activity that he has always developed from a humanistic perspective. Trained at the University of Barcelona and Edinburgh, he is the son of the respected psychiatrist Joaquín Fuster and Josefa Guirao. In the early 70's he moved to the

United States and since 1974 he has been working at the prestigious Mount Sinai Hospital in New York where he directs its extensive cardiology department [2, 3] In 2006 he was appointed president of the World Association of Cardiology after winning the Prince of Asturias Award for Technical and Scientific Research a decade earlier [4]. Many people met him talking about healthy food in the popular American children's series "Sesame Street", because food has always been one of his main concerns in the field of preventive medicine. Apart from his "muppet" called "Doctor Ruster", a transcript of "doctor Fuster", he has implemented initiatives on healthy dietary habits in Colombia, Kenya and other countries, some of them through his SHE (Science, Health and Education) Foundation, as a sign of his commitment to improving the quality of life in the most disadvantaged social sectors and in underdeveloped countries [5] (Fig. 31.2).

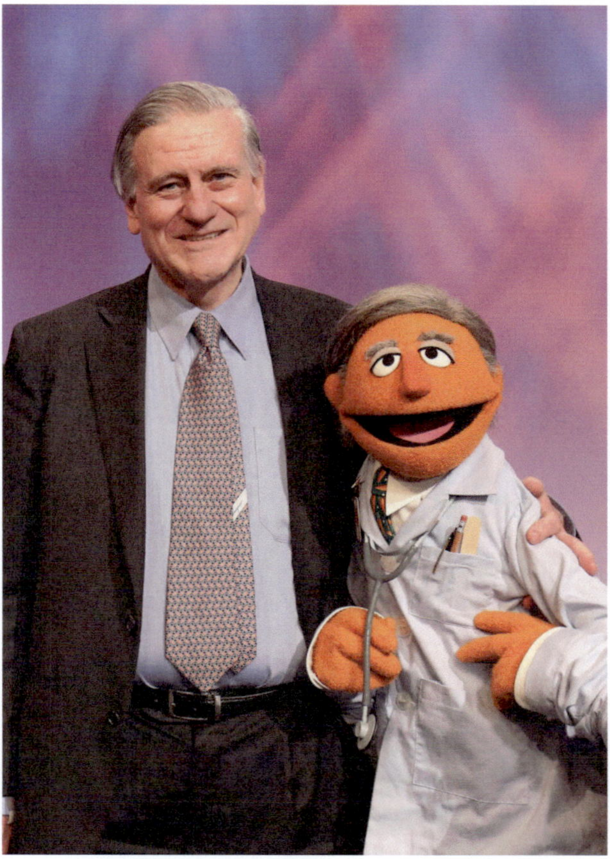

Fig. 31.2 Valentín Fuster with Dr. Ruster, his alter ego in Sesame Street. (Permission Sesame Street, USA)

When he was 16 years old, Dr. Fuster was awarded a grant to attend a seminar on neurology at the Menéndez y Pelayo International University in Santander. He confesses that he had no idea about the subject, but after a few hours sitting in the classroom he concluded that he wanted to be a researcher, which is why he believes that it is essential to motivate and encourage young people, hence the program of grants and scholarships proposed by the CNIC. After a lifetime dedicated to researching the heart, he confesses that he still has more and more to learn and that the more you investigate, the humbler you become. He continues to find it fascinating to understand how an organ that beats 60 times a minute has valves that open and close continuously and are not destroyed. And he has never found the answer to this. He says that every day in his New York practice he sees many executives working on Wall Street who live like crazy, constantly going from one place to another and constantly talking on the phone. The first thing he does is to convince them that half an hour of physical exercise a day is essential for their health and balance. The second is relaxation, meditation or yoga, and he believes that the combination of both factors serves to drastically reduce stress: moving and calming down, that is the key to vital balance for Dr. Fuster.

To Take Care or Not to Take Care: The Big Decision

The dilemma of each person is to ask himself if he is going to take care of himself or not. In this sense, for him, diet is only one of the components of health, together with exercise, monitoring blood pressure, cholesterol, glucose levels, avoiding obesity, not smoking and eating healthy. It is an absolutely personal decision, so much so that he affirms that chronological age has nothing to do with biological age and that the old age that each person will have is the inexorable result of the attention that he or she has paid to his or her health during the previous years. For example, he argues that Alzheimer's disease is directly related to the state of the cardiovascular system, as are hypertension, diabetes and hypercholesterolemia. He advises his patients to pay more attention to their brain than to their heart and instructs them that the two organs have a direct and essential relationship. He assures that he, as a physician, has to adopt a lot of sympathy towards people who do not take care of themselves and that it is counterproductive to enter into their lives and bad habits as a harsh judge because it simply does not work. In this way it is possible to unravel the causes that lead to a person's failure to avoid risk factors that compromise their health and future quality of life [6].

The Eight Keys to Balance

In Valentín Fuster's life there are eight keys to achieve a harmonious existence, and he defines them as four "T's" and four "A's" [7, 8].

In English, the first of these is "Time to reflect" every day; hence his 15 min of inner thought with which he has started each day for many years.

The second is "Talent", identifying which talent each of us has and exploiting it, something that is not the same for everyone.

The third is to "Transmit positivity," to be optimistic and see the good side of life. This attitude, he argues, is very important for the state of mind with which to face everyday reality.

And the fourth is "Mentoring", since everyone needs people to guide them. In fact, he has two people to whom he consults all his doubts and who provide him with guidance every day. One of them is 47 years old and was a former student of his whom he has entrusted with the task of warning him "the day he starts talking nonsense" to urge him to stop what he is doing. The other tutor is a 72-year-old who helps him with some of the decisions he has to make. "It is a monumental absurdity to think that we can do everything by ourselves," assures Dr. Fuster.

The first of the four "A's" is "Accept who you are", taking on what you have and your reality, which will always be different from that of another person, as close as it may be to us.

The second is "Altruism", something that acts as an engine that tells you that what you are doing is the right thing to do. It is about being thankful for what you have and also about helping others to the best of your ability.

The third is "Authenticity", basically everyone is the same person regardless of who they are talking to or where they are at any given time. The aim is not to differentiate according to class, economic or social status.

And the last one is "Attitude", based on being positive even in the midst of the most adverse situations that we may experience throughout our lives. "Always forward", "never give up"; this is the life purpose that Dr. Fuster has observed both in his personal life and throughout his professional career.

Patients and Students

He recognizes that doctors are less and less able to talk to patients. In his opinion, there is a need for training that can recover the traditional relationship between the family doctor and the patient. In view of this circumstance, he is optimistic and believes that this type of traditional humanistic medicine will make a comeback in the era of technology and artificial intelligence that surrounds us. The doctor believes that 50% of the conditions he sees every day in his office have an important psychological component that always aggravates the organic problems. Hence the importance of capturing the mental sensitivity of the patient and of practicing empathy with the patient, something fundamental for the achievement of his or her healing process. It happens that specialists have less and less time to interact, and that is something that has to change since the patients need to be comforted with a humanistic treatment by their doctors. The first thing Valentín Fuster tells the young residents who join his team every year is that they have to treat hospital administrative staff and secretaries exactly the same as the doctors in the centre. And the second thing is that in cardiology there are not first and second class patients, everyone is exactly the same "One day in the morning," he explains, "I was treating a homeless man and that same afternoon I had to treat the president of a country, and my students could not perceive any difference in my medical performance with each one of them". That is one of the keys to his conception of medicine.

Myocardial Infarction

On the leading cause of death in the world, Valentín Fuster explains: "In the 1960s, the causes of myocardial infarction were not known; that was the time when I did my doctoral thesis. In the 1970–80s, we began to learn why blood clots formed that obstructed the coronary arteries and caused these episodes. We learned that it was the consequence of something abnormal in the vascular wall, since ulcers are produced, and clots appear as a result of a cholesterol plaque that breaks. Magnetic resonance imaging helped us to find out what was happening inside the artery. It is essential to control cholesterol to avoid a heart attack. The important thing is to monitor all cardiovascular risk factors such as smoking, unhealthy diet, hypertension, glucose levels and others that we all know about but often do not put into practice". "In the last three decades we humans have extended life by six years due to new cardiovascular technologies, but this is so expensive that it is going to be impossible to continue on this path. We need to understand how we can prevent disease from appearing and enhance health." This is what Professor Fuster's team at Mount Sinai Hospital in New York is now working on every day. "I don't like the term prevention." He reasons, "I prefer to use the term health promotion, which seems much more correct to me" [8].

Health Education

Our protagonist tells us that Education, with a capital letter, is the key to everything: "Once I was at Laguardia airport, in New York, and I had a deadline to give a definitive name to our Foundation" [5]. In 15 min he thought of the three fundamental things to avoid disease: the first, Science, without which "we are going nowhere". The second is Health, and the third is Education. That is why he called it "Science, Health and Education" (SHE), for him the three fundamental words that give meaning to all his work. One of Dr. Fuster's concerns, within this education that is so decisive for enjoying good health, is children. He explains that from 3 to 6 years of age is a fundamental stage in the life of any person. In this sense, he understands that the cardiovascular problem is a question of behavior and for this reason it is necessary to act in childhood. It began in the United States and continued in Colombia, with 2000 children whom his teams trained in healthy habits, and they have continued afterwards, for more than a decade, verifying the fantastic effect that 70 h of health education had on their current condition. Now, a good part of them is going to undergo a new re-education program so that they know how to behave in the face of risk factors, tobacco, alcohol and drugs. The SHE Foundation currently works with 50,000 children worldwide.

The Magic of the "Polypill"

One of his best-known projects, and also one of his most beloved, is the "polypill". We are talking about a drug to prevent second heart attacks in which the patient is offered, in a single capsule, the three key components for this: acetylsalicylic acid, to prevent blood clots; a statin, to lower cholesterol; and, finally, an ACE inhibitor to control blood pressure by making the heart work less intensely. The advantage of this novel pharmacological presentation, which has consumed a great deal of research time, is that patients have everything they need in a single pill, thus avoiding absent-mindedness and forgetfulness, which could be very negative for them. It has already been approved by almost 60 countries and is a source of pride for Spain, because it is a project developed entirely by the CNIC. The polypill significantly reduces treatment costs, but to achieve this it was necessary to resort to private sponsorship. There were 12 years of intense work on the project with some ups and downs in its development, a period in which the fundamental collaboration of the Ferrer laboratories in Barcelona must be highlighted. For Fuster this project has been a lesson in life, to know that you should never give up if you really believe in something, although he recognizes that there were some very difficult moments when everything was on the verge of collapse. The project cost a total of 30 million euros, and it was not easy.

Tennis Lost: Medicine Won

All this is told by a scientist, a world-renowned physician, who, paradox of life, could have been a professional tennis player like Rafa Nadal. The story is fascinating and starts from a sporting defeat in Miami that became a personal victory for the health professional he is today (Fig. 31.3).

At the age of 15, he was on the verge of being selected for the prestigious Orange Bowl tournament in the capital of Florida. That summer he failed one subject in his high school (he explains that scientists have also failed at) and that forced him to study hard during the vacations and train less than necessary. In September, he finally passed at school, but when the coaches put him back to play, he was defeated in a match and that same day he decided to give up the racket. He had the intuition that he was not going to go forward in the sports field and considers that moment a priceless life lesson. At that time, he was in a moment of doubt. He wanted to study agricultural engineering, because he really liked the countryside, but it happened that in Barcelona, where he lived, there was no faculty to study it and he had to move to Valencia. At that moment, chance worked its magic and Dr. Pedro Farreras Valentí, a famous specialist in internal medicine whom he knew because he also played tennis at the same club, predicted: "You will be a doctor and not only that, but you will also be a great doctor". Encouraged by that resounding affirmation, he decided to study medicine. Later, Dr. Farreras suffered a heart attack, at the age of 47, and confessed to him that for him the most unknown part of the human body was the heart and, consequently, he should specialize in cardiology. When Valentín Fuster tells this story, which was fundamental in his life, he once again emphasizes the importance of mentors, something fundamental for anyone and which proved to be transcendental in his case.

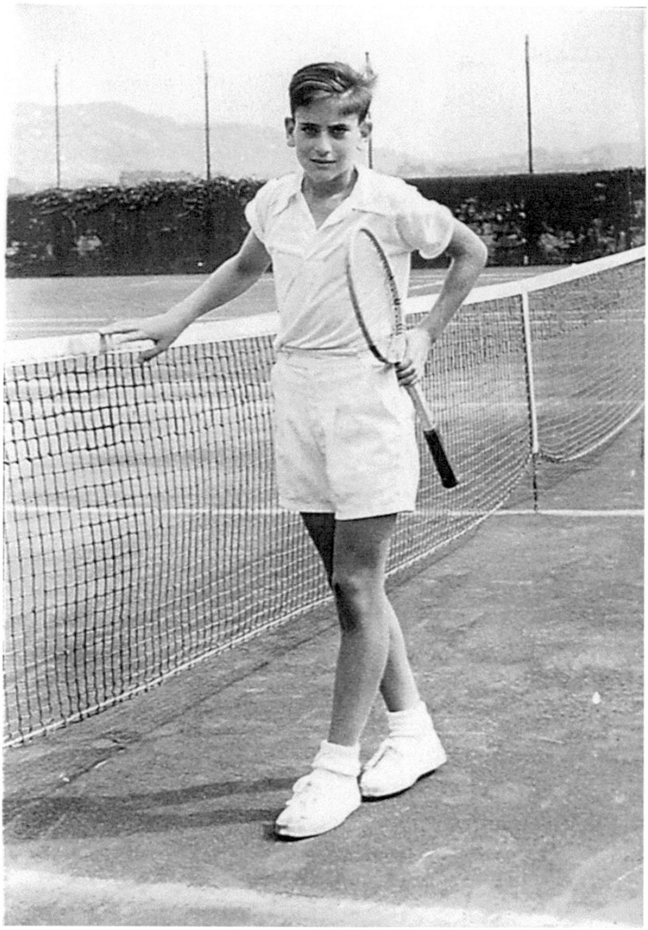

Fig. 31.3 Valentín Fuster playing tennis as a youngster

Prince of Asturias Award for Technical and Scientific Research

But there is more, in Liverpool, where he specialized after obtaining a grant from the Juan March Foundation, he worked with the pathologist Harold Sheehan, who, every morning, to train him, showed him slides in front of which he had to say the diagnosis of what the images showed. After projecting one of those photographs, Professor Sheehan confessed to him that he did not know anything about a specific one, it was an image

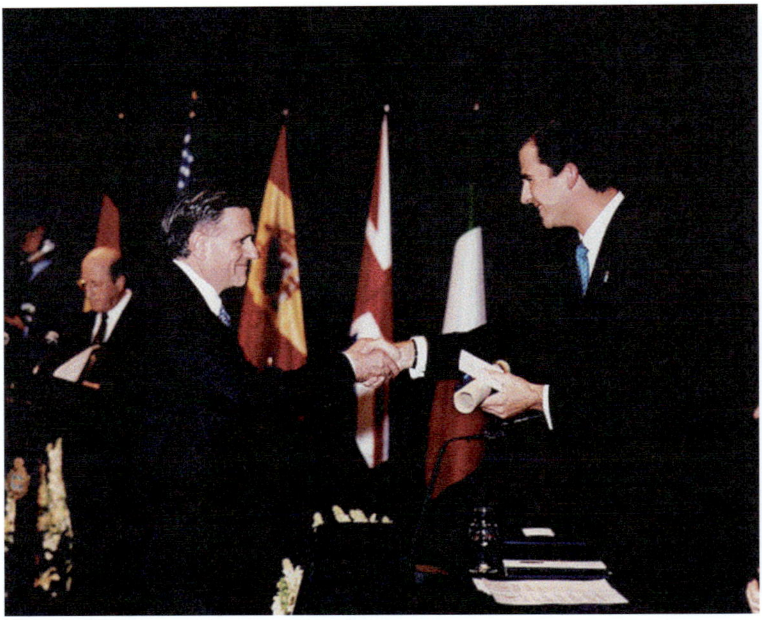

Fig. 31.4 Prize "Principe de Asturias" 1996. Receiving the Award from the then Prince Felipe de Borbon

of a clot causing a myocardial infarction, and that he then had to do his doctoral thesis on it. Valentín Fuster moved to Edinburgh and in his thesis, he demonstrated that the clot was the cause of heart attacks and not the consequence of them, as some doctors believed at the time. In 1996, as is well known, he was awarded the Prince of Asturias Prize for Technical and Scientific Research, (the highest prize given in Spain to national or international nominees in different fields) and, to date, he believes that the final reason for this award was that study in his youth that determined everything from then on in his professional career [4] (Fig. 31.4).

Regarding awards, he says that every time he has received one, and there have been many throughout his life, he comes home, and his wife always tells him that there are many people in the medical and scientific fields who deserve it more than he does. Of course, he appreciates it and likes it, he recognizes that it momentarily increases his self-esteem, but it doesn't go much further and after 10 days he has already forgotten the recognition. "What is important," he says, "more than stability, which is fickle by nature, is the fact that everyone knows at all times that they are doing what they really have to do". That for him is the closest thing to happiness.

The "M" Also Counts

One of his vital discoveries is, as he says, the "Ms":

- The first is the M for Mentoring, which is like the T for tutoring and boils down to the need to have someone to guide you in your career and in life.
- The second is the M for Method, something fundamental to achieve self-esteem and to know one's purpose. He affirms that the method was taught to him in his adolescence by the Jesuits and that acquiring it was one of the fundamental keys to everything he has done since then.
- The third M is Moral, values, something fundamental that begins in the family, an essential basis for vital harmony. He learned morals from his parents and continues to acquire them with his wife and his two children, one of them a musician and the second an architect. He talks to both of them every day on the phone without missing a single one.

Hobbies and Interests

As a fundamental hobby in his life, Valentín Fuster opts for writing. He confesses to being obsessed with putting his thoughts in black and white. And also reading. He is very fond of cinema and has even shot 400 h of personal films in the cities he has visited. In addition, he continues to practice cycling, which has always been his favorite sport. Every summer he sets himself a difficult test and so he has climbed the Tourmalet or the Col de Portet, a road as steep as it is dangerous in the French Pyrenees, with vertiginous precipices, which he climbed in the rain and in hellish weather until he reached the top.

His motivation in life has always been to get his own engine running. With that gesture a person becomes creative and within that scope it is important never get stuck, but to move forward and develop new talents and activities. With that creativity he feels the intimate satisfaction of feeling useful and of being able to help others with his medical science. Motivation is the basis of his existence, get going and keep going without fainting: "Always Move On" fueling his purpose. "When you get to a place or a position and you think you've achieved what you wanted, you start to die and go down," he explains, "at that point you start to get depressed," and the solution has to be found in how you motivate yourself. Everything is a circle, just like life itself".

The United States, His Vital Destination

Initially arriving in the country, he worked at the Mayo Clinic in Rochester for 12 years before moving to Mount Sinai in New York.

Valentín Fuster understands that this is a country that gives opportunities to those who know how to take advantage of them, and this is something he is deeply grateful for. He arrived thinking that he would be here for 1 year and he has been here for more than 50. He knows that it is a very competitive society in which you have to follow its system. "There you don't fight against your neighbor, but against yourself. The more you give to the country, the more it gives you back. It's a person-to-person nation where individualization has historical roots," he explains. Every day he sees between 15 and 20 patients in his practice and donates his science to them, but he also confesses that he learns from them. Sometimes the disease even leads to subsequent friendship, as happened to him with the economist and writer José Luis Sampedro, whom he treated in his office, where he arrived in a critical condition. After a lifetime dedicated to research, Dr. Fuster has a thorn in his side. He says that science in Spain has never been highly valued and that researchers hardly ever appear in the annual rankings of outstanding personalities. This is something that saddens him and, in his opinion, marks a notable difference with what happens, for example, in the United States, his adopted homeland. For him, this is one of the unfinished business that we have not yet passed either as a society or as a country.

Summary of Principal Contributions in the Field of Cardiovascular Diseases

Dr. Fuster has improved the prevention and treatment of myocardial infarction.

He has been also the one who developed the universal concept of health promotion to prevent cardiovascular disease and neurological degeneration. He has identified that platelets play a key role in coronary thrombosis and was the first researcher to use aspirin in heart disease, especially to prevent occlusion after bypass surgery. He has developed the polypill, mixture of acetylsalicylic acid, a statin and an ACE inhibitor of to prevent hypertension, as a single pill to prevent cardiovascular diseases [9].

Awards

We will only refer to some of the awards received, since, for example, he has been named Doctor Honoris Causa on 35 universities and has an index H 215 in Google Scholar, which makes him the most cited Spanish research scientist of all time. Gold Medal of the European Society of Cardiology (1992) Prince of Asturias Award for Technical and Scientific Research 1996): Gold Heart Award from the American Heart Association (2003).

World Heart Federation Lifetime Achievement Award: Recognition for his work in promoting cardiovascular health worldwide. Severo Ochoa Award for Biomedical Research: For his work in the field of prevention and treatment of cardiovascular disease. In addition, in 2022, the American College of Cardiology instituted the "Valentín Fuster Award in Science and Innovation," to be given annually to a single physician for the next several years, in honor of his legacy in cardiovascular research.

Books of V. Fuster (in English)

- "Fuster and Hurst's The Heart" [6]:
  This is a well-known and comprehensive reference book in cardiology, covering all major cardiovascular topics. The 15th edition, in particular, emphasizes practical patient care and includes updates on clinical trials and guidelines.

- "The Science of a Long Life":
  This book explores the science behind living a longer, healthier life, offering advice on diet, lifestyle, and stress management.

- "The Heart Manual":
  The Heart Manual: My Scientific Advice for Eating Better, Feeling Better, and Living a Stress-Free Life. Valentín Fuster and Josep Corbella. Harper Perennial Ed. 2010

- "Always Forward":
  This book shares personal and professional lessons learned by Dr. Fuster, including his groundbreaking research on heart attacks.

References

1. Valentín Fuster. Directorate General of the Carlos III National Center for Cardiovascular Research. CNIC. https://www.cnic.es/es/sobrecnic/direccion-general.
2. Valentín Fuster. Biografías y Vidas. https://www.biografiasyvidas.com/biografia/f/fuster_de_carulla.htm. El Circulo de la Motivación. Ed. Planeta; 2013.
3. Biografía de Valentín Fuster, Influyente 65YMAS. https://www.65ymas.com/comite-expertos/comite-salud/valentin-fuster-médico-cardiologia-espana_58537_102.html.
4. Valentín Fuster Carulla. Prince of Asturias Foundation. https://www.fpa.es/es/premios-princesa-de-asturias/premiados/1996-valentinfuster-carulla/?texto=trayec toria.
5. Dr. Valentín Fuster. Foundation for Science, Health and Education. https://fundacionshe.org/equipo/dr-valentin-fuster/
6. Fuster V, Narula J, Vaishnava P, Leon MB. Fuster and Hurst's The heart. 15th ed. McGraw Hill Medical; 2022.
7. Las ocho claves para vivir mejor. BBVA aprendemos juntos. https://aprendemosjuntos.bbva.com/especial/el-corazon-sirve-para-dar- cantidad-de-vida-el-cerebro-calidad-de-vida-valentin-fuster/.
8. A dialogue with Dr. V. Fuster: connecting heart, head and hands. Esade Alumni Inner Life & Leadership Club; 2024.
9. Valentín Fuster, MD, PhD: a conversation with the editor. Am J Cardiol. 2000;86:182–97.

32

Luis Rojas Marcos: The Restless Psychiatrist

Francisco Mateo Vallejo

Luis Rojas Marcos was born in Seville on a hot August day in 1943 (Fig. 32.1). His parents, María del Pilar and Alejandro—she, a Cantabrian from the Liendo Valley, and he, a pure-blooded Sevillian—were surprised by a hyperactive son who had a difficult childhood in lack of attention. The family had already another son 3 years earlier, Alejandro, who would become mayor of Seville in 1991 and one of the founders of the Andalusian Party after Franco's death. Luis remembers that, when he was 6 or 7 years old, he used to tour on the roofs of the houses adjacent to his own. He was tireless in all his activities, and his lack of attention caused him frequent problems at school and when studying. During the summers, when he would go to Liendo, his mother's village, he would not cease in his mischief either. When he was 9 years old, together with a friend from the village, he started setting fires in the forest, which led him to be locked up by the Guardia Civil in "la perrera", (the cell). His mother, probably hyperactive like him, was the person who supported him the most and knew how to perceive the need for some activity that could managing his hyperactivity, by instilling in him a taste for music by having him take piano lessons. However, the first teacher he had did not last long, because after only one lesson she left without getting paid in despair. In his native

F. M. Vallejo (✉)
Surgeon Specialized in Minimally Invasive Surgery for Gastrointestinal Cancer, Jerez de la Frontera, Cadiz, Spain

M. A. Cuesta, F. Mateo Vallejo (eds.), *Spain's Journey in Medicine*,
https://doi.org/10.1007/978-3-032-12221-6_32

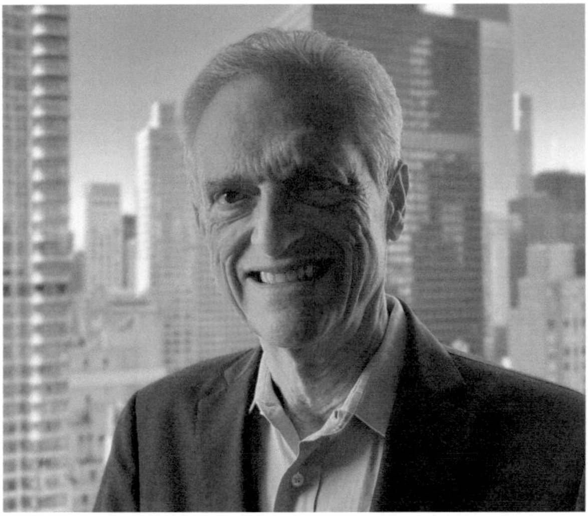

Fig. 32.1 Rojas Marcos in an interview. (Permission for all pictures by the Family of L. Rojas Marcos)

Seville, María del Pilar would tell him stories about her grandfather, a rural doctor in Santander who, when visiting homes to attend to his patients, would leave a few coins under the pillow when he saw that there was a lack of resources. These stories would mark her decision to study medicine. As he himself points out, he was a clear case of ADHD (Attention-Deficit-Hyperactivity Disorder), a pathology that had not yet been described and that condemned him to carry the label of a bad, naughty and hyperactive child. In an attempt to ingratiate himself with his family and with life, he joined three Nazarene brotherhoods, in the hope that God and his twin sister, now deceased, would protect him; however, he only managed to move faster than the rest of the procession and get out of line. Despite the fact that in the 50 s of the last century education was not accessible to many families, he began his studies in a prestigious school: the Jesuit school of Portaceli. There he did not stand out for his school grades, but on the contrary, for his failing grades, which relegated him to the back of the class as punishment. His situation was so complicated that, at the age of 14, after failing all subjects except Religión and Formación del Espiritu Nacional (Formation of the National Spirit), he was expelled from school. His parents then decided to transfer him to the Santo Angel School, known disparagingly as the "school of the cateados", (school for those who failed, the checked out), a place of pilgrimage for difficult students. Fortunately, there he found a teacher who knew how

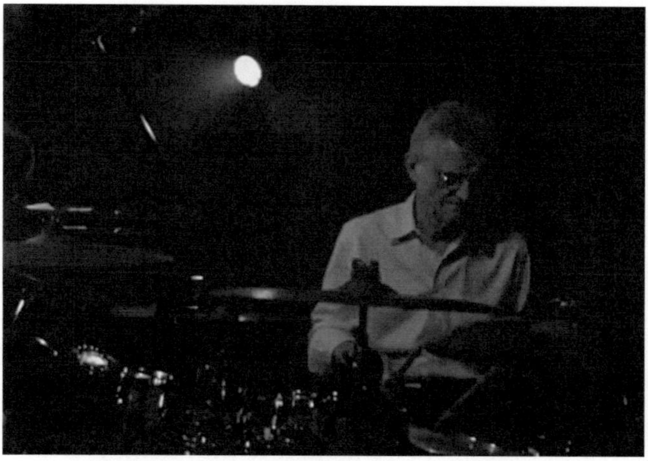

Fig. 32.2 Luis Rojas Marcos playing the drums. (Permission for all pictures by the Family of L. Rojas Marcos)

to adapt to his conditions and gave him the opportunity to improve in his studies: Doña Lolina. She forced him to sit in the front row, instead of the back row where he had been relegated until then, allowed him to leave class when hyperactivity made him restless and helped him focus on his studies. Thanks to her support, he began to pass subjects and courses, which also improved his relationship with his parents, giving him confidence and boosting his self-esteem. Following his passion for music, he learned to play the piano, guitar and drumming, and, at the of 15, he formed the Yungay quartet, where he played the drums—a musical instrument well suited to an ADHD! as he himself says. The other members of the quartet were Manolo Fombuena on vocals, Carlos Olmos on double bass and Jesús Domínguez on guitar (Fig. 32.2).

University Studies

After completing his secondary education, he began his medical studies at the University of Seville, where he graduated in 1968. During that time, he had the opportunity to speak with an American doctor who had come to the university looking for recently graduated doctors to specialize and work in the United States. This encounter, together with the political and social situation of Spain at the time, marked by Franco's dictatorship, as well as certain family disagreements and the lack of freedoms, led him to consider a change of scenery, emigrating to New York. He recalls, as he recounted in an interview, that although he had studied English in England, his level was only good enough to defend himself. When he arrived at the airport, accompanied by his family to see him off, he bought a book in a store entitled "Learn to speak English in a month". However, the reality was that it took him almost 2 years to make himself properly understood.

New York

He tells an anecdote that evidences his initial problems with the language: in the first weeks of his stay as an intern, while he was in the library of the "Good Samaritan" hospital, he heard over the loudspeakers: "Dr. Marcos, I see you" [1] (pronounced "ai sii iu"). He went out into the hallway, looked at the loudspeaker and replied, "I don't see you" [2]. At that moment, a fellow intern, Dr. Rodriguez, from Guatemala, who was passing by, explained to him: No, Luis, they want you to go to the ICU (Intensive Care Unit)—pronounced 'ai ci iou'—which is the intensive care unit, and it sounds the same. Although he did not know what to specialize in, he decided to study psychiatry, in part to know himself better and to understand many of the situations he had experienced. He specialized at Bellevue Hospital and New York University between 1969 and 1972. Among his teachers were Arnold Friedhoff and Murray Alpert, predecessors of what is now called [3] "evidence-based psychiatry" (EBP) and collaborated with them for several years on important pioneering research of today's "Biological Psychiatry", which his teachers developed [4]. In the 1970s, while attending classes taught by Stella Chess, a renowned specialist in child psychiatry, he received his first information about a disorder related to hyperactivity and behavior in certain groups of children. As he listened to her, he discovered that the description matched his own childhood behavior: children with a lot of energy and difficulty controlling it, but who were intelligent. It was then that he realized that the problems he had faced as a child were due to a condition that would later become known as Attention Deficit Hyperactivity Disorder (ADHD).

During his years of specialization, Luis noticed that the Hispanic immigrants who passed through his office spoke less when they were questioned in English, which led to their illnesses being diagnosed as more serious than they really were; even the recommended treatment might not be adequate. On the other hand, when they conversed with him in Spanish, they expressed themselves more clearly, described their ailments better and shared details that they would otherwise have omitted. These observations enabled him, in 1972, to obtain a grant from the National Institute of Mental Health to investigate the effects of the language barrier on sick immigrants with difficulty understanding and communicating in English. The publication of his studies in the American Journal of Psychiatry and his pressure on institutions contributed to New York City enacting a law requiring interpreters to be available in all hospital facilities [5–8], thus allowing physicians to communicate in patients' native language. Since the early 1970s, he had established a fruitful scientific collaboration between the universities of Bilbao and New York. Luis presented in 1975, his research on language in his doctoral thesis, entitled "La barrera del lenguaje" (The Language Barrier), directed by Professor Dr. José Guimón Ugarteche at the University of Bilbao (Spain). At the same time, he was attracted by the clinical orientation of the so-called American "cultural psychoanalysts" and trained at the Karen Horney Institute in New York. Undoubtedly, this experience influenced the humanistic and social perspective that he would later imprint on his career. In 1977, he received his M.D. in Medical Sciences from New York University. In 1981, he received one of his first recognitions when he was appointed Director of Psychiatric Services for New York's 's eleven general hospitals, emergency departments and outpatient clinics. In this position, he began working, among other activities, with people living on the streets, the "homeless," many of whom were from psychiatric institutions and living without a home due to the massive closure policies of those institutions [9, 10]. On October 29, 1987, an article was published in The New York Times entitled "Mentally ill Homeless Taken Off New York Streets," in which the administration of Mayor Edward Koch announced the beginning of a campaign to remove homeless people with serious mental illness from the streets, parks and roads of Manhattan, for the purpose of providing them with medical and psychiatric care, even against their will [11–13]. "Yesterday, four vans departed, each carrying a psychiatrist, a social worker and a nurse," the article recounted. "They were carrying a list of 50 homeless people who are deemed to need immediate hospitalization and pose a danger to themselves or others," city officials reported. Mayor Koch justified the move by arguing that "the pendulum swung too far," a reference to the deinstitutionalization process which, in its eagerness to prioritize the civil rights of people with mental illness, had drastically reduced the number of psychiatric patients in state hospitals: from 93,000 in 1955 to approximately 20,000 in 1987. The project, conceived by Rojas Marcos, was called Project Help: Homeless-Emergency-Liaison-Project. During its first year, it was able to care for more than 500 homeless people and hospitalize 298 patients requiring medical and psychiatric treatment. Over the years, and thanks to his advice, this initiative multiplied and spread to other states and countries. In New York, by 2023, there were 24 mobile interdisciplinary teams serving 12,800 patients annually. Following their model, numerous cities in the United States and Europe have developed mobile crisis units to assist people with mental illness in vulnerable situations. Shortly before the end of his term in 1989, Mayor Edward Koch sent Dr. Rojas Marcos a letter thanking him for his outstanding work in caring for the city and the mental health of its residents, with special recognition for his work on Project Help. On June 17, 1992, The New York Times published a story announcing that Mayor David N. Dinkins had appointed Dr. Rojas Marcos as New York City's Commissioner of Mental Health, thus becoming the top official responsible for municipal mental health, alcoholism and drug addiction services. Bronx Borough President Fernando Ferrer stated in the article, "Look, Luis Marcos is a first-rate psychiatrist. He's a first-rate government health care administrator. That he's Hispanic is good news. But he shouldn't be marginalized just because they had to choose a Hispanic." His comment was in response to pressure the mayor had received from the Hispanic community for the position to go to a Spanish speaking person. For his part, Dr. Rojas Marcos stated that his main objectives were to develop programs to reduce youth violence, to get homeless people with mental illnesses into clinics, and to ensure that minorities with limited English proficiency had better access to mental health care. In doing so, he was following up on previous efforts in translating services into native languages and serving the homeless. In relation to youth violence, he developed the Choose to de-fuse program to prevent violence in public schools. He argued that 90% of criminals had been victims or witnesses of constant aggression during their first 10 years of life, a crucial period for the development of empathy and compassion. Without these capacities, he asserted, an absence of guilt is generated that makes them capable of killing. Hence the need to address youth violence at its root in order to try to redirect their lives is very important. In relation to this problem, Dr. Rojas Marcos has reflected on the crisis of the family model in societies such as the American and Western societies in general. He points out that the incorporation of women into the world of work, together with the difficulties in sharing domestic tasks equitably, has generated uncertainty about who assumes the primary role in the education of children. Not so long ago, this responsibility fell primarily on the mother; however, today, with both parents working, the picture has changed without there being a clear definition of who assumes this task. Moreover, in cases of divorce, children often become a weapon of war, used as a tool to hurt the other parent instead of prioritizing their well-being. In December 1993, at the end of his term of office, Mayor David N. Dinkins sent him a letter of thanks in recognition of his projects and the anti-violence campaign he conducted during his tenure. In 1995, then-Mayor Rudolph Giuliani appointed him president of the New York Health and Hospital System, giving him responsibility for overseeing 16 municipal hospitals and the city's network of outpatient clinics. In a country where medicine is predominantly private, New York's public hospital system at the time had a staff of 43,000 employees and an annual budget of $5 billion. However, the public hospital network was in the red, and turnover in the presidency was high: few managed to stay in office for more than a year. By then, Rojas Marcos was recognized as a strong advocate for mental health and Medicaid programs which had experienced significant impulse [14]. However, as he pointed out, there were still many people without health coverage. Despite this challenge, he was confident that the health care corporation could achieve financial stability ensuring access to health for the most underserved. His first action was to drastically reduce personnel and optimize the efficiency of the system. Thanks to these measures, he managed to clean up the accounts and remain in office for several years, defying the trend of his predecessors, who rarely exceeded the first year in office. During his term as commissioner of the Department of Mental Health, and with the support of NAMI members [15], Assemblywoman Elizabeth Connelly and New York University psychiatry professor Howard Telson, Luis Rojas Marcos participated in the implementation of a pilot program for the institutionalization of psychiatric patients [16, 17]. This project, based at Bellevue Hospital, lasted 3 years. Upon completion of the program and the success of the program, Attorney General Eliot Spitzer, the Treatment Advocacy Center and the Mental Health Advocate formed a coalition to push for the passage of a state law. Thus was born the Kendra Law, which went into effect in November 1999 in New York State. This regulation allowed for the involuntary outpatients admission; a model known as assisted outpatient treatment. Its purpose was to ensure that certain psychiatric patients received regular treatment, thus preventing them from posing a danger to themselves or others. In case of non-compliance, the law provided for the possibility of compulsory confinement for up to 72 h. After several violent incidents involving psychiatric patients who had abandoned their treatment or failed to attend medical check-ups, the program began to be perceived not only as a public health measure, but also as a mechanism to reinforce public safety.

The September 11 Attacks

Luis Rojas Marcos witnessed firsthand the attacks of September 11, 2001 (Fig. 32.3). In the moments after the first impact, he was with a group of policemen and firemen in front of the Twin Towers, trying to communicate

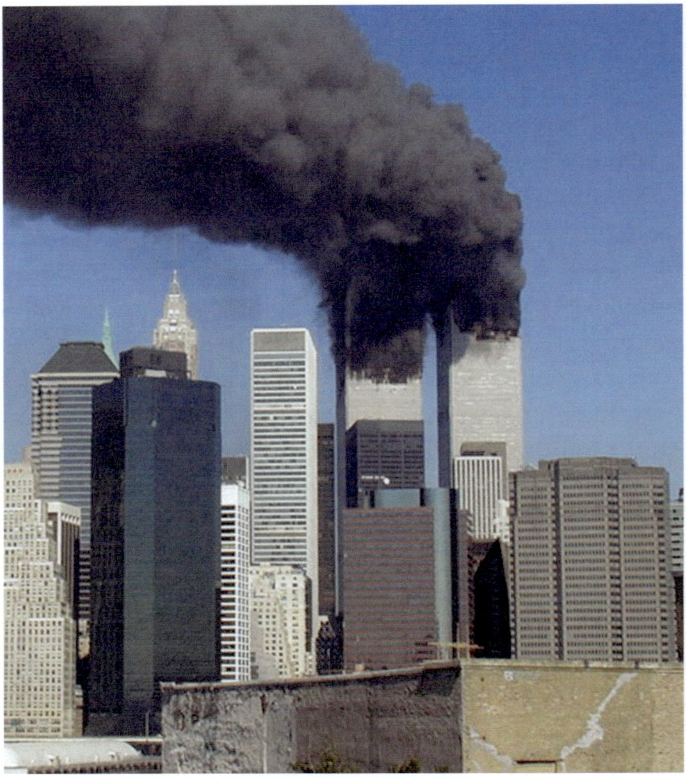

Fig. 32.3 The 9/11 attacks. (Permission for all pictures by the Family of L. Rojas Marcos)

with one of the hospitals he directed. With no telephone coverage, he was forced to move a few meters away. At that moment, a person offered to let him into a nearby building so he could use a landline phone. While he was making the call, the first tower collapsed, collapsing on the group of police and firefighters he had been with minutes before, causing the death of many of them. As a member of the city's Emergency Control Council and head of the Health System and Public Hospitals, Rojas Marcos played a key role in the medical and psychological care of the victims and their families during the difficult days and months following the attack. In 2013, he was appointed executive director of Physicians Affiliated of New York (PAGNY), a non-profit organization that serves six public network hospitals and ten jails. Under his leadership, the entity brings together 3500 professionals, including physicians, nurses and social workers, with a special focus on providing psychiatric assistance to people who are unable to access adequate services in their communities.

Academic Work

Dr. Luis Rojas Marcos has developed a brilliant academic career, since 2003 he has been Professor of Psychiatry at New York University. In 2005, the New York State Assembly appointed him to the Board of Medicine, the body charged with regulating the medical profession in that state. Three years later, he was appointed to the Council for Palliative Care Education. In addition, he is a Fellow of the New York Academy of Medicine and a Distinguished Life Member of the American Psychiatric Association. In Spain, Professor Rojas Marcos has been distinguished with honoris causa for the Ramón Lull, the Basque Country, and the Burgos Universities.

Personal Life

His first wife emigrated with him to New York from Seville, but, as he has said in interviews, she was unable to adapt to life in the United States and wanted to return. He, on the other hand, felt fully integrated there. This irreconcilable difference led to their divorce in 1977. After 6 years as single, he remarried in 1983. He became a U.S. citizen, although he has never denied his origins. Father of four children (Laura, Bruno, Joseph and Carolena) and grandfather of three grandchildren, he regularly travels to Spain to spend time with his family. The death of his son Joseph, at the age of 32, was for him "a devastating nonsense, for which I am looking for an argument to appease the grief and guilt. His memory has become a gaping hole in which, because he is absent, he is always present". To cope with his loss, he had to resort to all his vital principles.

He is passionate about music, writing essays, motorcycling and jogging. A firm believer in the power of "men sana in corpore sano," he became a regular participant in the New York City Marathon, in which he has competed for nearly three decades. However, the year after the COVID-19 pandemic, he assured that, at 78, it would be his last race. But not only did he manage to complete it, but in 2023 he surprised by bettering his personal record, placing second in the octogenarian category, with a time of 5 h, 47 min and 25 s. His daughter Laura, with whom he has a very special relationship, celebrated this on social networks with an emotional message: "My dearest father, your whole family is so proud of you! All of your children and grandchildren followed you excitedly every step of the way during the entire tour and we can't wait to get

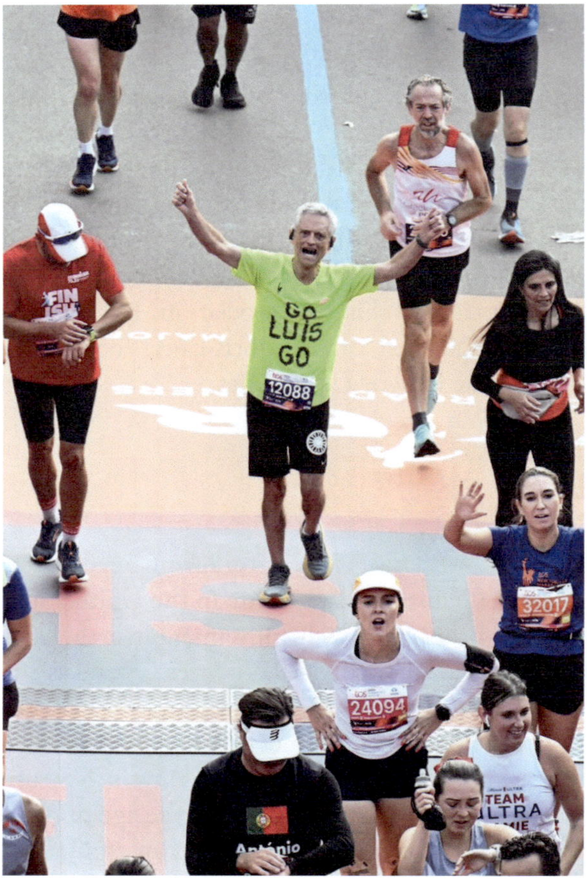

Fig. 32.4 Entering the finish line after the marathon. Luis Rojas Marcos is wearing a shirt with "Go Luis Go" (Permission for all pictures by the Family of L. Rojas Marcos)

together to celebrate this great achievement with you - we love you very, very much!" For his part, Luis Rojas Marcos himself shared in X: "Yesterday I crossed the finish line of the NY Marathon with difficulty (5h, 47m and 25s). As a slow winner, the satisfaction was immense. But the supportive shouts of the smiling spectators, GO Luis GO! became in my mind the indispensable source of vital energy" (Fig. 32.4).

It is curious that his brother Alejandro, in Seville, is also great athlete. At the age of 83, in 2024, he participated in the Hyrox World Championship, a demanding discipline that combines strength exercises with running.

Books

The literary activity of Luis Rojas Marcos has been very prolific, always with purpose of offering keys to confront the problems we face on a daily basis. As he himself expressed during his speech as Doctor Honoris Causa by the University of the Basque Country: "Working in the world of illness, I soon learned two lessons: to live a healthy and fulfilling life, it is not enough to cure illnesses; it is essential to study, know and strengthen those qualities of the human being that help us to stay healthy and overcome the adversity that life will inevitably present us with." Among these qualities, he placed special emphasis on several of them: Resilience, a combination of resistance and flexibility that allows us to adapt to life's challenges and adversities. The ability to make decisions, both about our own life and about the problems that arise. Improving self-esteem, the key to facing difficulties with greater confidence. Diversification of interests and areas in our life, which allows for greater emotional balance. And finally, but perhaps most importantly: positive thinking, optimism and a sense of humor, which are essential to face life with greater well-being. All these ideas have been reflected, in one or another, in his books.

The following is a brief summary of each of his works.

1. The city and all its challenges (1993) This book is aimed primarily at those who live in large cities and must face the challenges posed by the urban environment. In order to achieve safety and quality of life, it is essential that citizens understand the dilemmas that lie in their path and, after analyzing them, seek solutions and alternatives. According to Luis Rojas Marcos, the search for knowledge, a flexible attitude, candor and empathy are key tools for overcoming day-to-day problems.
2. The Broken Couple: Family, Crisis and Overcoming (1994) The anguish produced by the end of a relationship should be seen as a change, the beginning of a new stage and the opportunity to rediscover the illusion. Facing this process with optimism is essential to overcome one of the most difficult moments in life.
3. The Seeds of Violence (1995)—An in-depth analysis of violence in today's society, its causes, manifestations and the means to prevent it. After examining cruelty among people, the author proposes preventive strategies and reflects on altruism as an innate human tendency.
4. Beats at the end of the century (1996). This book compiles articles published by the author in which he addresses the main problems he observes

in contemporary society. Throughout its pages, he analyzes issues such as family conflicts, the situation of women in today's world and the challenges of the elderly, among other topics.

5. Antidotes to nostalgia (1999) We are often trapped in a melancholic and pessimistic state of mind that makes us reluctant to change and even blocks our ability to judge daily events objectively. Throughout his chapters, the author offers strategies to combat this state and regain a more balanced and positive outlook on life.
6. Our Happiness (2002) In this book, Rojas Marcos delves into the ability of human beings to seek and achieve happiness. Although happiness often seems to be hidden behind fear, depression and other pessimistic feelings, there are tools that help us find it. According to the author, the formula for happiness includes curiosity, introspection and self-knowledge. His conclusion is clear: in today's society, most people consider themselves happy for much of their time.
7. Beyond September 11 (2002) As a close witness to the tragedy, responsible for public hospitals and a member of the New York Emergency Council, Luis Rojas Marcos experienced the events of September 11 on the front line. His work as a psychiatrist, both during and after the attack, was crucial in people cope with its aftermath. In this book, he analyzes the emotional and social aftermath of the event: the psychological impact on citizens, the fear of new threats, the exaltation of patriotism, xenophobia and other collective feelings that emerged after the tragedy.
8. Our Uncertain Normal Life (2004) Throughout our lives, we face unexpected situations that alter our routine, generate uncertainty and affect our emotional stability. In this book, Rojas Marcos provides tools to regain balance and develop practical skills that allow us to enjoy life even in times of adversity.
9. The Power of Optimism (2005) For Rojas Marcos, optimism, positive thinking and a sense of humor are fundamental pillars for maintaining mental health and facing life's challenges. In this book, he explores the history of positive thinking and defines optimism as a transforming force that helps us achieve goals and overcome obstacles.
10. Self-esteem (2007) The author analyzes the factors that influence the construction of self-esteem: genetics, childhood, culture and personal experiences. In addition, he examines its relationship with depression, victimization and social interactions. Through this reflection, he stresses that our perception of ourselves is key to achieving happiness.
11. Live together (2008) Human relationships are full of challenges, both in the family, social and work environments. In this book, Rojas Marcos

analyzes the most frequent conflicts that arise in coexistence and offers strategies to strengthen bonds and prevent communication problems.

12. Heart and Mind: Keys Physical and Emotional Well-Being (2008) Together with renowned cardiologist Valentín Fuster, the author explores the interconnection between physical and mental health. Throughout the book, the author highlights the importance of listening to our body, adopting healthy habits and being physically active to improve our quality of life.
13. Overcoming Adversity: The Power of Resilience (2010) Resilience is one of the most valuable human capacities to face difficulties. In this book, Rojas Marcos explains how to strengthen this ability, adapt to problems and recover well-being after a crisis, transforming adversity into an opportunity for growth.
14. You Are Your Memory: Know Thyself (2011) In this book, the author takes us into the fascinating world of memory: how it is formed, how memories are stored in the brain and why we sometimes have difficulty remembering certain events. In addition, he analyzes how diseases, drugs, toxic substances or stressful situations can affect the ability to remember.
15. The Secrets of Happiness (2012) Once again, Rojas Marcos addresses happiness as the central axis of life. In this book, he defends optimism as a fundamental tool to give meaning to existence and argues that our primordial instinct is the search for happiness.
16. Everything I have learned (2014) Throughout 303 reflections, Rojas Marcos compiles ideas and lessons learned throughout his career, providing essential keys to better understand we and achieve a fuller and happier life.
17. We are what we talk about (2019) The author reaffirms one of his convictions: those who talk the most, live the longest. In this book, he explores the power of language and how communication influences our self-esteem, our social relationships and our physical and emotional well-being. Throughout its pages, he demonstrates that speech is closely linked to good health and greater satisfaction with life.
18. Optimism and health (2020) In this book, Rojas Marcos explains the importance of optimism in promoting a healthy and happy life. He clearly differentiates between optimism and pessimism and offers strategies to promote positive thinking to help us face daily challenges.
19. Being well here and now (2022) This book brings together and synthesizes many of the ideas that the author has developed in his previous publications, with the purpose of helping us to preserve our mental health

in times of uncertainty. By resilience, optimism, self-esteem and healthy relationships, Rojas Marcos provides us with tools to strengthen our well-being and bring us closer to happines.

Epilogue

It is difficult to determine, after reading his biography, whether Luis Rojas Marcos has lived only one life or several, given the impressive number of awards, books, articles and projects he has carried out over the years. Although I have tried to compile his entire trajectory, it is very likely that some information has escaped me or that I have overlooked some distinction awarded to him. In a society as demanding as the United States, achieving the prestige and influence that he has achieved requires exceptional talent, both personal and professional. To be a leading psychiatrist in a city like New York is no easy task. Rojas Marcos is, without a doubt, an admirable figure, and listening to him speak and reflect on fundamental issues such as depression, violence, separation or everyday fears is a real pleasure. His legacy extends through a prolific literary work in which, with an accessible and approachable language, he offers us keys to face many of the frustrations that affect us on a daily basis. His teachings, always impregnated with optimism and resilience, invite us to look at life with a more positive and adaptable attitude. A Sevillian, in short, world-renowned and renowned.

References

1. Dr. Marcos, I see you.
2. Dr. Marcos, don't see you.
3. EBP emphasizes the use of the best available data from rigorous scientific research to inform clinical practice.
4. Biological Psychiatry or Biopsychiatry is a branch of the Psychiatry that attempts to understand mental disorders in terms of the biological function of the nervous System.
5. Marcos LR, Alpert M, Urcuyo L, Kesselman M. The effect of interview language on the evaluation of psychopathology in Spanish-American schizophrenic patients. Am J Psychiatry. 1973;130:549–53.
6. Rojas Marcos L, Alpert M. Strategies and risks in the psychotherapy of bilinguals: the phenomenon of language independence. Am J Psych. 1976;122:1275–8.
7. Rojas Marcos L. Nonverbal behavior and thought processing. Arch Gen Psychiatry. 1979;36:940–3.

8. Rojas Marcos L. Adults' recollection of their language deprivation as immigrant children. Am J Psych. 1982;139:607–10.
9. Rojas Marcos L, Gil RM, Vazquez KM. Who will treat psychiatrically disturbed developmentally disabled patients? A health care nightmare. Hosp Community Psychiatry. 1986;37:171–4. 12
10. Rojas Marcos L. Mentally ill and homeless: the plight of freedom. Issues Ego Psychol. 1989;12:20–8.
11. Rojas Marcos L. Dysfunctions in public psychiatric bureaucracies. Am J Psychiatry. 1988;145:331–4.
12. Rojas Marcos L, Cohen NL. taking the suspected mentally ill off the streets to public general hospitals. N Engl J Med. 1986;315:1158–61.
13. Rojas Marcos L, Cohen NL, Nardacci D, Brittain J. Psychiatry takes to the streets: the New York City initiative for the homeless mentally ill. Am J Psychiatry. 1990;147:1557–61.
14. Medicaid is a program that helps cover medical expenses for people with low income and limited resources.
15. National Alliance on Mental Illness assisted living.
16. Rojas Marcos L. Who profits from deinstutionalization? Hosp Community Psychiatry. 1989;40:1221–4.
17. Salit SA, Rojas Marcos L. Have general hospitals become chronic care institutions for the mentally ill? Am J Psych. 1991;148:892–7.

33

Gabriella Morreale: Iodine and Thyroid Hormones in Brain Development

Juan Bernal

Gabriella Morreale de Castro was born in Milan on April 7, 1930, daughter of Eugenio Morreale and Emilia de Castro (Fig. 33.1). Due to her father's diplomatic activity, she spent part of her childhood in Vienna and Baltimore, where she attended elementary school, until 1941 when the family settled in Malaga, where she completed her high school studies [1]. In 1951, and in only 4 years, he obtained a degree in Chemical Sciences from the University of Granada, with Extraordinary Prize. Subsequently, she did postgraduate studies in the Laboratory of Physiopathology of Nutrition of the Faculty of Medicine, with Professor Eduardo Ortiz de Landázuri and in 1955 she obtained the degree of Doctor of Science, in the Chemistry section, under the direction of Prof. Enrique Gutiérrez Ríos, Professor of Inorganic Chemistry. In Granada she met her husband and lifelong collaborator, Francisco Escobar del Rey (Villaviciosa de Córdoba, 1923—Madrid, 2015), who was then Medicine student. The couple carried out postdoctoral studies at the Academic University Hospital of Leiden between 1955 and 1958 with Prof. Andries Querido, returning 1975 to that university for a sabbatical year as visiting scientists, sharing the Boerhaave Chair. In 1958, Gabriella and her husband moved to the Centro de

J. Bernal (✉)
Sols-Morreale Institute of Biomedical Research, Consejo Superior de Investigaciones Científicas and Universidad Autónoma de Madrid, Madrid, Spain

M. A. Cuesta, F. Mateo Vallejo (eds.), *Spain's Journey in Medicine*,
https://doi.org/10.1007/978-3-032-12221-6_33

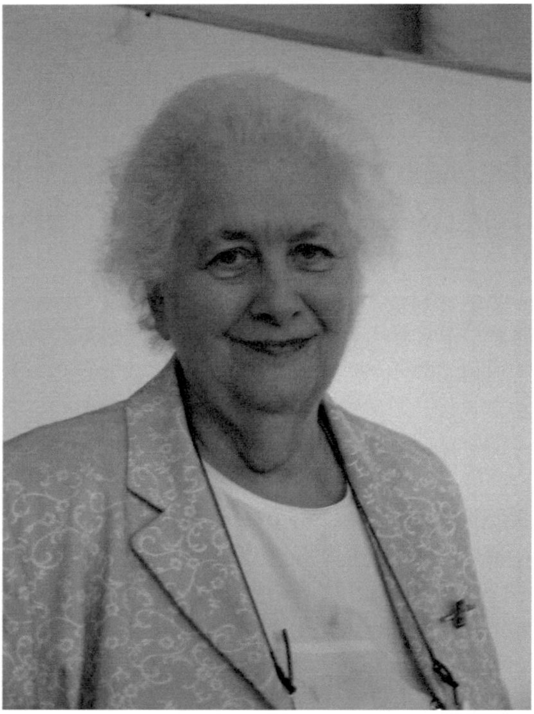

Fig. 33.1 Gabriella Morreale

Investigaciones Biológicas (CIB) of the Consejo Superior de Investigaciones Científicas (CSIC), where Gabriella had obtained in 1957 the position of Scientific Collaborator, joining the Instituto de Endocrinología y Metabolismo Gregorio Marañón with her own group. Subsequently, in 1968 she was promoted to Research Scientist and, in 1970, to Research Professor. Between 1975 and 1980 she was Director of the Institute. Gabriella's initial group at the CIB was the germ of the Department of Experimental Endocrinology of the Gregorio Marañón Institute, moving this de department in 1975 to the Faculty of Medicine of the Autonomous University of Madrid (UAM).

There, together with the Institute of Enzymology, directed by Alberto Sols, the Institute of Biomedical Research was founded in 1984, initially as a CSIC center and later, in 1988, as a joint CSIC-UAM center.

Gabriella carried out her research work at that Institute until 2010, the year she turned 80, passing away in Madrid on December 4, 2017. Currently, the institute bears her name together with that of Alberto Sols, as Instituto de Investigaciones Biomédicas Sols-Morreale (Fig. 33.2).

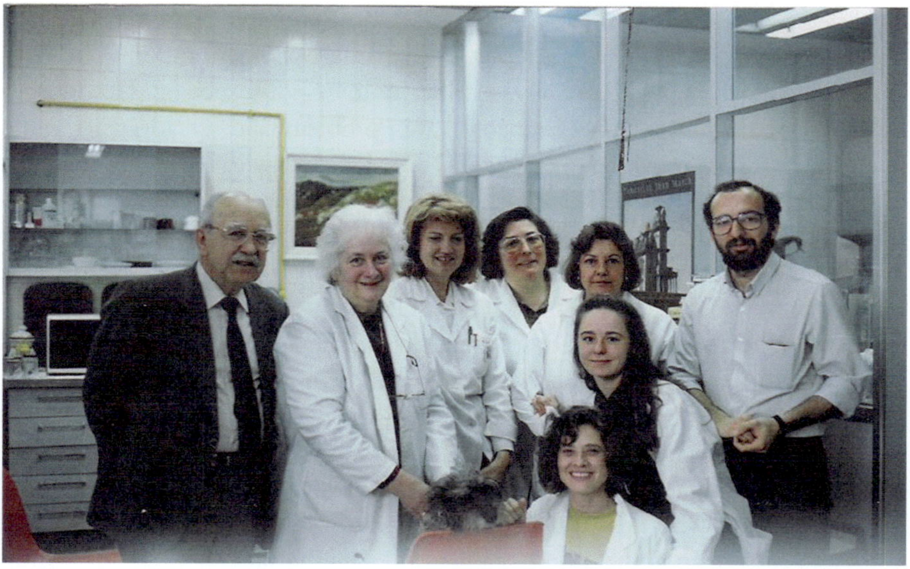

Fig. 33.2 Gabriella Morreale and Francisco Escobar in the Laboratory of the Faculty of Medicine of the UAM with collaborators, at eighties: María Jesús Presas, María Jesús Obregón, Socorro Durán, Arturo Hernández, Rosa Calvo and Elisabeth Subirat

Work

Gabriella's work decisively influenced research on the thyroid gland. Her discoveries were crucial in changing, in many cases, the course of thyroid hormone research. Without her contributions, current thyroidology, especially regarding the role of thyroid hormones in brain maturation and the relevance of maternal hormones in fetal development, would not be adequately understood. Moreover, her work has had a decisive impact on public health in our country, standing out in two areas: the eradication of iodine deficiency and the early detection of congenital hypothyroidism. Since Gabriella's doctoral thesis focused on the problem of endemic goiter, this line of research will be addressed first.

Eradication of Iodine Deficiency

During her training at the University of Granada, Gabriella became aware of the enormous public health problem represented by iodine deficiency. Her doctoral thesis, entitled "Cinética de la reacción $Ce^{4+} \rightarrow AsO_3^{3-}$ catalizada por yoduro", (Kinetics of the iodide-catalyzed $Ce^{4+} \rightarrow AsO_3^{3}$- reaction), laid the groundwork for developing a highly sensitive method for determining iodine concentration in water and biological fluid samples [2]. At that time, Spain was suffering from an endemic goiter disease, especially significant in regions such as Las Hurdes (Cáceres) and La Alpujarra (Granada). This problem had already caught the attention of Gregorio Marañón, who, in 1922, together with King Alfonso XIII, organized an expedition to Las Hurdes to closely observe the serious health situation. While in other regions of the world, such as the Swiss Alps, iodine supply had begun in 1920 with remarkable results, in Spain efforts were sporadic and limited, partly due to Marañón's doubts about the role of iodine deficiency, as he expressed in an article published in La Medicina Ibera on March 8, 1924. In this article he affirmed that the endemic goiter and cretinism was due to a hypoalimentary factor, but he expressed doubts about the hypothesis of iodine shortage as a direct cause "so much in vogue by contemporary Swiss authors". Thirty years later, it had yet to be demonstrated the role of iododeficiency. In La Alpujarra, Gabriella worked with Eduardo Ortiz de Landázuri, José Mora Lara and Enrique Gutiérrez Ríos to map the iodine levels in the region's water sources [3]. Using their novel method, they conducted screening population studies by analyzing iodine levels in serum and urine, confirming that the endemic goiter was a consequence of a nutritional deficiency of iodine. After these findings, between 1953 and 1958, they implemented a supplementation program, using iodized salt produced in the salt mines of Roquetas de Mar, which reached about 100,000 inhabitants of affected areas (La Alpujarra and Güejar Sierra). The results were spectacular, drastically reducing the incidence of goiter from 53% to 13%. In the late 1960s, the Escobars, from the Centro de Investigaciones Biológicas (CIB), undertook numerous studies in Las Hurdes, where iodine deficiency remained severe [4]. In a field study conducted by Dr. Escobar del Rey in 1968, it was found that most of the school children had grade III goiter and ioduria levels below 20 μg/L below the normal range of 100 μg/L). Of 350 adult individuals examined, 44 had cretinism. Given the lack of iodized salt, an attempt was made to remedy this problem by administering lipiodol, an iodized oil administered subcutaneously which provided a slow release of iodine over several years [5]. Finally, and thanks to the personal efforts of Gabriella and Francisco Escobar, in 1983 the production and marketing of iodized salt was regulated in Spain by Royal Decree 1424/1983, which allowed its use in homes and school canteens. This measure was decisive in normalizing iodine intake, not only in Las Hurdes, but also in other affected regions of the country. In 1998, the newspaper El Paí highlighted on its front page: "The Kings put an end to the black legend of Las Hurdes". Studies conducted in Las Hurdes, in collaboration with Professor Nicholas Bleichrodt of the Faculty of Psychology at the Vrije Universiteit of Amsterdam, provided crucial evidence to international public health organizations [6]. A psychometric analysis revealed that schoolchildren in this region, presumed to be normal, had lower mental development than children in socioeconomically comparable areas, but without severe iodine deficiency. These findings, confirmed by similar research in other regions of the world, were fundamental in supporting the World Health Organization's (WHO) global campaign to eradicate iodine deficiency in 2000.

Prevention of Intellectual Disability Caused by Congenital Hypothyroidism

Thyroid hormones are essential for normal brain development, with crucial functions from at least the second trimester of gestation, if not earlier. Congenital abnormalities in the development of the thyroid gland, especially agenesis, can cause serious disturbances in both physical and intellectual development. Congenital hypothyroidism is relatively common among low prevalence diseases, affecting approximately 1 out 2500 newborns. Fortunately, there is an extraordinarily effective and accessible therapeutic treatment: thyroxine. Administered chronically from the first days of life, it allows practically normal development in most, which underlines the importance of early detection of this disorder.

Early Detection of Congenital Hypothyroidism

Early detection of congenital hypothyroidism is performed by measuring TSH and/or thyroxine levels in blood samples obtained from the heel of neonates. This procedure, known as neonatal screening ("heel prick"), makes it possible to identify and treat those affected before severe symptoms develop. Starting in 1976, with a grant from the Real Patronato de Educación y Atención a Deficientes (Royal Board for Education and Care of the Disabled), Gabriella and her collaborators carried out a pilot study on newborns at the Hospital La Paz, from the laboratory of the Faculty of Medicine of the Universidad Autónoma de Madrid. In a first phase initiated after the pilot study, about 18,500 newborns were analyzed, 7 cases of congenital hypothyroidism were detected and received immediate treatment [7]. The program continued until 1985, when it was transferred to the autonomous communities, laying the foundations for the National Program for the Early Detection of Congenital Hypothyroidism. Up to that time Gabriella's team had studied more than 250,000 newborns, detecting more than

90 neonates with congenital hypothyroidism, who were treated in time to prevent permanent brain damage. In recognition of the implementation of the early detection program and her studies on the role of thyroid hormones in brain development, Gabriella, along with F. Escobar del Rey and A. Ruiz Marcos, received in 1982 the Primer Premio Reina Sofía de Investigación sobre Discapacidad Intelectual (First Queen Sofia Award for Research on Intellectual Disability). This award was shared with Magdalena Ugarte (see Chap. 34) and her team, recognizing their work in the advancement of research and treatment of congenital disorders.

The Importance of Tissue Conversion of Thyroxine (T4) to Triiodothyronine (T3)

Thyroxine, or T4, the main product secreted by the thyroid gland, was crystallized by Edward C. Kendall in 1924. This hormone, which contains four atoms of iodine, is essential for development and metabolism, but its biological activity depends on its transformation to T3 in tissues. During her postdoctoral stay in Leiden, Gabriella observed that the activity of T4 was linked to its metabolism in target tissues. When Gabriella and Francisco Escobar moved to the Centro de Investigaciones Biológicas (CIB) in 1958, they began to investigate this phenomenon in depth. In their studies, they demonstrated that drugs such as propylthiouracil (PTU), widely used to treat hyperthyroidism, not only blocked the thyroid gland by reducing the secretion of thyroid hormones, but they also inhibited the tissue deiodination of T4. Surprisingly, this inhibition decreased the biological activity of the hormone. This led to the hypothesis that T4, through a process of deiodination, was converted into a more active compound.

T4 deiodination is the process where the thyroid hormone T4 is converted into triiodothyronine (T3) or into reverse T3 (rT3).

The active metabolite turned out to be triiodothyronine, or T3, discovered a few years earlier in 1952. T3 is generated by the loss of the iodine atom of T4 at the 5′ position. It was then proposed that T4 is not the active hormone itself, but a prohormone which, in target tissues, selectively is deiodinated at that position generating T3, the active form of the thyroid hormone. These pioneering discoveries had a very significant international impact, so much so that Gabriella was invited to present her findings at the prestigious Laurentian Hormone Conference in 1966 [8]. It is now widely demonstrated that T3 is the true active hormone. Its generation occurs mainly in peripheral tissues from T4, thanks to the action of enzymes called deiodinases. T3 acts at the genomic level, regulating the expression of numerous genes following its interaction with specific nuclear receptors. Virtually all tissues are sensitive to T3, which plays an essential role in key processes such as development and metabolism, with particular relevance to the central nervous system [9]. Gabriella's work not only provided a more detailed understanding of these hormones, but also generated new hypotheses that transformed the approach to thyroid physiology. One crucial concept that emerged was the tissue regulation of T3 production, tailored to the specific needs of each tissue. This mechanism is particularly critical for brain development, as we will see in the next section. Furthermore, it was concluded that plasma T4 and T3 concentrations do not always accurately reflect the functional state of the thyroid system. For example, in conditions of iodine deficiency, serum T3 levels may be normal, while the brain is functionally deficient. Likewise, in pathologies such as thyroid hormone resistance syndromes or membrane transporter disorders (Allan-Herndon-Dudley syndrome), some tissues may exhibit characteristics of "hyperthyroidism" while others manifest a "hypothyroid" state, greatly complicating therapeutic management [10]. Ultimately, the findings of Gabriella and her team changed the way we understand thyroid hormone physiology, highlighting the importance of tissue control in T3 production to ensure a functional balance tailored to the individual needs of each tissue.

Placental Transfer of Thyroid Hormones and Their Importance for Fetal Brain Development

Until 1984, the prevailing idea was that the placenta was impermeable to thyroid hormones and that, therefore, fetal development occurred without their influence until the fetus's own thyroid gland began to produce them in significant quantities, towards the end of the third month of gestation. This concept was supported by research such as that of Delbert A. Fisher, Professor of Pediatrics at the University of California, and one of the foremost experts on this. In an article published in 1981 in the New England Journal of Medicine [11], Fisher stated: "The mammalian placenta is impermeable to the natural iodothyronines ". In another review in 1983, he stated: "There is now general agreement that thyroid function in the fetus is essentially independent of maternal thyroid status, providing indirect evidence that the placenta is relatively impermeable to the thyroid hormones". However, this view was challenged by G. Morreale and coworkers, who, using an extremely sensitive and specific method for measuring thyroid hormones-which remains a benchmark in the field-demonstrated the presence of these hormones in rat embryos 4–5 days before the onset of fetal thyroid function [12]. Furthermore, they detected T4 and T3 in human embryos as early as the fifth week of gestation, suggesting that maternal thyroid hormones play an important role in fetal development [13]. The maternal origin of these hormones was unequivocally confirmed by various experimental paradigms. In fact, in human fetuses at term up to 30% of circulating T4 is of maternal origin [14]. A key finding was that, although T3 can cross the placenta, it does not reach the fetal brain as efficiently as it does the adult brain, for reasons that are not yet well explained. In contrast, maternal T4 does and, once in fetal brain tissue, is converted to active T3 by the action of type 2 deiodinase. This implies that, in situations of fetal thyroid insufficiency, maternal T4 is the only source of T3 available to the developing brain [15], in which the temporal expression of deiodinases differs in different regions [16], depending on their asynchronous development.

This conceptual paradigm shift had profound implications.

First, it explains why treatment with thyroxine (T4), when initiated shortly after birth, is highly effective in cases of congenital hypothyroidism, yet ineffective in neurological cretinism. In congenital hypothyroidism, maternal T4 protects the fetal brain throughout gestation. In contrast, in neurological cretinism, maternal iodine deficiency prevents the availability of sufficient T4 to meet fetal requirements.

This conceptual change was clearly articulated in an article by Gabriella Morreale et al., published in the leading international journal of clinical endocrinology, *The Journal of Clinical Endocrinology and Metabolism* (November 2000), titled *"Is neuropsychological development related to maternal hypothyroidism, or to maternal hypothyroxinemia?"* [17]. The study proposed that, in cases of maternal thyroid insufficiency during pregnancy—particularly in the context of iodine deficiency—the critical factor for fetal neurodevelopment was not maternal hypothyroidism per se, but rather the serum levels of maternal T4.

Furthermore, it was demonstrated that maternal iodine deficiency does not need to be severe to adversely affect fetal brain development. During pregnancy, iodine requirements increase substantially, necessitating additional intake. If these increased needs are not met, maternal hypothyroxinemia may develop, a condition capable of impairing fetal brain development and leading to outcomes such as poor academic performance, attention deficits, hyperactivity, and other forms of "minimal brain damage."

Importantly, maternal hypothyroxinemia is not restricted to regions of endemic iodine deficiency; it can also occur in developed countries, where the general population's iodine intake is considered adequate, yet insufficient to meet the increased physiological demands of pregnancy (Fig. 33.3).

Gabriella's last public intervention was in 2009 on the occasion of receiving the Lissitzky Medal and Award at the European Thyroid Association congress in Lisbon. Her legacy lives on as a milestone in the history of endocrinology and public health. His unwavering commitment to research transformed the approach to thyroid disorders, establishing new frontiers in the eradication of iodine deficiency, the early detection of congenital hypothyroidism and the understanding of the conversion of T4 to T3 in different tissues and in the development of the fetus. The synthesis of scientific rigor and humanitarian vocation that characterized his career not only revolutionized clinical practice and health policies, but also laid the foundations for future generations of researchers and professionals. Today, the Sols-Morreale Biomedical Research Institute remains a living testimony of his legacy, inspiring us to continue the search for knowledge in the service of health and collective well-being. Throughout her scientific career, Gabriella Morreale de Castro received numerous awards. Among them, the following stand out:

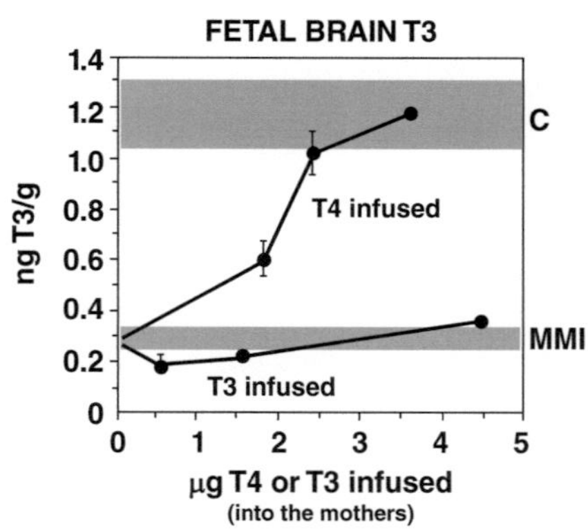

Fig. 33.3 Classic Gabriella Morreale experiment demonstrating the importance of maternal T4 for the development of the brain of the fetus. Pregnant rats treated with MMI (methimazol) that blocks hormone production in the fetal and maternal thyroid glands were used. The mothers were administered by continuous infusion with increasing doses of T3 or T4 throughout gestation. At the end of the experiment, T3 was measured in the brains of the fetuses of the different groups. It can be seen that T3 is very low in the brains of untreated fetuses (group MMI) compared to control (group C) and that only the administration of T4 is able to restore normal T3 concentrations in the fetal brains

- 1977. National Prize for Research in Medicine in Spain.
- 1982. First Prize Queen Sofía of Research on Prevention of Subnormality.
- 1985. European Thyroid Association Research Award.
- 1989. Severo Ochoa Award for Biomedical Research of the Ferrer Foundation.
- 1991. First Research Award and Lilly Medal of the Spanish Society of Endocrinology and Nutrition.
- 1994. Pitt-Rivers Lecture Award of the British Society of Endocrinology.
- 1997. Gregorio Marañón National Award for Medical Research.
- 1998. King Jaime I, Award Medical Research.
- Serge Lissitzky Career Award of European Thyroid Association (2009).
- Gold Cross of the Madrid Health Service of the Community of Madrid (2011). She was also appointed member of the Ordine del Merito della Repubblica Italiana by the President of the Republic in 1987, Honorary Academician of the Royal Academy of Medicine of Madrid in 1994, and in 2001 she received the Doctorate in Medicine Honoris Causa from the University of Alcalá de Henares.

References

1. Moreno JP, Obregón MJ, De Pablo F, Puertas F. Gabriella Morreale. Her life and her time. Ediciones de la Universidad Autónoma de Madrid (UAM Ediciones); 2019. ISBN 978-84-8344-701-7
2. Morreale de Escobar G. On the determination of iodine in biological media. Laboratory. 1954;10:1–24.
3. Morreale de Escobar G, Escobar del Rey F, Mora-Lara JR, Ortiz de Landázuri E. Scientific bases that advise the use of iodized salt in the prophylaxis of endemic goiter. Span Clin J. 1953;54:285–9.
4. Escobar del Rey F, Gomez Pan A, Obregon MJ, Mallol J, Arnao MDR, Aranda A, Morreale de Escobar G. A survey of schhool children from a severe goiter area in Spain. Q J Med. 1981;198:233–46.
5. Escobar del Rey F, Mallol J, Turmo C, Jiménez-Bustos JM, García-García A, Gómez-Pan A, Morreale de Escobar G. Endemic goiter in two areas of Guadalajara and its evolution after administration of iodized oil (Lipiodol). Endocrinology. 1987;34:53–60.
6. Bleichrodt N, García I, Rubio C, Morreale de Escobar G, Escobar del Rey F. Developmental disorders associated with severe iodine deficiency. In: Hetzel JD BS, Stanbury JB, editors. The prevention and control of iodine deficiency disorders. New York: Elsevier; 1987. p. 65–84.

7. Aranda A, Obregón MJ, Benlloch A, Saukkonen S, Durán-García S, Morreale de Escobar G, Escobar del Rey F. Pilot study for the early detection of congenital hypothyroidism in Spain. Endocrinology. 1981;28:85–90.
8. Morreale de Escobar G, Escobar del Rey F. Extrathyroid effects of some antithyroid drugs and their metabolic consequences. Recent Prog Horm Res. 1967;23:87–137.
9. Bernal J. Thyroid and Brain. Understanding the actions of thyroid hormones in brain development and function. Singapore: Bentham Science Publishers, Pte Ltd; 2024. ISBN 978-981-5274-23-3
10. Bernal J, Guadano-Ferraz A, Morte B. Thyroid hormone transporters--functions and clinical implications. Nat Rev Endocrinol. 2015;11:406–17.
11. Fisher DA, Klein AH. Thyroid development and disorders of thyroid function in the newborn. N Engl J Med. 1981;304:702–12.
12. Obregon MJ, Mallol J, Pastor R, Morreale de Escobar G, Escobar del Rey F. Lthyroxine and 3,5,3′-triiodo-L-thyronine in rat embryos before onset of fetal thyroid function. Endocrinology. 1984;114:305–7.
13. Contempré B, Jauniaux E, Calvo R, Jurkovic D, Campbell S, Morreale de Escobar G. Detection of thyroid hormones in human embryonic cavities during the first trimester of pregnancy. J Clin Endocrinol Metab. 1993;77:1719–22.
14. Vulsma T, Gons MH, de Vijlder J. Maternal-fetal transfer of thyroxine in congenital hypothyroidism due to a total organification defect or thyroid dysgenesis. N Engl J Med. 1989;321:13–6.
15. Calvo R, Obregón MJ, Ruiz de Oña C, Escobar del Rey F, Morreale de Escobar G. Congenital hypothyroidism, as studied in rats. Crucial role of maternal thyroxine but not of 3,5,3′-triiodothyronine in the protection of the fetal brain. J Clin Invest. 1990;86:889–99.
16. Kester MH, Martinez de Mena R, Obregon MJ, Marinkovic D, Howatson A, Visser TJ, Hume R, Morreale de Escobar G. Iodothyronine levels in the human developing brain: major regulatory roles of iodothyronine deiodinases in different areas. J Clin Endocrinol Metab. 2004;89:3117–28.
17. Morreale de Escobar G, Obregón MJ, Escobar del Rey F. Is neuropsychological development related to maternal hypothyroidism, or to maternal hypothyroxinemia? J Clin Endocrinol Metab. 2000;85:3975–87.

34

Magdalena Ugarte: Inherited Metabolic Diseases

Susana Pérez Holgueras

Magdalena Ugarte Pérez (Fig. 34.1) was born in Ceuta on September 10, 1941 [1]. She earned a degree in Pharmacy from the University of Granada, where she also completed her doctorate under the supervision of Federico Mayor Zaragoza, with whom she began the study of hereditary diseases from a metabolic perspective for the first time in Spain. In 1973 she moved to the Department of Biochemistry and Molecular Biology at the Universidad Autónoma de Madrid, where she became the first woman professor in the Department and director of the Centro de Diagnóstico de Enfermedades Moleculares (CEDEM) (Diagnostic Centre for Molecular Diseases), an international reference center dedicated to the early diagnosis and treatment of hereditary metabolic diseases. Throughout her long career, Magdalena Ugarte has directed 11 doctoral theses, has published more than 300 scientific articles and has received several awards and distinctions, among others the Reina

S. Pérez Holgueras (✉)
Science Culture Unit, Fundación madri+d, Regional Goverment of Madrid, Madrid, Spain

M. A. Cuesta, F. Mateo Vallejo (eds.), *Spain's Journey in Medicine*,
https://doi.org/10.1007/978-3-032-12221-6_34

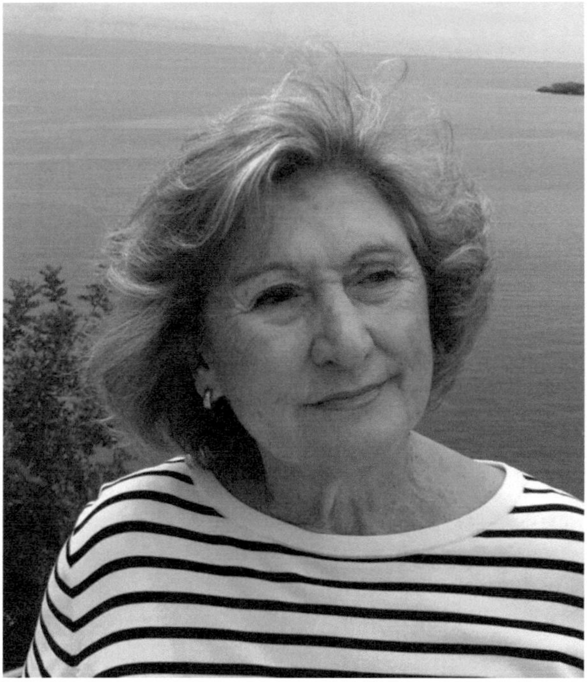

Fig. 34.1 Magdalena Ugarte | SEBBM

Sofía Award for Research on the Prevention of Subnormality (1982), the Encomienda of Alfonso X el Sabio (1982), the Royal National Academy of Pharmacy Award (1998) and the Spanis Assoctiation of Orphan and UltraOrphan Drug Laboratories Award (AELMHU, 2018) [2]. In addition, she has been a visiting professor in the Department of Human Genetics at Yale University between 1974 and 1975 [3]. Magdalena Ugarte is an indispensable figure in the research of inherited metabolic diseases in Spain. She has been a pioneer in neonatal screening and the driving force behind the "heel prick test" in Spain. Her work has improved the quality of life of thousands of patients suffering from rare diseases.

Neonatal Screening in Spain: First Steps

While studying Pharmacy in Granada, her professor Federico Mayor Zaragoza profoundly influenced Magdalena Ugarte's career [4]. He fostered her interest in biochemistry and supervised her doctoral thesis:

"Estudio de la L-glutamato deshidrogenasa NAD y NADP y de actividades enzimáticas relacionadas en Saccharomyces cerevisiae *(cepas normal y con deficiencia respiratoria inducida)"* (*Study of L-glutamate dehydrogenase NAD and NADP and related enzymatic activities in Saccharomyces cerevisiae, normal and induced respiratory deficiency strains*), defended at the University of Granada on June 15, 1968 [5].

After a research stay at Oxford University—where, while working with Hans Krebs, Mayor Zaragoza met Dr. Louis Wolf, a pioneer in rare disease detection—he challenged his team to begin early diagnosis of inherited metabolic disorders in Spanish newborns, starting with phenylketonuria (PKU).

Ugarte accepted, stating that preventing even a single case of PKU would justify the effort. She could not yet foresee the many cases her work would help prevent. Her decision was bold: in 1968 Spain lacked both a supportive research environment and a Ministry of Health, having only a General Directorate of Health within the Ministry of the Interior, led by Dr. García Orcoyen, a gynecologist unusually sensitive to the vulnerability of the newborn brain [2].

Inherited Metabolic Diseases

The Case of Phenylketonuria

Phenylketonuria (PKU) is the most common inherited disorder of amino acid metabolism. It is characterized by elevated concentrations of phenylalanine (Phe) in blood and tissues, resulting from deficiency of the enzyme **phenylalanine hydroxylase (PAH)**, which catalyzes the hydroxylation of Phe to tyrosine (Tyr) [6].

The concept of **hereditary metabolic disease** was introduced by the English physician **Archibald Garrod** at St. Bartholomew's Hospital, London, in 1902, when he described **alkaptonuria** (black urine disease) caused by impaired tyrosine catabolism and accumulation of homogentisic acid. By 1908, Garrod had identified four "inborn errors of metabolism": **albinism, alkaptonuria, cystinuria, and pentosuria** [7].

In 1934, Norwegian physician **Asbjørn Følling** investigated two intellectually disabled sisters and, using ferric chloride testing, identified **phenylpyruvic acid**—a compound not previously detected in nature—linking it to dietary phenylalanine and coining the term *phenylpyruvic oligophrenia* [8].

Følling's ferric chloride test marked the first diagnostic approach for PKU but was ineffective for early detection due to low metabolite levels in neonates [9].

By the 1950s, a **low-phenylalanine diet** was shown to prevent neurodevelopmental impairment, but early diagnosis remained elusive. In the 1960s, **Robert Guthrie** developed a simple and inexpensive **bacterial inhibition assay** using dried blood spots to measure phenylalanine concentrations—the **Guthrie test**—which enabled newborn screening for PKU and marked the beginning of systematic **neonatal screening programs** [10].

The CIAMYC Pilot Experience in Granada

In **Spain**, the first **neonatal screening program** for the early detection of **phenylketonuria (PKU)** was launched in **1967** at the **Department of Biochemistry, University of Granada**, with **Magdalena Ugarte as director.** In 1968, the **Centro de Investigación de Enfermedades Metabólicas y Cromosómicas (CIAMYC; Center for Metabolic and Chromosomal Disease Research)** began operating in a wing of the **Provincial Health Headquarters of Granada**.

The centerpiece of CIAMYC was an **amino acid chromatograph** used to analyze urine samples from all newborns in Granada province 15 days after birth. The screening could detect seven metabolic disorders associated with intellectual disability, including **galactosemia, cystinuria, and phenylketonuria** [7].

From its inception under Ugarte's leadership, CIAMYC combined **newborn screening** with **metabolic disease research**. Early identification of these conditions during the first days of life was—and remains—has been critical to preventing **irreversible neurodevelopmental impairment** that can occur if diagnosis is delayed.

CIAMYC implemented a simple home-sampling protocol: parents received instructions, two filter papers (10 cm long) to be soaked in the infant's urine about 15 days after birth, a form for basic data, and a prepaid envelope addressed to the center. The process was painless for the newborn and free of charge. Upon receiving samples, **Magdalena Ugarte** and her team analyzed them chromatographically; if abnormal values were detected, families were asked to provide fresh urine or blood for confirmation. When a metabolic defect was verified, a physician developed a treatment plan, aiming to initiate a **specialized diet within 2 months**, a critical window to prevent irreversible cognitive impairment.

Some therapeutic foods required importation from the United Kingdom, making treatment costly. Ugarte firmly advocated that **early diagnosis and prompt dietary intervention** could avert severe neurodevelopmental delay. Her team also identified that breast milk from mothers with **phenylketonuria** contained excessively high phenylalanine levels, posing a risk for affected neonates [11].

Despite its innovation, CIAMYC faced significant challenges. Many parents, unfamiliar with hereditary metabolic disorders, were reluctant to participate. In Granada city about 60% returned the urine samples; in the province, participation was much lower. Although the center's **chromatograph** could process 70,000 samples annually by 1972, only 6000 were analyzed due to limited funding. CIAMYC also used part of its modest budget to subsidize expensive therapeutic diets for affected families [11].

These experiences gave Ugarte a deep understanding of the real-life burden of metabolic disorders. She often recalled two sisters with **phenylketonuria**, aged two and four, as a driving force behind her work, and celebrated the diagnosis of Spain's **first asymptomatic PKU case** as proof that **prevention and early detection save lives**.

CIAMYC pursued a dual mission: to **expand early screening** across Spain and to **research the metabolic basis** of genetic disorders [4]. From **June 7–9, 1973**, Granada hosted the **First Symposium on the Detection and Treatment of Hereditary Metabolic Diseases**, with Ugarte serving on the organizing committee [12]. That same year, she began a **new and productive phase** at the **Universidad Autónoma de Madrid**.

A New Phase—Universidad Autónoma de Madrid (1973)

In **1973**, **Magdalena Ugarte** moved with **Federico Mayor Zaragoza** and his team to the **Universidad Autónoma de Madrid (UAM)** to expand **neonatal metabolic screening** in Madrid. She adopted the successful dual model from Granada, integrating **early diagnosis** with **basic research**. Clinical screening was conducted at the **Center for the Diagnosis of Molecular Diseases (CEDEM)**, while fundamental studies were pursued at the **Severo Ochoa Molecular Biology Center** by Ugarte's group, *Molecular Bases of Metabolic Diseases*. She was initially appointed **senior lecturer** and, in **1986**, became the **first female professor** in the Department of Biochemistry and Molecular Biology.

The Severo Ochoa Center is a joint research institute of the **Consejo Superior de Investigaciones Científicas (CSIC)** and UAM.

National Plan for the Prevention of Intellectual Disability

In **1976**, Spain created the **Real Patronato de Educación Especial** (now the **Royal Board on Disability**). That November, **Mayor Zaragoza** was tasked with developing a **National Plan for the Prevention of Intellectual Disability**, in which **Dr. Ugarte** played a key role. As part of this plan, **seven research agreements** were funded in **1979** to study metabolic disorders; Ugarte's group received **7,181,000 pesetas** (≈100,000 USD) [13].

In **1982**, the **Reina Sofía Award** for research on the prevention of intellectual disability was created. Its first edition honored **Magdalena Ugarte** (ex aequo with Gabriela Morreale, Francisco Escobar, and Antonio Ruiz) for her work *"Detection, prevention, and molecular etiology of intellectual disability caused by congenital metabolic disorders."* Meanwhile, in **1978**, Gabriela Morreale and Francisco Escobar launched Spain's first **congenital hypothyroidism screening program** at UAM's Faculty of Medicine [14].

This **interdisciplinary plan**, involving physicians, pediatricians, geneticists, and biochemists, gradually expanded **newborn screening** nationwide. Thanks to the efforts of scientists such as **Morreale** and **Ugarte**, neonatal screening became universal in Spain. Today, approximately **350,000 newborn screenings** are performed annually, with new conditions regularly incorporated into the **National Health System** [15, 16].

The Center for the Diagnosis of Molecular Diseases (CEDEM)

Founded in **1973** at the **Faculty of Sciences, Universidad Autónoma de Madrid (UAM)**, the **Center for the Diagnosis of Molecular Diseases (CEDEM)** is a **biochemical and molecular genetics laboratory** specializing in the **diagnosis and research of hereditary metabolic diseases (HMDs)**. Its mission includes **comprehensive prenatal and postnatal diagnosis**, treatment monitoring, and **carrier detection**. The CEDEM is part of the CIBERER.

The **Center for Biomedical Research Network on Rare Diseases (CIBERER)** and the **Research Institute of the University Hospital La Paz**

(IdiPAZ), collaborate closely with UAM research projects. It serves as a **national reference center** for research of rare diseases supporting **neonatal screening programs and diagnosis of endocrine-metabolic diseases** by providing **biochemical and genetic confirmation** of suspected cases. Moreover, the CEDEM analyzes **over 60 metabolites** in diverse biological fluids (blood, serum, urine, cerebrospinal fluid) and identifies variants in **more than 1000 genes** associated with HMDs [17].

Commitment to Rare Diseases and Orphan Drugs

Magdalena Ugarte's career has been deeply linked to **rare diseases** and the development of **orphan and ultra-orphan drugs**—therapies for conditions too rare to attract commercial investment without public support. From the 1970s, when dietary **phenylalanine restriction** was the only treatment for **phenylketonuria (PKU)**, Ugarte emphasized **prevention** as the first step in care. Her group has consistently aimed to **uncover the biochemical mechanisms** underlying this inherited diseases in order to develop targeted therapies.

Faced with untreatable disorders such as **congenital disorders of glycosylation**, Ugarte's team innovated by **patenting a chaperone protein** to correct misfolded enzymes and restore function. Over time, they contributed to the development of several **orphan drugs**, despite the limited profitability of such therapies. Progress in **mass spectrometry, genomics, proteomics, and metabolomics** has transformed their diagnostic and therapeutic capabilities.

From Madrid, Ugarte spearheaded the **national expansion of newborn screening** and built CEDEM into a leading **diagnostic and research hub** (Fig. 34.2). Her team has contributed to the **diagnosis of more than 5000 metabolic disorders**, integrating **genomic analysis** with **personalized therapies**. Among her notable contributions is the **clinical development and application of sapropterin (Kuvan)** for PKU.

Ugarte also founded and coordinated **REDEMETH** in 1995, the precursor to **CIBERER**, strengthening Spain's rare-disease research network. Her office remains filled with photographs of children whose lives have been improved by early detection and innovative treatments. Many scientists—such as **Belén Pérez Gómez** (deputy director of CEDEM and head of Molecular Genetics), **Pedro Ruiz-Sala**, and **Patricia Alcaide** (heads of Biochemistry)—continue her **scientific and human legacy**, advancing the vision she pioneered in the 1960s: **understanding HMDs and ensuring newborns a healthier future**.

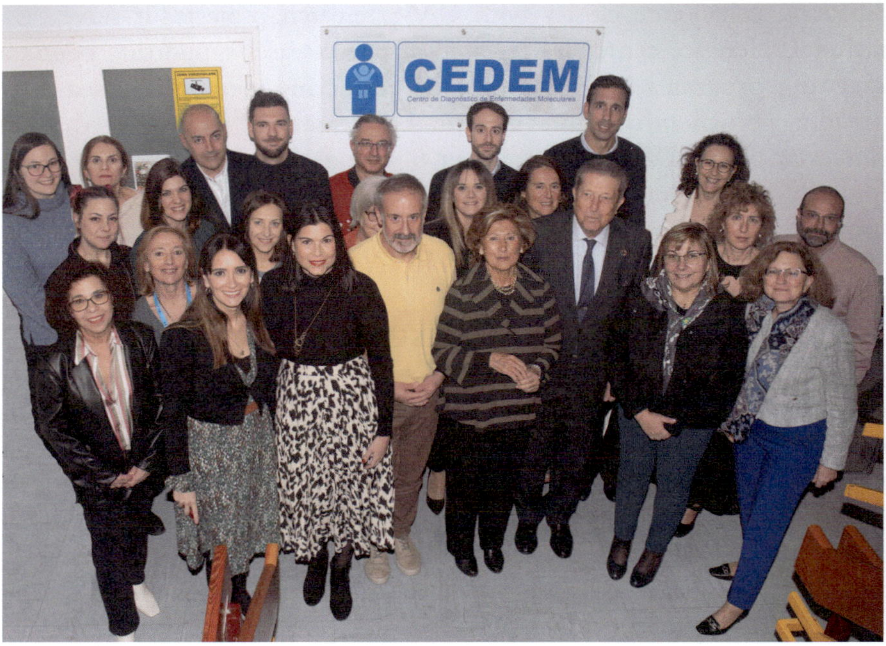

Fig. 34.2 Staff of the CEDEM. 2024. (Permission of the Centro de Diagnóstico de Enfermedades Moleculares—CEDEM)

References

1. Pérez González, Belén. Magdalena de Ugarte. Sociedad Española de Bioquímica y Biología Molecular (SEBBM) [Consultado el 23 de marzo de 2025]. Disponible en: https://sebbm.es/mujer-y-ciencia/magdalena-ugarte/
2. Entrevista a la profesora Magdalena Ugarte Pérez. Asociación Española de Laboratorios Huérfanos y Ultrahuérfanos. [Consultado el 23 de marzo de 2025]. Disponible en: https://www.youtube.com/watch?v=5GesNHYGY3E
3. De Pablo Dávila F, Suárez González T. La excelencia científica en pareja: tanto monta-monta tanto. Encuentros multidisciplinares. 2014;47:1–12.
4. Ugarte, Magdalena. Obituario. Federico Mayor Zaragoza. Academia Malagueña de Ciencias [Consultado el 23 de marzo de 2025]. Disponible en: https://academiamalaguenaciencias.wordpress.com/2025/01/18/obituario-federico-mayor-zaragoza
5. Pérez U, Magdalena. Estudio de la L-glutamato deshidrogenasa NAD y NADP y de actividades enzimáticas relacionadas en Saccharomyces Cerevisiae (cepas normal y con deficiencia respiratoria inducida) [Tesis doctoral]. Granada: Universidad de Granada; 1968.
6. Grupo de trabajo de cribado neonatal. Protocolo de cribado neonatal de la fenilcetonuria. Ministerio de Sanidad; 2021.

7. Mayor Zaragoza, Federico. 50 años de diagnóstico precoz de metabolopatías en España. En Pérez González, Belén (coord.). 50 años de cribado neonatal: cómo afrontamos el futuro. Fundación Ramón Areces; 2021, pp. 11–28.
8. Woolf LI, Adams J. The early history of PKU. Int J Neonatal Screen. 2020;6:59–62.
9. La fenilcetonuria (PKU) y la detección en recién nacidos. Eunice Kennedy Shriver National Institute of Child Health and Human Development [Consultado el 23 de marzo de 2025]. Disponible en: https://espanol.nichd.nih.gov/acerca/logros-cientificos/aportes/PKU
10. El Hospital Materno Infantil conmemora el 60 aniversario del cribado neonatal. Servicio Andaluz de Salud [Consultado el 23 de marzo de 2025]. Disponible en: https://www.sspa.juntadeandalucia.es/servicioandaluzdesalud/todas-noticia/el-hospital-materno-infantil-conmemora-el-60-aniversario-del-cribado-neonatal
11. Castillo JL. Seiscientos subnormales profundos pueden salvarse en España cada año. Patria. 1972:9–10.
12. Castillo JL. Clausurado el congreso de enfermedades metabólicas hereditarias. Patria. 1973:16–24.
13. Plan Nacional de prevención de la subnormalidad. Boletín Oficial de las Cortes Generales. Congreso de los Diputados; 1980. p. 1026-II.
14. Comité de la Calidad de la Asociación Española de Cribado Neonatal. Actividad de los programas de cribado neonatal en España. Revisión desde sus inicios hasta 2016. Ministerio de Sanidad; 2021. p. 13.
15. Couce ML, et al. Situación actual y nuevos pasos en el cribado neonatal en España. An Ped. 2025;102:503775.
16. Ministerio de Sanidad. Programa de cribado neonatal de enfermedades congénitas en prueba de talón [Consultado el 23 de marzo de 2025]. Disponible en: https://www.sanidad.gob.es/areas/promocionPrevencion/cribado/cribadoNeonatal/enfermedadesEndocrinoMetabolicas/home.htm
17. Centro de Diagnóstico de Enfermedades Moleculares [Consultado el 23 de marzo de 2025]. Disponible en: https://cedem.cbm.uam.es/

35

Francisco Martinez Mojica: Discoverer of the CRISPR Systems in Prokaryotes

Lluís Montoliu

We tend to think that the greatest scientific discoveries, the most spectacular and disruptive advances, always come from abroad (Fig. 35.1). That is why in our country we have an excessive tendency to praise the successes of foreign researchers while sometimes we tend to disdain or fail to recognize the contributions made by Spanish researchers. This could be the summary of the professional life of Francisco Juan Martínez Mojica, professor and microbiologist at the University of Alicante, who made one of the most surprising discoveries in molecular biology today, one that has changed the life of practically all experimental biology laboratories anywhere in the world.

Let's start at the beginning. Francis Mojica [1], the abbreviated name by which is known and cited, was born in Elche (Alicante) in 1963 and graduated in biology from the University of Valencia in 1986. His doctoral thesis, presented in 1993 at the University of Alicante, dealt with the response of halophilic archaea to environmental stress. This thesis was supervised by Francisco Rodríguez Valera and Guadalupe Juez Pérez. He made research stays at the Université Paris-Sud, in Paris and two postdoctoral stays at the

L. Montoliu (✉)
Department of Molecular and Cellular Biology, Spanish National Research Council (CSIC), National Centre for Biotechnology (CNB), Madrid, Spain, and Centre for Biomedical Network Research on Rare Diseases (CIBERER) of (ISCIII), Madrid, Spain

M. A. Cuesta, F. Mateo Vallejo (eds.), *Spain's Journey in Medicine*,
https://doi.org/10.1007/978-3-032-12221-6_35

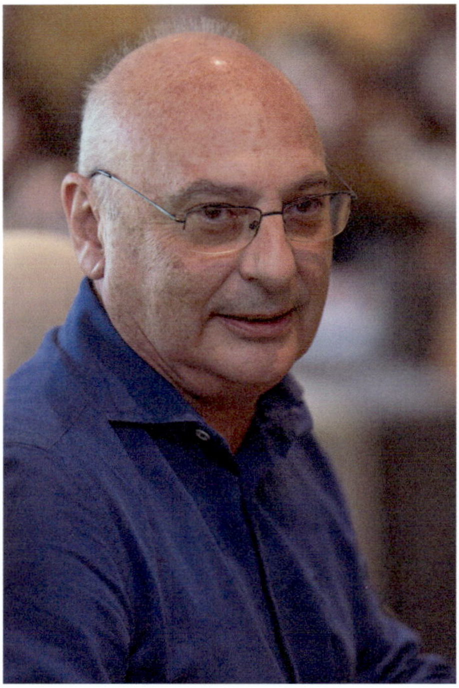

Fig. 35.1 Francisco Mojica

University of Utah (USA) and at the University of Oxford (UK) before returning in 1997 to the University of Alicante as professor of microbiology, where he founded the research group [1] of molecular microbiology focused on the study of CRISPR systems that his work led to the discovery of CRISPR systems. Between 1993 [2] and 2000 [3] he discovered curious clusters of small, repeated DNA sequences, separated by other, also short, sequences that were each distinct, in the genomes first of archaea and then of other prokaryotes.

Prokaryotes are unicellular organisms without a defined nucleus, and multiply by binary division., including the archaea, and Gram negative and positive bacteriae.

He was not the first to detect the presence of these unique sequences. They had already been described, without interpreting them or trying to understand what their function might be, by other Dutch and Japanese microbiologists, in 1991 and 1987, respectively [4]. Francis Mojica, on the other hand, was determined to try to understand how such a precise and apparently sophisticated genetic structure had withstood the onslaught of mutations for billions of years. He deduced, correctly, that the simplest explanation for why these sequences were found in most bacteria, both Gram+ and Gram-, and in most archaea was because they fulfilled a relevant function, yet to be discovered. In addition, the fact that these clusters of short DNA sequences appeared in the three main phylogenetic groups of prokaryotes: archaea, Gram+ bacteria and Gram- bacteria, which are evolutionarily very separate, implied that these sequences must surely have already existed in the common ancestor of all the groups of prokaryotes that we know today. In other words, these repeated sequences should be present practically from the origin of life, since the first prokaryotic cells appeared on our planet, something that we believe must have happened about three and a half billion years ago, out of the estimated four and a half billion years that the Earth has. Serendipity in science is at the basis of many discoveries.

Serendipity is the occurrence and development of events by chance in a beneficial way.

These are unexpected discoveries that make connections between apparently unconnected observations but which, after some unforeseen event, make sense and explain something complex that no one had been able to explain until then. This was undoubtedly what happened to Francis Mojica and his collaborators during the summer of 2003, ten years after having discovered DNA sequence repeats in the genome of the halophilic archae, the Haloferax mediterranei, isolated from the salt flats of Santa Pola (Alicante), and a couple of years after having proposed the acronym CRISPR (pronounced "crísper") to describe them [5], definitively resolving the dispersion of the myriad of names by which researchers referred to these curious sequences in their respective works. Indeed, CRISPR is the acronym for Clustered Regularly Interspaced Short Palindromic Repeats (Fig. 35.2).

Indeed, it was during the summer of 2003, on the campus of the University of Alicante, when Francis Mojica realized that these short unique sequences, separated by the same repetitive sequence, were actually fragments of the genome of viruses that infect bacteria and archaea, the bacteriophages. And he added an additional observation to that discovery. Those bacteria that

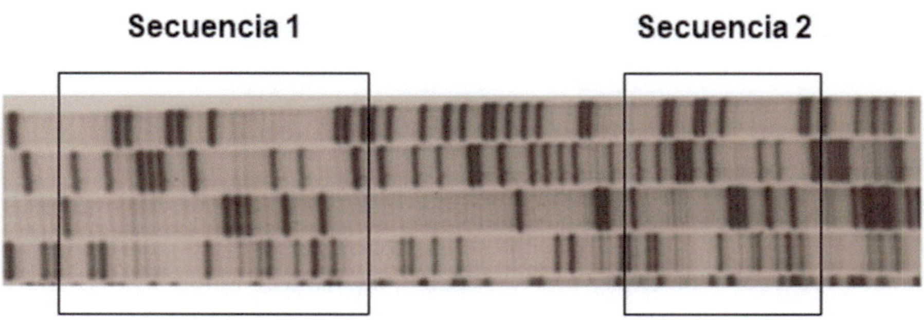

Fig. 35.2 CRISPR duplications in the genome of the arquea *Haloferax mediterranei*. (book in Spanish [18])

incorporated fragments of the genome of certain bacteriophages in their genome, turned out to be resistant to infection by those same viruses. In other words, he had found an ancestral, genetically based, adaptive defense system. The incorporation of new genome fragments from other viruses transformed the bacteria carrying those sequences into resistant to be attacked by those bacteriophages. Nothing less than a bacterial immune system was what Francis Mojica discovered in 2003. This was an experiment called to open the covers of prestigious scientific journals, due to its novelty and relevance. It did not. After submitting the work to the most important scientific journals, all of them rejected the manuscript. In short: they did not believe him. They did not believe that someone from Alicante, with only the help of predoctoral students, without international collaborations, could have discovered something as impressive as a new bacterial defense, which no one had been able to describe before. It could not be. After multiple failed attempts in several journals, the work was finally published in 2005 in the Journal of Molecular Evolution [6], a worthy journal but far from the most prestigious and famous journals. And then the magic that accompanies great scientific discoveries happened. It doesn't really matter so much "where" scientific results are published. What matters is that they are published, that they can be found by other interested researchers. Other scientists who are able interpret these results from another perspective and propose new applications derived from the initial description of a process. That is what happened with Mojica's seminal work. It was read by many other colleagues. In particular, Francis Mojica's work was rediscovered by two female researchers, Emmanuelle Charpentier, a French microbiologist, and Jennifer Doudna, an American biochemist, who had already been working on CRISPR systems. They met at a conference in San Juan de Puerto Rico in 2011 and agreed to collaborate on the description of a new application for CRISPR systems, until then only recognized as adaptive defense systems in prokaryotes. Charpentier and Doudna investigated the mechanism of action of CRISPR systems, integrating the results published by Mojica and other researchers who had described the different elements that these defense systems seemed to need to function.

In particular, small RNA molecules were needed to guide specific nucleases (like the Cas9), by sequence complementarity with DNA, to cut certain areas of the genome with great precision and robustness. When these double-stranded cuts were made in specific DNA sequences, something already happened: the repair of these cuts was activated. Repair could lead to both inactivation and editing of these DNA sequences, allowing to make specific changes to the genetic code. Thus, in their seminal paper published [7] in June 2012 in the journal *Science*, Charpentier and Doudna turned the adaptive immune system initially proposed by Mojica into a true gene-editing system, analogous in function to other previously described systems, such as meganucleases, zinc finger-associated nucleases (ZFNs), and TALE nucleases [8]. Charpentier and Doudna's article, derived from basic research conducted by Mojica in Alicante, revolutionized the biology and genetics laboratories around the world.

Their pioneering research led to the discovery and development of the CRISPR-Cas9 system, a transformative genome-editing technology frequently described as "molecular scissors" due to its capacity to introduce precise modifications in DNA sequences. They demonstrated that an adaptive immune mechanism in bacteria could be reprogrammed to recognize and cleave specific genomic targets. This innovation has fundamentally reshaped molecular biology, enabling unprecedented advances in functional genomics, biomedicine, agriculture, and the potential treatment of a wide range of inherited disorders.

Since January 2013, experimental evidence began to accumulate everywhere that it was possible to edit at will any gene of any genome of any living being, bacterium, yeast, plant or animal, including of course human cells [9]. The groundbreaking proposal made by Charpentier and Doudna to present the bacterial defense system described by Mojica as an extraordinarily versatile system to edit any genetic sequence of any organism had its highest reward with the awarding of the Nobel Prize in Chemistry in October 2020 to the two researchers [10], a well-deserved award, which however chose to forget Francis Mojica, the true discoverer of CRISPR systems and a fundamental element for understanding the subsequent technological evolution of these tools. Francis Mojica was left out of the Nobel Prize and Spain lost what was surely the closest opportunity to achieve the third Nobel Prize for researchers from our country, after the already classic ones of Santiago Ramón y Cajal, Nobel Prize in Physiology or Medicine in 1906 [11] (Chap. 10), shared with Camillo Golgi, and Severo Ochoa de Albornoz, Nobel Prize in Physiology or Medicine in 1959 [12] (Chap. 16), shared with Arthur Kornberg (Fig. 35.3).

We can speculate as to why Mojica was not awarded the Nobel Prize, given that without his initial contributions Charpentier and Doudna would not have been able to propose the use bacterial CRISPR systems as gene editing tools. But more likely (pending the release of the Nobel's Academy, 50 years later, in 2070),

the reason why the committee agreed to award the two researchers, about whom there was already an international consensus, and who had already received numerous previous awards, was that the committee decided to avoid

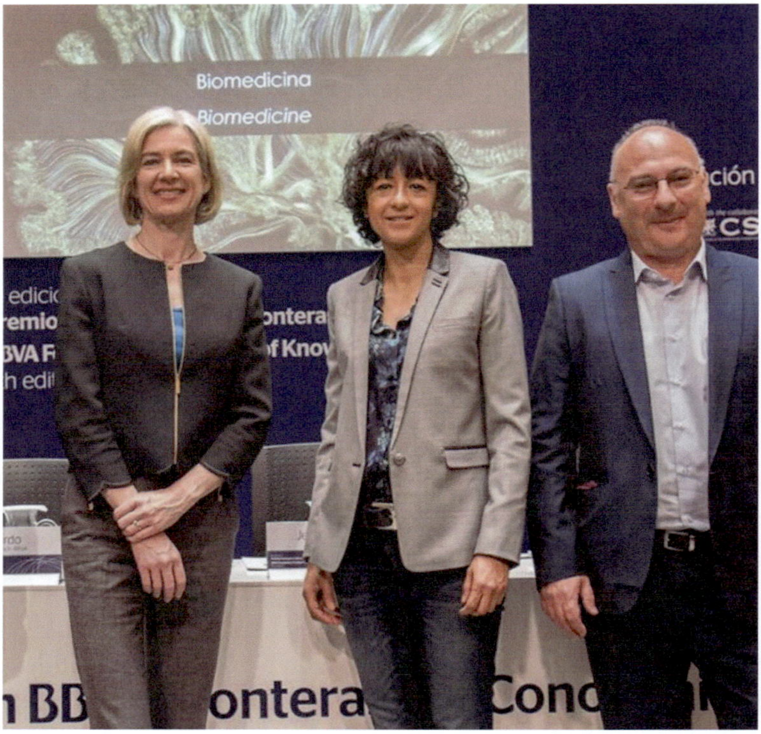

Fig. 35.3 Francis Mojica together with Jennifer Doudna and Emmanuelle Charpentier at the ceremony where the three received the Frontiers of Knowledge Award presented by the Foundation BBVA in 2017 (both were Nobel Prize Chemistry 2020). (Permission of the Foundation BBVA)

singling out a third researcher, given that not only Francis Mojica was proposed for that position but also several other key researchers in the structural and functional description of CRISPR systems, elements that were all indispensable to allow Charpentier and Doudna to carry out their successful experimental study. Surely the committee decided to keep the two awardees and avoid making a mistake by selecting another researcher for the possible third place among the several who had also been proposed, Mojica among them [13]. This is how history is written. However, Francis Mojica did receive numerous other awards, recognitions and distinctions, both nationally and internationally, which underlined and reminded the entire scientific community of the fundamental and primordial role he had played in the pioneering description of CRISPR systems, later transformed into gene editing tools, an application that was never on Mojica's research horizon, but that thanks to his experiments could flourish in the minds of other researchers who drew on Mojica's documentary sources.

Among the most outstanding awards received by Francis Mojica, alone and shared with other researchers, are the Frontiers of Knowledge award from the BBVA Foundation together with Charpentier and Doudna (2017) [14], the Albany Medical Center Prize (2017), the National Genetics Prize (2017), and the National Spanish Prize for Biotechnology 2021.Equally relevant are his contributions that, in the end, have been fundamental so that today all researchers in biology, biomedicine and biotechnology can benefit from using these CRISPR gene-editing tools.

Six Scientific Reasons

There are the six scientific reasons why Francis Mojica [15] deserves to be remembered.

First, for describing for the first time in 1993 the curious repetitions of DNA sequences in the genome of an archaeon, and for deciding to continue doing research on them, unlike his Dutch and Japanese predecessors, who, having described similar sequences in other prokaryotes (Gram+ and Gram-bacteria), did not continue investigating them, as Mojica did.

Secondly, for being the first to launch, in 1995, a first proposal to interpret the function of these repeated sequences by relating them to genome replication [16]. This proposal was not confirmed experimentally, but it is the first recorded attempt to understand what these clusters of small DNA sequences could be used for.

Thirdly, as I have already mentioned, for being the first to invent and propose the term CRISPR in 2001 to refer to these repetitive DNA structures in the genome of prokaryotes. This acronym was picked up in a 2002 publication by another Dutch microbiologist, and it is the first time CRISPR is used in scientific publications.

Fourthly, for being the first to make a first compilation of CRISPR sequences and systems in bacteria and archaea, a systematic review work that he published in 2000 and that surely put him on the track to correctly interpret the function of these CRISPR systems.

In the fifth place, this is Francis Mojica's greatest contribution to the description and understanding the reason of CRISPR systems. In 2005 he finally published after having discovered, in 2003, the raison d'être of these sequence repeats. This is Mojica's essential contribution that allows explaining these CRISPR systems as a true adaptive and genetically based immune defense system, which bacteria and archaea have been using to escape from viral infections.

And sixth and finally, Mojica described a control sequence, adjacent to the sequence complementary to the RNA guide that tells the nuclease where to cut, and which he also named with an acronym that has once again become popular: PAM (Protospacer Adjacent Motif). This sequence, present in the genome of the virus but not in the genome of the bacterium, explains why the bacterium does not self-digest its own genome if it carries target sequences from the viral genome. It is only in the presence of the adjacent PAM sequence, the control sequence, when the nuclease-associated Cas is activated. Mojica first described the PAM sequences in 2009 [17].

For all of the above, Francis Mojica deserves to be remembered as one of the most influential national and international contemporary scientist, whose basic research results led to the description of CRISPR gene editing tools that today are applied in countless situations, both in academic designs and in clinical approaches, including advanced gene therapies. There are many applications derived from the use of CRISPR in biology, biomedicine and biotechnology [18]. It is one of the greatest technological revolutions we have experienced in biology. And this revolution originated in Spain, in Alicante, at the hands of a now universal citizen of Elche: Francisco Juan Martínez Mojica.

References

1. https://cvnet.cpd.ua.es/curriculum-breve/es/martinez-mojica-francisco-juan/9438
2. Mojica FJ, Juez G, Rodríguez-Valera F. Transcription at different salinities of Haloferax mediterranei sequences adjacent to partially modified PstI sites. Mol Microbiol. 1993;9:613–21.
3. Mojica FJ, Díez-Villaseñor C, Soria E, Juez G. Biological significance of a family of regularly spaced repeats in the genomes of Archaea, Bacteria and mitochondria. Mol Microbiol. 2000;36:244–6.
4. Mojica FJM, Montoliu L. On the origin of CRISPR-Cas technology: from prokaryotes to mammals. Trends Microbiol. 2016;24:811–20.
5. Jansen R, Embden JD, Gaastra W, Schouls LM. Identification of genes that are associated with DNA repeats in prokaryotes. Mol Microbiol. 2002;43:1565–75.
6. Mojica FJ, Díez-Villaseñor C, García-Martínez J, Soria E. Intervening sequences of regularly spaced prokaryotic repeats derive from foreign genetic elements. J Mol Evol. 2005;60:174–82.
7. Jinek M, Chylinski K, Fonfara I, Hauer M, Doudna JA, Charpentier E. A programmable dual-RNA-guided DNA endonuclease in adaptive bacterial immunity. Science. 2012;337:816–21.
8. Fernández A, Josa S, Montoliu L. A history of genome editing in mammals. Mamm Genome. 2017;28:237–46.

9. Seruggia D, Montoliu L. The new CRISPR-Cas system: RNA-guided genome engineering to efficiently produce any desired genetic alteration in animals. Transgenic Res. 2014;23:707–16.
10. https://www.nobelprize.org/prizes/chemistry/2020/press-release/
11. https://www.nobelprize.org/prizes/medicine/1906/cajal/biographical/
12. https://www.nobelprize.org/prizes/medicine/1959/ochoa/biographical/
13. https://elpais.com/ciencia/2020-10-07/el-nobel-que-no-fue.html
14. https://www.premiosfronterasdelconocimiento.es/notas-prensa/premio-fronteras-del-conocimiento-biomedicina-charpentier-doudna-mojica-la-revolucion-la-edicion-genetica-2/
15. https://montoliu.naukas.com/2020/10/11/las-seis-razones-por-las-que-merece-ser-recordado-francis-mojica-en-la-historia-de-las-crispr/
16. Mojica FJ, Ferrer C, Juez G, Rodríguez-Valera F. Long stretches of short tandem repeats are present in the largest replicons of the Archaea Haloferax mediterranei and Haloferax volcanii and could be involved in replicon partitioning. Mol Microbiol. 1995;17:85–93.
17. Mojica FJM, Díez-Villaseñor C, García-Martínez J, Almendros C. Short motif sequences determine the targets of the prokaryotic CRISPR defence system. Microbiology (Reading). 2009;155:733–40.
18. "Editando genes: recorta, pega y colorea. Las maravillosas herramientas CRISPR", Lluís Montoliu, Editorial Pinolia, 4ª edición in Spanish, Madrid, 2025. ("Editing genes: cut, paste and color. The wonderful CRISPR tools", Lluís Montoliu, Pinolia (publisher), 4th edition, Madrid, 2025.)

36

Antonio Garcia-Bellido: The Genetic Basis of Development and Morphogenesis

Isabel Adrados Morán and Miguel A. Cuesta

Antonio García-Bellido y García de Diego was born on April 30, 1936, in Madrid, son of the historian and archaeologist Antonio García y Bellido, and grandson (on his mother's side) of the philologist Vicente García de Diego. He is a leading Spanish scientist specializing in developmental biology. His work focuses on research into the genetic basis of development and the morphogenesis (Fig. 36.1).

After obtaining his degree in Biological Sciences from the Complutense University of Madrid in 1958, he received his PhD grade with a thesis entitled "Phenogenetics of the locus furrowed ("fw") of the Drosophila melanogaster", while he was an assistant professor at the Faculty of Biological Sciences in Madrid.

In 1965, he started his work at the Spanish National Research Council (CSIC), initially as a collaborator and in 1970 as a staff scientist. At that time, the CSIC was staffed by leading Spanish scientists such as Alberto Sols, Julio Rodríguez Villanueva, Carlos Villar Palasí and Manuel Losada Villasante.

I. A. Morán
Professor of Anatomy and Embriology, Faculty of Medicine, Complutense University, Madrid, Spain

M. A. Cuesta (✉)
Department of Surgery, Amsterdam University Medical Centre (UMC), Amsterdam, The Netherlands

M. A. Cuesta, F. Mateo Vallejo (eds.), *Spain's Journey in Medicine*,
https://doi.org/10.1007/978-3-032-12221-6_36

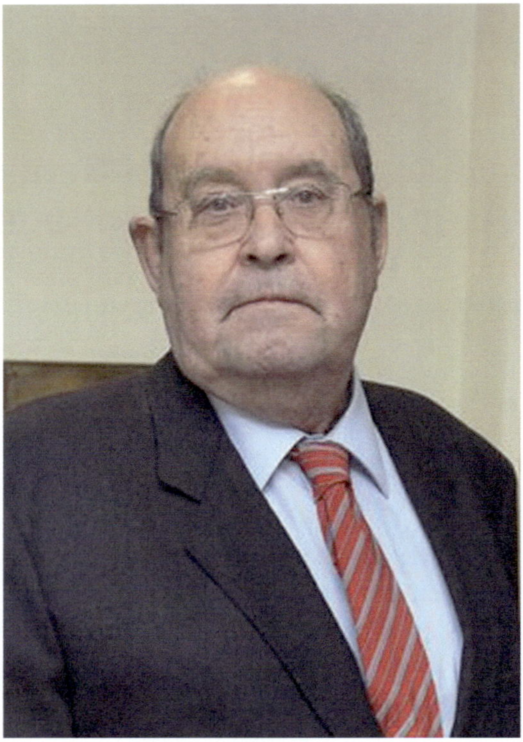

Fig. 36.1 Antonio García-Bellido

Afterwards, he alternated his work at the CSIC with stays in various departments abroad, such as at the University of Cambridge, where he was a fellow in the Department of Experimental Biology with Prof. W.B. Wigglesworth (1959–1960); as a research assistant (Forschung Assistent) at the Zurich Zoological Institute with Prof. E. Hadorn (1962–1965), and as a postdoctoral fellow (Gosney Postdoctoral Fellow) at the California Institute of Technology (CalTech) with Prof. A.H. Sturtevant and Prof. E.B. Lewis (1967–1969).

Upon his return, he was appointed director of the Developmental Genetics Section at the Institute of Biological Research of the CSIC, directing likewise the PhD Course in Developmental Genetics at the Complutense University of Madrid.

Throughout his career, he has been a visiting professor at several international institutions, including the Universities of Copenhagen (1976), Chicago (1977), the Division of Molecular Biology at the University of Sydney (1982),

CalTech in California (1990) and the University of Rome (1977), in many cases taking advantage of his sabbatical years.

He was professor emeritus linked to the CSIC and continued his work at the Centro de Biología Molecular Severo Ochoa in Madrid, of which he was a founding member. The Professor A. Garcia Bellido passed away on 11 November 2025.

His Life Project

From a young age, García-Bellido was torn between two passions: literature and biology. In the end, he chose biology, perhaps driven by the fascination awakened by a book that marked him in his adolescence: What is Life? by Erwin Schrödinger [1]. That book was, perhaps, the seed of his vocation. He always felt the need to explore, to live on the frontier of knowledge. He wanted to experience the thrill of research and the vertigo of big questions.

At the age of twelve, he built his first microscope and convert his home's coal storage into his first laboratory, where he devoted himself to studying cells. "To open the toy to see how it works," he said. Over time, his curiosity led him first to genes and then to morphogenesis.

But, as he acknowledges, there are still many questions to be answered: how a gene turns on a switch for an organ to develop and turn it off when its function is finished? How do organs acquire their shape and position in the body?

García-Bellido has become a reference in the research of developmental genetics and morphogenesis. His work addresses one of the great paradoxes of biology: how, from a single cell—the zygote—containing all the genetic information, specialized cells arise and organize themselves into perfectly differentiated tissues and organs. His work has been key in the advancement of Developmental Molecular Genetics (DMG), based importantly in the study of Drosophila melanogaster.

DMG combines developmental biology and molecular genetics to study how genes control the development of multicellular organisms.

His work is widely recognized and appears in fundamental textbooks such as Monroe W. Strickberger's Genetics and Bruce Alberts' Molecular Biology of the Cell [2, 3]. In addition, several of his articles have been considered "citation classics" by Current Contents and have been praised by numerous scientists in peer reviewed journals and books. Thanks to his tireless curiosity and dedication, García-Bellido has left a profound mark on science, clarifying some of life's most exciting mysteries.

What Are Developmental Genetics?

Developmental genetics studies how genes regulate cell growth and differentiation from the very first cell of the organism. It all starts with fertilization, when the zygote begins a process of segmentation in which it divides repeatedly by mitosis, using its own reserves for nourishment. Over time, this collection of cells undergoes a process called cellular determination, in which each group of cells acquires a specific identity.

At the beginning of development, all cells of the embryo are pluripotent, that is, they have the capacity to become any cell type. However, as the embryo grows and divides, each cell is determined to form a specific type, losing the ability to transform into another. During this process, cell differentiation and morphogenesis give rise to all the tissues and organs that will perform essential functions in the adult organism.

Stages of Embryonic Development

Early embryo development in animals goes through several key phases:

- Fertilization: Occurs when the male and female gametes fuse to form the zygote. This process includes different stages: approximation, oocyte activation, penetration and amphimixis (from the Greek anfi, "on both sides", and mixis, "mixture").
- Segmentation: The zygote undergoes multiple cell divisions by mitosis, giving rise to the morula and, subsequently, the blastula. During this phase, the internal cells will form the embryoblast, which will give rise to the embryo, while the external cells will give rise to the trophoblast, responsible for forming the placenta.
- Morphogenesis or Gastrulation: Cell displacements and differentiation organize the early embryo into three germinative layers: ectoderm, mesoderm and endoderm. These layers will be the basis of all tissues and organs of the body.
- Cell differentiation and Organogenesis: The formation of primary tissues (epithelial, connective, muscular and nervous) and, subsequently, of different organs.

Genetics plays a fundamental role in the regulation of embryonic development, since the activation and deactivation of certain genes guide each of these stages. Therefore, it is crucial to investigate the genetic mechanisms that control this process.

The Leloir Institute in Buenos Aires emphasizes that developmental biology integrates knowledge from various disciplines, such as biochemistry, cell biology, genetics, genomics, molecular biology and evolutionary biology. Its aim is to understand how cells organize and specialize to form functional structures in animals and plants.

This knowledge not only has applications in medicine, such as in the development of therapies based on cell reprogramming and tissue regeneration, but also in agriculture and food processing control of pests, contributing to the advancement of diverse scientific and technological areas.

Drosophila Melanogaster

Since 1909, when Thomas Hunt Morgan introduced it at Columbia University, Drosophila melanogaster (DM), commonly known as the fruit fly, has become the most widely used model for studying the genetic control of development in biomedical science. Its importance is such that in genetic research laboratories it is known as the "queen of genetics". This small fly has been key to countless discoveries, thanks to the wealth of information available on their genes, life cycle and rapid reproduction. The genetic principles derived from its study have proven to be applicable to many other organisms, including plants, animals and even humans (Fig. 36.2).

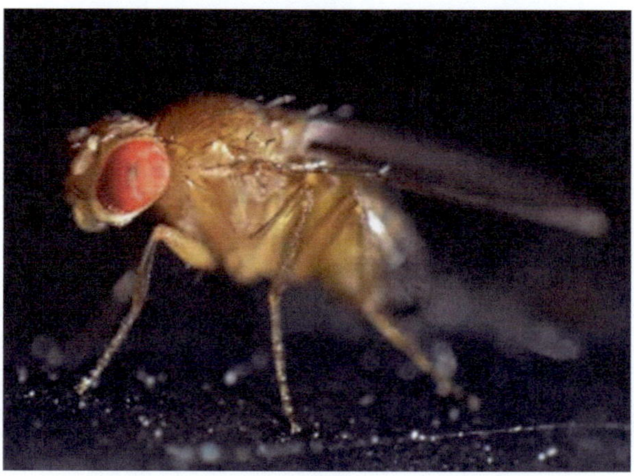

Fig. 36.2 Drosophila melanogaster (male)

For more than a century, its low cost, short reproduction time and the cutting-edge genetic tools that have been developed from their study have made Drosophila an indispensable organism in research. Today, with the incorporation of advanced molecular biology techniques, it continues to be an effective model, used in studies that range from the modeling of human diseases to the research of cell morphogenesis, cell behavior and aging. The body of Drosophila melanogaster is divided into three regions: head, thorax and abdomen. The thorax, in turn, is segmented into three parts, each with a pair of legs. The second thoracic segment includes the wings, while the third houses the halteres, small structures that act as sensory organs and help the fly maintain balance in flight.

The development of this body plan follows a series of welldefined steps. After fertilization, the early embryo goes through three essential phases:

1. The antero-posterior and dorso-ventral axes are established.
2. The orientation and number of segments that will make up the body are determined.
3. A specific genetic identity is assigned to each of these developments.

Questions in Developmental Biology

In 2001, researchers Manfred D. Laubichler and Gunter P. Wagner formulated four fundamental questions in the study of developmental genetics [4]:

- How does an initially homogeneous cell transform into an organism with multiple differentiated cell types?
- What are the mechanisms that organize this three dimensional development?
- What biological factors are responsible for guiding these processes in a casual way?
- How is genetic information related to phenotypic complexity resulting from this development?

Antonio García-Bellido's studies have been key to answering these questions. His innovative and original research methods have made it possible to understand the genetic mechanisms that regulate cell differentiation and organ morphogenesis.

His academic training was guided by some of the most influential scientists in his field. At Cambridge University he worked with V.B. Wigglesworth, in Zurich with Ernst Hadorn, and at the CalTech Institute in Pasadena with A.H. Sturtevant and Edward B. Lewis. Working with them, he acquired the conceptual foundations that would allow him to carry out pioneering studies in physiology, genetics and development, focusing on morphogenesis, the area that would mark his scientific career.

Thanks to his work, we now better understand how organisms evolve from a single cell to complex and specialized structures, a fundamental knowledge not only for biology, but also for medicine and biotechnology.

Work

The work of Antonio García-Bellido has pioneered the study of an epigenetic conception of development.

> Epigenetics studies the changes that activate or deactivate genes without altering the underlying DNA sequence, influenced by environmental factors and growth conditions.

His research career, always using the DM, started with studies on the genetic basis of cell recognition (1965–1969), based on the analysis of imaginal discs [5–7].

> Imaginal discs are epithelial structures, sac-like, that contains undifferentiated cells programmed to develop into specific adult body, such as eyes, legs and wings.

Between 1968 and 1973, he addressed the determination of genetic mosaic discs and the elaboration of blastodermal maps, followed by the clonal analysis of developing systems.

> Genetic mosaics in embryos are imaginal discs composed of cells with distinct genetic identities.
>
> Blastodermic maps are schematic representations of the blastoderm that indicate the speculative positions of future tissues, organs, and body structures.
>
> Clonal analysis is a technique used to trace the descendants of a single progenitor cell, providing insight into cell lineage and differentiation patterns.
>
> Cell lineage refers to the developmental trajectory of a cell, documenting its progression from a single progenitor to its final specialized cell type.

Based on these preliminary studies his most relevant finding was the discovery of the development of compartments, published in Nature New Biology in 1973, which earned him a Nobel Prize nomination in 1979.

Compartments are defined regions in an embryo that consist of cells sharing a common lineage and are separated by genetically determined boundaries. These boundaries prevent cell mixing between compartments and guide the spatial organization and patterning of a developing organ [8].

This breakthrough, it has been considered fundamental by Nobel laureates Francis Crick (discoverer of the structure of DNA) and Peter Lawrence (Prince of Asturias Award, 2007), and have laid the foundations of the Compartment Theory, key to understanding the morphogenesis.

In 1981, he formulated the theory of selector genes (Hox genes):

They are master regulatory genes that specify the identity and developmental fate of body segments along the anterior–posterior axis.

From 1984, he studied cellular interactions in morphogenesis, and, from 1989, he investigated the venation patterns and the control of cell proliferation (venation patterns refer to the arrangement of veins in a wing, which vary significantly between different species) [9–11].

Based on his research, García-Bellido has proposed several embryological models:

1. Compartment theory (1973): the organisms are organized in cellular compartments, regions where cells share a genetic identity and do not mix with those of other compartments. This explained how specific structures form in embryonic development and laid the foundation for understanding body segmentation in insects and other organisms.
2. Syntagm model: Proposes that genes are organized into functional modules called syntagms, which work together to define specific structures. This model helped to understand how different genes interact in development and allow cells to respond precisely to internal and external signals.
3. Entelechy model: It is a synthesis of the previous ones, integrating genetics and epigenetics in development. It suggests that the formation of an organism is a dynamic process in which compartments and syntagms interact with the cellular environment, ensuring that each structure develops in a coordinated and precise manner.

And based on these concepts, his main interest has been to formulate an unitary scientific explanation of morphogenesis, the biological process by which an initial cell, the zygote, develops into a complete organism.

> "When an embryo starts to grow and reaches the stage called morphogenesis or gastrulation, two big questions appear: where do the different organs come

from, and how are they arranged in the body? To answer these, the study of compartmentalization has been very important. This research combines two main genetic moments: some genes, through protein complex, organize cells into mosaics and then into compartments, and other genes set the boundaries that separate these compartments. After that, selector genes decide how the organs (ic. the wings) are arranged in space."

As he explained in an interview with the newspaper El País in 2006, on the occasion of his retirement:

> "We discovered that organisms are built in a modular way. They are independent modules (a group of protein complexes that perform a specific task), with borders that delimit them, that originate the organs, but that must communicate with each other."

This discovery arose from the study of the wing structure of Drosophila melanogaster, in collaboration with Ginés Morata and Pedro Ripoll.

> "The modular construction system is extensible to all of biology. It allowed us to understand that there are genes that define space, something unthinkable in the early 1970s. In the laboratory of the CSIC Biological Research Center, we identified genes that distinguished 'anterior' from 'posterior' and 'dorsal' from 'ventral'. In other words, space is genetically defined" [12, 13]

This knowledge has been key to understanding the role of different genes in the specification of embryonic territories of the DM:

- In the head-tail axis, with the segmentation of the body.
- In the dorso-ventral axis, with tissue differentiation.
- In the formation of appendages such as legs and wings.

The genes that determine these spatial differences have been conserved throughout evolution and are transferable between species as diverse as flies and humans, whose common ancestors date back 600 million years.

He has also been president of the European Organization of Developmental Biology.

In recognition of his work, he received the Principe of Asturias Award for Technical and Scientific Research in 1984 and the Ramón y Cajal National Research Award in 1995 (Fig. 36.3).

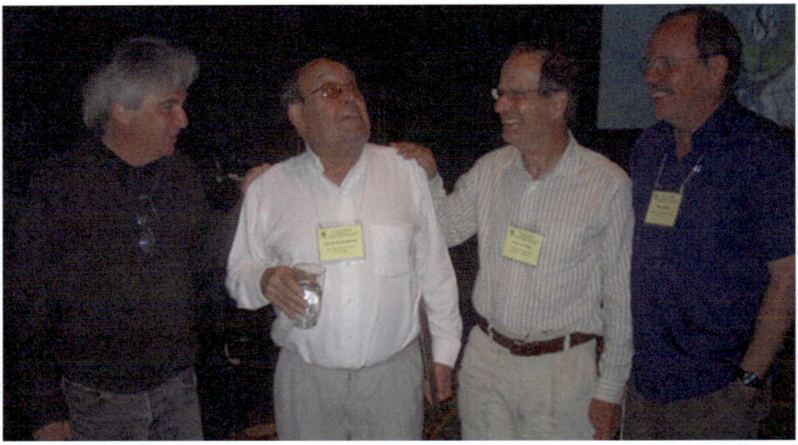

Fig. 36.3 Awarding of the SDB Prize in recognition of his entire career, 71st meeting Montreal, Canada. From left to right: Mike Levine, Garcia Bellido, Peter Lawrence and William McGinnis. (Permission of the SDB)

Interview with David Gubb

David Gubb's interviewed Antonio García-Bellido (published in the journal CIC Network (3, 2008) on the issue: "Scientists are going to have a great time in the next 100 years". Here, they discussed in depth about his career and scientific contributions in the field of developmental biology. Throughout the conversation, GarcíaBellido shares his views on genetics, embryonic development and evolution, and how his research has revolutionized our understanding of these processes.

He says that from his early formative years, he was greatly influenced by scientists such as Hadorn, Sturtevant and Lewis, who marked his interest in genetics and the study of Drosophila melanogaster. This fly became his key experimental model for understanding the mechanisms of development, a field that at its inception was at a very early stage in terms of molecular biology.

This fascination with the fundamental processes of life led him to develop innovative ideas and approaches that changed the course of research in biology.

One of the most significant contributions of García-Bellido was the concept of cellular compartments, which emerged from his work with genetic mosaics. This concept transformed the way scientists understood the organization of embryonic development. García-Bellido showed that multicellular organisms are not simply a jumble of undifferentiated cells but are organized into specific areas or compartments where cells follow specific genetic instructions. This revelation was crucial for understanding how tissues develop in an orderly fashion and how cells from different parts of the organism maintain their identity, without mixing with each other, which also advanced the understanding of diseases such as cancer and development defects.

In the interview, García-Bellido also delves into the relationship between evolution and development. Throughout his career, he was able to observe that the genes responsible for regulating the development of organisms are not only crucial for each species, but that they remain surprisingly conserved throughout evolution. Key genes in species such as Drosophila have homologues in mammals, which made it possible to connect the study of development with evolutionary processes. This approach helped to change the traditional view of evolution as a random process, to show that, in reality, evolution works from already existing genetic modules, modifying and reusing them in different contexts to form new structures.

Another important aspect discussed is the role of homeotic genes, those that regulate the formation of body structures throughout development. García-Bellido explains how the study of these genes helped to understand how organisms generate specific body patterns and how alterations in these genes can lead to mutations that generate evolutionary changes or malformations in organisms.

Beyond the technical aspects, García-Bellido devotes an important part of the interview to reflect on the future of biology and the role of basic research. In this regard, he stresses the importance of funding fundamental research without the pressures of immediate applications or commercial results. His defense of independent science emphasizes that true innovation in biology comes from studies that initially may not have clear practical applications, but in the long term open up new possibilities for medicine, biotechnology and other fields. In conclusion, the interview with Antonio García-Bellido provides a comprehensive overview of his thinking and discoveries, which have left an indelible mark on developmental genetics and evolutionary biology.

References

1. Schrödinger E. What is life? Wat ist Leben? 1944.
2. Genetics. Monroe W. Strickberger.
3. Alberts B. Molecular biology of the cell.
4. Laubichler MD, Wagner GP. How molecular is molecular developmental biology? A reply to Alex Rosenberg's reductionism Redux: computing the embryo. Biol Philos. 2001;16:57–8.

5. García-Bellido A. Pattern reconstruction by dissociated Imaginal Disk cells of Drosophila melanogaster. Dev Biol. 1966;14:278–306. (First indication of cell specificity and recognition properties of individual Cells. New perspective on development: from the cell to the cellular ensemble).
6. García-Bellido A, Merriam JR. Cell lineage of the Imaginal Discs in Drosophila Gynandromorphs. J Exp Zool. 1969;170:61–76. (Classic blastoderm fate mapping. Paves the way for identification of Genetic hotspots of action).
7. García-Bellido A, Merriam JR. Parameters of the wing imaginal disc development of Drosophila melanogaster. Dev Biol. 1971;24:61–87. (First description of the clonal development of a imaginal disc).
8. García-Bellido A, Ripoll P, Morata G. Developmental compartmentalization of the wing disk of Drosophila. Nat New Biol. 1973;245:251–3. (Discovery of the compartments in the wing of the DM).
9. Botas J, Moscoso del Prado J, García-Bellido A. Gene-dose titration analysis in the search of trans- regulatory genes in Drosophila. EMBO J. 1982;1:307–10. (Search of regulatory genes).
10. Gubb D, Garcia Bellido A. A genetic analysis of the determination of cuticular polarity during development in Drosophila melanogaster. J Embryol Exp Morphol. 1982;68:37–57.
11. García-Bellido A, de Celis JF. Developmental genetics of the venation pattern of Drosophila. Annu Rev Genet. 1992;26:275–302. (Definition of the genetic parameters of wing morphogenesis).
12. Baena-López LA, Baonza A, García-Bellido A. The orientation of cell divisions determines the shape of Drosophila organs. Curr Biol. 2005;15:1640–4. (Description of the role of the orientation of cell division in defining the shape of an organ).
13. Baena-López LA, García-Bellido A. Control of growth and positional information by the graded vestigial expression pattern in the wing of Drosophila melanogaster. PNAS. 2006;103:13734–9. (Description of the function of the Vestigial gen in the growth control during the development).

37

Minimally Invasive Surgery (MIS) in Spain and Its Diffusion to the World

Miguel A. Cuesta

Endoscopic or minimally invasive surgery is defined as the set of surgical procedures that, unlike conventional techniques, avoid the classic access through large incisions in the abdominal or thoracic wall. Instead, trocars are inserted through small incisions, allowing the introduction of a visualization system and the necessary surgical instruments. This technique, also known as laparoscopic surgery, was conceived and introduced in Germany in 1985 by Dr. Erich Muhe and in France in 1989 by Dr. Philippe Mouret.

Laparos in old Greek is abdomen and scopy to see or observe

However, its antecedents go back several decades. In 1901, George Kelling first introduced an endoscope into the abdominal cavity of a dog, calling this technique laparoscopy. Even before this milestone, experiments had already been conducted to visualize organic cavities that communicate with the exterior, such as the bladder, the uterus and the larynx, by means of complex systems of mirrors and illumination (see Chap. 7). The need to insufflate gas into the abdominal cavity for exploratory purposes was also described by Kelling, although its original purpose was neither diagnostic nor therapeutic,

M. A. Cuesta (✉)
Department of Surgery, Amsterdam University Medical Centre (Amsterdam UMC), Amsterdam, The Netherlands

M. A. Cuesta, F. Mateo Vallejo (eds.), *Spain's Journey in Medicine*,
https://doi.org/10.1007/978-3-032-12221-6_37

but to stop intra-abdominal bleeding by hyperpressure. One of the main challenges faced by the pioneers of this technique was the risk associated with the blind introduction of needles or trocars into the abdominal cavity. In response to this limitation, Otto Goetze designed a needle in 1918 that allowed pneumoperitoneum to be performed more safely. Subsequently, Janos Veress perfected this design by incorporating a spring mechanism that automatically retracted the puncture tip into a sheath after passing through the abdominal wall. It should be noted that Veress' original purpose was to perform therapeutic pneumothorax in tuberculosis patients. In 1929, the German gastroenterologist Heinz Kalk developed an optical system with 135-degree lenses and pioneered the laparoscopic approach by using two trocars: one for the laparoscope and the other for inserting instruments. His studies were mainly focused on liver and biliary tract pathologies. In turn, in 1934, internist J. C. Ruddock designed a grasper with integrated electrocoagulation capability, which constituted a fundamental advance in control of bleeding during minimally invasive procedures. During World War II, important technical advances were made in aspects such as intra-abdominal pressure, optical quality and light sources. In 1952, N. Fourestier built a laparoscope with a quartz rod capable of conducting cold light from an external source into the peritoneal cavity, which significantly improved visibility without causing an increase in temperature. A year later, in 1953, the British Harold Hopkins revolutionized endoscopic imaging by introducing the rod lens system, which offered sharper, brighter images with greater chromatic fidelity. However, the real transformation of laparoscopy took place in the mid-1960s with the contributions of Kurt Semm, who developed new techniques and instruments that made it possible to perform the first surgical interventions on the adnexa [1, 2]. His main objective was to reduce the surgical trauma, avoiding laparotomic incisions and the numerous complications they entail. Over time, laparoscopy has spread to multiple medical specialties, such as thoracoscopy and arthroscopy, profoundly revolutionizing all surgical approaches. Unlike traditional open surgery, this minimally invasive techniques minimize blood loss, respects the anatomical planes and favors a faster, less painful recovery with better cosmetic results for the patient. Cholecystectomy for cholelithiasis represented a turning point in the evolution of minimally invasive surgery. In the late 1980s, open cholecystectomy was considered an intervention with a disproportionate level of trauma for the treatment of a benign pathology, the gallstones. The pathophysiologic consequences, postoperative pain, prolonged hospitalization—ranging from seven to ten days—as well as the esthetic impact of the surgical wound, and complications like abdominal wall hernia, whether through a subcostal or median incision, motivated the search for less invasive alternatives. This concern was especially relevant in relatively young patients, mostly women around 40 years of age, frequently with a certain degree of obesity. Before the rise of laparoscopy, other therapeutic alternatives were explored, such as stone's dissolution by percutaneous injection of solvent substances followed by aspiration, and lithotripsy -inspired in the treatment of ureteral lithiasis. However, the results obtained were unsatisfactory, which led to the abandonment of both techniques. In parallel, minimally invasive surgery began, in the eighties, to consolidate in Europe, particularly in Germany and France. In this context, two pioneers faced the challenge of cholecystectomy with different but complementary approaches. In Germany, Erich Mühe introduced a wide tube into the right hypochondrium to remove the gallbladder, with the aim of minimizing the surgical wound, in line with Germanic surgical tradition [3]. For his part, the French surgeon Philippe Mouret, in Lyon—considered the true pioneer of this technique—used his extensive experience in gynecological laparoscopy to approach cholelithiasis in an innovative way. During a gynecological laparoscopic intervention on a patient who also had gallstones, Mouret directed the laparoscope into the right hypochondrium after resolving the pelvic pathology and managed to perform the cholecystectomy by the same route, avoiding the open surgery that had initially been planned [4]. This event marked the true beginning of the laparoscopic revolution. The enthusiasm was quickly shared by French surgeons such as Jacques Dubois and François Perissat, who played a key role in the development of laparoscopic surgery.

International Expansion

In 1992, François Perissat organized in Bordeaux the first congress of the European Association for Endoscopic Surgery (EAES), which was well attended consolidating the recognition of laparoscopy as the new surgical paradigm.

Introduction in Spain

When the news reached Spain that Mouret, Dubois and Perissat had successfully performed the first cholecystectomies by laparoscopy, showing notable advantages for the patients, numerous Spanish surgeons came to their centers in France with the purpose of learning these innovative techniques. On December 14, 1989, Enric Laporte performed the first laparoscopic cholecystectomy in

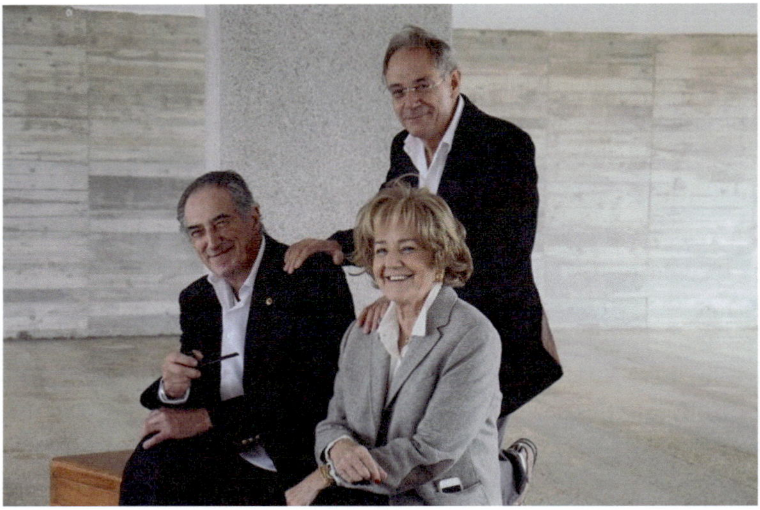

Fig. 37.1 Pioneers of Minimally Invasive Surgery in Spain: Enric Laporte, Elizabeth Vincent and Salvador Pascual. (Permission Enric Laporte)

Spain, at the Hospital H. Adria-CS Vall d'Hebron in Barcelona. The next step was to invite these French experts to national and regional congresses held in Spain, where they shared their experiences, offered specialized training and performed laparoscopic interventions for different pathologies. An outstanding example was the participation of Philippe Mouret and Namir Katkhouda at the Hospital La Fe in Valencia in November 1991 (Figs. 37.1 and 37.2).

Once the success of laparoscopic cholecystectomy was confirmed -despite the important complication represented by a high rate of common bile duct injuries, close to 1%-, the development of techniques for the safe approach to the Calot's triangle like the critical view of safety, CVS, introduced by Strasberg et al. significantly reduced this major complication, making the laparoscopic approach more and more widespread [5]. This advance allowed a rapid expansion of the laparoscopic approach, initially in benign surgical pathologies such as appendicitis, acute abdomen, hernias, abdominal wall corrections, esophageal hiatus procedures and Nissen fundoplication. The next great challenge was to apply the minimally invasive approach to colon and rectal cancer surgery. The first laparoscopic procedure for colon cancer in Spain was performed in Valencia, in the Department of Surgery (David Rodero) of the Hospital La Fe, by Miguel A. Cuesta, during the above mentioned surgical course held in November 1991. Since then, the use of these techniques—both for benign digestive surgery and for the treatment of colorectal cancer—began to spread progressively in specialized centers in

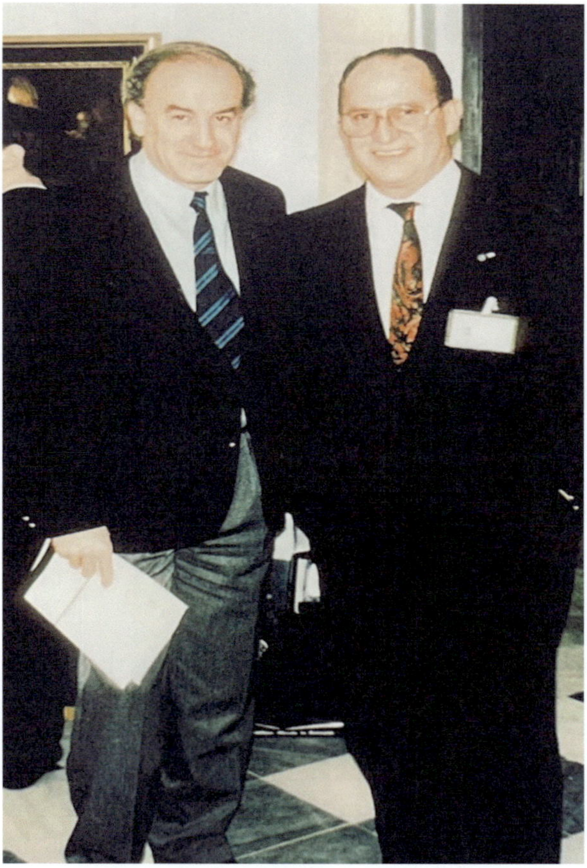

Fig. 37.2 1993. Philippe Mouret and Miguel A. Cuesta in a meeting in Puerto de Santa María (Cadiz)

various cities, such as Barcelona, Madrid, Valencia, Cádiz, Castellón, Seville, Santiago de Compostela, among others. Little by little, and thanks to pioneering courses such as that of Salvador Pascual in El Puerto de Santa María, David Rodero at the Hospital La Fe in Valencia, and Salvador Morales Méndez at the Hospital Virgen del Rocío in Seville, as well as others specifically focused on colorectal surgery -such as the one organized at the Hospital de Bellvitge in Barcelona, under the direction of Joan Martí Ragué, and the one held since 1994 in Baiona by Enrique Casal- laparoscopic colorectal surgery began to consolidate throughout Spain. This minimally invasive approach was soon also applied to bariatric surgery, in the treatment of morbid obesity, as well as to gastric oncological surgery and liver surgery, thanks to the pioneering work of Santiago Azagra. In this context, the

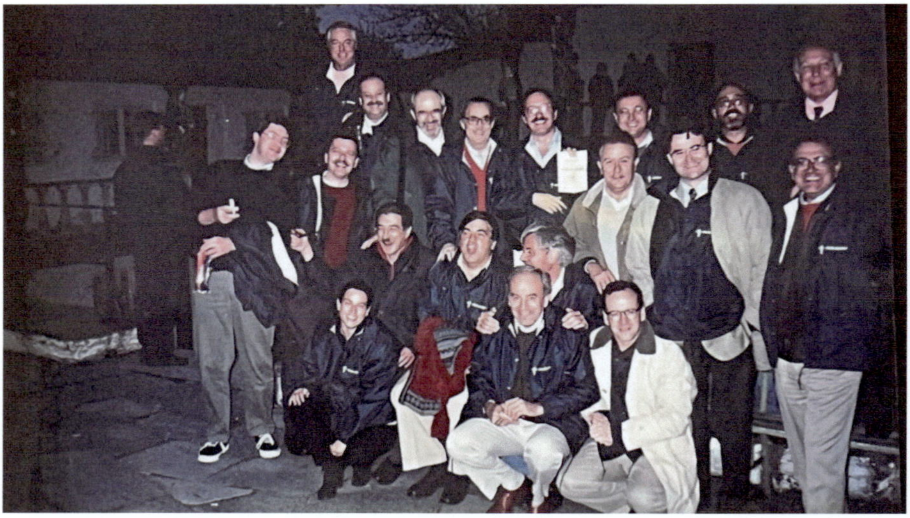

Fig. 37.3 1996. A Group of Spanish Surgeons during the EAES Congress in Trondheim, Norway

Spanish Association of Surgeons (AEC) created the section of Cirugía Minimamente Invasiva (CMI) Minimally Invasive Surgery Section (MIS), which since then has developed an intense work, organizing its own sessions at national congresses and consolidating itself as a reference in the field. Centers such as the Hospital Clínic in Barcelona, with Antonio de Lacy; the Hospital de Sant Pau, with Eduardo Targarona; the Hospital Virgen del Rocío in Seville, with Salvador Morales Méndez, among others, not only brought this discipline to an internationally recognized level of excellence, but also promoted unparalleled teaching work, attracting the attention and recognition of specialists from other countries (Figs. 37.3 and 37.4).

The remarkable international projection of Spanish minimally invasive surgery (MIS) has been possible thanks to several decisive factors:

- The organization of highly prestigious, courses in which live surgical procedures are performed and transmitted to the outside world.
- Training of young surgeons and residents from Europe and Latin America through stays in Spanish hospitals.
- The outstanding participation of Spanish surgeons in leading international congresses, such as those organized by the European Association for Endoscopic Surgery (EAES) and the Society of American Gastrointestinal and Endoscopic Surgeons (SAGES) in the United States.
- The performance of highly relevant clinical studies, such as the randomized study in Barcelona, led by Antonio de Lacy, which compared the open and

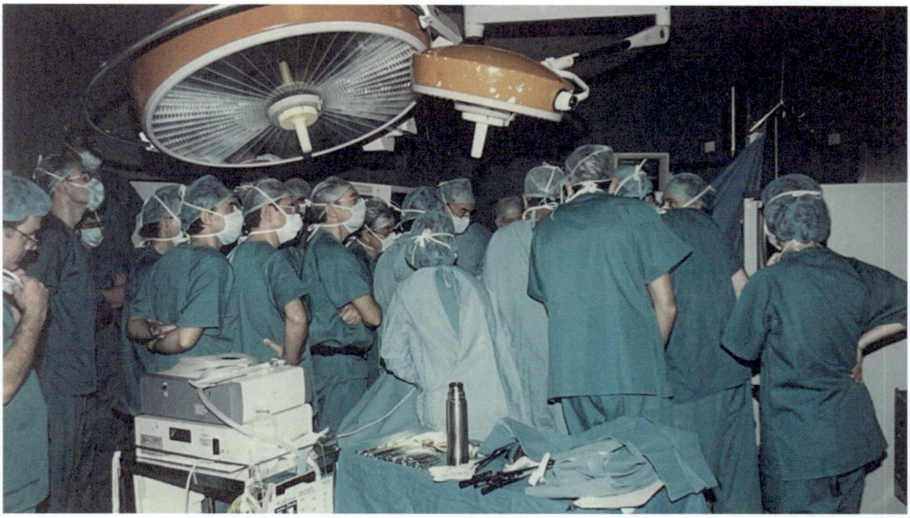

Fig. 37.4 A MIS intervention in the late 1990s with many participants around the surgeons (Miguel A. Cuesta)

the laparoscopic approach in the treatment of colon cancer, and which had a significant impact worldwide [6].

- The presidency of the EAES was held by three Spanish surgeons: Antonio de Lacy (2007-2009), Eduardo Targarona (2015–17) and Salvador Morales Conde (2021–23).

In 1994, Elizabeth Vincent organized the second international congress of the European Association for Endoscopic Surgery (EAES) in Madrid, an event that marked a milestone in the international projection of Spanish laparoscopic surgery. Years later, in 2004, Barcelona hosted the 12th EAES congress, under the presidency of Antonio de Lacy, and in 2019, the 27th EAES congress hosted in Seville with Salvador Morales Conde as president, These congresses definitively consolidate Spain as a reference in this discipline.

Courses and Congresses

Currently, two major training courses on minimally invasive surgery stand out on the national scene: the one organized in Seville by Salvador Morales Conde and the one in Valladolid, coordinated by Miguel Toledano and David Pacheco (Fig. 37.5).

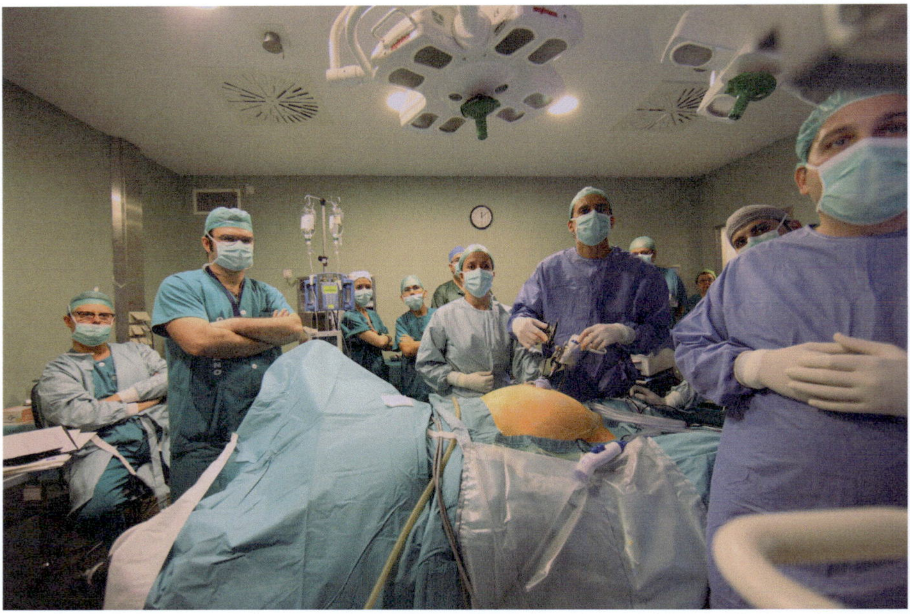

Fig. 37.5 Salvador Morales Conde performing a Live Surgery during one of the latest courses in Seville

These courses are considered the most complete nationally and are among the best in the world. They combine advanced theoretical training in MIS with live surgery, and in recent years have incorporated robotic-assisted surgery (RAMIS), which further enhances their prestige and technical level.

Studies and Scientific Evidence

In the search for solid scientific evidence, Antonio de Lacy has been a pioneer in publishing the renowned Barcelona Study, the first randomized clinical trial comparing open surgery with the laparoscopic approach in the treatment of colon cancer. Published in The Lancet in 2002, this work demonstrated the clear advantages of laparoscopy and had a decisive international impact on the global expansion of this technique. Eduardo Targarona also made a significant contribution through a randomized study that evaluated the hand-assisted versus laparoscopic approach in the treatment of colon cancer and organized the first Guideline for MIS in Spain in 2010 [7] Subsequently, several Spanish surgeons actively participated in international clinical trials of great relevance, such as the COLOR I, II and III studies, which compare the open and laparoscopic approaches in colon and rectal cancer [8, 9]. Likewise, other Spanish specialists, dedicated to esophagogastric surgery, have played a fundamental

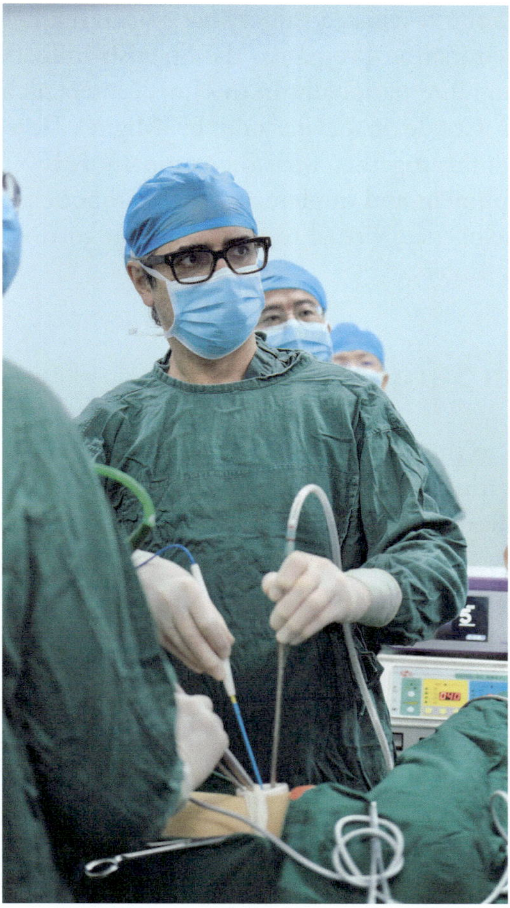

Fig. 37.6 Diego González Rivas performing a Pulmonary resection by a thoracoscopic assisted single port. (Permission Foundation Gonzalez Rivas, La Coruña)

role in international clinical trials, such as the TIME study (in esophageal cancer, [10]) and the STOMACH study (in total gastrectomy for gastric cancer, [11]), both focused on the comparison between open surgery and the laparoscopic approach. At present, different Spanish groups are working -or have worked- with the aim of further reducing surgical trauma, through techniques such as NOTES (minimally invasive surgery through natural orifices) and single-port approach. In the latter field, Diego González Rivas, a world pioneer in the performance of lung surgery for lung cancer by means of a single port, stands out. Currently, his work using the robot is considered outstanding. He has extended these techniques all over the world and his authority and influence is huge [12] (Fig. 37.6).

More recently, robotic-assisted surgery has gained relevance, and thanks to training and dissemination programs, the Spanish influence of MIS group continues to expand internationally. In this line, centers such as the one led by Salvador Morales Conde in Seville and by Miguel. Toledano and David Pacheco in Valladolid, together with the company ABEX, are actively promoting the development and implementation of robotic platforms that integrate artificial intelligence, virtual reality and other cuttingedge technologies in this new era of surgery.

Four Spanish Surgeons Abroad

The contribution to the development of minimally invasive surgery in Spain and worldwide of four Spanish surgeons working abroad should also be highlighted. Their dedication to teach and then to contribute knowledge, through courses and congresses, often performing live surgery, has had an important influence.

These specialists have not only represented with excellence the countries in which they work, but have also spread the spirit, technical competence and pride of Spanish surgery throughout the world. Many of them have frequently traveled to international centers to teach advanced surgical techniques, thus contributing to the creation of a true school of training with global influence.

Juan Santiago Azagra Soria (Fig. 37.7)

Born in Cascante, Navarra, on July 24, 1955, he attended high school at the San Francisco Javier Jesuit school in Tudela (Navarra). Subsequently, he emigrated to Belgium for political and socioeconomic reasons, where he began his medical studies at the Free University of Brussels, obtaining his degree with Grand Distinction. He specialized in General Surgery, acquiring a comprehensive training as a surgeon in all areas of the discipline. He developed his professional career mainly in Brussels, at the Brugmann Academic Hospital, under the tutelage of renowned surgeons, including Louis Clerckx, head of the Department of General Surgery at the Hospital de La Hestre. Later, he continued his work at the CHU de Tivoli, in La Louvière, where he decided to focus his career on Digestive Surgery. In 1986, he became head of the Department of Digestive, Oncological and Minimally Invasive Surgery at the André Vésale University Hospital in Charleroi, where he also served as a teaching professor. In 2003, moved to Luxembourg with his wife, surgeon Martine

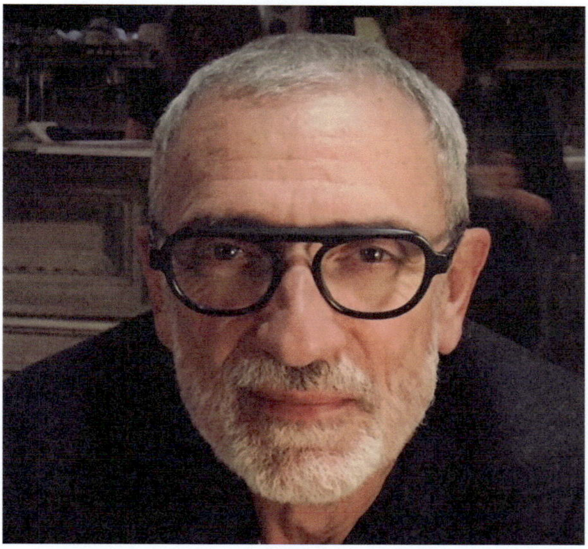

Fig. 37.7 Juan Santiago Azagra Soria

Goergen, to become head of the Department of Visceral, Vascular and Thoracic Surgery and of the UMADE (Multidisciplinary Unit of Digestive and Endocrine Diseases) at the Centre Hospitalier de Luxembourg. Currently, he is mainly involved in abdominal robotic surgery. Dr. Azagra is internationally recognized as an innovative surgeon, having pioneered procedures such as laparoscopic liver surgery and total gastrectomy for gastric cancer [13, 14]. He is a founding member of several scientific surgical societies, honorary member of numerous national and international associations, and honorary consultant to universities and hospitals in different countries. He devotes much of his time to the conceptualization and improvement of minimally invasive surgical approaches, using laparoscopy and robotic surgery techniques. He considers teaching surgery to be his "true vocation". In addition to his medical career, he is passionate about music—especially rock, including metal and blues—plays electric guitar, and enjoys traveling and sports.

Julio García Aguilar (Fig. 37.8)

He is currently Chief of the Colorectal Surgery Department at Memorial Sloan Kettering Cancer Center in New York, holding the Bennot C. Schmidt Chair in Oncologic Surgery and is Professor of Surgery at Weill Cornell Medical College. He studied Medicine at the Faculty of Medicine of the

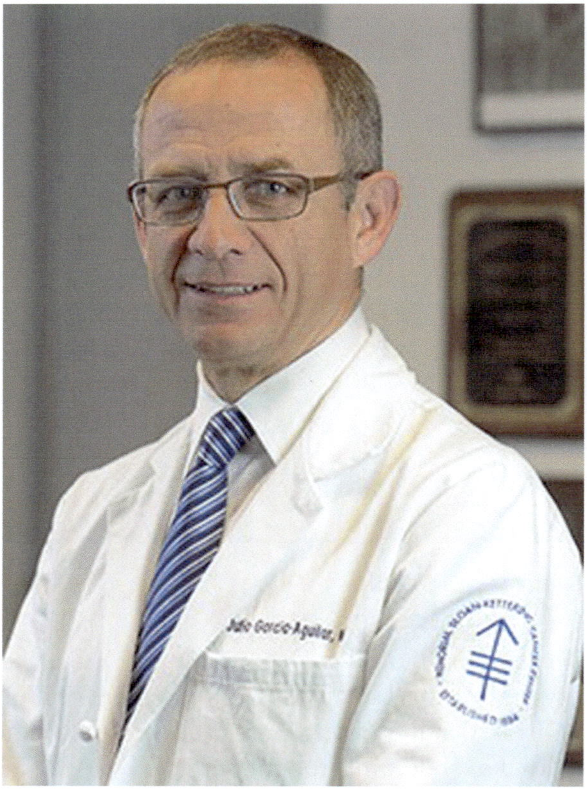

Fig. 37.8 Julio García Aguilar

Universidad Complutense of Madrid, where he also completed his residency in General Surgery at the Hospital Clínico San Carlos. Subsequently, he completed his training in General Surgery under the tutorship of Dr. William Silen at Beth Israel Deaconess Medical Center, Boston, being specialized in colorectal surgery at the University of Minnesota. After a period of practice in Madrid, he returned to the United States in 1996, again joining the University of Minnesota, this time under the mentorship of Dr. David Rothenberger. After 6 years, he was appointed Chief of the Colorectal Surgery Department at the University of California, San Francisco Medical Center, and later became Chief of the Department of Surgery at the City of Hope Medical Center in Duarte, California. In 2012, after a decade at that institution, he moved to New York, where he was appointed Director of the Colorectal Surgery Dpt. at Memorial Sloan Kettering. Dr. García-Aguilar has stood out for his pioneering work in surgical innovation and for his committed teaching work with surgical residents, fellows in colorectal surgery and numerous international visitors who have collaborated with him. He has an inquisitive mind, unconventional, constantly questioning established practices and seeking answers to complex questions through clinical research and translational basic science. He is recognized worldwide as an expert in the treatment of rectal cancer, which is reflected in his authorship of more than a hundred scientific publications and in the frequent invitations he receives to give international conferences [15]. He is married and father of two children. His hobbies include reading, cycling in groups and visiting his hometown, Escalona in the province of Toledo, where his parents and lifelong friends live.

Miguel Ángel Cuesta (Fig. 37.9)

Miguel A. Cuesta is currently Professor Emeritus of General and Gastrointestinal Surgery at the Amsterdam University Medical Center (Amsterdam UMC), The Netherlands, where he has developed the minimally invasive oncological surgery of the digestive tract. Born in Guadalajara on January 17, 1947, he studied Medicine at the University of Navarra (Pamplona) and completed his residency in Surgery at the VUmc (University Hospital of the Vrije Universiteit of Amsterdam), with Prof. Dr. G. den Otter. After almost a decade of professional practice as a general and digestive surgeon at the Residencia Virgen de la Salud in Toledo, he returned to the VUmc in Amsterdam, where he oriented his career towards academic surgery and

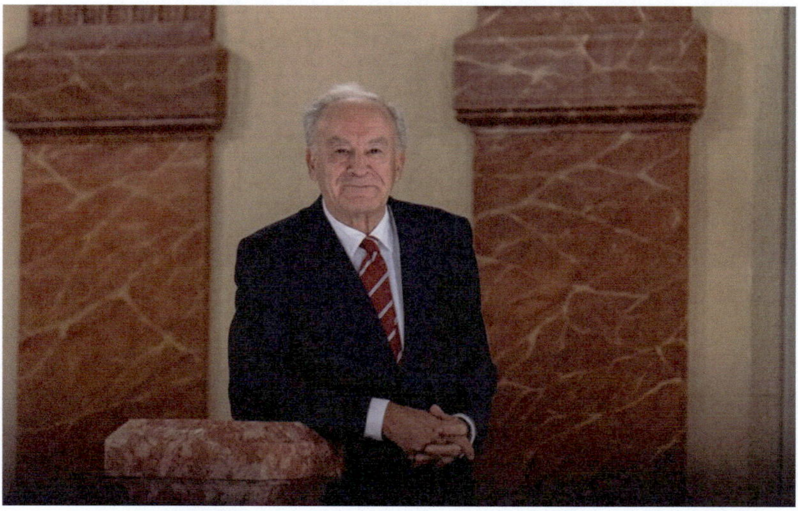

Fig. 37.9 Miguel A. Cuesta

technological innovation. His research work has focused on the development and implementation of Surgical Oncology of the Digestive Tract in minimally invasive (MI) laparoscopic techniques. With a rigorous approach based on scientific evidence, he has participated as Principal Investigator and collaborator in ten randomized clinical trials, in which minimally invasive techniques have been compared with conventional ones. These studies have also explored the impact of neoadjuvant treatments (chemotherapy or radiotherapy prior to surgery) in combination with MI surgery, particularly in cases of esophageal and gastric cancer. The results have consistently demonstrated the advantages of minimally invasive surgery on the short term in the surgical approach of digestive cancer with at the long term similar oncological outcome. Miguel Cuesta has carried out intense international teaching work, providing training and performing live surgery in countries such as India, Brazil and several European countries, focusing on the treatment of esophageal, gastric and colorectal cancer. He is the author of more than 360 scientific publications indexed in PubMed (under the name cuesta ma) and has served as editor-in-chief of five books specialized in minimally invasive surgery of the Gastrointestinal Cancer (among them the first book, in 1993, on Minimally Invasive Surgery in Gastrointestinal Cancer, [16]) in addition to a work dedicated to the treatment of surgical complications. He is currently married to Carmen Padules González. Among his many national and international distinctions, the appointment as Knight of Honor (Ridder in de Orde van de Nederlandse Leeuw) by the King of the Netherlands, Willem-Alexander, in 2018 stands out. In November 2021, he received in Barcelona the Career Achievement Award of the European Society for Minimally Invasive Surgery (EAES).

Alberto Martínez Isla (Fig. 37.10)

Alberto Martínez Isla was born in La Coruña on October 14, 1959. He studied Medicine at the Faculty of Santiago de Compostela and later obtained his doctorate in Surgery at the Universidad of Salamanca. He completed his specialization in Digestive Surgery at the Hospital Puerta de Hierro in Madrid. In 1995 he moved to the Hammersmith Hospital in London as Senior Registrar under the supervision of Professor Robin C.N. Williamson. In 1998 he was appointed Consultant Surgeon at the London Northwest Healthcare NHS Trust and is currently working at St. Mark's Hospital. His field of specialization focuses on laparoscopic biliary tract and esophageal hiatus surgery. He has made an important contribution in the field of laparoscopic biliary

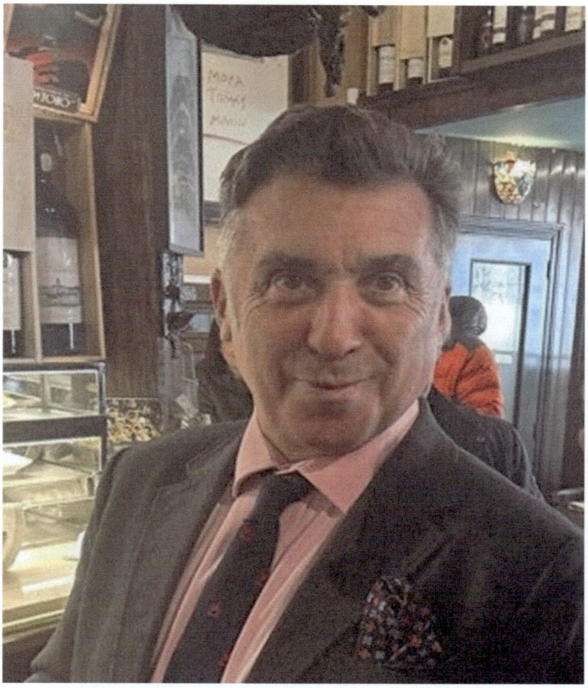

Fig. 37.10 Alberto Martínez Isla

surgery, being a pioneer worldwide in performing, in a single session, cholecystectomy together with the resolution of common bile duct lithiasis [17]. This innovative procedure has been spread and adopted globally. He has also excelled in the surgical treatment of gastroesophageal reflux. He is the author of numerous scientific articles and books specialized in this discipline, including his latest work entitled Laparoscopic Common Bile Duct Exploration.

References

1. Delgado Gomis F. Cirugía laparoscópica. Cir Esp. 2000;68(4):297–8.
2. Alkatout I, Mechler U, Mettler L, et al. The development of laparoscopy. A historical overview. Front Surg. 2021;8:799442.
3. Mühe E. Die erste cholecystecktomie durch das laparoskop. Langenbecks Arch Klin Chir. 1986;369:804.
4. Blum CA, Adams DB. Who did the first laparoscopic cholecystectomy? J Min Access Surg. 2011;7:165–8.

5. Strasberg SM. Biliary injury in laparoscopic surgery. Part I. Processes used in determination of standard care in misidentification injuries. J Am Coll Surg. 2005;201:598–603.
6. Lacy AM, García Valdecasas JC, Delgado S, et al. Laparoscopy-assisted colectomy versus open colectomy for treatment of non-metastatic colon cancer: a randomized trial. Lancet. 2002;359:2224–9.
7. Targarona E, Feliu X, Salvador JL. Cirugía Endoscópica. Guías Practicas de la Asociación Española de Cirujanos. Ed Aran; 2010. ISBN:978-84- 92977-17-8.
8. The Colon Cancer Laparoscopic or Open Resection Study Group. Survival after laparoscopic surgery versus open surgery for colon cancer: long-term outcome of a randomised clinical trial. Lancet Oncol. 2009;10:44–52.
9. Bonjer HJ, Deijen CL, Abis GA, Cuesta MA, et al. A randomized trial of laparoscopic versus open surgery for rectal cancer. N Engl J Med. 2015;372:1324–32.
10. Biere SSAY, van Berge Henegouwen MI, Maas KW, et al. Minimally invasive versus open oesophagectomy for patients with oesophageal cancer: a multicentre, open-label, randomised controlled trial.
11. van der Wielen N, Brenkman H, Seesing M, et al. Minimally invasive versus open gastrectomy for gastric cancer. A pooled analysis of two European randomized controlled trials. J Surg Oncol. 2024;129:911–21.
12. González-Rivas D, Manolache V, Bosinceanu ML, et al. Uniportal pure robotic-assisted thoracic surgery-technical aspects, tips and tricks. N Ann Transl Med. 2023;11:362.
13. Azagra JS, Goergen M, Gilbart E, Jacobs D. Laparoscopic anatomical (hepatic) left lateral segmentectomy-technical aspects. Surg Endosc. 1996;10:758–61.
14. Azagra JS, Goergen M, De Simone P, Ibañez-Aguirre J. Minimally invasive surgery for gastric cancer. Surg Endosc. 1999;13:351–7.
15. Yuval JB, Thompson HM, Garcia-Aguilar J. Organ preservation in rectal cancer. J Gastrointest Surg. 2020;24:1880–8.
16. Cuesta MA, Nagy AG, editors. Minimally invasive surgery in gastrointestinal cancer. Churchill Livingstone; 1993.
17. Martínez-Isla A, Navaratne L, editors. Laparoscopic common bile duct exploration. Springer; 2022. ISBN: 978-3-030-93202-2.

38

Rafael Yuste Rojas: Discovering Our Brain. The "BRAIN Project" and the Neurorights

Francisco Mateo Vallejo and Estrella Mateo Torres

The Brain, That Great Unknown

It may seem incredible, but despite the fact that we are in the first quarter of the twenty-first century, our knowledge about the brain is still limited. Although it is the main organ of the central nervous system, and responsible for controlling and coordinating most of the body's functions—including thought, memory, emotions, movement and sensory perceptions—what we know about it is largely focused on its anatomy and the characteristics of some of its cells. However, as far as its functioning is concerned, we have barely taken the first steps. Over the centuries, this organ has been the subject of study by anatomists, neurohistologist, philosophers, neurophysiologists, psychologists and theologians, who have tried to understand whether the mind, emotions and feelings constitute a unity at the cerebral level. At the cellular level the brain is composed mainly of neurons and glia and communicates through electrical and chemical impulses. We have about 100 billion neurons each connected, at a minimum, with at least 100,000 million other neurons.

F. M. Vallejo (✉)
Surgeon Specialized in Minimally Invasive Surgery for Gastrointestinal Cancer, Jerez de la Frontera, Cádiz, Spain

E. M. Torres
Specialist in Anaesthesia and Resuscitation, Madrid, Spain

M. A. Cuesta, F. Mateo Vallejo (eds.), *Spain's Journey in Medicine*,
https://doi.org/10.1007/978-3-032-12221-6_38

The complexity of the brain network is so great that we could compare it to three times the internet system of the whole earth [1].

Ramon y Cajal used to say that it was like an “impenetrable jungle”. And despite being in the XXI century we know very little of how these functions are developed and not being able to know how it works we cannot know the treatment of conditions that originate in it such as schizophrenia, depression, etc. Currently, there are basically two specialties dedicated to the study of the brain: neuroscience and neurotechnology. Neuroscience studies our central nervous system to understand the functioning and responses of our brain in search of “why” we react in one way or another. Neurotechnology, on the other hand, develops methods and techniques for neuroscience, to measure and manipulate brain activity. And thus enabling knowledge of the mind at an unprecedented level of detail. However, as we will see below, the specialties that are now being applied to the study of this field have increased significantly.

Biography of Rafael Yuste

“This is important, since the brain is not just another organ of the body, since it generates the human mind. From the brain activity comes all the mental and cognitive activity of the person; that is, everything we are: memory, thoughts, imagination, emotions, decisions... If the brain could be understood, the human being would understand himself inside, scientifically”. These words are pronounced by an outstanding Spanish researcher who is at the top of the study of the brain: Dr. Rafael Yuste Rojas (Fig. 38.1).

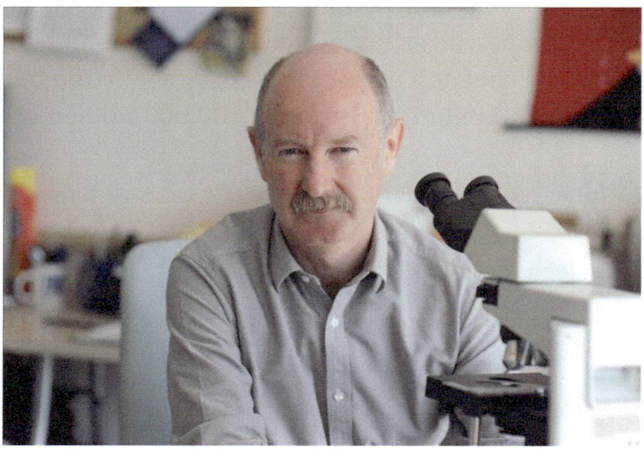

Fig. 38.1 Rafael Yuste

Born in Madrid on April 25, 1963, he spent his childhood in the Argüelles neighborhood. He studied at the Colegio Decroly, near his home. As he himself says: "My father gave me two books by Ramón y Cajal: "Reglas y consejos sobre investigación científica" (Rules and advice on scientific research) and "Los tónicos de la voluntad" (The tonics of the will), and his reading captured me. My mother had also given me another book entitled "Microbe Hunters" de Paul de Kruif, which describes the history of nineteenth century bacteriologists and how they discovered that infectious diseases were caused by bacteria. From then on, I knew that I would dedicate myself to look through the microscope to study Cajal's neuronal circuits. He finished his high school studies at the Instituto Ramiro de Maeztu, where he studied the entrance at the university (COU). He was hesitating between studying music, of which he is very fond, or beginning his medical studies, finally opting for the latter. Between 1981 and 1987, he studied medicine at the Universidad Autónoma de Madrid and at the Fundación Jiménez Díaz, where he became interested in the study of the brain, influenced by the work of Cajal. During his rotation in the Department of Psychiatry at the Rodriguez Lafora Hospital in Madrid, he came into contact with schizophrenic patients and experienced the helplessness of not being able to do anything for them. As with other psychic or neurological conditions, such as dementia, depression, Alzheimer's, mental retardation, epilepsy or paralysis, the cause of these disorders remains largely unknown. To understand their causes and develop effective treatments, it is essential to first decipher how the brain works, especially that of the cerebral cortex. Without a thorough understanding of brain physiology, the diseases that affect it can never be successfully addressed. In 1985 and 1986, he worked in the molecular biology laboratory of Dr. Sydney Brenner in Cambridge, one of the fathers molecular genetics and the deciphering of the genetic code. In 2002, Dr. Brenner would culminate his career by winning the Nobel Prize of Medicine or Physiology. During his time in his laboratory, Yuste became passionate about basic research, and he decided to pursue a career in neurobiology. However, the cutbacks implemented by Margaret Thatcher forced him to move to the United States in 1987. There he worked at Rockefeller University in New York, under the direction of the Swedish neurobiologist Torsten Wiesel, winner of the 1981 Nobel Prize in Medicine together with the Canadian David H. Hubel, for his discoveries on information processing in the visual system. During his time at the university, until 1992, he developed the technique of "calcium imaging" to measure neuronal activity. This is based on the principle that when an electrical signal depolarizes a neuron, calcium channels are activated, allowing Ca^{2+} ions to enter the cell. By staining neurons in the brain with a calcium-sensitive dye, it is possible to detect neuronal activity by microscopy. His research was reflected in his doctoral thesis, directed by T. Wiesel and Lawrence Katz, entitled "Optical Studies of Calcium Dynamics in Developing Neocortical Neurons". This work became one of the fundamental pillars of modern neurobiology. To perfect this technique, Yuste moved to the Bell Laboratories at AT&T, under the supervision of David Tank and Winfried Denk, between 1992 and 1996 and in 1996 he joined the Department of Biological Sciences at Columbia University where he was appointed professor in 2006. From 2005 to 2013 he was also an investigator at the Howard Hughes Medical Institute (HHMI). Founded in 1953, HHMI is a biomedical research and philanthropic organization with a community of researchers, educators, students and practitioners whose mission is to discover the fundamentals of biology. From 2004 to 2021, he codirected the Kavli Neurological Research Institute at Columbia University. From 2012 to 2014 he was a visiting researcher at the Allen Institute for Brain Science in Seattle. From 2014 to the present he is the director of the Center for Neurotechnology at Columbia University and since 2019 he is a visiting researcher at the Donostia International Physics Center (DIPC) institute in San Sebastian.

Science Project

His research is focused on understanding how sets of neurons that are activated in certain circumstances function as if they were modules. These modules are the fundamental building blocks responsible for sensory perception and behaviour and possibly also for what we understand as thoughts and emotions. This initiative represents an unprecedented effort in understanding the human brain, with the potential to revolutionize both science and medicine. As Dr. Yuste explained in an interview: How can we understand the work being done on this issue of brain functioning? Let me give you an example: when we look at a TV with millions of pixels, we perceive a clear and coherent image. However, if we focus on each pixel in isolation, we do not distinguish anything, and it is impossible to understand the whole scene on the screen. The same is true for the brain. If we study the activity of a single neuron, we cannot decipher what happens in the brain as a whole or even in a specific set of neurons. For this, we need methods that allow us to observe their global functioning and understand their dynamics as a whole. How can we see the TV screen of a brain by looking at the activity of all the neurons, looking at all the pixels at once? How can it be done? It is a complex challenge. We need techniques that do not alter the composition of a tissue with extremely delicate properties, where millions of neurons are organized in three dimensions, closely interconnected. To intervene in neuronal circuits, we use methods such as infrared laser light, a non-invasive tool that allows us to access the brain without damaging it. We currently have techniques capable of activating or inhibiting neurons, either individually or in groups, although, for now, we can only apply them to the most superficial layer of the cerebral cortex, up to approximately two millimeters below the skull. Neurons transmit information via nerve impulses, known as action potentials: electrical waves that travel along the cell membrane. Through genetic engineering, we can insert ion channels and light-sensitive pumps, called microbial opsins, into neurons. When we project a beam of light with a specific wavelength, only the cells that have incorporated these opsins respond, becoming electrically activated or silenced. Upon receiving the light pulse, the opsins open, depolarizing the neuron and propagating the signal to the cells with which it is connected. This technique, known as optogenetics, allows us to activate or deactivate neurons with extraordinary precision, simply by illuminating a region of the brain. Thanks to this technology, we can identify which neurons or neuronal groups are responsible for specific functions and behaviors, opening up new possibilities for understanding how the brain works. In September 2011, together with about twenty neurobiologists and other scientists gathered in Buckinghamshire, England, he proposed a large-scale project to improve calcium imaging and develop new cellular neuroimaging techniques. Their goal was to overcome current limitations, which only allowed two dimensional movies of the activity of a limited number of neurons, and instead record high-resolution 3D maps of brain activity in organisms, starting with simple animals such as Hydra or the worm C. elegans. and ending with the human brain. The initiative was warmly welcomed by some of the participants, but also rejected by others who considered it impossible, very complex and with very complicated results. Nevertheless, among the group of scientists who supported him was George Church, Professor of Genetics at Harvard Medical. Church is known for his contributions to genomic sequencing, interpretation of biological data, synthetic biology and genomic engineering. Yuste also received support from Miyoung Chun, vice president of the Kavli Institute. That same evening Yuste and four other scientists, delighted with the idea, drafted a project to develop technologies that could measure the activity of entire neural circuits.

The Brain Project

Rafael Yuste thus became the father of the BRAIN project (Brain Research through Advancing Innovative Neurotechnology's) [2], an initiative born in 2011, when the draft of the project was sent to the White House Office of Science and Technology. The same day they sent it, they replied saying that they loved it and from there, after five meetings at the White House, it was announced in February 2013 by the then US President Barack Obama, in his State of the Nation address, and launched on April 2, 2013, with the staging reserved for major occasions [3]. This project, conceived to be developed over a decade, officially began in 2016. Its funding, provided by the U.S. Congress, which has always supported this project, has been raised mainly by the National Institutes of Health (NIH), which in its first year provided 110 millions of dollars for the initiative. The second year, Congress gave more money than requested, because of the importance they attached to it. Under President Trump, funding increased again, thanks to senators and congressmen, who manage the budgets. Under President Biden, even more was invested. In total, more than six billion dollars are foreseen over 12 years, financing more than five hundred and fifty laboratories inside and outside the USA. Over the years, other agencies, such as the National Science Foundation (NSF) and the Defense Advanced Research Projects Agency (DARPA) have also contributed resources. Yuste also led the internationalization of the BRAIN Initiative, with the creation of the Brain International Initiative in 2017, incorporating projects. That emerged as a result of BRAIN in countries such as China, Japan (Brain/Minds), South Korea, Australia, Canada (CanadaBrain) and Israel, also incorporating the European Union through the Human Brain project, which complements the U.S. initiative.

The primary objectives of the BRAIN project are to accelerate the development of technologies to map brain circuits, measure the dynamic patterns of activity within those circuits, and understand how their interactions give rise to our unique cognitive and behavioral capacities.

Associated with these goals is the aim of developing techniques to deliberately alter neuronal activity within these circuits, in order to modulate it in the brains of patients and thereby correct functions impaired by disease.

> "If we can only observe activity without repairing it, we will not be able to do much for these patients: we may diagnose their problems with extraordinary precision, but we will remain powerless to cure them. Techniques are needed to access the brain, repair faulty connections, and redirect abnormal brain activity in order to restore function—which lies at the core of the pathophysiology of mental disorders. Additionally, computational tools must be developed to ana-

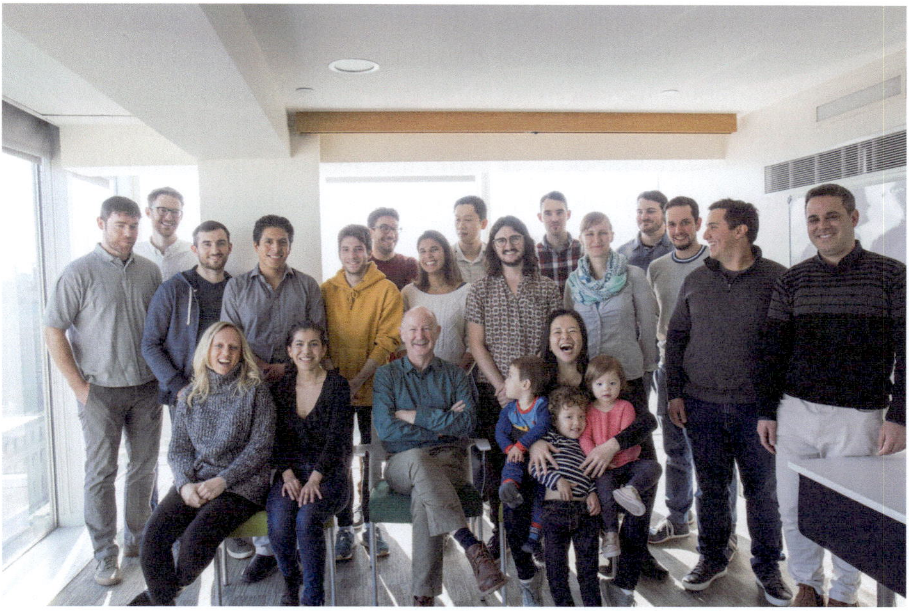

Fig. 38.2 Rafael Yuste with his team

> lyze the data effectively. We are dealing with data from millions of neurons changing at millisecond timescales. This represents a major challenge—one of the most difficult in science." [4] (Fig. 38.2)

Seven priority research areas have been developed to achieve the objectives of the BRAIN project [5]:

- Identify and provide experimental access to different types of brain cells to determine their function in health and disease.
- Mapping connected neurons in local circuits and brain systems.
- Produce a dynamic image of the brain at work.
- Link brain activity to behavior, developing tools to modify the dynamics of neural circuits.
- To foster collaboration between researchers in statistics, physics, mathematics, engineering and computer science to understand the biological basis of mental processes.
- Developing technology to understand the brain and treat its disorders.
- Integrate all the results to discover how patterns of neural activity are converted into cognition, emotion, perception, and action in health and disease [6]. To this end, interdisciplinary teams have been formed that bring

together experts in various fields, such as neuroscience, physics, chemistry, engineering, computer science and mathematics. Increasingly more sophisticated techniques have been included to perform this work, such as short-wave magnetic resonance imaging, nanotechnology, scanning electron microscopy of serial block faces (SBF) and focused ion beam (FIB), automated tape ultramicrotomy [6] and two-photon holographic microscopy, a technique patented by himself [7].

Neurorights

This breakthrough in neurotechnology research is associated with a series of ethical and social consequences that should not be overlooked. Summoned by Yuste, a group of twenty-five representatives from all BRAIN projects around the world, academics, clinicians, bioethicists, entrepreneurs and AI specialists gathered in 2017 at Columbia University, Morningside Campus, to discuss these issues and their impact on human rights. Because, to the extent that the brain generates the mind, accessing and modifying brain information affects the very essence of being human. From this was born the concept of NeuroRights or brain rights, which was published in an article in Nature Magazine in 2017, "Four ethical priorities for neurotechnology's and AI" [8]. These neuro-rights are [9]:

The first neuroright is the right to mental privacy, which implies that the contents of the mind will not be deciphered without the person's consent. We are talking about ensuring the right to privacy of thoughts, emotions, memories, and so on. All this may be unraveled by neurotechnology in the future, and although it may seem like science fiction, the truth is that work is already being done with animals.

The second neuroright is the right to our personal identity; this the capacity we possess to have a personality, a conscience. Something so obvious that throughout history it has not deserved special protection. However, these aspects of the human being are also generated by the brain, so that the ability to alter it has direct consequences on the person and the self. We now know that in Parkinson's patients in whom a new neurotechnology has been used, which consists of stimulating certain brain nuclei by means of an electrode, their relatives have noticed changes in their personality when the electro stimulator is turned on. We can consider this experience as a preview of what is to come, from which we deduce clearly the human right character of one's own psychological or mental identity.

The third neuroright is the right to free will, to the ability to make free decisions, which, as in the previous cases, can be manipulated. In the field of animal experimentation, sensory perceptions can be activated that condition their actions. Obviously, we are faced with another human right, since the person would be deprived making decisions of his own free will, and these decisions could be controlled from the outside through neurotechnology.

The fourth neuroright is linked to the applications of these neurotechnology's to the general public. We can venture a future in which human beings try to increase our cognitive and mental capacities with neurotechnology's. Just to give an example, the direct connection to the Internet through a brain-computer interface, to external databases, AI algorithms, etc., which will allow us to improve ourselves as a species and with a habituation as simple as that of the GPS application in the cell phone. This opens up an obvious possibility of a fracture in society, so that there will be two types of human beings: those who are cognitively augmented and those who are not. We cannot make the mistake of considering it, once again, as something very distant without laying the groundwork to channel it for the benefit of humanity.

The fifth of the neuro-rights has to do with the use of biased information through the neurotechnology applications we use.

Already today, the information we receive through social networks and other media is biased; however, we have the ability to evaluate it in relation to our own opinion or personality, despite the influence it may have on it. The problem with neurotechnology's is that introducing biased data directly into the brain implies that it will assume this information as its own, which translates into a much bigger problem, since what is actually being assumed is a series of intentionally predetermined and premeditated biases. This can lead to a direct modification of the way of thinking of the citizens, with the consequences of all kinds that we can imagine and that raise the fundamental need for the neurotechnology to be used to be free of biases that interfere with the human mind. NeuroRights constitute a platform in order to address the fit of these neurotechnology's in society. Since 2017 Yuste has been working on it; and constituted in 2021 the NeuroRights Foundation to spread the idea in different countries and international organizations. In this regard, it is worth mentioning the outstanding example of Chile, which, thanks to the direct involvement of Yuste, working intensively with the Senate of the Republic and the Government of President Sebastián Piñera, on October 25, 2021, enacted in the Official Gazette of the Republic a constitutional amendment to Article 19 that protects brain activity, and the information derived from it, thus becoming a pioneering initiative in the field of neuro-rights. Chile was followed by the state of Rio Grande do Sul in Brazil, with a similar constitutional amendment, and the U.S. states of Colorado and California, where Yuste and his team sponsored laws protecting mental privacy. Yuste has also collaborated with the United Nations, holding discussions with its secretary general, António Guterres, and his team. They are involved in the regulation of human rights in the field of neurotechnology's. In fact, Guterres' agenda for the UN for the next few years of his mandate includes a mention of the need to update the Universal Declaration of Human Rights, which has not been amended since 1948, especially in aspects such as frontier technologies, and particularly neurotechnology's, which is a real challenge. Rafael Yuste's team, in response to a request from the Office of the UN Secretary General, conducted a legal study that concluded that the existing treaties are not sufficient to meet this challenge. They even detected a problem of terminology, as there is not even a language in the current regulations that can describe what is happening in this field. Some neuro-rights, such as the right to free will, could be protected with minor amendments to some international treaties, however, in others, such as that of personal identity, there is a notable void, since the need for such a problem has never before been addressed in the sense of providing a response to such a problem. The recommendation put forward by the NeuroRights Foundation is that, through an international treaty sanctioned by the Security Council, a report should be drawn up to provide a solution on neurotechnology and NeuroRights. The aim is to establish global regulation before the first problems arise. Finally, Yuste has collaborated with the Government of Spain, through the Secretary of State for Artificial Intelligence, which has promulgated the Charter of Digital Rights. This Charter, in which Professor Tomás de la Quadra Salcedo has participated as a drafter, extends the discussion of fundamental rights to all digital technologies, including the five neuro-rights already mentioned, but also covering potential problems arising from technologies such as the internet, social networks, surveillance technologies, robotics and the metaverse. Although it is an indicative document, with no legal value, it can be interpreted as a "soft law", stimulating discussion and creation of bills and constitutional amendments. The discussion of neuro-rights in recent years takes us into a world that seems like the science fiction of Isaac Asimov's books and the mythical obligations or laws of I, Robot. NeuroRights protect people's minds, and as more possibilities of neurotechnology are discovered, the more important it becomes to protect them from wrongdoing. Neurotechnology's are, in principle, neutral in nature, and can be used for good—to understand the brain, or the treatment of patients with brain diseases, or to open up new avenues for the economy, for example—or for bad, in relation to all the risks that have been mentioned. We must ensure that this new revolution, which will modify the human species, is positive in this sense, and to this end we must articulate a series of legal measures that, as guardrails, to channel its development and application and led us to the desire objective that will benefit all of us.

Personal Life

Married in 1993 to Stephanie R. Golob, who he met on a blind date, they were partly united by their love of music, since, like him, she used to sing in a choir. They have two daughters together. Rebecca was born in 1997 and Clara in 2003. Stephanie is Associate Professor of Political Science at Baruch College, City University of New York, where she teaches courses on globalization, Latin American politics and transitional justice. She has participated as a member of an international research team, based at the Consejo Superior de Investigaciones Científicas (CCHS-CSIC), studying the legal and political impact of mass grave exhumations after atrocities in a comparative perspective (http://politicasdelamemoria.org). Her research on the role of domestic and international law in the politics of historical memory in Spain has most recently appeared in the volume Memory Laws and Historical Justice: The Politics of Criminalizing the Past (Palgrave, 2022) [10].

In the spring of 1996 they both joined the New Amsterdam Singer (NAS). Founded in 1966, the New Amsterdam Singers is a critically acclaimed 60-voice choir performing in and around New York City under the direction of Clara Longstreth. Rafael sings bass, while Stephanie is a contralto and after moving to the Upper West Side, they discovered that NAS was rehearsing around the corner from their first apartment, at 113 th and Broadway. Both were admitted to NAS and have continued singing ever since, balancing family life with choir.

Awards

Among others, he has received many awards: In 2002. New York City Mayor's Young Investigator for Excellence in Science and Technology Award. In 2013 he received the Pioneer Award from the National Institutes of Health. (INS) of the United States.

In 2018 the Eliasson Global Leadership Award of the Tallberg Foundation. This award honors established leaders with a well-established record of achievement and whose work is embedded in a global worldview.

Recognized as one of the most important researchers in the world by Nature magazine in 2012.

In 2015, she received the XLVII Jiménez Díaz Memorial Lecture Award for her research work granted by the Conchita Rábago de Jiménez Díaz Foundation.

2015. Academician of the Royal Academy of Medicine of Spain.

2020. In celebration of the centenary of the Cajal Institute of the Spanish National Research Council (CSIC).

Doctor Honoris Causa from the Universidad Carlos III de Madrid (UC3M) in 2022 and from the Autonomous University of Mexico in 2025.

Books

1. THE BRAIN, THE THEATER OF THE WORLD

In this book Yuste makes a fascinating journey through modern neuroscience. He uncovers how the brain organizes itself to create the human mind. He describes the scientific discoveries made by pioneering brain researchers, as well as the ideas of consciousness, personality and feelings of such renowned philosophers as Plato, Kant and other writers who, without knowledge of neuroscience, made theories that are now being confirmed.

2. DENDRITIC SPINES

Based on the study of small protrusions found in the branches of nerve cells, known as dendrites, the author explains how they play a crucial role in the communication between neurons and in synaptic plasticity. He links their function to the computational logic of neural circuits. He concludes with a speculative chapter on the computational function of spines, searching for the ultimate logic of their existence in the brain and offering a proposal that will undoubtedly stimulate debate and drive future research.

3. LECTURES IN NEUROSCIENCE

Starting from the basic elements of neuroscience, the author, through a plain and easy to understand language, guides us through the functioning of the brain. He describes how the brain is organized and develops, how neurons operate and form neural circuits, and how these circuits function as neural networks to generate behaviors and mental states. It offers readers insight into the functioning of sensory and motor systems and the neurobiological basis of our perceptions, thoughts, emotions, memories and consciousness. Sprinkled with anecdotes and illustrations, this book is accessible to readers with no previous experience in the subject.

Epilogue

In the age in which we live, considering ourselves superior beings who have traveled to space and descended to the depths of the seas, it is almost unthinkable that we are still not able to know how our brain works. But the reality is there, and we have to understand that the journey to know how it works is still going to be a long one. However, in recent years there has been considerable progress thanks to a number of researchers who have launched a series of techniques to understand how they work. Among them we have to highlight a compatriot, who following the steps of Ramón y Cajal, is considered the father of these studies and who is laying the foundations for their realization: Professor Rafael Yuste. He is a source of pride for Spaniards, and it is said that he could be a possible candidate for the Nobel Prize in the near future. He has been able, through his knowledge, techniques, tenacity and enthusiasm, to bring together a plethora of professionals throughout the world to work in the same direction, gaining ground in the knowledge of the brain. Brain mapping, knowledge of brain circuits and groups of neurons that work in common for a given function is allowing researchers not only to know the function of each area of the brain, but also to plan possibilities of interconnection between machine and brain, possibilities of applying specific treatments for brain ailments whose origins were not known until recently, and even the ability to modify certain brain functions on demand. All this may sound like science fiction, but it is just around the corner.

References

1. Yuste R. Neurotechnology, by accessing the center of our mental activity, bypasses all the filters we have in the body. CNIC Journal. Centro Nacional de Investigaciones Cardiovasculares Carlos III; 2023. https://www.cnic.es/es/noticias/rafael-yuste-neurotecnologia-al-acceder-al-center-our mental-activity-bypasses-all.
2. Brain research through the advancement of innovative neurotechnology's.
3. Tovar D. Rafael Yuste: "I was shocked when Obama used the words, I wrote in the draft of the BRAIN project". Diario de Avisos. Tenerife newspaper; 2021.

https://diariodeavisos.elespanol.com/2021/02/rafael-yuste-me-quede-de-piedra-cuando-obama-utilizolas-palabras-que-que-escribi-en-el-borrador-del-proyecto-brain/.
4. New Neurotechnology's and their impact on Science, Medicine and Society. Conference given at the Ramón Areces Foundation. February 21, 2019. https://www.fundacionareces.es/fundacionareces/es/actividades/las-nuevas-neurotecnologias-y-suimpacto-en-la-ciencia-medicina-y-sociedad.html.
5. Jorgenson LA, et al. The BRAIN initiative: developing technology to catalyze neuroscience discovery. Philos Trans R Soc Lond B Biol Sci. 2015;370:20140164. https://doi.org/10.1098/rstb.2014.0164. Accepted: 23 December 2014.
6. BRAIN. A Scientific Vision. NIH BRAIN Initiative Reports; 2025.
7. Yuste R. Research area I: optical methods for neuroscience leader. Neuro Technology Center Columbia University. https://ntc.columbia.edu/rafael-yuste/.
8. Yuste R, Goering S, Arcas B, et al. Four ethical priorities for neurotechnology's and AI. Nature. 2017;551:159–63. https://doi.org/10.1038/551159a.
9. Neurotechnology and Human Rights. Reception speech as Doctor Honoris Causa by the Carlos III University. 2020. https://www.uc3m.es/ss/Satellite/UC3MInstitucional/es/TextoDosColumnas/1371353404778/?d=Touch.
10. Golob S. Faculty profiles. Baruch College. The City University of New York. https://baruch.cuny.edu/profiles/faculty/Stephanie-Golob.

39

Juan C. Izpisúa Belmonte: The Scientist Who Studies Cellular Aging in Order to Rejuvenate It

Miguel A. Cuesta

Juan Carlos Izpisúa Belmonte was born in Hellín, Albacete (Spain) on December 16, 1960, into a humble family. He says it all the time: he owes everything to his mother (Fig. 39.1). She was a nougat seller at the fair in Albacete, insisting that her son should study, that he should go further than she did. Working from sunrise to sunset or working as a hotel bellboy, the early orphan had to face a difficult childhood and adolescence. But from an early age, his passion for science drove him to study Biology. At one of the entrances to Hellín, you can read a graffiti that reads: "Utopia is that which has not been tried to be realized". A phrase that probably reflects the dreams of his youth. "What a beautiful sentence!" exclaimed Juan Carlos Izpisúa as he read it. "I would sign it right now." He also mentioned another quote, this time from Jonas Salk, sponsor of his university in California and creator of the polio vaccine: "Hope lies in dreams, in the imagination and in the courage of those who dare to turn them into reality" (Fig. 39.2).

Following his vocation for Biology, Juan Carlos studied Pharmacy at the University of Valencia, where he obtained the extraordinary prize. Subsequently, he completed a master's degree in pharmacology at the same university before receiving his PhD in Biochemistry and Pharmacology from the University of Bologna and the University of Valencia, specializing in the field of

M. A. Cuesta (✉)
Department of Surgery, Amsterdam University Medical Centre (UMC), Amsterdam, The Netherlands

M. A. Cuesta, F. Mateo Vallejo (eds.), *Spain's Journey in Medicine*,
https://doi.org/10.1007/978-3-032-12221-6_39

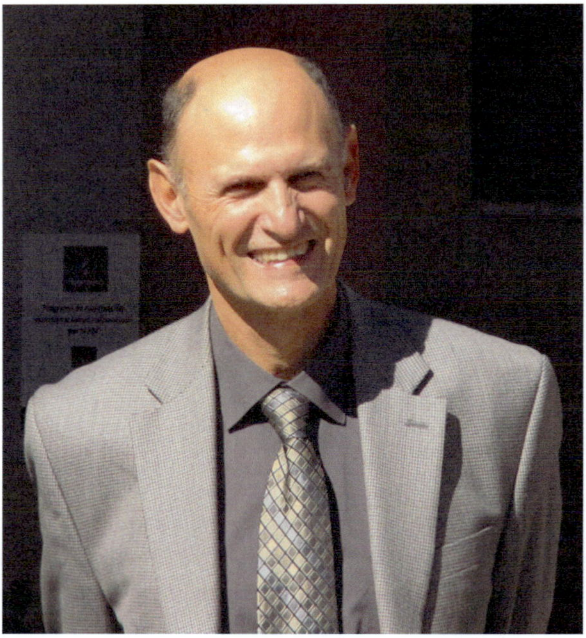

Fig. 39.1 Juan Carlos Izpisúa Belmonte. (Faro de Hellín, Albacete)

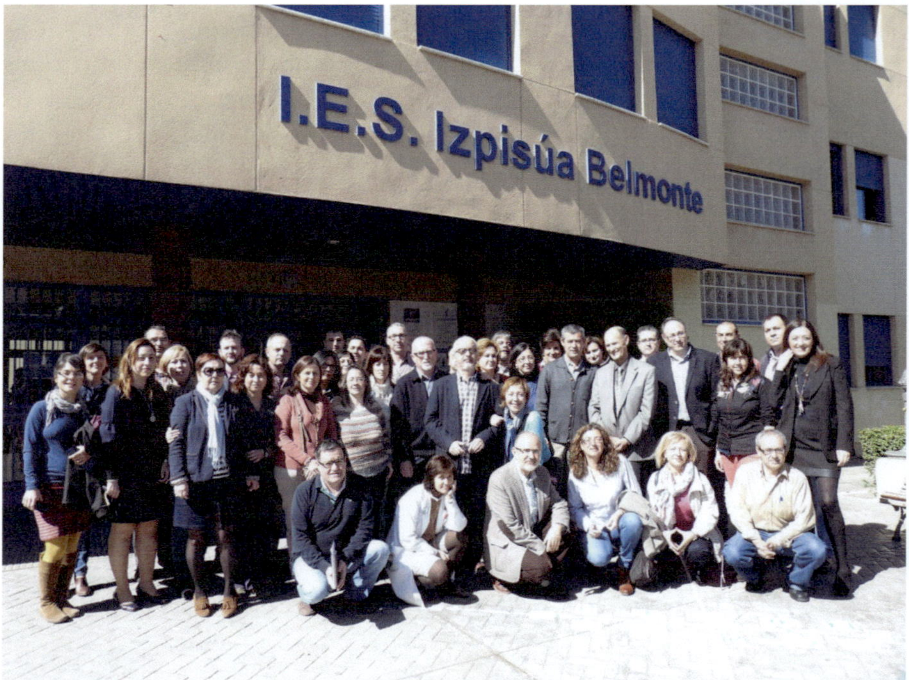

Fig. 39.2 Juan C. Izpisúa in front of his former High School in Hellín (Albacete, Spain) with the Current teaching staff. (Faro de Hellín, Albacete)

Developmental Biology. After conducting postdoctoral research at the European Molecular Biology Laboratory (EMBL) in Heidelberg, Germany, and at the University of California, Los Angeles (UCLA), he participated in 2004 in the creation of the Center for Regenerative Medicine in Barcelona, of which he was director until January 2014.

Regenerative medicine is a branch of medicine dedicated to study the processes of reprogramming, regeneration, or replacement of human cells, tissues or organs, with the aim of restoring their normal functioning. The methods used in this discipline are based on molecular biology and tissue engineering, and seek, as far as possible, to correct damaged tissues and organs by stimulating natural regeneration to achieve optimal recovery. Regenerative medicine also focuses on the study and growth of tissues and even organs in the laboratory, to be implanted when the body itself can no longer regenerate them. This growth can start from the own cells, which facilitates their compatibility and avoids organ rejection. However, the use of animal cells and even whole animals as incubators to create new organs that could be transplanted into humans is also being investigated.

This branch of medicine relies on various techniques for its research, including the use of pluripotent stem cells, cell therapies, the induction of cell and tissue regeneration by means of certain molecules or factors, cell reprogramming, and the transplantation of cultured tissues and organs in vitro, as well as tissue engineering, both in vitro and in vivo.

Cellular reprogramming aims to rejuvenate the cellular aging process.

Move to United States

In 2014, he moved to the United States to join the Gene Expression Laboratory at the Salk Institute for Biological Studies in La Jolla, California, holding the Roger Guillemin Chair. In 2022, he move to ALTOS Labs in San Diego, California, under a highly advantageous research contract aligned with his scientific aspirations. This institute brings together an elite group of scientists whose main objective is to study aging and promote well-being over the years through cellular rejuvenation. He is currently director of this laboratory and professor of Developmental Biology at the Catholic University of Murcia, Spain.

The cause of many diseases, including those associated with aging (cardiovascular diseases (like heart disease and stroke), neurodegenerative diseases (such as Alzheimer's and Parkinson's), musculoskeletal conditions (like osteoarthritis and osteoporosis), and metabolic disorders (such as Type 2 diabetes) is the deterioration of cellular health. Restoring and maintaining cellular health is one of the most ambitious challenges and important issues of our time. I joined ALTOS Labs because of its radical yet humble approach, its unconventional structure, and its pioneering vision for programming cellular health to overcome human disease for the benefit of all.

During his time at the Salk Institute, his work has first helped to understand the cellular and molecular mechanisms responsible for embryonic development from the moment of fertilization to the formation of an adult organism composed of millions of cells. These studies are having a significant impact on the development of novel treatments for diseases and have contributed to the creation of new frontiers for biomedical science in fields such as organ and tissue regeneration and anti-aging. When reviewing the titles and results of some of his research on these diverse topics, the words that come to mind are utopia, dreams and even science fiction. His work has been published in the most prestigious scientific journals, such as Cell or Nature, and has made headlines in social media around the world. His collaboration with Nobel laureate Shinya Yamanaka (Nobel Prize of Physiology or Medicine, 2012) has been fundamental in his dedication to the reversal of cellular aging, focus of his current research. In his seminal paper, "Induction of Pluripotent Stem Cells from Mouse Embryonic and Adult Fibroblasts" S. Yamanaka described the four Yamanaka factors (Oct4, Sox2, Klf4, and c-Myc). The paper details the process of reprogramming somatic cells, like fibroblasts, into induced pluripotent stem cells (iPSCs) by introducing these four factors [1] (Fig. 39.3).

Among the most relevant studies of Izpisua Belmonte is the one published in 2009 with Yamanaka: "Induced pluripotent stem cells and reprogramming: seeing the science through the hype" [2]. This study seeks to illustrate the personal perspectives of four experts on the subject of cellular reprogramming and its possible applications in medicine.

" No one can have overlooked the impact that induced pluripotent stem (iPS) cells have had in the few years since somatic cells were first reprogrammed to pluripotency. Four pioneering iPS cell researchers offer their personal perspectives on these and other current issues under debate. In addition to expressing hope for improved understanding and treatment of human diseases, they call for caution regarding safety concerns and advocate for the establishment of iPS cell banks".

In 2016 he garnered worldwide attention for his research on how to reverse cellular aging, in a paper titled: "In Vivo Enhancement of Aging-Associated Traits by Partial Reprogramming" [3], stating in its conclusion:

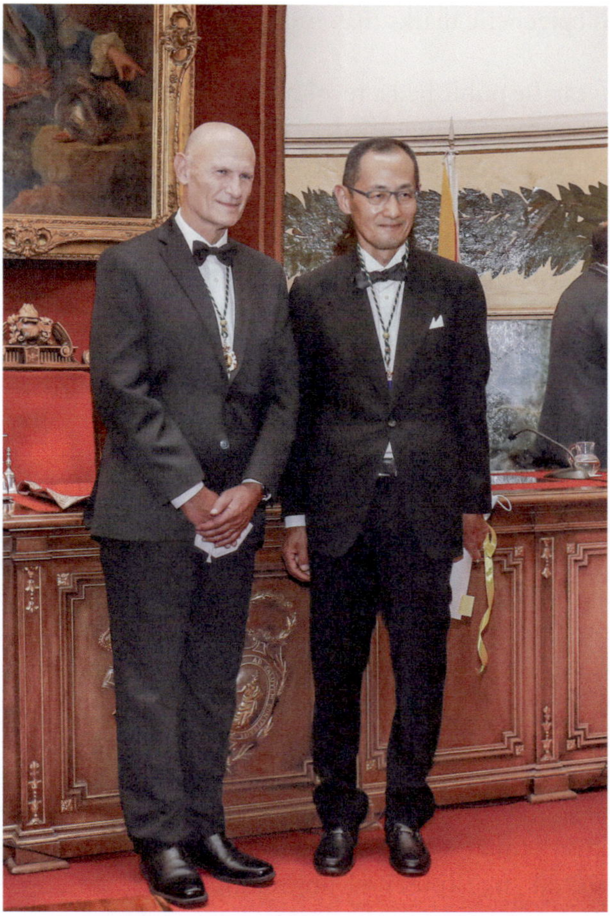

Fig. 39.3 Juan C. Izpisúa Belmonte with Prof. Shinya Yamanaka in RANM de course 2022-2023, Madrid. (Permission Banco Imágenes RANME)

"Aging is the major risk factor for many human diseases. In vitro studies have shown that cellular reprogramming to pluripotency reverses cellular aging, but alteration of the aging process through reprogramming has not been directly demonstrated in vivo. Here, we report that partial reprogramming through short-term cyclic expression of Oct4, Sox2, Klf4, and c-Myc (OSKM or Yamanaka's 4 factors) improves cellular and physiological features of aging and prolongs lifespan in a mouse model of premature aging. The amelioration of age-associated phenotypes by epigenetic remodeling during cellular reprogramming highlights the role of epigenetic dysfunction as a driver of mammalian aging. Establishing in vivo platforms to modulate age-associated epigenetic marks may provide further insights into the biology of aging."

That same year, he published a revolutionary study on a subject he has been working on for some time, entitled: "Human Organs from Animal Bodies" [4]. It is based on solving the lack of transplantable organs by using pigs as "incubators".

In 2017, he published in Nature [5], together with an international team of researchers, where they managed to correct pathogenic mutations in human genes. To do so, they use the CRISPR-Cas9 technique, described in 2003 by Spanish researcher Francis Mojica (see Chap. 35) and use for genetic engineering by Jennifer Doudna y Emmanuelle Charpentier (Nobel Prize Physiology or Medicine, 2020).

CRISPR-Cas9 uses a specially designed RNA molecule to guide an enzyme, called Cas9, to a particular DNA sequence. Cas9 then cuts the DNA strands at that location and removes a small piece. This creates a space in the DNA where a new piece of DNA is placed.

Since 2016, Juan Carlos Izpisúa's main research focus has been on partial cell reprogramming to revert aging. His studies began with mice and, subsequently, have sought ways to apply them to human cells in the laboratory. *"I am optimistic that, with cellular rejuvenation, we could alter the rate of progression of aging and, therefore, increase the duration of health,"* he said in an interview on the subject. To advance this line of research, Izpisúa has the backing of Altos Labs, the best-funded biotech company in history. Founded in January 2022, Altos Labs hired Izpisúa as a director and received an initial investment of approximately $3 billion. This capital comes from large fortunes in the technology sector and other investors, which could include Jeff Bezos, founder of Amazon. The media and social networks have described the creation of Altos Labs as an ambitious attempt to use the most advanced technology and bring together the best scientists in the quest to prolong life and even achieve immortality reversing cellular aging.

However, almost all researchers and analysts agree, that human experiments involving cellular reprogramming, whether at Altos Labs or in other laboratories, will encounter limitations in their development. Research is expected to focus on specific diseases related to aging, such as diabetes, arthritis, stroke, glaucoma, and dementia, among others. Aging itself will not be addressed, as the FDA does not consider it a disease, which prevents initial approval of drugs and therapies aimed at treating it. However, many believe that if effective treatments to slow it down were discovered and scientifically validated, its use would be inevitable.

Interest in Cell Regeneration

Interest in cell regeneration and rejuvenation has grown enormously. In 2023, Izpisúa attracted such a large audience at a conference in Boston that the authorities were forced to suspend the event for exceeding the allowed capacity and violating the building's fire safety code [6]. In addition, several articles have been published in the press about his work [7–10]. Nevertheless, many biologists warn against excessive expectations—what they call hype—and advise waiting for the publication of results in prestigious scientific journals before drawing definitive conclusions. Even so, Izpisúa has established himself as a key figure in one of the most promising fields of biomedicine today: regenerative medicine. His work could lead to the discovery of new molecules and gene- and cell-targeted treatments to prevent and cure aging diseases in both adult and embryonic stages. In addition, his research could induce regenerative responses in vivo, enabling tissue and organ regeneration in humans. In the long-term, their work could not only broaden our understanding of aging and its associated diseases, but also pave the way to healthier living and, potentially, greater longevity. During his work at the Salk Institute, in 2022, a spectacular news item appeared in the press: "The therapy of cellular rejuvenation safely reverses signs of aging in mice". Scientists at the Salk Institute, together with Genentech, a member of the Roche group, demonstrated that it is possible to safely and effectively reverse the aging process in middle-aged and elderly mice, partially restoring their cells to more youthful states. The study, entitled "In vivo partial reprogramming alters age associated molecular changes during physiological aging in mice," was published in Nature Aging in 2022 by his team [11], concluding:

> Partial reprogramming by expression of reprogramming factors (Oct4, Sox2, Klf4, and c-Myc), Yamanaka's 4 factors, for short periods of time restores a youthful epigenetic form in aged cells and extends the lifespan of a mouse model of premature aging. However, the effects of long-term partial reprogramming in aging mice are unknown. Here, we performed several partial reprogramming regimens, including different times of onset, during the physiological aging. Long-term partial reprogramming led to rejuvenating effects in different tissues, such as kidney and skin, and at the organism level; the duration of treatment determined the magnitude of the beneficial effects. Overall, our observations indicate that partial reprogramming protocols can be designed to be safe and effective in preventing age-related physiological changes. Furthermore, we conclude that long-term partial reprogramming regimens are more effective in delaying aging phenotypes than short-term reprogramming.

In other words, this cell therapy is able to clearly reverse the signs of aging in mice. *"We are elated to be able to apply this approach across the lifespan to delay aging in healthy animals. The technique has been shown to be safe and effective in mice,"* said Juan C. Izpisua. *"In addition to addressing age-associated diseases, this strategy could provide the biomedical community with a new tool to restore tissue and organismal health by improving cell function and resilience in various diseases, such as neurodegenerative diseases."* As organisms age, not only do their appearance and health transform, but every cell in their bodies carries a molecular clock that keeps track of the passage of time. Isolated cells of older people or animals have distinct patterns of chemicals in their DNA, known as epigenetic markers, compared to younger individuals. The term epigenome comes from Greek and means "on" the genome, referring to the mechanisms that regulate gene expression without altering the DNA sequence.

Just as the genome is the instructions we inherit from our parents, epigenetics refers to how your behaviors, age and environment can cause changes that affect the way your genes function or express themselves. Unlike genetic changes (mutations), epigenetic changes are reversible and do not alter the sequence of DNA bases, but they can change the way your body reads a DNA sequence.

Conceptual Discoveries

His conceptual discoveries and methodologies on aging and regenerative medicine, can be summarized as:

- The identification of some of the key cellular and molecular bases that explain how an organism with millions of cells develops from a single cell embryo after fertilization.
- The development of new methodologies for the differentiation of human stem cells into different cell types and organs, such as kidney and heart
- The study of human aging and its associated diseases, as well as the discovery of new drivers of rejuvenation.
- Research on the potential of induced pluripotent stem cell (iPSC) technology to generate patient-specific cells corrected for diseases, with possible application in cell therapies.
- The development of methodologies to culture embryos, including non-human primates, and the creation of synthetic mammalian embryos.
- The generation of technologies that allow the differentiation of human cells within embryos of different species, which could facilitate the production human tissues and organs.

Juan Carlos Izpisúa Belmonte and His Program at ALTOS Labs

My work program is both philosophical and evolutionary: *"I try to understand how human beings develop and how that knowledge can contribute to curing diseases,"* he explains. *"It's as if, throughout our lives, we were writing a manuscript. We keep adding marks and, over time, our cells find it difficult to read it correctly, which causes their malfunction and leads to the appearance of diseases and aging. We have observed that the introduction of just four genes (the so-called Yamanaka factors)* [1] *in an experimental organism allows its organs to rejuvenate, regenerate and, in some cases, even prolong its life. The key is to better understand the interaction between the environment and our genome in order to modify it and prevent devastating diseases such as neurodegenerative, cardiovascular or cancer." "We find ourselves in a fascinating moment for humanity, in which human beings have the ability change their destiny and reinterpret the reading, and even the writing, of that manuscript that is life." "We are born with a genome inherited from our parents, composed of millions of genes (or letters). However, sometimes there are mistakes in this genetic code. For example, a change in a gene from GGC to GGT - referring to DNA bases guanine, guanine, cytosine to guanine, guanine, thymine - can cause progeria (a premature aging disease), and today we are already able to correct these mutations. However, only 1% of human diseases are due to specific mutations. The vast majority do not have a genetic origin point, but that aging is the underlying factor common to many of them"* (Fig. 39.3).

Aging and Its Impact on Health

From the of 40–45, aging becomes the main cause of virtually all diseases that lead to mortality: heart disease, cancer, respiratory pathologies, cerebrovascular diseases, diabetes, influenza, kidney failure, sepsis, hypertension, Alzheimer's disease and Parkinson's disease. The longer we live, the greater the probability of developing these diseases, even if they are not associated with specific genetic mutations. How do they appear and what can we do to reverse these diseases? It is necessary to go deeper at the cellular level. In the early stages of life, cells show high levels of plasticity, regeneration and resilience to stress, dysfunction and injury, key characteristics for human health. There are two main types of cells: young cells, which are healthy and resilient, and aged cells, which are fragile and less functional. Resilience is defined as the ability of an organism to resist or recover quickly from adverse conditions. The young cells have a high buffering capacity against stress, whereas aged cells show a much reduced capacity. What is buffer capacity? It is the ability of a cell or organism to respond to stress while maintaining its resilience. Can we increase the buffering capacity of elderly cells? Is it possible to enhance the resilience of aging cells to delay or even reverse the onset of disease?

A New Approach to Medicine

The goal of the new medicine will be to restore cellular health and improve buffering capacity through cellular reprogramming, with the aim of reversing diseases. ALTOS Labs is currently developing technologies to reprogram and rejuvenate adult and diseased cells, returning them to states similar to those observed in the early stages of life. This strategy has the potential to revolutionize medical therapies and offer new solutions to combat aging and human diseases. There are three main factors that cause a healthy cell to become fragile:

1. Changes in metabolism associated with aging.
2. Decreased energy levels.
3. The mitochondria do not produce the ATP necessary for cell function, which can lead to cell death. The genome of a cell is coiled and very long, almost two meters long, and has two different types of chromatin: the closed chromatin of healthy cells and the open chromatin of unhealthy cells.

The main function of chromatin is to package, with the help of certain proteins, long DNA molecules into more compact and dense structures that can fit into the cell nucleus. This prevents from tangling together and also plays an important role during cell division, preventing DNA damage and regulating gene expression and DNA replication.

Changes in chromatin can have multiple consequences for cellular health. In 2006, Shinya Yamanaka published an article in Cell [1] in which he described how, in mice, by adding four proteins—known as the four Yamanaka factors—to an adult cell, the cell could be reprogrammed. One year later, he described the same phenomenon in human adult cells. Four years later, Izpisúa's team discovered the correlation between chromatin conformation, aging and disease. When chromatin is closed, in its heterochromatin form, it represents a young and healthy epigenome. In contrast, open chromatin, or euchromatin, is associated with an aged and diseased epigenome. But how can we reverse this process, is it possible to modify it, from open to closed chromatin, and in what way? A clear example is progeria, a disease of accelerated aging caused by a mutation. In mouse models, two possible solutions are possible: correcting the mutation or modifying the buffering of the epigenome. In both cases, a change in the phenotype of the mouse is achieved, resulting in rejuvenation. By administering the Yamanaka factors for a couple of days a week, the mutation persists, but the aged and diseased mouse undergoes a transformation, resembling a younger animal. In both kidneys and skin, the epigenetic patterns of the treated animals reflect characteristics similar to those of younger healthy individuals. Modifying the chromatin conformation in an aged cell not only makes it more resilient and functional, but also represents an innovative strategy known as partial reprogramming treatment (PRT).

And we have more examples in mice of the importance of partial reprogramming in the improvement of various diseases. For example, in the case of the genetic mutation of leptin, which causes obesity, the administration of Yamanaka's factors allows rejuvenating the mouse, reducing the fat content in the liver and restoring its response to glucose. Regardless of the disease, chromatin is modified, increasing cellular buffering capacity and resilience. This causes the disease to take longer to manifest itself or, in some cases, to be reversed. It should be noted that it is not the genome that is altered, but the epigenome. As for the availability of organs for transplantation, it is well known that this is one of the main limitations of the healthcare system. More than 100,000 people in the U.S. are on the waiting list for a transplant, and one person dies every hour waiting for an organ (see Chap. 26). Many organs are discarded due donor age or other factors. Currently, in collaboration with a leading Transplant Unit, innovative ex vivo perfusion work is being carried out on kidneys and other organs of questionable viability prior to transplantation. The aim is to rejuvenate these organs and improve their quality so that they can be used, significantly increasing the number of organs available for transplantation. One of the key challenges of this cell reprogramming therapy is that, with aging, not all cells in the body deteriorate; many remain healthy. So the question arises: how do we get the reprogramming factors to reach only the damaged cells without affecting healthy cells? What is the ideal dosage and how do we administer it? We are investigating these aspects," says Izpisúa, "and developing new genes and markers to specifically target the four Yamanaka factors to the affected cells.

Is it possible to reverse aging and promote rejuvenation?

Our purpose is clear: to make people healthier. Our mission is to restore cellular health and strengthen the body's resilience through cellular reprogramming in order to reverse disease and disability throughout the human lifespan. Currently, we are working with human cells to increase their buffering capacity. These cells are studied in isolation in Petri dishes, but the next step is to transfer the research to humans, taking all the necessary safety measures to avoid any damage. What are the risks of this process? A crucial issue is the administration and dosage of the factors in the cells. If treated with the four Yamanaka factors, it is possible to convert unhealthy cells into embryonic cells resulting in the loss of their identity and function. For example, if an unhealthy heart cell is indiscriminately reprogrammed with the 4 factors, it could be transformed into an embryonic cell and lose its function completely, which would prevent the heart from continuing to beat. This clearly not the goal. Therefore, the way these factors are administered, and their dosage is a fundamental aspect of our studies, to rejuvenate the cells, not to revert to embryonic cells. Moreover, it is likely that there are other factors beyond Yamanaka's, which opens up new lines of research for the future. Our work, like that of other laboratories with the same vision, consists of generating knowledge. However, it will be the industry that will be in charge of transferring these discoveries to the market. Of course, we should not forget that there are other very important key factors to mitigate the effects of aging on health, such as exercise, intermittent fasting and nutrition, among others.

Legacy

When we analyze Juan C. Izpisúa Belmonte, he seems to us to be a character of the future. He is a visionary, not only because of his personal, career, but also because of his current role in the highest spheres of science, especially in partial cellular reprogramming programs to reverse aging. Once these cells are reprogrammed, the body could rejuvenate itself and reverse many of the associated diseases to aging, which constitute the majority of them. Although these programs could extend life, their greatest contribution would be to significantly improve quality of life, and that is fundamental. When reviewing the titles and results of some of his research in these various fields, the words that come to mind are utopia, dreams, even science fiction. He is like a prophet anticipating new changes in the evolution of the human being.

Awards

Izpisúa Belmonte has received numerous awards and distinctions, including those awarded by the National Institutes of Health of the United States, the Presidential Career Award from President Bill Clinton, and the Pew Scholar Award. In October 2018, Time magazine included him in its list of the 50 most influential people in healthcare. Likewise, his work has been selected twice by Science magazine as the "Breakthrough of the Year": in 2008, for his research in cell reprogramming, and in 2013, for the generation of mini-organs.

References

1. Takahashi K, Yamanaka S. Induction of pluripotent stem cells from mouse embryonic and adult fibroblast cultures by defined factors. Cell. 2006;126:663–76.
2. Izpisua Belmonte JC, Ellis J, Hochedingler K, Yamanaka S. Induced pluripotent stem cells and reprogramming: seeing the science through the hype. Nat Rev Genet. 2009;10:878–82.
3. Ocampo A, Reddy P, Martínez-Redondo P, et al. In vivo amelioration of age-associated hallmarks by partial reprogramming. Cell. 2016;167:1719–33.
4. Izpisua Belmonte JC. Human organs from animal bodies. Sci Am. 2016;315:32–7.
5. Ma H, Marti-Gutierrez N, Park S-W, et al. Correction of a pathogenic gene mutation in human embryos. Nature. 2017;548:413–9.
6. Regalado A. Police got called to an overcrowded presentation on "rejuvenation" technology "technology". MIT Technolog Review; 2023.
7. Wade N. NYT aging. The New York Times; 2016.
8. Artificial embryos draw closer with Salk Institute work in mice San Diego Union-Tribune; 2019.
9. Wade N. New prospects for growing human replacement organs in animals. The New York Times; 2017.
10. Researchers have created embryos that are part-human and part-monkeys. They could one day provide organs for transplant. The Economist; 2021.
11. Browder KC, Reddy P, Yamamoto M, et al. In vivo partial reprogramming alters age-associated molecular changes during physiological aging in mice. Nat Aging. 2022;2:243–53.

40

Josep Baselga: The Doctor Who Wished to Change the World of Oncology

Miguel A. Cuesta and Carmen Padules González

Josep Baselga Torres was born on July 3, 1959, in Barcelona. From a doctor's family, his father, Manuel Baselga was a pioneer in Occupational Medicine in Spain, and his mother Esther Torres, was a nurse. He studied high school with the Jesuit Fathers in Sarriá, where he shaped his personality and his vision of the world, based on service to others and the demand for intellectual rigor. He left with the ambition to transform the world and make it a better place, based on the values he had learned with the Society of Jesus. He studied Medicine at the Autonomous University of Barcelona, specializing in Internal Medicine at the Vall d'Hebron Hospital [1] (Fig. 40.1).

M. A. Cuesta (✉)
Department of Surgery, Amsterdam University Medical Centre (UMC), Amsterdam, The Netherlands

C. P. González
Registered Nurse and Researcher, Madrid, Spain

M. A. Cuesta, F. Mateo Vallejo (eds.), *Spain's Journey in Medicine*,
https://doi.org/10.1007/978-3-032-12221-6_40

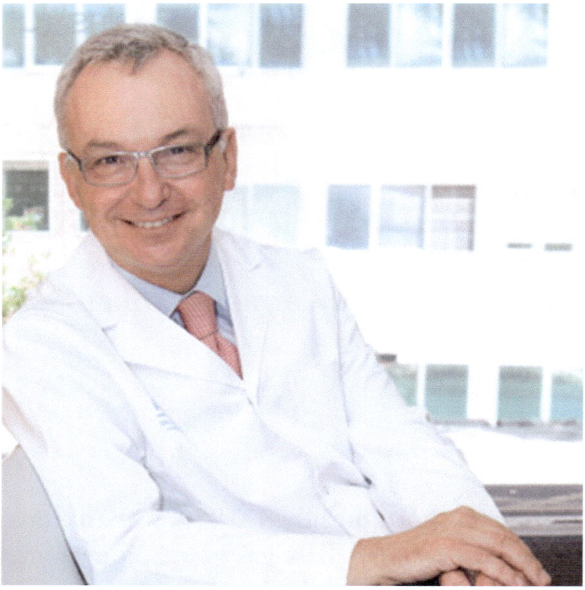

Fig. 40.1 Josep Baselga

Move to New York

In 1985, he moved to New York to complete his training, first at King's County Hospital in Brooklyn, where he met his future wife, Silvia Garriga, and then in Oncology at Memorial Sloan Kettering Hospital in New York. York, a hospital that Valentín Fuster had recommended him years before to do oncology as a specialty, putting him in contact with Carlos Cordón, a pathologist at that hospital. When he arrived there, he spent several months in Cordón's house, where at night they talked about how to treat cancer in the future, aware of the great difference between what they idealized and the bad results they obtained. During those years, he was part of the medical staff of the Breast Medicine Unit. There he studied with John Mendelsohn the role of monoclonal antibodies directed specifically against cellular proteins associated with breast and lung cancer. In those years, he led the development of a new treatment for breast cancer, Trastuzumab (or Herceptin®), synthetized by the company Genentech.

> Trastuzumab is a humanized monoclonal antibody developed to target the cell membrane receptor HER2, which is overexpressed on some cancer cells, including 30% of breast cancers.

(*) In the early 1990s, at The Memorial, he had a patient with metastatic breast cancer who had exhausted all treatments available at the time. Baselga treated her with Trastuzumab as part of a clinical trial. Upon seeing her again in his office and observing that the metastases had shrunk significantly, he got excited and went to tell his boss, Larry Norton, to explore the patient: -Larry, you have to see this! -he said. -I'm not impressed," Norton replied. -What do you mean you're not impressed? -Baselga protested, "this patient is getting better! -Look, Pepe, what is happening to you is normal. You're young, you're enthusiastic, a patient improvement... It's normal that you think it's extraordinary, you're a good boy. But no, I'm not impressed. Baselga placed on the table a photo he had taken of the patient before treatment, with extensive skin lesions that had disappeared. -Do you think it's my enthusiasm that has brought this about? -All right," Norton conceded at last, Agreed, not bad".

But not all patients reacted with the drug, so it was necessary to identify the group that responded positively. The key was the HER-2/c-erbB-2 oncogene, which encodes the HER2 receptor located in the cell membrane.

> The implication of the HER-2/c-erbB-2 oncogene in the pathogenesis of breast cancer established a major shift in the paradigm for its treatment (1987 by Slamon et al)

A period of biological research began on this family of receptors and how to target them. Trastuzumab acts by blocking the protein that produces this gene. Due to the variability in the drug's efficacy, the Genentech company was on the verge of abandoning the project, until Dr. Baselga convinced them, by showing his data, that there was a group of patients in whom the treatment would be very effective. Finally, the company decided to go ahead with Trastuzumab, which was approved in the U.S. in 1998 and in Europe in 2000.

Return to Barcelona

In 1996, after eleven years in New York, he returned to Barcelona, where he was appointed full professor at the Autonomous University of Barcelona and director of the Oncology Department at the Vall d'Hebron Hospital until 2010. There he distinguished himself for his ability to treat breast cancer patients with experimental drugs in the development phase. *"I had my ideas about how I should organize an oncology service in the era of molecular biology to bring research advances to patients,"* he told Josep Corbella. During this period, the Institute of Oncology at Vall d'Hebron Hospital became, and still is, an international leader in cancer research, treatments and clinical protocols.

There, he proposed to Dr. Josep Tabernero, whom he knew from his time as a resident, to join the group, sharing both a passion for medicine, rigor in reasoning and a high level of self-demand. All with an overriding idea let's cure cancer, let's make it chronic! Dr. Tabernero says in Josep Corbella's book: *"They told me I was wrong. I had a stable job at the Sant Pau hospital and at Vall d'Hebron everything was still to be done. But I was convinced by his enthusiasm. He was someone who wanted to change things. He had clear ideas about what he wanted to achieve, and he explained it with an energy and enthusiasm that did not leave you indifferent. I thought we could do important things".*

These were times in which the fundamental change undergone by Medical Oncology must be highlighted. In the eighties of the last century, oncology was a specialty in which the oncologist's work consisted practically of accompanying the cancer patient with a cycle of chemotherapy in the last stages of life. However, since the 1990s, figures such as J. Baselga transformed this specialty, stating that his ambition was to cure cancer. Cancer became the next bastion of medicine to be solved, since the first oncogenes had been discovered. Baselga's personality was already characterized by his immense eagerness to discover new drugs, based on the biology of the cancer cell, which could cure the patient. This was reflected in his professional life, where he communicated with patients with absolute clarity and spoke empathetically about the disease and its possible treatment, which is, after all, the real work of the physician. His rhythm of work, based on the development of biology, biochemistry and laboratory work, was first implemented in basic and clinical protocols, prior to its general acceptance in clinical practice, always supported by industry. He conveyed a sense of urgency (*): *"Cancer doesn't wait, patients can't wait". "Think big," he said.* He always lived his career in this way, creating a style that endures to this day: close collaboration between the pharmaceutical industry and the oncologists. Speaking about collaboration with industry in an interview (*) he said: *"Look, we doctors need industry to develop the drugs we need to treat cancer. If industry doesn't do it, nobody will. And the pharmaceutical companies need us to guide them".* Josep Corbella, noticing that Baselga treated patients and also worked with the pharmaceutical industry, raised the question of conflicts of interest. His response was that conflicts of interest must exist, but that the bottom line is to think about what is best for patients. *"The best thing is for physicians and industry to collaborate. If you are an expert, it is normal for the industry to consult you;*

if they don't consult you, you are not an expert. Conflicts of interest must be made public and be transparent." Unlike radiotherapy and chemotherapy, which attack both diseased and healthy cells, molecular therapies act selectively against tumor cells. Cancer had to be defeated without damaging healthy cells. From his passion for biology, Baselga dedicated a large part of his career to understanding how cancer cells work and to finding their vulnerable points in order to attack them with drugs. His scientific life is linked to kinases. *"For me, biology is almost poetry, it's an aesthetic pleasure," he said.*

Tyrosine kinases are a family of enzymes belonging to the protein kinase group that catalyze the transfer of a phosphate group from ATP to a specific amino acid: tyrosine within a protein. Tyrosine kinases play a key role in cell proliferation, survival, adhesion and motility and have also been shown to mediate the transformation of malignant cells. In general, mutations in kinases lead to a loss or gain of cellular function that can cause cancer.

In 2001, Baselga, along with Dr. Dennis J. Slamon of UCLA, who had discovered the clinical significance of the HER2 receptor, present at high levels in approximately 30% of breast cancers, led the first randomized clinical study of the drug in metastatic breast cancer, publishing it in the New England Journal of Medicine [2]. The findings demonstrated that Trastuzumab, along with chemotherapy, could significantly extend the life of patients with HER2-positive metastatic breast cancer compared with traditional chemotherapy. He had the idea that tumors should be classified according to their genetic profile, rather than according to the organ where they originated. He instilled in the oncologists at Vall d'Hebron the need to become more professional, to work with more rigor and less resignation, all with a high level of demand. He transformed the center, turning it into one of the best in Europe, a prestige that has been growing ever since with Dr. J. Tabernero. From the UITM (Research Unit of Molecular Therapies "La Caixa" at Vall d'Hebron), created in 2007, 7800 patients have been investigated in those years in successive trials of drugs in advanced development. Many of these studies were phase I and II, experimental treatments for which neither the efficacy of the drugs, many of them monoclonal antibodies, nor the side effects were known. Thirty of these studies have been used as new clinical treatments against cancer (Fig. 40.2).

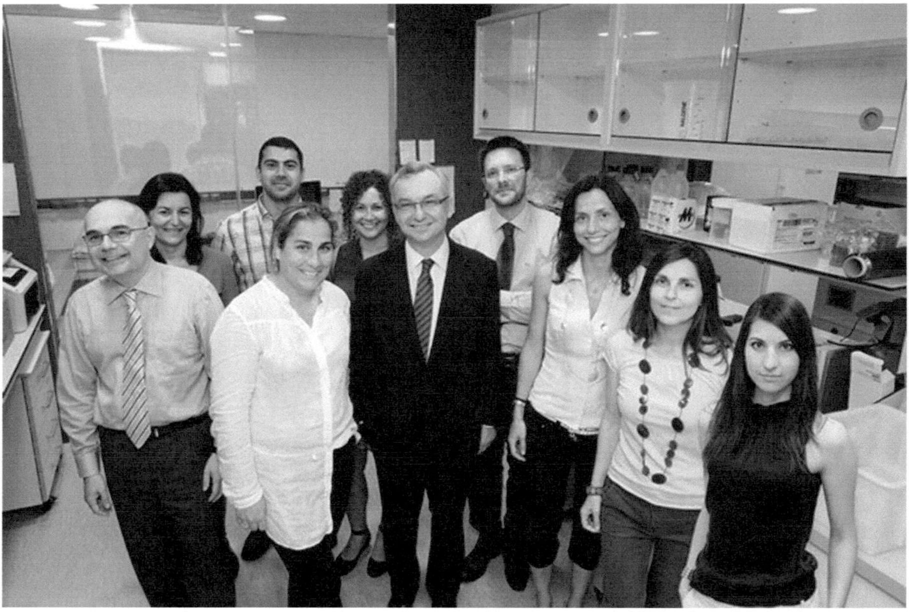

Fig. 40.2 Dr. J. Baselga visiting Dr. J. Tabernero (on the left) and colleagues at the VHIO. (Permission VHIO)

Again to United States

In March 2010, because of his scientific career and prestige, he was appointed head of the Division of Hematology and Oncology at the General Hospital of Massachusetts (the Mass General) in Boston, where he continued his great ambition in basic and clinical research at an accelerated pace, as an oncologist focused on the development of new drugs targeting specific molecules in breast cancer, and their use in clinical treatments, which was a revolution in the treatment of these tumors.

At Mass General, Josep Baselga remained a key figure in the clinical development of monoclonal antibodies, which included drugs such as Cetuximab, Pertuzumab, Olaparib and Lapatinib. As with Trastuzumab, Baselga had to convince the pharmaceutical industry to move forward with these drugs in clinical trials. Antoni Ribas, Professor of Medicine at UCLA, in a conversation with Josep Corbella, told him about Baselga: *"He was a pioneer in understanding the clinical implications of basic science. This led him to lead the development of a new generation of treatments." "Baselga saw the future before it happened."* Among the many studies carried out during this stage, the Cleopatra multicenter study, published in 2012, stands out for its importance. The action of Pertuzumab was considered very similar to that of Trastuzumab, although both were known to act on the HER2 receptor in a complementary manner.

> The HER2 receptor is located on the outside of the cell membrane. When activated, by binding to another receptor (HER2 or HER3, forming a dimer), it signals the cell to divide. Trastuzumab blocks the HER2-HER2 interaction, while Pertuzumab blocks the HER2-HER3 interaction.

In this study published in 2012 [3], both drugs were used together with great efficacy, publishing the results of that study, conducted while he was still at Mass General, on 800 patients (N Engl J Med. 2012.) The study, in clinical phase, was randomized, doubleblind and placebo-controlled, and was signed as principal investigator by José Baselga.

The study, funded by F. Hoffmann-La Roche/Genentech, concluded that the combination of Pertuzumab, Trastuzumab and Docetaxel, compared with placebo, when used as treatment for HER2-positive metastatic breast cancer, significantly prolonged progression-free survival, without an increase in cardiac toxic effects.

To New York: The Memorial

His prestige was growing, and, in 2013, he was appointed Physician-in-Chief at Memorial Sloan Kettering Hospital and Professor of Medicine at Weill Cornell Medical College in New York, probably the most important cancer hospital in the world. He was also president of the American Association for Cancer Research and editor of the journal *Cancer Discovery*. Although the decision to change was difficult at first, he was confident in his choice because, although the Mass General was intellectually stimulating, the position of medical director at Memorial represented a major influence in the world of medical oncology. He continued to work and mentor many oncologists by his influence and authority, investigating and treating breast cancer patients with clinical treatments supported by evidence from randomized studies, while evaluating new experimental monoclonal drugs, alone or in combination with others, targeting the various cancer cell-specific molecules [4].

He easily obtained external financing for all its projects (*):

-How it? -I asked, "How do you get everyone to finance you? - You have to put yourself in the shoes of the people you are asking to donate money," he told

J. Corbella. Understand how they think and what motivates them and make them see that their donations will be useful. I thought human beings are naturally generous. His research focus extended to many fields in oncology, such as the study of drug resistance in some cancers, as well as toxicity complications (especially cardiac) caused by these treatments. He also studied drugs that could target tumors derived from the PI3K mutation, as well as treatments with the same monoclonal drugs in patients with non-metastatic breast cancer who had undergone surgery (early breast cancer). Dr. Baselga was also selected as one of the principal investigators of the Stand Up to Cancer "Dream Team" to lead PI3K pathway research in breast cancers.

A "Dream Team" is a scientific task force, a collaboration of top researchers from different institutions who come together to develop new approaches to a specific cancer. By combining their knowledge and resources and working together toward common goals, they are able to move faster and bring therapies and treatments from the laboratory to industry, thus benefiting patients.

2017 was a very productive year in terms of his publications in scientific journals, collaborating on 54 articles. In a review article published that year, entitled "Advances in the management of HER2 positive early breast cancer" in Crit Rev Oncol Hematol [5], they summarized it this way:

HER2-targeted therapy has transformed the prognosis for both early and metastatic HER2-positive breast cancer, beginning with trastuzumab and continuing with the development of several novel HER2-targeting agents. The biology of HER2-positive breast cancer is complex, with multiple interactions between signaling pathways. These interactions promote resistance to trastuzumab and may affect the chances of successful treatment, but also offer opportunities for new approaches to treating HER2-positive disease. Newly developed agents and treatment strategies, such as the combination of pertuzumab and trastuzumab, as well as extended HER2 inhibition with trastuzumab followed by neratinib, have further improved the results seen with trastuzumab, reducing the relapse rate in HER2-positive early breast cancer. With the introduction of any new therapy or regimen, it is critical to pay careful attention to the risks versus benefits of therapy. When a novel treatment approach offers a significant improvement over current standards, some additional toxicity may be tolerated. Without however, we must ensure that these advances do not significantly affect the patient's quality of life. Attention to patient education, prophylaxis against adverse events and proactive management is essential to minimize any unwanted effects associated with HER2-targeted therapy."

At the end of the article, the author clearly elaborates on their conflict-of-interest statement, fully clarifying any possible controversy on the matter." Medical journals, although they ask many questions on this subject, do not require that the amounts received from the industry for the grant or for the advice be specified. However, it is essential and mandatory to clearly inform the hospital and the university where you work about these matters.

News in the New York Times

On September 8, 2018, the New York Times published on its front page, "Top Cancer Researcher Fails to Disclose Financial Ties to Industry in Top Scientific Journals" [6]. The story, published in collaboration with the nonprofit journalistic organization ProPublica, revealed that he had failed to make public in his publications, in prestigious journals such as The New England Journal of Medicine and The Lancet, payments in the millions of dollars received from medical and pharmaceutical companies in exchange for his studies and results. The conflict arose with about sixty scientific articles published under his name between 2013 and 2017. The article mentioned that, at a scientific meeting that same year, he had presented two clinical trials sponsored by the Roche company, the results of which many attendees did not consider positive, without disclosing his relationship with Roche. Since 2014, he had received more than $3 million in consulting fees and for his involvement in a company that was acquired. The news was shocking; readers might think he put his profit motive before his duty as a physician. Although the story did not speak corruption, readers would come to that conclusion on their own. The article made an important ethical point: "Ethicists are concerned that external links may condition how studies are designed and how medications are prescribed to patients". Regarding the three million dollars mentioned, it was eventually discovered that they were not payments from the industry to modify or alter protocols or results, but came from the sale of a company (Seragon) to Roche. Dr. Baselga had advised this company, which had paid him in stock. When this company was sold to Roche, the sale of those shares generated the three million dollars. Later, Forbes magazine would denounce the flaws and manipulation of the New York Times article, but it was too late. It seemed like revenge, but by whom? How was it possible that such a person could be the medical director of a hospital? like the Memorial? Social networks caught fire and many people who knew nothing about him sank him. Four days after the news broke, he had to resign. It was the worst experience of his life, a revenge that sank his academic career. One can speculate as to who could have moved this news. When you work and are responsible, not only in your hospital as medical director, but also with your great influence in the world of oncology, you make supporters, but also enemies, who are disadvantaged in their own careers. (*) José Baselga, as Jean Charles Soria, who worked a lot with him, used to say, was like St. Paul: if you shared his vision, you counted on him. It was nothing personal, but did not stray from his path. He probably left some victims along the way. If I had to investigate who threw the stone and hid the hand, that's where I would start looking. The people who had worked with him could not explain it to themselves. The news did not represent at all the doctor they knew, who was always at the side of the patients. It was disproportionate, too hard for a person who had given so much. He had a very hard time; it left a deep impression on him. Trying to reason his response to the New York Times, Baselga analyzed the 178 publications in which he had collaborated in some way, sometimes as lead author, and of those, only in 17 should he have disclosed his conflicts of interest, and he didn't. Why not? He had nothing to lose by being transparent, which is what he had always advocated. It would have been the right thing to do (*). Josep Corbella clarifies: he was never interested in the small print. He thought big, was impatient and was bothered by minor details. When you publish so much and you also have a very complicated agenda, you don't write the articles personally, even if you supervise them, especially the results. Conflict of interest statements usually always come at the end, sometimes days later, and you don't give them the importance they should have. You never thought this could destroy you. His scientific papers have been reviewed again and none of them have been retracted in their conclusions. The methodology is correct and the results are valid. Due to the controversy caused by this news, on Thursday, September 13, 2018, Baselga in resigning from his position at the Memorial, expressed concern that "keeping me in office with these allegations would all become too much of a distraction for the hospital and its remarkable team of physicians, researchers and staff." Dr. Baselga also took "full responsibility for failing to make appropriate notifications in scientific and medical journals and at professional meetings." He noted that he had already "updated his conflicts of interest in successive medical journals and will continue to do so until the record is complete." In addition, he stated that his involvement in pharmaceutical companies. and biotechnology, as well as its consulting activities, had been public and were reported and reviewed by Memorial Sloan Kettering.

Recruited BY AstraZeneca

In January 2019, three months later, he was recruited due to his prestige and scientific rigor, as well as his innovative vision for the future of cancer treatment, by the pharmaceutical company AstraZeneca as head of R&D (research and development) in oncology, where he worked until his death [7]. During this time, he first led this company's partnership with the Japanese pharmaceutical company Daiichi Sankyo to develop a new cancer treatment, Trastuzumab Deruxtecan (T- DXd), an antibody-drug conjugate that appeared to be very aggressive against tumor cells that have HER2 receptors, helping to selectively destroy these cells. Once again, as on previous occasions, a company, in this case AstraZeneca, hesitated to make decisions on a drug that initially seemed aggressive. The company initially decided not to partner with the Japanese company until Baselga, studying the drug from another perspective, convinced them to do so. T-DXd has been shown to be an effective drug in patients with metastatic breast cancer disease with a high level of HER2. It has also been shown to be effective in breast cancer with low HER2 expression. In addition, other studies have been initiated with the use of this drug for the treatment of other cancers expressing HER2- such as some lung, stomach and colorectal cancers. These studies are currently underway. Later, during the COVID-19 pandemic, AstraZeneca developed one of the most promising vaccines against the SARS-CoV-2 virus. After many ups and downs, in late December the first clinical trial results were positive, and in January 2021 it was licensed by the European Union for use.

On his passing in March 2021, Josep Corbella wrote: "Josep Baselga, a key figure in the progress of oncology in Spain since the 1990s and in the development of molecular therapies that have saved thousands of lives worldwide, has died at the age of 61 victim of Creutzfeldt- Jakob disease, a rapidly progressive degenerative neurological disorder. His motto was that" research breakthroughs must reach patients as soon as possible. "Over a career spanning more than 30 years, he succeeded in translating an ever-deepening understanding of the molecular mechanisms of cancer into clinical advances that have improved the treatment of multiple tumor types."

Dave Fredrickson, head of AstraZeneca's business area, wrote a farewell letter to José (as he was called in the USA and signed his articles) after his death: "Thank you, José. You have taught me to think more about patients, reminding me that there is no cancer that is easy to treat, that rare cancers are not so rare, and that the side effects are not minor if you are the one suffering from them. José, you are not perfect (you would laugh at this). You empathetically

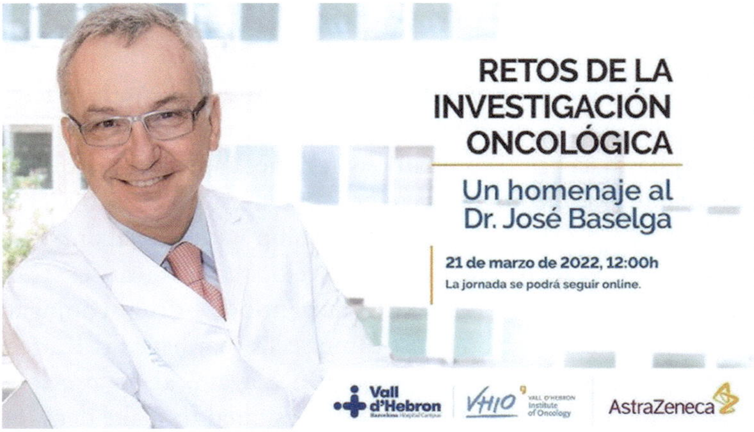
RETOS DE LA
INVESTIGACIÓN
ONCOLÓGICA
Un homenaje al
Dr. José Baselga
21 de marzo de 2022, 12:00h
La jornada se podrá seguir online.
Vall d'Hebron
VHIO
AstraZeneca

Fig. 40.3 Challenges in Oncological Research. Tribute to Dr. José Baselga in the VHIO (Vall d'Hebron Institute of Oncology), March 2022. (Permission VHIO)

acknowledge with empathy when you have made a mistake and work to adapt when you feel you need to change. You push me to be more ambitious, daring and creative. You always encourage me with urgency. You never settle for good enough. Sometimes you exhaust me with your insistence, but because of it we achieve greater clarity, and you know how to bring out the best in me, yourself and our teams. You make all of us better." (Fig. 40.3)

José Baselga has been, due to his drive and intellectual recognition, one of the most fascinating oncologists in the world in the last thirty years. His studies and treatments, based on tumor cell biology and the use of monoclonal antibodies and selective tyrosine kinase inhibitors against tumor cells, especially in breast cancer, have had a worldwide scope. He has contributed to change the paradigm about breast cancer and other types of cancer, confirming the idea that cancer can be cured and chronified. He was a role model for many, many oncologists and, despite being involved in a conflict unrelated to his career as a scientific oncologist, he recovered and was rehired by a major pharmaceutical company, where he once again excelled, tragically passing away due to a rare disease in 2021, at the age of 61.

(*) quotes from the book "Baselga, el médico que quería cambiar el mundo", Josep Corbella, author (cited in the references).

Awards

During his professional career, he received numerous awards, among which are:

- 1994–1997 Career Development Award. American Society of Clinical Oncology (ASCO).
- 2005 Annual Award. European Society of Medical Oncology (ESMO).
- 2008 American Association for Cancer Research (AACR)- Trueta Medal and International Prize of Catalonia.

He also served as president of the European Society for Medical Oncology (ESMO) and the American Association for Cancer Research (AACR).

References

1. Corbella J. Baselga, the doctor who wanted to change the world. Barcelona: Editorial Navona SL; 2022.
2. Slamon DJ, Leyland-Jones B, Shak S, et al. Use of chemotherapy plus a monoclonal antibody against HER2 for metastatic breast cancer that overexpresses HER2. N Engl J Med. 2001;344:783–92.
3. Baselga J, Cortés J, Kim S-B, et al. Pertuzumab plus Trastuzumab plus Docetaxel for Metastatic Breast Cancer. N Engl J Med. 2012;366:109–19.
4. Swain SM, Baselga J, Kim S-B, et al. Pertuzumab, Trastuzumab, and docetaxel in HER2- positive metastatic breast cancer. N Engl J Med. 2015;372:724–34.
5. Baselga J, Coleman RE, Cortés J, Janni W. Advances in the management of HER2 positive early breast cancer. Crit Rev Oncol Hematol. 2017;119:113–22.
6. Top cancer researcher fails to disclose corporate financial ties in major research journals. The New York Times, Charles Ornstein and Katie Thomas, 8/09/2018.
7. AstraZeneca signs Spaniard Baselga as global head of cancer R&D. Cinco días newspaper. Accessed March 7, 2019. 11.

41

Highlights of the Spanish Healthcare System: Primary Care and Its Community Dimension Within NHS

Juan José Rodríguez Sendín

Introduction and Background (Fig. 41.1)

Following the decisive impetus that the World Health Organization (WHO) gave to Primary Health Care (PHC) at the Alma-Ata Conference in 1978, some influential health systems around the world—such as those of the United States and Germany—questioned the social and economic effectiveness and cost-efficiency of models based on a strong PHC approach. In Spain, PHC had always been present, although with a model different from the current one, which began to take shape in the 1980s by incorporating the principles set forth in Alma-Ata, specifically through Royal Decree 137/1983 on Basic Health Structures (Estructuras Básicas de Salud, EBS). General Medicine was transformed into the specialty of Family and Community Medicine (Medicina Familiar y Comunitaria, MFC), and the first Primary Care Teams (Equipos de Atención Primaria, EAP) and Health Centers (Centros de Salud, CS) were established [1, 2].

Today, it is widely acknowledged that the difference in quality, effectiveness, and efficiency among health systems is largely determined by the strength

J. J. R. Sendín (✉)
Family Medicine and Communitarian Medicine, General Council of the College of Physicians of Spain (CGCOM), National Commission of Deontological Ethics (CGCOM), Madrid, Spain

M. A. Cuesta, F. Mateo Vallejo (eds.), *Spain's Journey in Medicine*,
https://doi.org/10.1007/978-3-032-12221-6_41

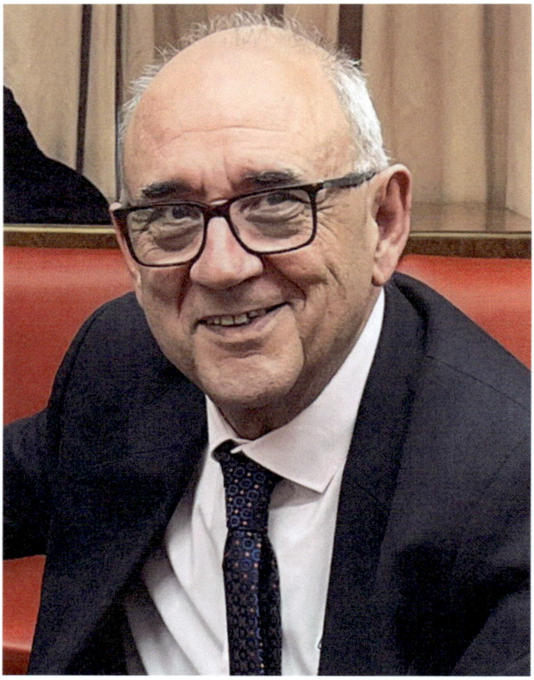

Fig. 41.1 Juan José Rodríguez Sendín

of their PHC models. A seminal study by Barbara Starfield of Johns Hopkins University, Baltimore, United States, documented the state of primary care worldwide in a book. In her view, population health depends directly on the general practitioner, as this is the only professional who focuses on the person rather than solely on the disease[3].

PHC has evolved differently across European countries, not only in terms of organizational design but also regarding financing models, service delivery, and development strategies. The establishment of EAPs—comprising administrative staff, nurses, social workers, pediatricians, and family physicians—has created a socio-healthcare framework which, when properly managed, operates on the basis of shared values and commitment, achieving excellent health outcomes, high user satisfaction, and significantly lower costs compared to other models.

The reform of PHC (RAPS, Reforma de la Atención Primaria de Salud) refers to an evolutionary process aimed at adapting structures and resources to contemporary needs as a necessary response to an initially deficient situation. The current state of PHC is the result of political, administrative, and labor-related changes, as well as an expansion of social protection, but it has not emerged from a long-term, systematically planned process with clearly defined objectives and resources allocated to achieve them.

Current Situation of Primary Care in Spain

Primary Health Care (PHC) in Spain constitutes a fundamental epidemiological framework, responsible for addressing the health needs of the individual and of that primary socializing unit—the family—and the environment in which it lives. It operates by adapting to the social and health realities of the communities it serves, with which its professionals must, or should, coexist, understand, and ultimately become experts in. This continuity and longitudinally of care throughout the life of the individual, their family, and their community environment cannot be provided by hospitals. Consequently, PHC and its professionals play an essential role not only in clinical care but also in the broader health and social spheres, with significant implications for the protection of the rights and needs previously mentioned. Many of the persistent challenges faced by the Spanish National Health System (SNS) require the intervention of PHC.

During the first decade of the twenty-first century, numerous voices emerged denouncing what was perceived as a barrier to the development of PHC, as the dangerous deterioration of working conditions and the decline in investment became evident. Increasing bureaucratization consumed the time available for direct patient care, and professionals struggled to understand—let alone justify—the reasons behind the system's visible decline. In response, a framework for discussion and planning was established: the Strategic Framework for the Improvement of Primary Health Care in Spain 2007–2012 (AP21). This framework outlined 44 strategies aimed at addressing and providing concrete solutions to the deficiencies and challenges identified. However, the economic crisis—accompanied by a parallel crisis of values—ultimately undermined the strategy and further exacerbated the very problems it sought to resolve [4, 5].

Public spending cuts severely and indiscriminately affected the health sector, with particularly profound consequences for PHC human resources. The austerity measures implemented between 2008 and 2015, which reduced healthcare expenditure from 6.9% of GDP in 2008 to 5.9% in 2015, had a direct impact on staffing levels and working conditions, the renewal of medical technology, and—most critically—PHC budgets and workforce availability. Positions were eliminated, vacancies went unfilled, and precarious working conditions were imposed, as later recognized by a ruling of the Court of Justice of the European Union (September 15, 2016).

These cuts were accompanied by a rise in prescription drug units and an inability to contain hospital pharmaceutical expenditure, largely driven by the exorbitant cost of new medications. The increase in drug spending effectively displaced other budgetary lines: while medication invoices must be paid, professional staffing and technological renewal were neglected. Under conditions of job insecurity, lack of continuity, and excessive workloads, physicians cannot provide patients with adequate consultation time; what can be offered instead are prescriptions and diagnostic tests. Under such circumstances, it is impossible to maintain high-quality services or ensure that the right care is delivered appropriately.

To speak of PHC within the SNS is to speak of solidarity, justice, and excellence; it is a way of conceptualizing public health services and understanding civic relationships based on equality. It implies prioritizing obligations toward the patient above other values—such as financial considerations—and addressing citizens' health needs even when they lack the means to afford care. Discussing the SNS and PHC is, fundamentally, to speak of deep respect for the dignity of every human needing assistance, of professional integrity and optimal working conditions, and of the tireless defense of these values by healthcare professionals. For this reason, and despite the damage caused by indiscriminate austerity measures and recent health policies, public opinion regarding the SNS remains generally positive—particularly in relation to PHC.

The Primary Care Professional

Between 80% and 90% of the health problems commonly presented by the population can be effectively and efficiently resolved within Primary Health Care (PHC), at a lower cost and with fewer risks for the patient than in even the most well-equipped hospital centers. To achieve this, patients require good accessibility and continuous follow-up by an accessible physician, freely chosen, who—regardless of the additional health services that may be required from other professionals—can guarantee initial care and diagnostic guidance, continuity of care over time, and a comprehensive, integrative perspective that should not be interrupted, not even at the threshold of a hospital.

In general, the population perceives their PHC physician and nurse as their primary advisors—not only regarding health matters but also in other areas of life. People desire a physician who is reliable, trustworthy, stable, easily accessible, and professionally competent; one who can understand and assess the patient's needs, provide timely and individualized responses, and, at the same time, maintain up-to-date and sufficient knowledge. Such a physician must be able, from a position of professional autonomy, to recognize when external assistance is required, to safeguard their patients and the population, and to guide them against potential excesses or unnecessary interventions related to their health or family environment.

The societal need for PHC professionals has been, and will continue to be, a key factor in the development of primary care and will shape its future according to what it is capable of offering and returning to the society it serves. In PHC, daily clinical practice is defined largely by the chronic patient—those with comorbidities and multiple conditions. Additionally, it now includes survivors of serious illnesses that were once fatal, such as cancer, cardiovascular disease, and HIV/AIDS, as well as highly vulnerable chronic patients who require many years of continuous health care.

The central question is not whether solutions to major health and social care challenges lie in one professional qualification or another, nor whether specialist X or specialist Y holds the answer. Rather, it is about determining who best responds to what society and each citizen truly need: what care, how it should be provided, where, and when. PHC must be able to offer and guarantee the necessary care to meet these expectations.

Global and Integrated Health Management

Every activity or organizational structure ultimately exists to fulfill a specific function that defines its very nature. The comprehensive and integrated management of health constitutes the essence of Primary Health Care (PHC). This nature, along with the obligations it entails, defines the professional role and provides the fundamental rationale for its existence. Although the central focus of healthcare is the individual—treating disease, alleviating suffering, and reducing disability—the overarching goal of the National Health System (SNS) is to promote and improve the health of the population. This population-based mission represents the community dimension of healthcare, a responsibility largely entrusted to and historically assumed by PHC.

PHC is defined by globality, continuity of care, and accessibility. *Globality* involves a comprehensive, integrated approach to all aspects of an individual's health (transversality) throughout the life course—from birth to death (longitudinally)—including the individual, their family, and the community in which they live. This approach encompasses biological, emotional, and social dimensions, considering personal and family life events, ways of living, and individual concerns, while ensuring continuity, accessibility, and personalized attention. PHC activity is provided wherever the healthcare need arises—most often in clinics, urgent care, or the patient's home. Home visits, in particular, represent a unique opportunity to observe and assess the circumstances and environment in which the patient lives. For the clinician, entering a patient's home is not only a professional privilege but also a valuable source of insight, granting access to the intimate realities of the patient and their family.

Globality also implies coordinated care across all members of the Primary Care Team (Equipo de Atención Primaria, EAP), collaboration with patients and communities, and integration with other services and sectors. Owing to the longitudinal nature of their practice, PHC professionals must understand the communities they serve and the social determinants of health within them, becoming de facto experts in the social and community context in which they work. They must manage their time efficiently, organize their activities, and coordinate with the rest of the healthcare team. Their primary concerns evolve dynamically in response to societal changes and emerging health problems. They play a key role in protecting patients from false promises of cure, overdiagnosis, excessive medicalization of life, health-related sectarian practices, and pseudoscientific interventions—educating relentlessly on the dangers of unnecessary medication use.

The continuity of care—maintaining the same physician over extended periods—enables closer, more personalized relationships. Such continuity allows the physician to know the patient thoroughly, having diagnosed, treated, and followed them over time. This facilitates more accurate diagnoses, more effective treatments, and reduced risks of drug interactions or adverse effects. It also enables earlier problem detection, more efficient consultations, and reduces unnecessary testing and specialist referrals, which are more common when the physician has little prior knowledge of the patient. Continuity over time in primary care has been linked to reduced mortality, fewer low-birth-weight infants, higher vaccination coverage, and improved appropriateness of specialist referrals.

Mental health care for both individuals and communities acquires particular relevance within Family and Community Medicine (MFC) and PHC, as it addresses conditions and circumstances that cause profound suffering and carry significant social impact—reflecting the tensions and pressures of contemporary society. Dissatisfaction, anxiety, depression, anguish, and fear are frequent. Detecting these conditions is not always straightforward, as they rarely present in isolation and are often intertwined with socioeconomic, cultural, and biological factors. No one should underestimate the cultural, economic, and even political components involved in the genesis of mental illness—components that PHC must address to the extent possible. The help required by patients and their families can only be provided by a trusted physician—one who is their first and last point of contact for all matters concerning their health and that of their family, and who has accompanied them through much of their life.

In summary, the integrated management of health is a fundamental objective of PHC and its professionals. Within the SNS, PHC constitutes an essential instrument for fulfilling the constitutional right to health protection. The SNS requires a well-resourced PHC, with sufficient human and technological capacity to meet the healthcare needs of 80–90% of the population's demands. It also requires general hospitals with robust teaching, research, and clinical care capabilities for all citizens in their health area; a comprehensive and well-distributed emergency and urgent care network; and specialized high-complexity units such as those for transplants, severe burns, and spinal cord injuries. Without all these components—or by neglecting and underfunding the complex networks that sustain them—it is impossible to build an excellent health system in Spain. Abandoning these foundational structures, or denying them effective governance and management tools, poses a serious risk to citizens' interests, professional development, and the core values of modern, socially oriented medicine.

The Speciality of Family and Community Medicine

For decades, numerous authors—albeit with slight variations—have defined the competencies required for the practice of medicine in Primary Health Care (PHC), where understanding the social, economic, and health context of the served community is of paramount importance.

Every professional is expected to possess the training, attitude, and commitment that will make them a healthcare provider capable of serving the world. This requires interdependent learning and education grounded in critical reasoning and an ethical conduct sustained by the core values of professionalism. PHC is responsible for caring for individuals, their families, and the environments in which they live, doing so before, during, and after the onset of illness, without any other condition or prerequisite.

Within Family and Community Medicine (MFC) practice, clinical, diagnostic, and therapeutic challenges rarely occur in isolation. They are embedded in a multidisciplinary context and shaped by economic, social, and cultural determinants that also frame the accompanying organic conditions. PHC remains the discipline best positioned to monitor and manage clinical and epidemiological information. This reality requires that PHC professionals operate within a healthcare system that grants them full autonomy, enabling their work to be both more effective and qualitatively more meaningful.

PHC itself must drive the changes that affect it—its educational and scientific initiatives, its institutional participation, and its capacity to influence the policies and factors that shape its practice. However, since PHC is not fully integrated as a core discipline in undergraduate medical education, future physicians are unlikely to choose what they do not know. As Dr. Ciril Rozman once reflected—an opinion still relevant today and often cited when advocating for stronger PHC recognition:

> *"I was fortunate to receive a generalist education. Those who currently edit an Internal Medicine textbook cannot compete with a primary care physician (...) I have never ceased to be a general practitioner, and I do not know how I will leave this message behind when I am gone."*

Barbara Starfield, in the aforementioned seminal book *The Situation of Primary Care in the World*, argued that the health of the population depends directly on primary care physicians, as they are the only professionals who focus on the person rather than the disease. She also observed that in societies with a strong primary care system, the main beneficiaries are children, even more so than adults. Perhaps even more noteworthy is that, according to the conclusions of her study, Spanish Primary Care ranked fifth worldwide—alongside Denmark and ahead of leading nations such as Canada, Australia, and Sweden, and notably outperforming Germany, Belgium, and the United States, which Starfield classified as having "poor" primary care models.

The Future of Primary Care

The objectives of the National Health System (SNS), Primary Health Care (PHC), and Family and Community Medicine (MFC) must never be confused or distorted, lest their origins and fundamental principles be forgotten. If the services provided by the SNS and its professionals were to shift away from patient-centered care and instead become instruments aimed primarily at maximizing economic outcomes at the expense of health, we could no longer speak of true PHC or MFC. Both have clearly defined purposes and competencies that would be lost if health promotion and the provision of high-quality care to all individuals—regardless of their social or economic status—were abandoned. Such a deviation would directly contradict the very model of the SNS that Spain has established for itself.

Multiple studies have demonstrated the close relationship between patient safety and the quality of care, highlighting how both overuse and underuse of services can severely undermine clinical practice and compromise patient safety. Determinants of quality include patient-centeredness, safety of the care environment, accessibility, appropriateness, continuity, efficacy, effectiveness, efficiency, and timeliness of care—precisely the core attributes that define the essence of PHC and MFC.

The typical patient seen today within the SNS is increasingly chronic, polymedicated, elderly, fragile, and economically vulnerable. Such individuals require physicians who are trustworthy, well-trained, stable, easily accessible, and capable of providing individually tailored responses. At the same time, these physicians must possess sufficient and up-to-date knowledge to practice with professional autonomy, safeguard their patients and communities, and guide them against potential excesses or unnecessary interventions.

End-of-life care holds particular relevance within PHC. When patients approach the end of life or when cure is no longer a realistic expectation, they have the right to receive comprehensive, active, and continuous care aimed at maximizing their quality of life, rather than prolonging survival at any cost. This care must address the physical, psychological, social, and spiritual needs of both the patient and their family, while respecting their wishes and preferences.

Final Considerations

To renew the prestige and effectiveness it once achieved, as a model for many other Health systems in the world, Primary Health Care (PHC) requires an innovative, dynamic, and scientifically grounded orientation, with clear accountability and a continuous pursuit of the best responses to both individual and collective health needs. Its quality must be embedded within a professional doctrine whose ultimate goal is to serve and satisfy those it exists to help.

PHC urgently needs a new impetus to reaffirm and revitalize the National Health System (SNS) and its fundamental principles. It is essential to provide PHC with modernization, transparency, and adequate funding to meet the expectations and responsibilities assigned to it by society. This renewal must include a selective and purpose-driven increase in budgetary resources.

Moreover, the SNS requires a third wave of decentralization, transferring management and decision-making power closer to the service level and care delivery points—a move that, in the case of PHC, represents a commitment to shared responsibility for the future.

Spanish PHC needs a genuine, selective, and immediate action plan that is reliable, financially explicit, and publicly committed. Faced with growing fragmentation of service provision and increasing complexity of demand, the SNS must restore PHC to its role as the foundational and distinctive element of the health system.

References

1. WHO. Alma Ata Conference, 1978.
2. Ministerial Order of 19 December 1983 to "Regulate the development of training in Primary Health Care in the speciality of Family and Community Medicine" (BOE 23 December 1983).
3. Starfield B. Primary care: concept, evaluation and policy. Oxford University. Press Inc.; 1992.
4. Gómez Asorey C, Palacios Castaño JA. Situation and development of general medicine and the speciality of family and community medicine in Spain. UD1 distance training and refresher course in general and family medicine. 1st part. WTO-FSE Madrid; 2000.
5. National Commission for the Speciality of Family and Community Medicine. Official programme of the speciality of family and community medicine. Madrid: Ministry of Health and Consumer Affairs; 2005.

42

From Rodés to Llovet. The Road to Excellence in Hepatology

Roger Corcho

Joan Rodés

Cars are manufactured in Barcelona, but above all, livers are researched. Institutions such as Hospital Clínic de Barcelona, Hospital Vall d'Hebron or the University of Barcelona lead cutting-edge research with international projection in this field. Their physicians and researchers have been recognized and awarded worldwide and their publications are among the most cited by the scientific community. Medical care in liver diseases is also at the forefront, with centers capable of offering the most advanced therapies. "We can now offer our patients the same opportunities, in the diagnostic and therapeutic field, as those that can be offered in the best place in the civilized world" [1] stated Professor of Medicine Miquel Bruguera in an article published in 2013. Barcelona has established itself as one of the world capitals of Hepatology. This scenario was unthinkable in 1968, when Dr. Joan Rodés inaugurated the first Hepatology Unit in Spain at the Hospital Clínic. Although at that time the delay in the treatment of liver diseases was considerable in comparison with Europe or the United States, from then on everything began to change. By the end of the twentieth century, Hospital Clínic had already established itself as a reference center both research and medical care, a position it has maintained to the day (Fig. 42.1).

R. Corcho (✉)
Philosopher, and Science Popularizer, Barcelona, Spain

M. A. Cuesta, F. Mateo Vallejo (eds.), *Spain's Journey in Medicine*,
https://doi.org/10.1007/978-3-032-12221-6_42

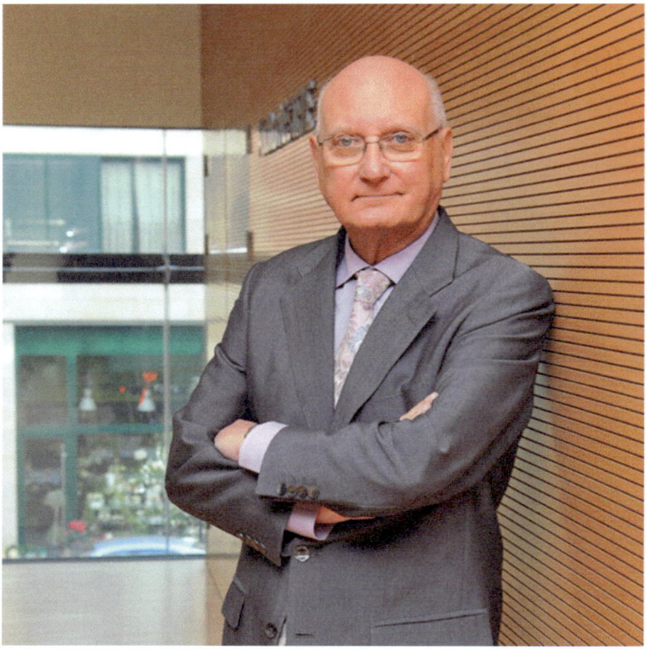

Fig. 42.1 Joan Rodés Teixidor. (Permission Clinic Hospital, Barcelona)

Numerous physicians and scientists have participated in this transformation, but there is consensus in highlighting the role of Joan Rodés in the creation of research institutions, his involvement in obtaining funding, and above all his ability to instill a rigorous and committed way of working. His achievements also include the creation, in 1996, of the Institut d'Investigacions Biomèdiques August Pi i Sunyer (IDIBAPS), a center linked to the Hospital Clínic that integrates the research work of the University of Barcelona and also has the support of the Consejo Superior de Investigaciones Científicas (CSIC). Doctors who worked with Rodés agree in highlighting his unwavering commitment to science, a requirement that he transmitted to all his collaborators. The epidemiologist Pedro Alonso, for example, recalls that, when he was hired, Rodés said to him: "You will be judged by the quality of your work and your research, and I don't care if it is on malaria, mosquitoes or whatever". He was a man who was clear in that the specialty should be professionalized, and he knew how to do it. At the meetings of the Spanish Association for the Study of the Liver, he proposed in 1985 that they should be held annually—so that contacts between specialists could be intensified—and that they should always take place in Madrid, in order to facilitate access to all participants and to avoid the temptation to organize itinerant meetings for tourist purposes [2]. With these decisions, he marked the path to excellence.

Clinical Research

Perhaps Rodés' most important contribution is related to his understanding of scientific progress. From the outset, it was clear to him that treating liver patients would be the driving force behind research, and that this, in turn, would contribute to improving the treatments available. This was a virtuous circle that Dr. Llovet also emphasized in an article: "to ensure that healthcare activity would allow the development of clinical research at the highest level so that, at the same time, it would have an impact on the quality of the healthcare activity itself" [3]. Only from the first line of care can it be observed that same treatment has very different outcomes depending on the patient. It is then that the different variables that influence the evolution of a disease can be identified. Even if a therapy has been effective in the laboratory, its true usefulness can only be gauged when it is tested on real patients in clinical trials. On the other hand, the most widespread conception among scientists and physicians is to consider patients as passive elements who simply benefited from the advances achieved in the laboratory, without playing any other role in the progress of knowledge. For Rodés, this model was based on "a great misunderstanding about the sources of scientific knowledge" that was contributing to a widening gap "between research and practice, between knowledge and utility, between knowing and doing". As he defended in the article *"The forgotten clinical research"* -signed together with other colleagues-, "practice itself (clinical and experimental clinical experience) is an unquestionable source of knowledge". Specific circumstances have a decisive influence on patients, but it is precisely these variables that tend to be neutralized in controlled laboratory settings. For this reason, Rodés argued that developing the best therapies necessarily requires the active involvement of patients. The following reflection summarizes his point of view: "Attentive clinical observation, curiosity, critical scientific thinking and the will to resolve questions, together with the desire to improve the condition of patients and the service offered, remain basic elements of research and scientific and medical progress" [4]. A medical innovation tested in the laboratory does not in itself represent an advance in knowledge. Progress can only be assured when it is possible to quantify real and beneficial effects on patients. Without clinical trials, any hope placed in a newly applied therapy must be held in abeyance until it confronted with clinical reality. Several generations of scientists have been able to develop fruitful careers with results and international projection thanks to the use the infrastructure and teachings that Dr. Rodés promoted. The contributions to the treatment of hepatocellular carcinoma (HCC) have been especially notable, and among those who have excelled most in this field is Dr. Josep Maria Llovet.

Dr. Llovet Against Hepatocellular Carcinoma

Josep M. Llovet is Director of the Liver Cancer Program and Professor of Medicine (Division of Liver Diseases) at the Icahn School of Medicine at Mount Sinai Hospital in New York (Fig. 42.2). He is also Professor of Medicine-Liver Oncology at the University of Barcelona and ICREA (Catalan Institution for Research and Advanced Studies), and at IDIBAPS-Hospital Clínic de Barcelona. He was the founder and president of the International Liver Cancer Association and contributed to the development of more than ten clinical guidelines and clinical trial design related to clinical management of liver cancer. He was coordinator of the 2012 Clinical Practice Guidelines of the European Association for the Study of Liver Diseases (EASL), president of the Hepatobiliary Neoplasia Special Interest Group of the American Association for the Study of Liver Diseases and a member of the EASL Education Committee. He has published more than 345 articles in peer-reviewed journals (with more than 145,000 citations), more than 55 book chapters and has given more than 675 lectures. He is editor-in-chief of JHEP Reports and associate/senior editor of the Journal of Hepatology and Clinical Cancer Research. Llovet has been one of the most highly cited researchers in

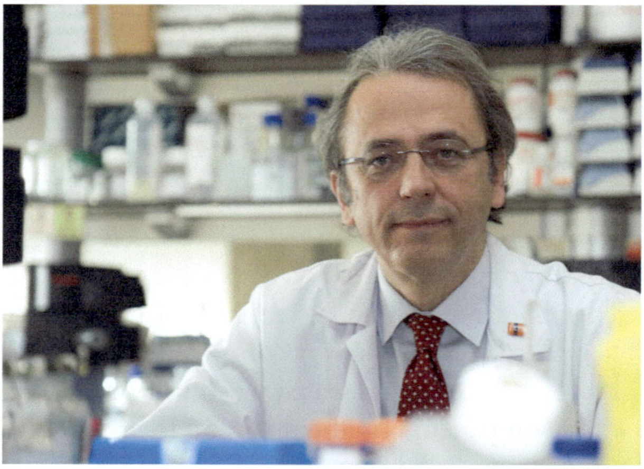

Fig. 42.2 Josep M. Llovet. (Permission Clinic Hospital, Barcelona)

Clarivate Analytics since 2014 [5]. He has devoted his career to the study of the pathogenesis and treatment of liver cancer. He received the Landon International Award from the American Association for Cancer Research (2009) and the Hans Popper International Award (2012) and has received competitive funding from the National Cancer Institute, the European Commission and other entities for more than 100 research projects.

The liver can be affected by different types of cancer, but there is one—hepatocellular carcinoma—that directly affects the hepatocytes and is particularly prevalent: it is diagnosed each year in around half a million people worldwide. It is also one of the most lethal cancers in existence. It is a very aggressive disease that affects mostly men—90% of those affected—and its incidence is higher in developing and poor countries.

> HCC is significantly linked to chronic hepatitis B (HBV) and hepatitis C (HCV) infections. Vaccination against HBV is a crucial primary strategy that can reduce significantly the incidence of HCC.

For a long time, it hardly made headlines or aroused clinical interest commensurate with its impact. As a consequence, the development of treatments had lagged behind other types of cancer. This situation began to change thanks to researchers at Hospital Clínic-IDIBAPS (Fundació de Recerca Clínic Barcelona-Institut d'Investigacions Biomèdiques August Pi I Sunyer) such as Llovet, who decided to focus their careers on identifying more effective and less aggressive therapeutic strategies to combat this disease. Among the advances promoted from Hospital Clínic for the treatment of this disease, a key clinical tool stands out: the Barcelona Clinic Liver Cancer Classification (BCLC). This system classifies patients affected by hepatocellular carcinoma according to their prognosis and was a milestone. Llovet and his team were also pioneers in identifying two treatments that transformed the clinical management of this disease: chemoembolization and the use of the drug Sorafenib.

Barcelona Classification: a Clinical Model for the World

Although certain treatments for hepatocellular carcinoma have been shown to be effective, not all patients respond in the same way. As the hepatologists at Hospital Clínic were taught, research cannot be separated from clinical practice. Therefore, knowing the main factors that influence the outcome of a therapy is as relevant as the therapy itself. Without this knowledge, the physician will not be able to determine precisely which option is best for each patient at each stage of the disease. The risk of allocating scarce and costly resources to ineffective treatments is, in this context, very high. At Hospital Clínic, Drs. Jordi Bruix and Josep Llovet and other collaborators identified three decisive factors in assessing whether a treatment would be effective. The first, and most obvious, is the size of the tumor and its degree of dissemination at the time of diagnosis: the larger and more widespread it is, the more limited the therapeutic options will be and the less effective they will be. In the early stages, some surgical interventions—such as resection or liver transplantation—can completely eliminate the disease and offer a real chance of cure, provided the right clinical conditions are met. But when the cancer is already advanced, these options should be discarded and other alternatives, such as chemotherapy, should be considered. The second factor is the functionality of the liver. Even if it is affected by the tumor, if it retains enough healthy tissue it can continue to filter the blood. A functional liver can significantly improve the prognosis, even in advanced stages. Finally, the hepatologists noted that the patient's general clinical condition also plays a role: the results were very different if the patient had maintained an active life despite the cancer, or if the disease had weakened him to the point of being unable to get out of bed. Clinical studies, especially if they are randomized, require a great deal of effort, but the knowledge they can generate is pure gold. Thanks to the work of Bruix and Llovet, that empirical experience became an algorithm that guides to this day the practice of hepatologists around the world. Presented in 1999 and known as the Barcelona Classification -or by official name, Barcelona Clinic Liver Cancer (BCLC)-, this tool was able to rigorously associate the most effective therapies to each of the stages of the disease. Although the Barcelona Classification distinguishes between very early, initial, intermediate, advanced and terminal stages of the disease, Llovet and his collaborators insisted that this was not its main purpose. As he explained in one of his articles, "physicians caring for patients with hepatocellular carcinoma not only have to establish the tumor stage and prognosis of the patients but should also be able to select the best treatment option for each patient following a well-established treatment program" [6]. The aim was not, therefore, to create a scoring system aimed solely at stratifying patients according to their prognosis, but to propose a clinical staging tool that would directly link tumor stage with the most appropriate therapeutic strategy. The aim was to ensure that each patient would receive the most relevant treatment according to his or her specific clinical circumstances. Compared to other stratification systems, the Barcelona Classification stood out for its practical applicability: it required only a rigorous clinical examination, a good diagnostic imaging and a few laboratory tests common in patients with cirrhosis. It was a tool designed to facilitate clinical management of the patient and ease the burden of responsibility on physicians in making complex therapeutic decisions. But the most important thing was that it worked: several international groups found that following its recommendations increased patient survival. After its clinical implementation, the algorithm was rapidly adopted by medical centers around the world and remains, to this day, the reference guide for the treatment of hepatocellular carcinoma. The guide has been updated periodically to incorporate new scientific advances. A first revision was presented in 2009, followed by another in 2018, and the most recent to date appeared in 2022. The BCLC system has sometimes been criticized for being too rigid and not contemplating borderline situations or more complex therapeutic combinations. However, this simplification has been a deliberate sacrifice in favor of ease of use and clinical applicability. In each update, it has been emphasized that the guide should be understood as an orientative scheme, not as an inflexible prescription book. It is not intended to replace clinical judgment, especially in those cases where the particularities of the patient require a different decision from standardized recommendations (Fig. 42.3).

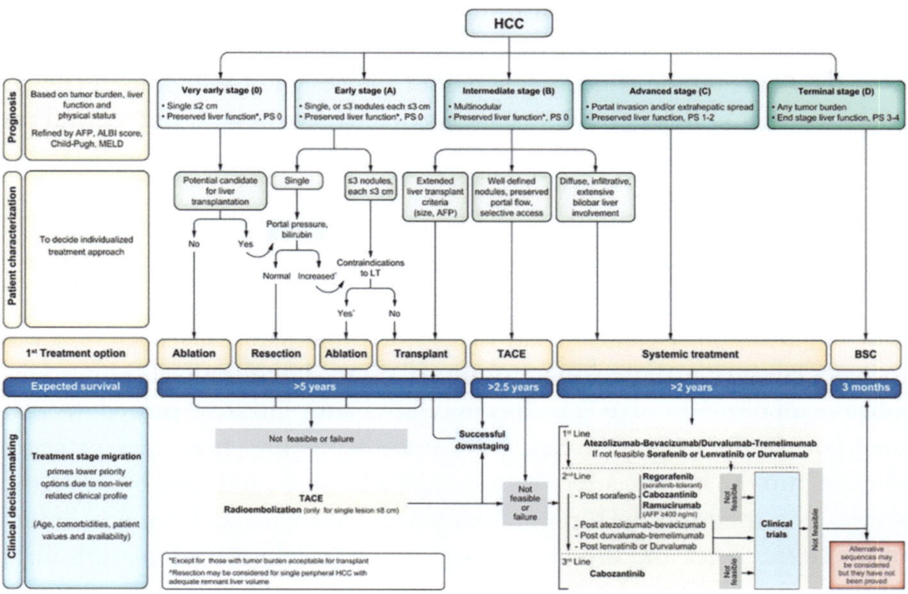

Fig. 42.3 BCLC Algorithm for treatment of HCC of the update of 2022. LT is hepatic transplantation; BSC best supportive care and TACE Transarterial Chemoembolization

Scientific Truth, the Only Tool Against Cancer

As with any type of cancer, in hepatocellular carcinoma there is no room for half-measures: does the therapy prolong the patient's life? does it improve his or her quality of life? does it outperform existing treatments in terms of efficacy? Dr. Llovet was confronted again and again with these questions, with a clear conviction: without a well-designed clinical trial, none of them could be answered with certainty. For a trial to have impact, be recognized by the scientific community and be integrated into clinical practice, its design must be impeccable. Strong management skills are essential to coordinate multiple institutions and bring together eligible patients, often from different parts of the world, and it is also crucial to secure public or private funding to sustain the study for as many years as necessary. In addition, to avoid any doubt about the results, it is essential that the investigators responsible for the study have unquestionable prestige. When pharmaceutical companies participate, they also demand the utmost rigor, since they cannot risk years of work or million-dollar investments for the sake of a poorly executed study. This level of excellence is precisely that achieved by Llovet and his staff, who has been internationally recognized for his ability to design solid, well-executed randomized clinical trials oriented to the real needs of medical practice. He embodies the figure of the trialist in the Galilean sense of the term: one who seeks scientific truth with rigor, method and evidence. Since 2008, he has been the main author of the guidelines for the design of randomized clinical trials on hepatocellular carcinoma, used as a reference in both Europe and the United States [7].

Arterial Chemoembolization

One of Llovet's first clinical trials that gained international recognition was the one dedicated to the technique of arterial chemoembolization (Transarterial Chemoembolization, TACE). This is a minimally invasive procedure that does not require surgery: it consists of introducing the chemotherapy agent directly into the hepatic artery by means of a catheter, and then blocking the artery. This interrupts the supply of oxygen and nutrients to the tumor, inducing necrosis. Since the drug remains concentrated in the tumor site for a longer period of time, the procedure promotes apoptosis—i.e. programmed cell suicide—of the cancer cells. Unlike systemic chemotherapy, the rest of the body is not exposed to its toxic effects. Arterial chemoembolization was proposed as an alternative therapy for patients in the intermediate stage of hepatocellular carcinoma, when the tumor can no longer be removed, but it is still possible to halt its progression. In contrast to the merely palliative treatments practiced at the time, which only sought to alleviate pain, this technique offered an active option with the capacity to extend life expectancy. In 2002, Llovet presented the results of a 4-year study comparing chemoembolization with palliative treatment, which showed a significant improvement: survival increased from 16 to 26 months [8], lapse of time after which cancer progression is reactivated. Supported by a meta-analysis published in 2003 [9], Llovet concluded: "The results of this study and the meta-analysis provide sufficient evidence to propose chemoembolization as a standard treatment in patients with HCC, intermediate stage [10]. Since then, this approach has been adopted by most hospitals in the world.

Sorafenib, the First Treatment for Advanced Cancer

The clinical study on the drug Sorafenib was undoubtedly the one that consolidated Llovet's international prestige and placed him among the 1% of the most cited scientists in the world. In 2008 the results of the international SHARP (Sorafenib HCC Assessment Randomized Protocol) trial were presented, in which 602 patients from America, Europe, New Zealand and Australia participated. The study was led by Llovet and Bruix from the Hospital Clínic in Barcelona, with the collaboration of Mount Sinai in New York and the pharmaceutical company Bayer, developer of the drug. The trial demonstrated, for the first time, that the treatment could increase survival in patients with advanced hepatocellular carcinoma. Until then, no therapy had been approved that offered tangible benefits to this group of patients, for whom neither surgery nor chemoembolization was indicated. As Peter Galle described it, the situation with these cancers was one of "therapeutic nihilism" [11], a perception that began to be reversed thanks to this drug. The results were significant: if the average survival of these patients was around 8 months, Sorafenib raised it to almost 11 months. Three months may not seem long, but it represents a relative increase of, which is remarkable in the context of terminal disease. And in terms of scientific research, this drug opened the door to new research. Sorafenib, inhibitor of the tyrosine kinase, treatment could cause adverse effects, such as diarrhea or skin reactions, although in many cases these were preventable [12]. However, in some patients the

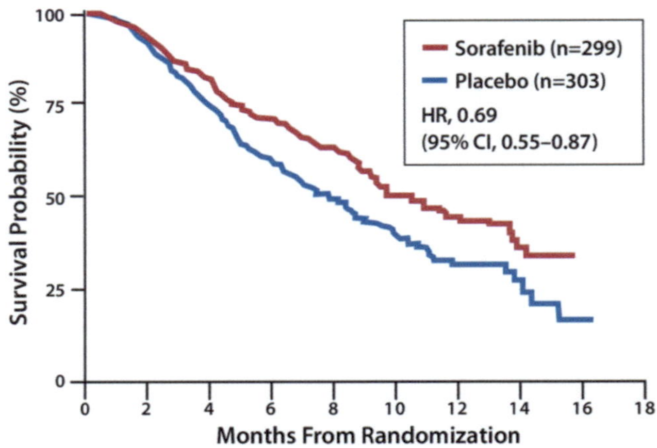

Fig. 42.4 SHARP trial: 299 patients treated with placebo, and 299 patients treated with Sorafenib. The Kaplan-Meier survival curve shows that patients treated with Sorafenib achieved a longer survival tan placebo

treatment had to be stopped. This situation inevitably opened up the debate as to whether its high cost was justified, an issue on which opinions varied depending on the perspective: suffering from the disease is not the same as managing healthcare resources (Fig. 42.4).

The Present and Future of Research Lies in Combination Therapies

Currently, research is focused on exploring combination therapies that also activate the immune system, a line of work in which Llovet continues to play an active and decisive role. For example, sorafenib was the standard first-line treatment for advanced hepatocellular carcinoma for more than a decade, from its approval in 2007 until around 2020, when the combination of atezolizumab and bevacizumab-a therapy that focuses on preparing the immune system to attack the cancer-was found to give better results in terms of survival. Sorafenib is still considered, however, as a valid therapeutic option in case of contraindications given that only 30% of patients respond to this treatment. Llovet and his team at the Hospital Clínic-IDIBAPS are studying the molecular factors involved in this resistance in so many patients [13].

Another result of this line of research combining different treatments has been improving therapy for arterial chemoembolization, a breakthrough that has required two decades of research. In 2025, the team of the Clinic in

Barcelona published in The Lancet the results of the LEAP-012 study [14], which evaluated the combination of chemoembolization with two additional drugs. On the one hand, the Lenvatinib, a cell proliferation inhibitor that also prevents the formation of new blood vessels (angiogenesis); on the other, Pembrolizumab, an immunotherapeutic drug designed to reactivate the immune system's response to possible micrometastases. This simultaneous three-pronged attack on the cancer was able to extend patient survival by an additional 4.6 month, a clinically significant improvement that opens a new therapeutic avenue and renews expectations for those suffering from this disease. The scientific trajectory of Dr. Llovet and the other hepatocellular carcinoma researchers has shown that every week of life gained in the face of cancer requires enormous effort but is also invaluable. And it is precisely the small victories that indicate that progress is being made in the right direction. That is why it is essential to continue researching.

References

1. Bruguera M. History of hepatology in Catalonia. Gastroenterol Hepatol. 2013;36:484–91.
2. Bruguera M. Brief history of the congresses of the Spanish Association for the Study of the Liver (1967-2015). Gastroenterol Hepatol. 2016;39:324–8.
3. Llovet JM. Les aportacions científiques de Joan Rodés i la Unitat d'Hepatologia de l'Hospital Clínic. Ann Med. 1998;82:98–100.
4. Vianney Pons JM, Rodés J, Andreu A, Arenas J. The forgotten clinical research. Med Clin. 2013;140:91–2.
5. Josep Llovet MD. Profiles. Mount Sinai- New York. https://profiles.mountsinai.org/josep-llovet.
6. Llovet JM, Brú C, Bruix J. Prognosis of hepatocellular carcinoma: the BCLC staging classification. Semin Liver Dis. 1999;19:329–38.
7. Llovet JM, Ducreux M, Lencioni R, et al. Trial design and endpoints in hepatocellular carcinoma: AASLD consensus conference. Hepatology. 2012;56:1314–24.
8. Llovet JM, Real MI, Montaña X, et al. Arterial embolization or chemoembolization versus symptomatic treatment in patients with unresectable hepatocellular carcinoma: a randomized controlled trial. Lancet. 2002;359:1734–9.
9. Llovet JM, Bruix J. Transarterial chemoembolization for unresectable hepatocellular carcinoma: meta-analysis of randomized controlled trials. Australas Radiol. 2003;230:491–7.
10. Varela M, Llovet JM. Chemoembolization in the treatment of hepatocellular carcinoma: clinical trials and clinical practice. CGH. 2004;3:175–7. https://www.elsevier.es/index.php?p=revista&pRevista=pdfsimple&pii=70000200&r=8.

11. Galle PR. Sorafenib in advanced hepatocellular carcinoma - we have won a battle, not the war. J Hepatol. 2008;49:871–3.
12. Reig M, Mantilla A, Bustamante J, et al. Management recommendations for sorafenib in patients with hepatocellular carcinoma. Gastroenterol Hepatol. 2010;33:741–52.
13. Cappuyns S, Piqué-Gili M, Esteban-Fabró R, et al. Single-cell RNA sequencing-derived signatures define response patterns to atezolizumab + bevacizumab in advanced hepatocellular carcinoma. J Hepatol. 2024;82:1036–49.
14. Kudo M, Ren Z, Guo Y, et al. Transarterial chemoembolization combined with Lenvatinib plus Pembrolizumab versus dual placebo for unresectable, non-metastatic hepatocellular carcinoma (LEAP-012): a multicentre, randomized, double-blind, phase 3 study. Lancet. 2024;403:1234–45.

MIX
Papier aus verantwortungsvollen Quellen
Paper from responsible sources
FSC® C105338

If you have any concerns about our products,
you can contact us on
ProductSafety@springernature.com

In case Publisher is established outside the EU,
the EU authorized representative is:
Springer Nature Customer Service Center GmbH
Europaplatz 3, 69115 Heidelberg, Germany

Printed by Libri Plureos GmbH
in Hamburg, Germany